T0320336

BIOPHARMACEUTICS MODELING AND SIMULATIONS

BIOPHARMACEUTICS MODELING AND SIMULATIONS
Theory, Practice, Methods, and Applications

KIYOHIKO SUGANO
Asahi Kasei Pharma Corp.
Shizuoka, Japan

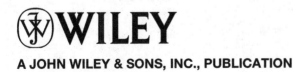

A JOHN WILEY & SONS, INC., PUBLICATION

Copyright © 2012 by John Wiley & Sons, Inc. All rights reserved

Published by John Wiley & Sons, Inc., Hoboken, New Jersey
Published simultaneously in Canada

No part of this publication may be reproduced, stored in a retrieval system, or transmitted in any form or by any means, electronic, mechanical, photocopying, recording, scanning, or otherwise, except as permitted under Section 107 or 108 of the 1976 United States Copyright Act, without either the prior written permission of the Publisher, or authorization through payment of the appropriate per-copy fee to the Copyright Clearance Center, Inc., 222 Rosewood Drive, Danvers, MA 01923, (978) 750-8400, fax (978) 750-4470, or on the web at www.copyright.com. Requests to the Publisher for permission should be addressed to the Permissions Department, John Wiley & Sons, Inc., 111 River Street, Hoboken, NJ 07030, (201) 748-6011, fax (201) 748-6008, or online at http://www.wiley.com/go/permission.

Limit of Liability/Disclaimer of Warranty: While the publisher and author have used their best efforts in preparing this book, they make no representations or warranties with respect to the accuracy or completeness of the contents of this book and specifically disclaim any implied warranties of merchantability or fitness for a particular purpose. No warranty may be created or extended by sales representatives or written sales materials. The advice and strategies contained herein may not be suitable for your situation. You should consult with a professional where appropriate. Neither the publisher nor author shall be liable for any loss of profit or any other commercial damages, including but not limited to special, incidental, consequential, or other damages.

For general information on our other products and services or for technical support, please contact our Customer Care Department within the United States at (800) 762-2974, outside the United States at (317) 572-3993 or fax (317) 572-4002.

Wiley also publishes its books in a variety of electronic formats. Some content that appears in print may not be available in electronic formats. For more information about Wiley products, visit our web site at www.wiley.com.

Library of Congress Cataloging-in-Publication Data:

Sugano, Kiyohiko.
  Biopharmaceutics modeling and simulations : theory, practice, methods, and applications / Kiyohiko Sugano.
       p. ; cm.
  Includes bibliographical references and index.
  ISBN 978-1-118-02868-1 (cloth)
  I. Title.
  [DNLM: 1. Biopharmaceutics–methods. 2. Computer Simulation. 3. Drug Compounding–methods. 4. Models, Theoretical. QV 38]

615.7–dc23

                                        2012007296
Printed in the United States of America

ISBN: 9781118028681

10 9 8 7 6 5 4 3 2 1

To Hitomi

CONTENTS

PREFACE

"Science is built of facts the way a house is built of bricks; but an accumulation of facts is no more science than a pile of bricks is a house."

—Henry Poincare

The aim of this book is to provide a systematic understanding of biopharmaceutical modeling. Probably, this is the first book challenging this difficult task.

Biopharmaceutical modeling demands a wide range of knowledge. We need to understand the physical theories, the physiology of the gastrointestinal tract, and the meaning of drug parameters. This book covers the wide range of scientific topics required to appropriately perform and evaluate biopharmaceutical modeling. In this book, oral absorption of a drug is mainly discussed. However, the same scientific framework is applicable for other administration routes such as nasal and pulmonary administrations.

Oral absorption of a drug is a complex process that consists of dissolution, precipitation, intestinal wall permeation, and gastrointestinal transit. In addition, drug metabolism can also occur in the intestinal wall and the liver before drug molecules enter into systemic circulation.

Historically, a reductionist approach has been taken to understand the oral absorption of a drug. Each process of oral absorption was reduced to its subprocesses up to the molecular level. However, understanding each piece of the puzzle is insufficient in understanding the whole picture of oral absorption. It is critically important to reconstruct the whole process of oral absorption and understand the interrelationship between each piece that comprises oral absorption of a drug.

In the field of biology, computational systems biology has been emerging since the millennium [1]. In systems biology, the interactions between biological molecules are investigated in both reductionist and constitutive approaches to understand the quantitative relationship between a disease state and each molecular process. In this book, a similar approach is applied for the oral absorption of a drug.

In the first section of this book, the whole picture of oral absorption is discussed. As the central dogma of oral drug absorption, the interplay of dissolution rate, solubility, and permeability of a drug is discussed in a comprehensive manner without using mathematics. Even though the discussion in the first section is only a conceptual and qualitative outline, correct understanding of this central dogma will be of great benefit for drug discovery and development. The central dogma of oral drug absorption is the basis of the biopharmaceutical classification system (BCS), which is widely used in drug discovery and development [2].

We then move forward to each theory that comprises the entire oral absorption model. In this book, the entire mathematical framework is called the "gastrointestinal unified theoretical framework (GUT framework)." The concept of "concentration" is first discussed in detail, as it is critically important for understanding biopharmaceutical modeling. Then, theories of solubility, dissolution, precipitation, membrane permeation, and drug metabolisms are discussed. Each theory is described based on the unified definition of drug concentration and then incorporated into the GUT framework.

We then move forward to the physiological and drug property data that is used for biopharmaceutical modeling. The quality of biopharmaceutical modeling heavily relies on the quality of input data. The input data are roughly categorized into drug property and physiological parameters. These data are reviewed from the viewpoint of their use in biopharmaceutical modeling.

Before moving on to the discussions about practical applications of biopharmaceutical modeling in drug research, the validity of biopharmaceutical modeling is critically reviewed. A step-by-step approach has been taken to validate the biopharmaceutical modeling employing Occam's razor as a leading principle.

As the applications of biopharmaceutical modeling in drug research, biopharmaceutical classification system, dose/particle size dependency prediction, selection of solid form and enabling formulation, food effect prediction, etc. are then discussed.

Next, the strategy to use biopharmaceutical modeling in drug research and regulatory application is discussed. Introduction of good simulation practice for biopharmaceutical modeling would be an emergent issue for regulatory application.

Many figures and tables are provided to make it easy to understand biopharmaceutical modeling. In addition, more than 900 references are cited. I hope that readers will enjoy reading this book and that this book will be a helpful reference for biopharmaceutical modeling.

I would like to thank Mr. Jonathan Rose of John Wiley & Sons, Inc. for giving me this opportunity to write a book about biopharmaceutical modeling.

I would like to thank Dr. Takashi Mano and Dr. Ravi Shanker for carefully reading my manuscript and giving me valuable advice. They also supported the investigation of biopharmaceutical modeling at Pfizer. I also thank Dr. Brian

Henry, Dr. Mark McAllister, and Ms. Nicola Clear for their kind support at Pfizer. The scientific discussion with the Pfizer biopharmaceutics group members improved my understanding of this subject. The suggestions from Prof. Steve Sutton, Dr. Kazuko Sagawa, and Ms. Kelly Jones about *in vivo* physiology are greatly appreciated. Ms. Joanne Bennett kindly lectured me about the cell culture models. I would like to thank Dr. Claudia da Costa Mathews, Dr. Hannah Pearce, Dr. Sue Mei Wong, Mr. Simon Pegg, Mr. Neil Flanagan, Mr. Mike Cram, Mr. Unai Vivanco, Ms. Sonia Patel, and Mr. Richard Manley for investigating the enabling formulations and physchem screening. I would like to thank the Pfizer Pharmaceutical Science members for supporting and inspiring me to pursue the sciences and practical drug research work. I would like to thank Dr. Tomomi Mastuura for her instructions about pharmacokinetics. I would like to thank Dr. Stefan Steyn for implementation of biopharmaceutical modeling in early drug discovery.

Thanks also goes to the Pfizer Nagoya Pharm R&D members. Mr. Shohei Sugimoto, Dr. Toshiyuki Niwa, Dr. Naofumi Hashimoto, Mr. Akinori Ito, Dr. Takashi Kojima, Mr. Omura Atsushi, and Mr. Morimichi Sato kindly taught me solid-state chemistry and enabling formulations. I would like to thank Mr Arimich Okazaki, Mr. Yohei Kawabata, Ms. Keiko Kako, Dr. Sumitra Tavornvipas, Ms. Akiko Suzuki, Ms. Tomoko Matsuda, and Ms. Shiho Torii for kindly working together toward progress of the science at the Nagoya site.

I would like to thank Dr. Ryusuke Takano of Chugai Pharm. for his excellent works on biopharmaceutical sciences. I also would like to thank the Chugai physicochemical and pharmacokinetics group members, especially Mr. Hirokazu Hamada, Dr. Noriyuki Takata, Dr. Akiko Koga, Mr. Ken Goshi, Dr. Kazuya Nakagomi, Mr. Ro Irisawa, Ms. Harumi Onoda, Dr. Hidetoshi Ushio, Dr. Yoshiki Hayashi, Dr. Yoshiaki Nabuchi, Dr. Minoru Machida, and Dr. Ryoichi Saito. They brought me up as an industrial scientist. I would like to thank Dr. Ken-ichi Sakai and Mr. Kouki Obata for working with me toward progress of the sciences at Chugai.

I would like to thank Dr. Alex Avdeef for finding a young scientist at a rural countryside in Japan and introducing him to the world. I greatly appreciate the kind support from the UK physicochemical scientist community, especially, Dr. John Comer, Dr. Karl Box, Dr. Alan Hill, Dr. Nicola Colclough, Dr. Toni Llinas, Dr. Darren Edwards, and other scientists. Their kind support made my UK life enjoyable and fruitful. I would also like to thank Prof. Amin Rostami-hochaghan, Dr. David Turner, Dr. Sibylle Neuhoff, and Dr. Jamai Masoud of SimCYP. I would like to thank Prof. Per Artursson, Dr. Manfred Kansy, Dr. Bernard Faller, Dr. Edward Kerns, and Dr. Li Di for discussions about PAMPA. I would like to thank Dr. Lennart Lindfors for constructive discussions.

I greatly appreciate the mentorship of Prof. Katsuhide Terada and Prof. Shinji Yamashita. I also would like to thank Dr. Makoto Kataoka and Dr. Yoshie Masaoka for the collaboration works.

Finally, I would like to express my greatest thanks to my wife, Hitomi. Without her dedicated support, I could not have gone through the tough task of writing a book like this. I sincerely dedicate this book to her.

KIYO SUGANO

REFERENCES

1. Amidon, G.L., Lennernas, H., Shah, V.P., Crison, J.R. (1995). A theoretical basis for a biopharmaceutic drug classification: the correlation of *in vitro* drug product dissolution and *in vivo* bioavailability. *Pharm. Res.*, 12, 413–420.
2. Kitano, H. (2002). Computational systems biology. *Nature*, 420, 206–210.

LIST OF ABBREVIATIONS

API	Active pharmaceutical ingredient
A to B	Apical-to-basal
BA	Absolute bioavailability
BCS	Biopharmaceutical classification system
B to A	Basal-to-apical
CER	Ceramide
CFD	Computational fluid dynamics
CHO	Cholesterol
CM	Carrier mediated
CNT	Classical nucleation theory
CSSR	Critical supersaturation ratio
DDI	Drug–drug interaction
DRL	Dissolution-rate limited
DSC	Differential scanning calorimeter
DTA	Differential thermal analysis
FFA	Free fatty acid
FaSSIF	Fasted stated simulated intestinal fluid
FeSSIF	Fed stated simulated intestinal fluid
FIH	First in human
GET	Gastric emptying time
GI	Gastrointestinal
GUT framework	Gastrointestinal unified theoretical framework
HH	Henderson–Hasselbalch
IVIVC	*In vitro* (dissolution)–*in vivo* correlation
LCT	Long-chain triglyceride
LHS	Left-hand side

MCT	Medium chain triglyceride
MMC	Migrating motor complex
NBE	Nernst–Brunner equation
NS	Navier–Stokes
PAMPA	Parallel artificial membrane permeation assay
PC	Phosphatidylcholine
PDE	Particle drifting effect
PE	Phosphatidylethanolamine
PG	Phosphatidylglycerol
PI	Phosphatidylinositol
PK	Pharmacokinetics
PL	Permeability limited
PLM	Polarized light microscopy
PPS	Prediction process step
PS	Phosphatidylserine
PXRD	Powder X-ray diffraction
RHS	Right-hand side
RPM	Revolution per minute
SC	Stratum corneum
SEDDS	Self-emulsifying drug delivery system
SITT	Small intestinal transit time
SL-E	Solubility–epithelial membrane permeability limited
SL-U	Solubility–UWL permeability limited
SPIP	Single-pass intestinal perfusion
TC	Taurocholic acid
TG	Thermal gravity
USP	United state pharmacopeia
UWL	Unstirred water layer
A_H	Hydrogen-donor strength
AUC	Area under the curve (subscript indicates administration route, etc.)
$A_{blood\,vessel}$	Surface area of the blood vessel in the villi
Acc	Accessibility to villi surface
C_D	resistance coefficient
CF_{SSR}	Steady-state reduction correction factor
CL_h	Hepatic clearance
$CL_{h,int}$	Intrinsic hepatic clearance
CL_{perm}	Permeation clearance
$CL_{subepithelial}$	Permeation clearance of subepithelial space
CL_{tot}	Total clearance
CR	Controlled-release function
C_{active}	Effective concentration for active transport
C_{bile}	Concentration of bile acid
C_{bm}	Concentration of bile-micelle bound drug

$C_{dissolv}$	Dissolved drug concentration
$C_{dissolv,ss}$	Steady-state concentration
C_{nc}	Number of critical cluster per volume
C_p	Plasma concentration
C_{pd}	Particle-drifting coefficient
$C_{subepithelial}$	Concentration of drug in subepithelial space
C_{tot}	Total drug concentration
$C_{u,z}$	Concentration of unbound drug with charge z
C_{water}	Concentration of water (55.6 M)
DF	Degree of flatness of intestinal tube
$D_{albumin}$	Diffusion coefficient of albumin-bound drug
D_{bm}	Diffusion coefficient of bile-micelle-bound drug
D_{eff}	Effective diffusion coefficient
Disp	Dispersion coefficient for GI transit
$D_m(x)$	Local diffusion coefficient at position x in membrane
D_{mono}	Diffusion coefficient of monomer drug
Dn	Dissolution number
Do	Dose number
D_{oct}	Octanol–water distribution coefficient
Dose	Dose amount (subscript indicates administration route, etc.)
D_{paddle}	Paddle diameter
D_{vessel}	Diameter of vessel
F	Absolute bioavailability
Fa	Fraction of a dose absorbed (subscript indicates administration route, etc.)
Fa_{DRL}	Fa for the dissolution-rate-limited cases
Fa_{NI}	Fa calculated by numerical integration using the S1I7C1 model
Fa_{PL}	Fa for the permeability-limited cases
Fa_{SL}	Fa for the solubility-permeability-limited cases
Fa_{SS}	Fa calculated with steady-state approximation
$Fa_{min. limit}$	Minimum value of $Fa_{PL,}$ Fa_{SL}, and Fa_{DRL}
Fa_{sfo}	Fa calculated as sequential first-order processes of dissolution and permeation
F_{cn}	Frequency of addition of another molecule to critical cluster
Fg	Fraction not metabolized in intestinal epithelial cells
Fh	Fraction not metabolized in hepatic first pass
GIP	Position in GI tract
Gz	Graetz number
H_{paddle}	Height of paddle from vessel bottom
H_{viili}	Height of villi
J_{max}	Maximum flux by carrier-mediated transport
J_{nc}	Primary nucleation rate per volume per time
J_{perm}	Permeation flux

K_a	Dissociation constant
K_{bm}	Bile micelles–water partition coefficient
K_m	Michaelis–Menten constant
$K_{org}(x)$	Local partition coefficient at position x in membrane
K_{sc}	Partition coefficient into stratum corneum
K_{sp}	Solubility product
K_w	Ionic product for water
$K_{transit,k}$	First-order transition kinetic constant
L	Representative length
L_{GI}	Length of GI tract
N_A	Avogadro number
$N_{API,GI,k}$	Number of API particle bins in GI position k
N_n	Number of nuclei
N_p	Number of particles in one dose
P_{CM}	Carrier-mediated transcellular permeability
PE	Plicate expansion
P_{UWL}	UWL permeability in the GI tract
P_{WC}	Permeability by water conveyance
P_{app}	Apparent permeability of *in vitro* membrane permeation assay
P_{eff}	Effective intestinal membrane permeability
P_{ep}	Epithelial membrane permeability
P_{oct}	Octanol–water partition coefficient
P_{para}	Paracellular pathway permeability
$P_{plicate}$	Plicate surface permeability
P_{trans}	Transcellular pathway permeability
$P_{trans,0}$	Intrinsic transcellular pathway permeability of undissociated species
Q_{GI}	Flow rate along small intestine
Q_h	Hepatic blood flow
Q_{villi}	Villi blood flow
Q_{in}	Infusion rate
R_{GI}	Radius of GI tract
RK	Renkin function
R_{MW}	Apparent pore radius of paracellular pathway based on MW selectivity
RPM_{min}	Minimum agitation speed
R_{SA}	Ratio of drug particle surface area in UWL and villi surface area
Re	Reynolds number
R_{mucus}	Nominal pore radius of mucus layer
R_{para}	Apparent pore radius of the paracellular pathway
S_0	Intrinsic solubility of undissociated drug
$S_{0,rp}$	Solubility of particles with radius r_p

$S_{0,\infty}$	Solubility of particles with infinitely large particle size
SA_{API}	Particle surface area of API
SA_{GI}	GI surface area for absorption (based on smooth tube)
SA_p	Surface area for one particle
SRn	Steady state reduction number
S_{blank}	Solubility in a blank buffer (without micelles)
Sc	Schmitt number
$S_{cocrystal}$	Intrinsic solubility of cocrystal
$S_{dissolv}$	Solubility in a biorelevant media (unbound + micelle bound)
Sh	Sherwood number
Sh_{disk}	Sherwood number for rotating disk
Sh_p	Sherwood number for particle
Sh_{tube}	Sherwood number for tube
$Sn_{T_{si}}$	Saturation number at time T_{si}
Sn_{ini}	Initial saturation number (Sn_{ini})
S_{salt}	Intrinsic solubility of salt
$S_{surface}$	Solubility at solid surface
T_{DO1}	Time when drug amount remaining in small intestine gives $Do = 1$
T_m	Melting point (Kelvin)
Tn_{exss}	Extended steady-state duration number
U	Flow speed
U_e	Microeddy effect velocity
Ur	Urinary excretion fraction
$U_{rel,tot}$	Relative flow velocity
U_t	Terminal sedimentation velocity
VE	Villi expansion
V_{GI}	GI fluid volume
Vc	Velocity of intestinal fluid
V_{me}	Velocity representing microeddy effect
V_p	Volume of one particle
V_{rel}	Relative velocity between fluid and particle
V_t	Terminal (sedimentation) slip velocity
Vx	McGowans molecular volume
$W_{channel}$	Width of channel between villi
W_{villi}	Width of villi
X_{bm}	Bile-micelle-bound drug amount
$X_{dissolv}$	Dissolved drug amount
$X_{u,z}$	Amount of unbound drug with charge z
Z_{ch}	Zel'dovich number
Z_{para}	Paracellular pathway charge
d_{disk}	Disk diameter
d_p	Particle diameter

d_{tube}	Tube diameter
f_{PSB}	Volume percentage of each particle size bin in one dose
f_{bm}	Fraction of bile-micelle-bound molecule
f_n, f_0	Fraction of undissociated species
$f_{subepithelial}$	Unbound fraction of drug in subepithelial space
f_u	Bile-micelle-unbound fraction
f_{up}	Plasma unbound fraction
f_z	Fraction of charged species
g	Gravitational acceleration constant
h	Unstirred water layer thickness
h_{HJ}	Criteria value for Hintz–Johnson model
h_{UWL}	Unstirred water layer thickness in the intestine
h_{WF}	Criteria value for Wang–Flanagan model
h_{fam}	Thickness of firmly adhered mucus layer
$h_{UWLvitro}$	UWL thickness in *in vitro* permeability assay
$h_{subepithelial}$	Thickness of subepithelial space
k_B	Boltzmann constant
k_{abs}	Absorption rate coefficient
k_{deg}	Degradation rate constant
k_{diss}	Dissolution rate coefficient
k_{el}	Elimination rate
k_{mass}	Mass transfer coefficient
k_{perm}	Permeation rate coefficient
l_{tube}	Tube length
m.p.	Melting point (Celsius)
m_{atom}	Number of atoms in molecule
r_{mono}	Molecular radius
r_p	Particle radius (at time t)
$r_{p,PSB}$	Particle radius for particle size bin
$r_{p,ini}$	Initial particle radius
$r_{p,ini,PSB}$	Initial particle radius for particle size bin
$r_{p,nc}$	Critical radius of nuclei
v_{atom}	Relative volume of atom
v_m	Molecular volume
z	Molecular charge
ΔC	Concentration gradient
ΔG_{nc}	Energy barrier for nucleation
ΔH_m	Enthalpy of melting
ΔS_f	Entropy of fusion
ΔS_m	Entropy of melting
Π	Particle shape factor
β	Lump constant (β) of foreign particle number, sticking provability, etc
γ	Interfacial tension between solid surface and fluid

ε	Agitation strength (Energy input per time)
η	Kolmogorov's minimum eddy scale
λ_{disso}	Dissociation resistance from solid surface (in length dimension)
λ_{nc}	Interfacial attachment resistance (in length dimension)
μ	Viscosity of fluid
ν	Kinematic viscosity of fluid
ρ_f	Density of fluid
ρ_p	True density of drug
ψ_{cn}	Interfacial reaction rate correction factor

CHAPTER 1

INTRODUCTION

"The eternal mystery of the world is its comprehensibility. The fact that it is comprehensible is a miracle."

—Albert Einstein

The aim of this chapter is to discuss the whole picture of oral absorption of a drug in a comprehensive and descriptive manner without using any mathematical equation.

1.1   AN ILLUSTRATIVE DESCRIPTION OF ORAL DRUG ABSORPTION: THE WHOLE STORY

The oral absorption of a drug is a sequential process of dissolution and intestinal membrane permeation of a drug in the gastrointestinal (GI) tract (Fig. 1.1).

After dosing a drug product (e.g., tablet and capsule), the formulation disintegrates to release solid particles of active pharmaceutical ingredient (API) ① in Fig. 1.1). The released API particles then dissolve into the GI fluid as molecularly dispersed drug molecules ②. The maximum amount of a drug dissolved in the GI fluids is limited by the solubility of the drug in the fluids. In some cases, after an initial API form (such as a salt form) being dissolved, a transient supersaturated state is produced, and then, another solid form (i.e., a free base or an acid) can precipitate out in the intestinal fluid via nucleation ③. The dissolved

Biopharmaceutics Modeling and Simulations: Theory, Practice, Methods, and Applications,
First Edition. Kiyohiko Sugano.
© 2012 John Wiley & Sons, Inc. Published 2012 by John Wiley & Sons, Inc.

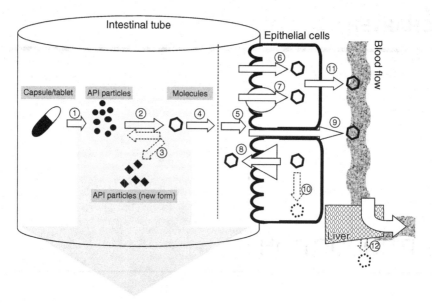

Figure 1.1 Schematic presentation of oral drug absorption processes: disintegration, dissolution, permeation, and transit.

drug molecules are conveyed close to the intestinal wall by the macromixing of the intestinal fluid (④) and further diffuse through the unstirred water layer (UWL), which is adjacent to the epithelial cellular membrane (⑤). The drug molecules then permeate the apical membrane of the epithelial cells mainly by passive diffusion (⑥) but in some cases, via a carrier protein (a transporter) such as PEP-T1 (⑦). If the drug is a substrate for an efflux transporter such as P-gp, a portion of the drug molecules is carried back to the apical side (⑧). Some drugs pass through the intercellular junction (the paracellular route) (⑨). In the epithelial cells, the drug could be metabolized by enzymes such as CYP3A4 (⑩). After passing through the basolateral membrane (⑪), the drug molecules reach the portal vein. The drug molecules in the portal vein then pass through the liver and reach the systemic circulation (⑫).

1.2 THREE REGIMES OF ORAL DRUG ABSORPTION

The central dogma of oral drug absorption is the interplay between solubility, the dissolution rate and permeability of a drug. On the basis of the central dogma, the three rate-limiting steps of oral absorption can be defined. Crystal clear understanding of these regimes is the first step toward understanding biopharmaceutical modeling [1]. Figure 1.2 shows the schematic presentation of the rate-limiting steps in the oral absorption of a drug [2].

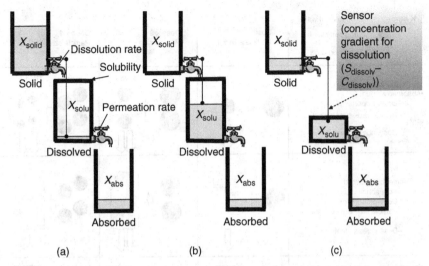

Figure 1.2   Rate-limiting steps in oral absorption of a drug represented by the bucket model [2]. (a) Dissolution rate limited; (b) permeability limited; and (c) solubility–permeability limited.

- Dissolution rate-limited absorption (DRL) (Fig. 1.2a)
  - In this case, the dissolution rate of API is much slower than the permeation rate. Once the API is dissolved, the drug molecules instantly permeate the intestinal membrane and get absorbed into the body. The dissolved drug molecules does not accumulate in the intestinal fluid as it is rapidly removed by the intestinal membrane permeation. Therefore, the dissolved drug concentration ($C_{dissolv}$) in the intestinal fluid is maintained well below the saturated solubility of a drug ($S_{dissolv}$). In this case, the rate of drug absorption is determined by the dissolution rate. The fraction of a dose absorbed (Fa%) is not dependent on the dose strengths of a drug (Figs. 1.2a, 1.3), whereas particle size reduction will be effective in increasing Fa% (Fig. 1.4).

- Permeability-limited absorption (PL) (Fig. 1.2b)
  - In this case, the API dissolves immediately and completely in the intestinal fluid; however, the permeation of the drug is slow. Owing to the slow permeation clearance, the dissolved drug molecules accumulate in the intestinal fluid. The dissolved drug concentration does not reach its saturated solubility when the administered drug amount (Dose) is smaller than the solubilization capacity of the intestinal fluid (Dose $< S_{dissolv} \times V_{GI}$ (intestinal fluid volume)) (Fig. 1.2b). In this case, the rate of drug absorption is determined by the permeation rate. Fa% is not dependent on the dose strength and particle size of a drug (Fig. 1.4).

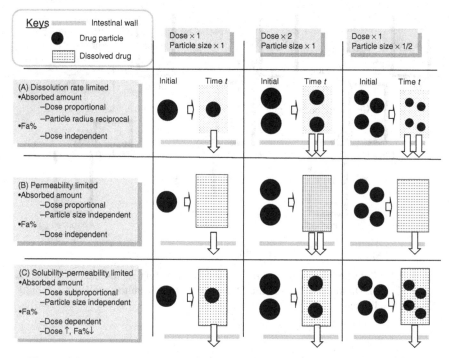

Figure 1.3 The effect of dose and particle size in each rate-limiting step cases.

- Solubility-permeability-limited absorption (SL) (Fig. 1.2c)
  - When the dissolution rate of a drug is much faster than the permeation rate and the solubilization capacity of the intestinal fluid is smaller than the dose strength (Dose $> S_{dissolv} \times V_{GI}$), the dissolved drug molecules accumulate in the intestinal fluid and the dissolved drug concentration reaches the saturated solubility of the drug. In this case, the total absorption flux is determined as the maximum amount of dissolved drug ($= S_{dissolv} \times V_{GI}$) multiplied by the permeation rate of the drug (Fig. 1.2c). This case is further categorized by the rate-limiting step in the permeation process, that is, solubility–epithelial membrane permeability limited (SL-E) and solubility-UWL permeability limited (SL-U) cases [3]. Fa% decreases as the dose strength increases (Fig. 1.4).[1] Particle size reduction will not be effective in increasing Fa% for SL-E cases but could be effective for SL-U cases (Section 4.7.2).

The balance of the dissolution rate coefficient (k_{diss}), the permeation rate coefficient (k_{perm}) and the ratio of dose strength to the solubilization capacity of the

---

[1]In some cases, this dose subproportionality in oral absorption can be cancelled out by supraproportionality in systemic elimination clearance (Section 5.5.3).

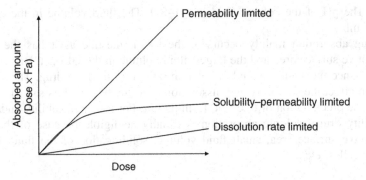

Figure 1.4 Typical dose–absorbed amount relationship.

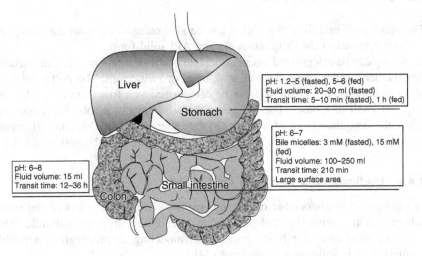

Figure 1.5 Gastrointestinal tract and key characteristics.

GI fluid (Dose/$S_{dissolv} \times V_{GI}$) determines the regime of oral drug absorption. The last parameter is called the dose number (Do). The dose number is one of the most important parameters in biopharmaceutical modeling.

1.3 PHYSIOLOGY OF THE STOMACH, SMALL INTESTINE, AND COLON

The GI tract can be roughly divided into the stomach, the small intestine, and the colon (Fig. 1.5). In humans, the pH of the stomach fluid is 1.2–2.5 in the fasted state but 5–6 in the fed state. The fluid volume in the stomach is ca. 30 ml. The pH of the intestinal fluid is 6.0–7.0 and is maintained relatively constant. The fluid volume in the small intestine is ca. 100–250 ml. Bile acid concentration in the small intestine is ca. 3 mM in the fasted state and 10–15 mM in the fed state. The pH of the colonic fluid is 6.0–8.0. The fluid volume in the colon is ca. 15 ml.

Drug absorption mainly occurs in the small intestine as it has the largest absorptive surface area and the largest fluid volume in the GI tract. Bile micelles can enhance the solubility and dissolution rate of a lipophilic drug. The stomach pH can affect the solubility and dissolution of a free base and its salt. It can also affect the precipitation of free acid from its salt. For low permeability and/or low solubility drugs, colonic absorption is usually negligible because of the small absorptive surface area, small fluid volume, solidification of the fluid, lack of bile micelles, etc.

1.4   DRUG AND API FORM

The patterns of oral drug absorption can be also categorized from the viewpoint of the properties of the drug molecule and API solid form.

A drug can be categorized as undissociable or dissociable ones. The dissociable drug is then further categorized as acid, base, or zwitterions. The API solid form of an acid, base, and zwitterion can be categorized as a free form or a salt form (e.g., HCl salt of a base). For PL cases, the difference of a solid form does not affect the oral absorption of a drug. On the other hand, for DRL and SL cases, the solid form of a drug has a significant impact on the oral absorption of a drug.

1.4.1   Undissociable and Free Acid Drugs

In the case of undissociable drugs and free acid drugs, the effect of the stomach pH on the solubility and dissolution rate of the drug is negligible. This is the simplest cases for biopharmaceutical modeling. A practically reasonable predictability is anticipated (Chapter 8) [4].

1.4.2   Free Base Drugs

Free base drugs dissolve better in the low pH environment of the stomach than in the small intestine. However, as the stomach contents move into the small intestine, the pH is neutralized and the solubility of the drug is decreased. The drug particles, which once reduced its size by dissolution in the stomach, regrows in the small intestine (the dissolved drug molecule moves back to the solid surface of the free base particles) [5]. The biopharmaceutical modeling for this case is simpler compared to the salt cases. A practically reasonable predictability is anticipated (Chapter 8) [6].

1.4.3   Salt Form Cases

In the case of salts, the oral absorption process is much more complex. A salt form drug usually dissolves rapidly in the GI fluid. However, once the dissolved drug concentration hits the critical supersaturation concentration, the free form drug precipitates out as a solid. To represent this phenomena in biopharmaceutical modeling, a nucleation theory has to be taken into account [7]. However, little is known about the nucleation of drug molecules in the GI environment. Therefore, the extent and duration of supersaturation in the GI tract is currently not quantitatively predictable from *in vitro* data. A similar scenario can be applied for cocrystalline, amorphous solid form, and supersaturable formulations. To improve the biopharmaceutical modeling in the future, this area requires significant investigations.

1.5   THE CONCEPT OF MECHANISTIC MODELING

The mechanistic modeling approach is pursued in this book. To enable computational simulation, the processes that consist of drug absorption must be reduced down to the molecular level mechanisms. The network of theoretical equations connects the overall processes of drug absorption from the molecular level mechanism to the plasma concentration (C_p) time profile of a drug in humans (can be further connected to pharmacological effects via pharmacokinetic–pharmacodynamic (PKPD) modeling). The whole network of theoretical equations of oral drug absorption is called the gastrointestinal unified theoretical (GUT) framework in this book. As described above, oral drug absorption consists of four main processes, dissolution, permeation, nucleation, and GI transit. These processes are further reduced down to the molecular level mechanisms. Ideally, all processes of oral drug absorption should be described by mechanistic mathematical equations that have physical meanings at the molecular level. Therefore, the GUT framework shares the same philosophy of the "analysis"–"synthesis" approach employed by systems biology and physiologically based pharmacokinetic (PBPK) modeling.

Empirical multivariant statistical models (e.g., artificial neural network) are one of the other modeling approaches. Multiple drug parameters are used as input parameters and connected to outcome values using linear or nonlinear empirical equations. There are many investigations applying this approach for the prediction of oral drug absorption [8–11]. However, in the GUT framework, this approach is not pursued unless otherwise inevitable.

The "analysis" (reductionist) approach is rather a traditional approach in the history of science since Galileo's era, and this approach has been incredibly successful. This approach revealed many mysteries of astronomy, physics, chemistry, and finally, biology. However, an analytical understanding of each part does not mean the understanding of relationship between each part and their role on the total performance. For example, understanding of enzyme-level activity is not sufficient (but necessary) to understand how our brain works. With the aid of computational power, the "synthesis" approach has become available. We can now understand the relationship between primary processes and simulate the total performance. In computational systems biology, the networks of enzyme reactions and their effect on the phenotype is described by mechanistic mathematical

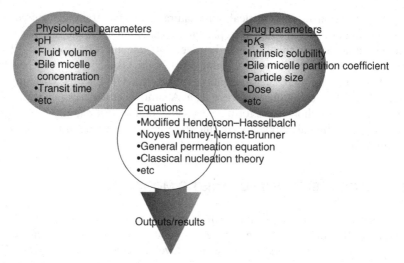

Figure 1.6 Physiological and drug parameters and theoretical equations.

models. By pursuing this approach, we will be able to model the disease state and find a clue to cure the patient. In this book, we pursue the same approach with systems biology. However, in addition to biological processes, the drug substance and formulation perspectives must be taken into account in biopharmaceutical modeling. By using the mechanistic modeling approach, we will be able to control the total bioperformance of a drug by designing the molecular structure, API form, and formulation of the drug.

The mechanistic biopharmaceutical modeling consists of theoretical model equations, physiological parameters, and drug parameters (Fig. 1.6). All of these factors significantly affect the performance of biopharmaceutical modeling. The physiological and drug parameters are often thought to have less error than the mechanistic model equations. However, this notion is incorrect. The physiological data in the literature have large variation and some physiological parameters have not been obtained yet. In addition, a drug parameter can have a large error (variation) when an experiment is not properly performed. Even in the case of solubility measurement, it often has more than twofold variation for low solubility drugs. Therefore, in addition to the theoretical models, the physiological and drug parameters are also discussed in Chapters 6 and 7.

The first step to construct the GUT framework is the unification of the concept of dissolved drug concentration (C_{dissolv}) [7]. We will start the next chapter with defining the dissolved drug concentration.

REFERENCES

1. Yu, L.X. (1999). An integrated model for determining causes of poor oral drug absorption. *Pharm. Res.*, 16, 1883–1887.

2. Sugano, K., Okazaki, A., Sugimoto, S., Tavornvipas, S., Omura, A., Mano, T. (2007). Solubility and dissolution profile assessment in drug discovery. *Drug Metab. Pharmacokinet.*, 22, 225–254.

3. Sugano, K., Kataoka, M., Mathews, C.d.C., Yamashita, S. (2010). Prediction of food effect by bile micelles on oral drug absorption considering free fraction in intestinal fluid. *Eur. J. Pharm. Sci.*, 40, 118–124.

4. Sugano, K. (2011). Fraction of a dose absorbed estimation for structurally diverse low solubility compounds. *Int. J. Pharm.*, 405, 79–89.

5. Johnson, K.C. (2003). Dissolution and absorption modeling: model expansion to simulate the effects of precipitation, water absorption, longitudinally changing intestinal permeability, and controlled release on drug absorption. *Drug Dev. Ind. Pharm.*, 29, 833–842.

6. Sugano, K. Computational oral absorption simulation of free base drugs. (2010). *Int. J. Pharm.*, 398(1–2), 73–82.

7. Sugano, K. (2009). Introduction to computational oral absorption simulation. *Expert Opin. Drug Metab. Toxicol.*, 5, 259–293.

8. Wessel, M.D., Jurs, P.C., Tolan, J.W., Muskal, S.M. (1998). Prediction of human intestinal absorption of drug compounds from molecular structure. *J. Chem. Inf. Comput. Sci.*, 38, 726–735.

9. Turner, J.V., Maddalena, D.J., Agatonovic-Kustrin, S. (2004). Bioavailability prediction based on molecular structure for a diverse series of drugs. *Pharm. Res.*, 21, 68–82.

10. Klopman, G., Stefan, L.R., Saiakhov, R.D. (2002). ADME evaluation. 2. A computer model for the prediction of intestinal absorption in humans. *Eur. J. Pharm. Sci.*, 17, 253–263.

11. Tian, S., Li, Y., Wang, J., Zhang, J., Hou, T. (2011). ADME evaluation in drug discovery. 9. Prediction of oral bioavailability in humans based on molecular properties and structural fingerprints. *Mol. Pharm.*, 8, 841–851.

CHAPTER 2

THEORETICAL FRAMEWORK I: SOLUBILITY

"Everything should be made as simple as possible, but not simpler."

—Albert Einstein

Figure 2.1 shows the network of equations, which consist of the gastrointestinal unified theoretical framework (GUT framework) [1]. The GUT framework is discussed in the following four sections. This framework is constructed based on the unified definition of "dissolved drug concentration (C_{dissolv})" and "fraction (f)" of each molecular species.

2.1 DEFINITION OF CONCENTRATION

Even though the definitions of concentration look trivial and often being omitted in the literature, clear understanding of this point is important for biopharmaceutical modeling.[1]

---

[1]The readers of this book may think that this kind of basic definition should not be cited in a book for advanced scientists. However, a lot of misunderstandings about oral absorption actually come from the confusion of the concepts of concentration. Another often observed confusion is among "fraction (f)," "concentration (C)," and "solubility (S)." The concept of these terms is critically important for biopharmaceutical modeling and should be clearly understood.

Biopharmaceutics Modeling and Simulations: Theory, Practice, Methods, and Applications,
First Edition. Kiyohiko Sugano.
© 2012 John Wiley & Sons, Inc. Published 2012 by John Wiley & Sons, Inc.

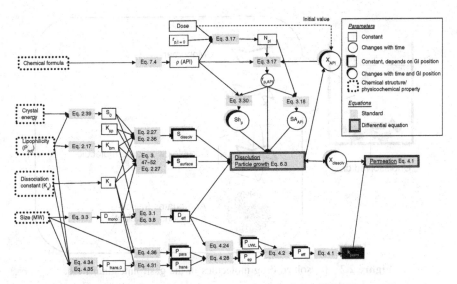

Figure 2.1   Network of equations consisting of the GUT framework.

2.1.1   Total Concentration

Total concentration of a drug (C_{tot}) is the amount of a drug substance in a fluid, regardless of the substance being undissolved solid or dissolved molecules. For example, when 100 mg of a solid drug is diluted to 1 ml with a fluid, the concentration is 100 mg/ml, regardless of whether the drug is completely dissolved or not in the fluid. This point is often miscommunicated by a formulation scientist and a biologist. Biologists often tacitly assume complete dissolution in the assay media, whereas a formulation scientist uses this expression for a suspension formulation.

2.1.2   Dissolved Drug Concentration

"Dissolved drug concentration ($C_{dissolv}$)" is used in this book to express the concentration of dissolved drug molecules in the fluid. Drug molecules can exist in various states in a fluid (Fig. 2.2). After adding a solid compound to a blank medium, if it looks transparent to the eye, we often say it is "dissolved" and the medium is typically called a *solution*. However, the molecule can exist in this transparent solution as (i) a monomer (a single molecule surrounded by solvent molecules), (ii) a dimer or higher self-aggregate, (iii) complexes with large molecules (such as cyclodextrin), (iv) the micelle included state, or even (v) nanoscale particles. In the literature, with the exception of the last case, these are referred to as *solubilized* (the last example is often referred to as *nanosuspension*). We use this definition of "solution" in this chapter unless otherwise noted. In this book, undissociated monomer molecules, dissociated monomer molecules, and bile-micelle-bound molecules are considered in the theoretical

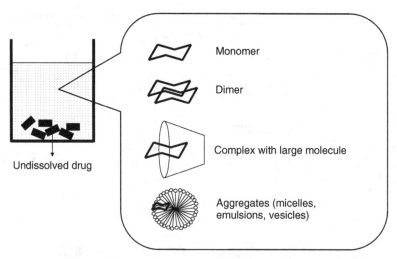

Figure 2.2   Dissolved drug molecules in the gastrointestinal fluid.

framework unless otherwise noted. The dissolved drug concentration (C_{dissolv}) in the gastrointestinal (GI) fluid is expressed as the sum of each species as

$$X_{\text{dissolv}} = \sum_{z} X_{u,z} + X_{\text{bm}} \qquad (2.1)$$

$$C_{\text{dissolv}} = \frac{X_{\text{dissolv}}}{V_{\text{GI}}} = \sum_{z} C_{u,z} + C_{\text{bm}} \qquad (2.2)$$

where X is the amount of drug (weight or mole) and C is the concentration (X/V_{GI}). The subscripts u, z (expressed as $+, -, ++, --, \ldots$ in the following sections), and bm indicate unbound monomer molecules, charge of molecules, and bile-micelle-bound monomer molecules, respectively. V_{GI} is the fluid volume in a GI position.

2.1.3   Effective Concentration

The effective concentration for a reaction, such as dissolution and permeation, depends on the "availability" of the molecular state for the reaction. For example, the dissolution of drug particles can be carried out as both the unbound monomer and the bile-micelle-included state. On the other hand, passive transcellular permeation across the intestinal epithelial membrane occurs mainly for unionized unbound monomer molecules (pH partition and free fraction theories) (Fig. 2.3).

The effective concentration of a reaction is expressed as the fraction of the dissolved drug concentration. For example, concentration of the undissociated

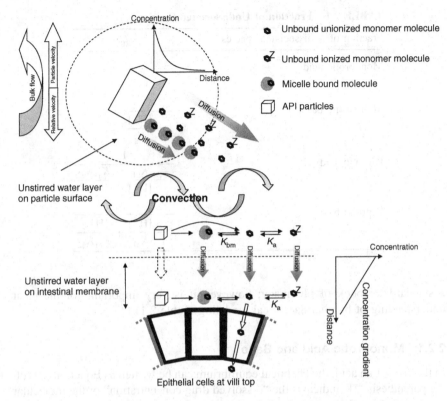

Figure 2.3 Schematic representation of dissolution and permeation.

unbound monomer molecule is expressed as

$$C_{u,0} = f_u f_0 C_{dissolv} \qquad (2.3)$$

where f_u is the fraction of unbound monomer molecules and f_0 is the fraction of undissociated molecules. This expression is the same as that for plasma concentration and unbound fraction used in pharmacokinetics (PK).

2.2 ACID–BASE AND BILE-MICELLE-BINDING EQUILIBRIUMS

The fraction of undissociated monomer molecule (f_0) is determined by the dissociation constant (pK_a) of a drug and pH of the fluid. The famous Henderson–Hasselbalch (HH) equation is derived from the acid–base chemical equilibrium equation.[2] The derivation of the HH equation is often omitted in

---

[2]The acid–base and bile-micelle-binding equilibrium is achieved immediately compared to the timescales of other processes of oral absorption. In general, the reaction rates of these dynamic equilibriums are more than one order faster than the other processes such as dissolution and permeation. Therefore, pseudoequilibrium approximation is appropriate.

TABLE 2.1   Fraction of Undissociated Species

Fraction of undissociated species	(f_0)
Monoprotic acid	$\dfrac{1}{1+\dfrac{K_a}{[H^+]}}$
Monoprotic base	$\dfrac{1}{1+\dfrac{[H^+]}{K_a}}$
Diprotic acid	$\dfrac{1}{1+\dfrac{K_{a1}}{[H^+]}+\dfrac{K_{a1}K_{a2}}{[H^+]^2}}$
Diprotic base	$\dfrac{1}{1+\dfrac{[H^+]}{K_{a1}}+\dfrac{[H^+]^2}{K_{a1}K_{a2}}}$

a standard textbook of pharmacy; however, it is very important for the clear understanding of biopharmaceutical modeling (Table 2.1).

2.2.1 Monoprotic Acid and Base

In the case of an acid, the chemical equilibrium can be written as Equation 2.4 (cf. the parenthesis "[]" indicates the "dissolved drug concentration" of the molecular species (Section 2.1)).

$$[AH] \overset{k_a}{\rightleftharpoons} [A^-] + [H^+] \tag{2.4}$$

$$K_a = \frac{[A^-][H^+]}{[AH]} \quad cf. K_a = 10^{-pK_a}, [H^+] = 10^{-pH} \tag{2.5}$$

where $[H^+]$, $[AH]$, and $[A^-]$ are the concentrations of proton, the undissociated, and the ionized (anion) drug molecules, respectively. This equation is based on the law of mass action. In addition, this equation describes the definition of K_a. K_a is the pH at which the concentrations of undissociated and dissociated species become equal (i.e., $[A^-]/[AH] = 1$). The fraction of the undissociated (unionized) molecular species (f_0) in the total monomer concentration ($C_{u,0} + C_{u,-}$) is then written as

$$f_0 = \frac{\text{Undissociated monomer}}{\text{Total monomer}} = \frac{[AH]}{[AH] + [A^-]} = \frac{1}{1+\dfrac{[A^-]}{[AH]}} = \frac{1}{1+\dfrac{K_a}{[H^+]}} \tag{2.6}$$

Figure 2.4 shows the relationship between pH, pK_a, and f_0 for an acid with $pK_a = 4.5$. When the pH is lower (so the fluid is acidic, the proton concentration

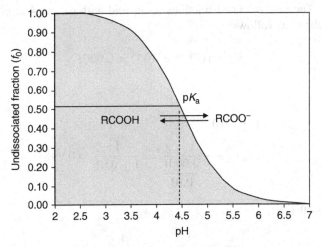

Figure 2.4   The relationship between pH, pK_a, and f_0 for an acid with $pK_a = 4.5$.

is higher), the equilibrium is pushed to the left-hand side of Equation 2.4 and the fraction of undissociated molecules increases, whereas when the pH is higher (the fluid is alkaline, the proton concentration is lower), the equilibrium is pushed to the right-hand side of Equation 2.4 and the fraction of anion molecule increases.

In the case of a base,

$$[BH^+] \overset{K_a}{\rightleftharpoons} [B] + [H^+] \tag{2.7}$$

$$K_a = \frac{[B][H^+]}{[BH^+]} \tag{2.8}$$

Therefore,

$$f_0 = \frac{1}{1 + \dfrac{[H+]}{K_a}} \tag{2.9}$$

Note that the position of the undissociated and the charged drug[3] concentrations in the equation is swapped as for an acid case. When the pH is higher (the fluid is alkaline, the proton concentration is lower), the fraction of undissociated molecules increases ($[H^+]/K_a$ becomes smaller in Equation 2.9).

---

[3]This is "proton-associated (proton bound)" species. Conceptually, this proton binding can be treated in the same manner as bile-micelle binding. This community of concept helps us to understand the theoretical scheme.

Example The undissociated fractions of an acid with pK_a of 4 at pH 2, 4, and 6 are calculated as follows:

$$K_a = 10^{-pK_a} = 10^{-4} = 0.0001$$

At pH 2,

$$[H^+] = 10^{-pH} = 10^{-2} = 0.01$$

$$f_0 = \frac{1}{1 + \dfrac{0.0001}{0.01}} = \frac{1}{1 + 0.01} = 0.99$$

Similarly, at pH 4,

$$f_0 = \frac{1}{1 + \dfrac{0.0001}{0.0001}} = \frac{1}{1 + 1} = 0.5$$

And at pH 6,

$$f_0 = \frac{1}{1 + \dfrac{0.0001}{0.000001}} = \frac{1}{1 + 100} = 0.01$$

2.2.2 Multivalent Cases

For a divalent acid,

$$[AH_2] \overset{K_{a1}}{\rightleftharpoons} [AH^-] + [H^+], [AH^-] \overset{K_{a2}}{\rightleftharpoons} [A^{2-}] + [H^+] \tag{2.10}$$

$$K_{a1} = \frac{[AH^-][H^+]}{[AH_2]}, K_{a2} = \frac{[A^{2-}][H^+]}{[AH^-]} \tag{2.11}$$

The fraction of the undissociated molecular species is then given as

$$f_0 = \frac{[AH_2]}{[AH_2] + [AH^-] + [A^{2-}]} = \frac{1}{1 + \dfrac{[AH^-]}{[AH_2]} + \dfrac{[A^{2-}]}{[AH_2]}}$$

$$= \frac{1}{1 + \dfrac{[AH^-]}{[AH_2]} + \dfrac{[AH^-]}{[AH_2]}\dfrac{[A^{2-}]}{[AH^-]}} = \frac{1}{1 + \dfrac{K_{a1}}{[H^+]} + \dfrac{K_{a1}K_{a2}}{[H^+]^2}} \tag{2.12}$$

An equation for a divalent base can be derived similarly.

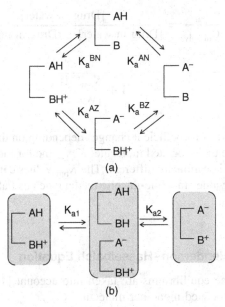

Figure 2.5   (a) Micro pK_a and (b) macro pK_a.

Zwitter ionic cases are much more complex, as both of undissociated and zwitter ionic species are of charge neutral (Fig. 2.5) [2]. To calculate the fractions of undissociated and zwitter ionic species (f_0 and f_{+-}, respectively), the microscopic pK_a value have to be obtained. However, there is no simple experimental method to determine the microscopic pK_a (Section 7.2).

2.2.3 Bile-Micelle Partitioning

The bile-micelle partitioning is another important equilibrium of drug molecules in the intestinal fluid. Drug molecules bound to bile micelles behave differently from unbound ones during dissolution and permeation of the drug. Therefore, the bile-micelle-unbound fraction (f_u) has to be explicitly taken into account for biopharmaceutical modeling. The bile-micelle binding can be treated in a similar way to acid–base equilibrium.[4] Since it is difficult to define the concentration of micelles, the bile-micelle partition coefficient (K_{bm}) is usually defined based on the bile acid concentration ([M]) [3].

$$K_{bm} = \frac{[D-M]/[M]}{[D]/[Water]} \tag{2.13}$$

---

[4]"Bile binding" is a like "proton binding of a base."

$$f_u = \frac{C_u}{C_{dissolv}} = \frac{[\text{Drug in water}]}{[\text{Drug in water}] + [\text{Drug in micelles}]}$$

$$= \frac{1}{1 + \dfrac{[D - M]}{[D]}} = \frac{1}{1 + \dfrac{K_{bm}[M]}{[\text{Water}]}} \tag{2.14}$$

The bile-micelle partition coefficient changes depending on the molecular charge, that is, $K_{bm,0}$ for the undissociated molecule, $K_{bm,-}$ the for monoprotic anion, and $K_{bm,+}$ for monoprotic cation are different. The K_{bm} values can be back-calculated from the solubility values in a bile-micelle media (such as FaSSIF, Section 7.6.2) and its blank media.

2.2.4 Modified Henderson–Hasselbalch Equation

Finally, when all the equilibriums are taken into account [4–6], the fraction of the unbound undissociated monomer molecule ($C_{u,0}/C_{dissolv}$) for acid is

$$\frac{C_{u,0}}{C_{dissolv}} = f_0 \times f_u = \frac{[AH]}{[AH] + [A^-]} \times \frac{[AH] + [A^-]}{[AH] + [A^-] + [A - M] + [A^- - M]}$$

$$= \frac{[AH]}{[AH] + [A^-] + [A - M] + [A^- - M]}$$

$$= \frac{1}{1 + \dfrac{[A^-]}{[AH]} + \dfrac{[AH - M]}{[AH]} + \dfrac{[A^-]}{[AH]}\dfrac{[A^- - M]}{[A^-]}}$$

$$= \frac{1}{1 + \dfrac{K_a}{[H^+]} + \dfrac{K_{bm,0}[M]}{[\text{Water}]} + \dfrac{K_a}{[H^+]}\dfrac{K_{bm,-}[M]}{[\text{Water}]}} \tag{2.15}$$

Similarly, for a monoprotic base,

$$\frac{C_{u,0}}{C_{dissolv}} = f_0 \times f_u = \frac{1}{1 + \dfrac{[H^+]}{K_a} + \dfrac{K_{bm,0}[M]}{[\text{Water}]} + \dfrac{[H^+]}{K_a}\dfrac{K_{bm,+}[M]}{[\text{Water}]}} \tag{2.16}$$

These equations are called *modified HH equation* in this book. The pH solubility profile of dipyridamole in a biorelevant media containing bile micelles is shown in Figure 2.6 [1, 3].

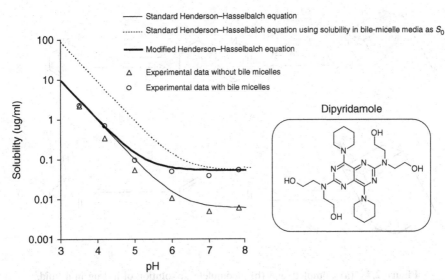

Figure 2.6 pH solubility profile of dipyridamol in biorelevant media containing bile micelles [3].

2.2.5 K_{bm} from Log P_{oct}

K_{bm} can be roughly calculated from the octanol water partition coefficient (P_{oct}) as [3]

$$\log K_{bm,0} = 0.74 \log P_{oct} + 2.29 \tag{2.17}$$

The bile-micelle partition coefficients of monocation and anion ($K_{bm,+}$ and $K_{bm,-}$, respectively) can be estimated as [7, 8]

$$\log K_{bm,+} \approx \log K_{bm,0} - 1 \tag{2.18}$$

$$\log K_{bm,-} \approx \log K_{bm,0} - 2 \tag{2.19}$$

2.3   EQUILIBRIUM SOLUBILITY

2.3.1   Definition of Equilibrium Solubility

The solubility of a drug is defined based on the equilibrium state between the dissolved drug molecules and the undissolved solid drug molecules (Figs. 2.7 and 2.2).[5] At equilibrium, the chemical potential at the solid surface (free

---

[5]Please also refer to Section 7.6.1 for detailed definitions of solubility.

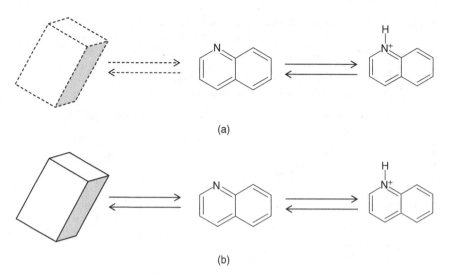

(a)

(b)

Figure 2.7   (a) Complete and (b) incomplete dissolution of a drug in a fluid.

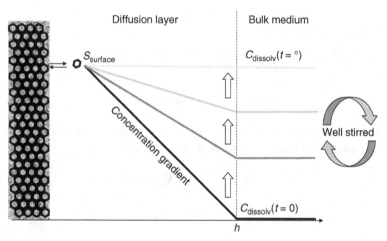

Figure 2.8   Detachment of a molecule from the solid surface and concentration gradient in the diffusion layer.

energy/mole) is equal to that in the fluid. When we look at the solid surface at a molecular level, there is a dynamic equilibrium determined by the balance of detaching and attaching rates (Fig. 2.8). The term *thermodynamic solubility* is also used in the literature but not used in this book.

To measure the solubility of a drug, the amount of the drug (Dose) added to the fluid must exceed the solubilization capacity of the fluid, that is, solubility × fluid volume.[6] The dose number (Do) is defined as (in a broad sense)[7]

$$Do = \frac{Dose}{Solubility \times Fluid\ volume} \qquad (2.20)$$

For the Do > 1 cases, when a solid drug is added to the fluid, a portion of the added drug remains undissolved in the fluid. For example, when 10 mg of a drug with an equilibrium solubility of 1 mg/ml is added to 2 ml of the fluid, Do is 5(= 10 mg/(1 mg/ml × 2 ml). In this case, 2 mg gets dissolved and 8 mg remains undissolved. When Do < 1, the drug completely dissolves in the fluid (Fig. 2.7). For example, when the above drug is added to 20 ml of the fluid, Do is 0.5 (= 10 mg/(1 mg/ml × 20 ml).

The concept of the dose number can be expanded and generally defined when a solid material is added to a fluid. The dose number determines whether a portion of the solid drug remains undissolved in the fluid and participates in the equilibrium network of drug molecules in the fluid (Fig. 2.7). In the absence of the undissolved drug in the fluid (i.e., Do < 1, the drug is completely dissolved in the fluid), the equilibriums in the solution are sufficient to describe the concentration of each molecular species in the fluid, for example, pH equilibrium and bile-micelle-binding equilibrium. However, in the presence of undissolved drug material (i.e., Do > 1), the equilibrium between the solid drug (remaining undissolved) and the dissolved drug have to be additionally taken into account.

2.3.2 pH–Solubility Profile (pH-Controlled Region)

The typical pH–equilibrium solubility profile of a monobasic compound is shown in Figure 2.9. The pH–solubility profile can be divided into "pH" and "common ionic effect" controlled regions. The pH–solubility profile of a drug in a simple buffer (without solubilizers such as micelles) is controlled by the pK_a, intrinsic solubility (S_0), and solubility product (K_{sp}) of a drug, as well as the pH and the common ion concentration in the fluid. The smaller value of the pH-controlled or common-ion-controlled solubility determines the actual solubility of a drug experimentally observed.

The pH–solubility curve in the pH-controlled region is derived as follows. In the case of an acid, when an excess amount of a solid drug coexists in a fluid at a pH where no dissociation occurs (i.e., pH ≪ pK_a of the drug), the equilibrium between the solid and the dissolved drug is written as

$$\langle AH \rangle \rightleftharpoons [AH] \qquad (2.21)$$

---

[6]Whether an excess undissolved solid drug exists in the fluid or not is very important in biopharmaceutics. The dose number is the central parameter that governs the biopharmaceutical characteristics of a drug.

[7]In the regulatory context, the minimum solubility in the GI physiological pH range and the fluid volume of 250 ml is used to calculate the dose number. However, the dose number has wider and deeper implication in biopharmaceutical modeling, hence, used as a generalized concept in this book.

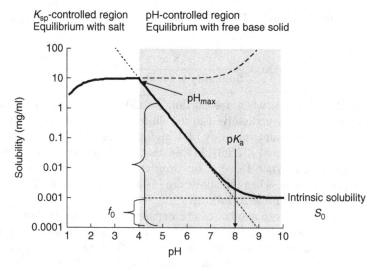

K_{sp}-controlled region   pH-controlled region
Equilibrium with salt   Equilibrium with free base solid

Figure 2.9   Typical pH–solubility profile of a base.

where $\langle AH \rangle$ represents the solid form of the undissociated drug (cf. [] indicates the "dissolved drug concentration" (Section 2.1). When the system is at equilibrium in this pH region, [AH] equals the intrinsic solubility of the undissociated drug (S_0).

As the pH goes up, the acid molecules start to dissociate. Therefore, we add a pH–pK_a equilibrium:

$$\langle AH \rangle \rightleftharpoons [AH] \tag{2.22}$$

$$[AH] \overset{K_a}{\rightleftharpoons} [A^-] + [H^+] \tag{2.23}$$

As far as the solid form of the undissociated acid coexists in equilibrium with [AH] (i.e., Do > 1), the concentration of the dissolved free acid ([AH]) remains constant and equals to S_0. As described in Section 2.2.1, [A$^-$] can be determined by pK_a, pH, and [AH].

$$[A^-] = \frac{K_a}{[H^+]}[AH] \quad \left(cf. \ K_a = \frac{[A^-][H^+]}{[AH]} \right) \tag{2.24}$$

Therefore, the total dissolved drug concentration in a buffer ($S_{buffer} = $ [AH] + [A$^-$]) when [AH] is in equilibrium with the solid undissociated acid can be described as

$$S_{buffer} = [AH] + [A^-] = S_0 + \frac{K_a}{[H^+]}S_0 = S_0 \left(1 + \frac{K_a}{[H^+]} \right) = \frac{S_0}{f_0} \tag{2.25}$$

When we rewrite this,

$$S_0 = f_0 S_{\text{buffer}} \quad \text{or} \quad f_0 = \frac{S_0}{S_{\text{buffer}}} \tag{2.26}$$

Example The solubility of an acidic drug ($pK_a = 4, S_0 = 0.001$ mg/ml) at pH 6.0 can be calculated as

$$S_{\text{buffer}} = \frac{S_0}{f_0} = \frac{0.001}{0.01} = 0.1$$

In Figure 2.10, the concept of concentration, fraction, and solubility are illustrated.

- Complete Dissolution Case (Do < 1)
  - When the added solid drug is completely dissolved in the fluid at all pH (Do < 1), the dissolved drug concentration does not depend on pH ([AH] + [A$^-$] = added drug amount/fluid volume), however, the fractions (ratios) and the concentrations of undissociated and dissociated species changes (Figs. 2.10a and 2.4).
- Incomplete Dissolution Case (Do > 1)
  - When an excess amount of solid drug is added (D > 1), [AH] is in equilibrium with the solid of undissolved free acid (AH). Therefore, [AH] remains constant (as S_0, which is independent of pH), but the ratio of [A$^-$] and [AH] increases as pH increases. Therefore, as pH increases, dissolved drug concentration (= [AH] + [A$^-$]) becomes higher (Fig. 2.10b).[8]

2.3.3 Solubility in a Biorelevant Media with Bile Micelles (pH-Controlled Region)

As discussed in Section 2.2.4, the bile-micelle-binding equilibrium can be treated in a similar way to acid–base equilibrium. The solubility of undissociable acid and base drugs in a biorelevant media with bile micelles (S_{dissolv}) can be written as

$$S_{\text{dissolv}} = \frac{S_0}{f_u} = S_0\left(1 + \frac{K_{\text{bm}}[\text{Bile acid}]}{[\text{Water}]}\right) \qquad \text{Undissociable} \quad (2.27)$$

$$S_{\text{dissolv}} = \frac{S_0}{f_u f_0} = S_0\left(1 + \frac{K_a}{[\text{H}^+]} + \frac{K_{\text{bm},0}[\text{Bile acid}]}{[\text{Water}]}\right.$$
$$\left. + \frac{K_a}{[\text{H}^+]}\frac{K_{\text{bm},-}[\text{Bile acid}]}{[\text{Water}]}\right) \qquad \text{Monoprotic acid} \quad (2.28)$$

[8]The ratio of undissociated and dissociated species (of dissolved drug) is the same, regardless of Do.

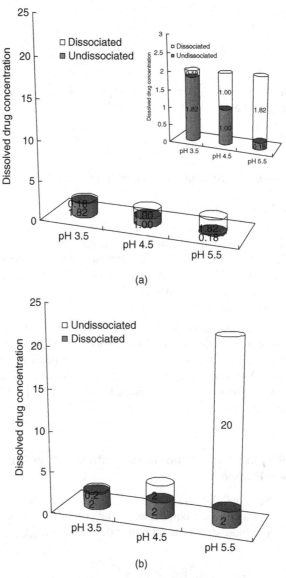

Figure 2.10   Fraction, concentration, and solubility. (a) Do <1 at all pH and (b) Do >1 at all pH. (a) 2 mg of a drug (acid, $pK_a = 4.5$, $S_0 = 2$ mg/mL) added to 1 mL. (b) An excess amount added.

$$S_{\text{dissolv}} = \frac{S_0}{f_u f_0} = S_0 \left(1 + \frac{[\text{H}^+]}{K_a} + \frac{K_{\text{bm},0}[\text{Bile acid}]}{[\text{Water}]} \right.$$

$$\left. + \frac{[\text{H}^+]}{K_a} \frac{K_{\text{bm},+}[\text{Bile acid}]}{[\text{Water}]} \right) \qquad \text{Monoprotic base} \quad (2.29)$$

2.3.4   Estimation of Unbound Fraction from the Solubilities with and without Bile Micelles

From Equation 2.29, the unbound fraction (f_u) can be back-estimated from the solubilities in the media with and without bile micelles $(S_{dissolv}$ and S_{buffer}, respectively).

$$f_u = \frac{S_{buffer}}{S_{dissolv}} = \frac{S_0/f_0}{S_{dissolv}} \tag{2.30}$$

This method is practically useful as S_{blank} and $S_{dissolv}$ is usually available during drug discovery.

It should be emphasized that, as in the same manner with acid–base equilibrium, when the fluid is in equilibrium with excess amount of a solid drug (i.e., Do > 1), even when bile-micelle concentration is increased, the concentration of unbound drugs remains constant (and equals S_{blank}), whereas $C_{dissolv} (= S_{dissolv})$ is increased and the fractions of unbound drugs is decreased. On the other hand, when the drug is completely dissolved in the fluid (i.e., Do < 1), both the concentration and the fraction of unbound drugs are decreased as bile-micelle concentration is increased. This point is important especially when considering the food effects on oral absorption of a drug, as the food intake increases the bile-micelle concentration in the GI tract (Sections 12.2.2.1 and 12.2.3.1).

2.3.5   Common Ionic Effect

The solubility of a salt is described by the solubility product (K_{sp}). In the case of a salt of base drug,

$$< BH^+X^- > \overset{K_{sp}}{\rightleftharpoons} [BH^+]_{sat} + [X^-] \tag{2.31}$$

$$K_{sp} = \frac{[BH^+]_{sat}[X^-]}{\langle BH^+X^- \rangle} \tag{2.32}$$

where the subscript "sat" indicates the saturated species (species of equilibrium maker), and $\langle BH^+X^- \rangle$ is the activity of the solid part of the salt and is defined as 1. Therefore,

$$K_{sp} = [BH^+]_{sat}[X^-] \tag{2.33}$$

When we consider the case that the fluid pH is adjusted by an acid, HX (e.g., HCl) and ionic strength is adjusted by a salt, MX (e.g., NaCl), because of the charge neutrality in the fluid, the sum of the anions $(= [X^-] + [OH^-])$ equals the sum of the cations $(= [H^+] + [BH^+] + [M^+])$.

$$[X^-] + [OH^-] = [BH^+]_{sat} + [H^+] + [M^+] \tag{2.34}$$

By inserting this charge neutrality equation into the solubility product equation,

$$K_{sp} = [BH^+]_{sat} \left([BH^+]_{sat} + [H^+] + [M^+] - \frac{K_w}{[H^+]} \right) \qquad (2.35)$$

where K_w is the ionic product of water ($K_w = [H^+][OH^-] = 1 \times 10^{-14}$ M^2). This equation is a quadratic equation of $[BH^+]_{sat}$ and can be solved as

$$[BH^+]_{sat} = \frac{-\left([H^+] + [M^+] - \frac{K_w}{[H^+]} \right) + \sqrt{\left([H^+] + [M^+] - \frac{K_w}{[H^+]} \right)^2 + 4K_{sp}}}{2}$$

$$(2.36)$$

The dissolved drug solubility is the sum of B and BH$^+$. Therefore, using the HH equation for mono bases,

$$S_{dissolv} = [BH^+]_{sat} + [B] = [BH^+]_{sat} \left(1 + \frac{[B]}{[BH^+]_{sat}} \right)$$

$$= [BH^+]_{sat} \left(1 + \frac{K_a}{[H^+]} \right) \quad pH < pH_{max} \qquad (2.37)$$

where pH_{max} is the pH of the maximum solubility, the system changes from the pH-controlled region to the common-ion-effect-controlled region. Similar equation can be derived for acid drugs.

In the pH-controlled region (acid: pH < pH_{max}, base: pH > pH_{max}), the slope of the logarithmic pH–solubility plot is 1. Therefore, one unit shift of pH or pK_a results in 10-fold change in solubility. The maximum solubility of the pH–equilibrium solubility profile is limited by the solubility product. In the common-ion-effect-controlled region, the equilibrium solubility of a drug depends largely on the concentration of the counterions (common ion effect) but less on the pH (concentration of H_3O^+). Therefore, the species of the counterion is an important factor when we measure the pH–equilibrium solubility profile (K_{sp} is different among the counterion species such as Cl$^-$, CH$_3$SO$_3{}^-$).

Na$^+$ and Cl$^-$ are most often used, as they are the major ionic species in the physiological condition.

In this book, the intrinsic solubility of a salt (S_{salt}) is defined as

$$S_{salt} \equiv \sqrt{K_{sp}} \qquad (2.38)$$

2.3.6   Important Conclusion from the pH–Equilibrium Solubility Profile Theory

From the theories of the pH–equilibrium solubility profile, it is concluded that, regardless of the initial solid form (free or salt) used for a solubility measurement, the pH–equilibrium solubility profile becomes identical in the pH-controlled region.[9] Figure 2.11 shows some experimental data [10]. For example, even when we start with an HCl salt of a base, as the pH is titrated above the pH_{max}, the free base precipitates out and $S_{dissolv}$ is determined based on the equilibrium with the solid of the free base (not HCl salt). In other words, the pH–equilibrium solubility profiles measured from a free base and its salt become identical when the pH is well maintained by the buffer. This situation is very different from the equilibrium solubility in an unbuffered media (i.e., pure water), as the initial pH can be shifted by the added drug. In this case, the final pH and the equilibrium solubility become different depending on the starting solid material. In drug discovery, a strong buffer (e.g., 50 mM phosphate buffer) is often used for the solubility measurement. Therefore, an identical (or very similar) solubility value is usually reported for a free drug and its salt.

Even though the equilibrium solubility measured from a free form and a salt form becomes the same in a buffer, the bioavailabilities of a free base and its salt are usually significantly different. This suggests that the equilibrium solubility in a buffer at a pH cannot be simply used for biopharmaceutical modeling of a salt (as it is identical to a free base).[10] The reasons that salt formation increases the oral absorption of a poor solubility drug are (i) salt formation increases the dissolution rate (by increasing the solid surface solubility), and/or (ii) a supersaturated concentration can be produced in the gastrointestinal fluid after the dissolution of a salt (Sections 3.3 and 11.1) (the dissolved drug molecules at the transient supersaturated concentration are absorbed before the dissolved drug concentration settle down to the equilibrium solubility (which is identical to that of the free base form)). The difference in the dissolution and precipitation mechanisms between a free form and a salt should be taken into account in biopharmaceutic modeling.[11,12]

2.3.7   Yalkowsky's General Solubility Equation

The intrinsic solubility of a drug (free form) in water is determined by the hydration energy of a drug molecule and the sublime energy (Fig. 2.12). Yalkowsky's

---

[9]We are assuming that the precipitated free form has the same solid form with the other free form. When the pH titration method is used without enough equilibrium time, the pH–*apparent* solubility curve can deviate from the theoretical HH curve. When the drug forms aggregate, equilibrium to the aggregate state must additionally be taken into account [9].

[10]This is one of the most often observed mistakes in biopharmaceutical modeling.

[11]In some literature, this important aspect was unremarked.

[12]For appropriate modeling for a salt, a nucleation theory is required.

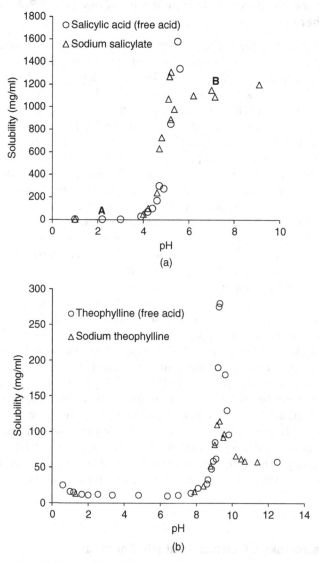

Figure 2.11   pH solubility profile of (a) salicylic acid and (b) theophylline measured from the free acids and the sodium salts. (a) The pH–solubility profiles of salicylic acid (free acid, circle) and sodium salicylate (triangle). Points A (pH 2.3) and B (pH 6.9) represent the pH values and concentrations of saturated solutions of salicylic acid and its sodium salt in pure water. (b) The pH solubility profiles of theophylline (free acid, circle) and sodium theophylline (triangle). *Source:* Adapted from Reference 10 with permission.

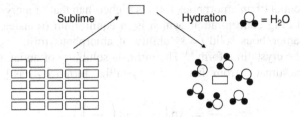

Figure 2.12   Sublime and hydration.

general solubility equation is a simple but very useful equation [11, 12].

$$\log S_0(\text{M}) = -\log P_{\text{oct}} - 1.1\frac{\Delta S_f(\text{m.p.} - 25)}{1364} + 0.54 \qquad (2.39)$$

$$\Delta S_f = 13.5 + 2.5(n - 5) \qquad (2.40)$$

where ΔS_f is the entropy of fusion, n is the number of nonhydrogen atoms ($n > 5$) in a flexible chain, and m.p. is the melting point of a drug. This equation can be further simplified to

$$\log S_0(\text{M}) = -\log P_{\text{oct}} - 0.01(\text{m.p.} - 25) + 0.50 \qquad (2.41)$$

In this equation, the $\log P_{\text{oct}}$ reflects the hydration energy, and the melting point reflects the crystal lattice energy. Roughly speaking, a change in m.p. of 100°C will change the solubility 10-fold. This equation cannot be applied for enantiotropic polymorph cases (Section 7.5.2.4). The average error of this equation is 0.42 log units [13].

Equations 2.40 and 2.41 can be used to diagnose the main reasons for poor solubility. When high lipophilicity is the main reason, micelle solubilization would be effective to increase the solubility of a drug [14–16]. When high melting point is the reason, structural modification to reduce the lattice energy would be effective, for example, introducing a steric barrier for molecular stacking or removing an intermolecular hydrogen bond in the crystalline.

As the solubility measurement is not straightforward and the experimental data is sometimes accompanied with an artifact error, cross validation of the experimental solubility value with the predicted value by this equation is important[13] (Section 7.6).

2.3.8   Solubility Increase by Converting to an Amorphous Form

An amorphous solid form is often used to enhance the bioavailability of a poor solubility drug (Section 11.1.2.3). We can define the solubility of an amorphous form of a drug in the same manner as that for a crystalline form. As the

---

[13] A decomposition temperature is often misleadingly reported as the melting point of a drug.

chemical potential of an amorphous form is higher than that of a crystalline form, the dissolved drug concentration, which is in equilibrium (transiently) with the undissolved amorphous solid (= solubility of amorphous form), is also higher than that of the crystalline form.[14] The intrinsic solubility of an amorphous form ($S_{0,A}$) can be estimated from that of the crystalline form ($S_{0,C}$) as [17]

$$\frac{S_{0,A}}{S_{0,C}} = \exp\left(\frac{\Delta S_m}{R} \ln\left(\frac{T_m}{T}\right)\right) \tag{2.42}$$

where R is the gas constant, T is the absolute temperature, and ΔS_m is the entropy of melting. ΔS_m can be calculated using $\Delta S_m = \Delta H_m/T_m$, where ΔH_m is the enthalpy of melting and T_m is the melting temperature. ΔH_m and T_m can be measured by differential scanning calorimeter (DSC) (Section 7.5.3.3).

2.3.9   Solubility Increase by Particle Size Reduction (Nanoparticles)

The solid surface energy increases as the surface area increases. Therefore, theoretically, particle size reduction increases the solubility of a drug. According to the Ostwald–Freundlich equation (Kelvin equation), the increase in solubility by particle size reduction can be estimated as

$$\frac{S_{0,r_p}}{S_{0,\infty}} = \exp\left(\frac{2\gamma v_m}{r_p RT}\right) \tag{2.43}$$

where S_{0,r_p} and $S_{0,\infty}$ are the solubility of particles with radius r_p and that of an infinitely large particle (larger than several micrometers), respectively, γ is the interfacial tension between the solid surface and the fluid and v_m is the molar volume of a drug. A simple calculation scheme for γ from $S_{0,\infty}$ has been reported [18].

$$\gamma = \frac{k_B T}{(v_m/N_A)^{2/3}} \times 0.33 \times \left(-\ln\left(\frac{S_{0,\infty}}{55.6}\right) - 5\right) \tag{2.44}$$

where N_A is the Avogadro constant (6.022×10^{23} mol^{-1}) and k_B is the Boltzmann constant (1.38×10^{-23} J/K). v_m can be estimated as [19]

$$v_m(\text{cm}^3/\text{mol}) = 3.85 \sum_{\text{atom}} m_{\text{atom}} \cdot v_{\text{atom}} \tag{2.45}$$

where m_{atom} is the number of atoms in the molecule and v_{atom} is the relative volume of the atom, which is 1 for H, 2 for the first short period in the periodic table (LiF), 4 for NaCl, 5 for KBr, and 7.5 for RbI.

---

[14]An amorphous form converts to a crystalline. However, the induction time before crystallization to occur can be long enough to achieve a transient equilibrium with the amorphous solid.

It is theoretically suggested that the increase in solubility by particle size reduction is less than 15% even at approximately 150 nm range [20]. This theoretical suggestion was recently confirmed by careful experiments [20]. The filtration and centrifuge methods are often used in solubility measurements to separate the fluid from the undissolved drug. However, these methods lead to overestimation of the solubility of nanoparticles because of the incomplete separation of nanoparticles from the fluid. A few alternative methods have been introduced to measure the solubility of nanoparticles (Section 7.6.3.4).

2.3.10 Cocrystal

The solubility of a cocrystal can be defined in the same manner as that for a salt [21].

$$\langle DC \rangle \xleftrightarrow{K_{sp}} [Drug]_{sat} + [Coformer] \tag{2.46}$$

$$K_{sp} = \frac{[Drug]_{sat}[Coformer]}{\langle DC \rangle} \tag{2.47}$$

where the subscript "sat" indicates the saturated species and <DC> is the activity of the solid cocrystal and is defined as 1. Therefore,

$$K_{sp} = [Drug]_{sat}[Coformer] \tag{2.48}$$

The intrinsic solubility of a cocrystal ($S_{cocrystal}$) is then defined as

$$S_{cocrystal} \equiv \sqrt{K_{sp}} \tag{2.49}$$

Cocrystal solubility always refers to intrinsic solubility in pure solvent as defined by this equation.

REFERENCES

1. Sugano, K. (2009). Introduction to computational oral absorption simulation. *Expert Opin. Drug Metab. Toxicol.*, 5, 259–293.
2. Pagliara, A., Carrupt, P.A., Caron, G., Gaillard, P., Testa, B. (1997). Lipophilicity Profiles of Ampholytes. *Chem. Rev.*, 97, 3385–3400.
3. Glomme, A., März, J., Dressman, J., Predicting the intestinal solubility of poorly soluble drugs, in: *Pharmacokinetic Profiling in Drug Research*, B., Testa, S., Krämer, H., Wunderli-Allenspach, G., Folkers (Eds.) Wiley-VCH, Zurich, 2006, pp. 259–280.
4. Rippie, E.G., Lamb, D.J., Romig, P.W. (1964). Solubilization of weakly acidic and basic drugs by aqueous solutions of polysorbate 80. *J. Pharm. Sci.*, 53, 1346–1348.
5. Dressman, J.B., *PhysChem Forum 5*, 2007.

6. Jinno, J., Oh, D.M., Crison, J.R., Amidon, G.L. (2000). Dissolution of ionizable water-insoluble drugs: the combined effect of pH and surfactant. *J. Pharm. Sci.*, 89, 268–274.

7. Avdeef, A., Box, K.J., Comer, J.E., Hibbert, C., Tam, K.Y. (1998). pH-metric logP 10. Determination of liposomal membrane-water partition coefficients of ionizable drugs. *Pharm. Res.*, 15, 209–215.

8. Miyazaki, J., Hideg, K., Marsh, D. (1992). Interfacial ionization and partitioning of membrane-bound local anesthetics. *Biochim. Biophys. Acta, Biomembr.*, 1103, 62–68.

9. Avdeef, A., Voloboy, D., Foreman, A., Dissolution and solubility, in *Comprehensive Medicinal Chemistry II Volume 5 ADME-Tox Approach*, B., Testa, H., vande Waterbeemd (Eds.) Elsevier, Oxford, 2007, pp. 399–423.

10. Serajuddin, A.T.M., Jarowski, C.I. (1985). Effect of diffusion layer pH and solubility on the dissolution rate of pharmaceutical acids and their sodium salts. II: Salicylic acid, theophylline, and benzoic acid. *J. Pharm. Sci.*, 74, 148–154.

11. Yang, G., Ran, Y., Yalkowsky, S.H. (2002). Prediction of the aqueous solubility: comparison of the general solubility equation and the method using an amended solvation energy relationship. *J. Pharm. Sci.*, 91, 517–533.

12. Yalkowsky, S.H., Valvani, S.C. (1980). Solubility and partitioning. I: Solubility of nonelectrolytes in water. *J. Pharm. Sci.*, 69, 912–922.

13. Jain, N., Yalkowsky, S.H. (2001). Estimation of the aqueous solubility I: application to organic nonelectrolytes. *J. Pharm. Sci.*, 90, 234–252.

14. Wassvik, C.M., Holmen, A.G., Draheim, R., Artursson, P., Bergstroem, C.A.S. (2008). Molecular characteristics for solid-state limited solubility. *J. Med. Chem.*, 51, 3035–3039.

15. Wassvik, C.M., Holmen, A.G., Bergstrom, C.A., Zamora, I., Artursson, P. (2006). Contribution of solid-state properties to the aqueous solubility of drugs. *Eur. J. Pharm. Sci.*, 29, 294–305.

16. Zaki, N.M., Artursson, P., Bergstrom, C.A. (2010). A modified physiological BCS for prediction of intestinal absorption in drug discovery. *Mol. Pharm.*, 7(5), 1478–1487.

17. Lindfors, L., Forssen, S., Skantze, P., Skantze, U., Zackrisson, A., Olsson, U. (2006). Amorphous drug nanosuspensions. 2. Experimental determination of bulk monomer concentrations. *Langmuir*, 22, 911–916.

18. Lindfors, L., Forssen, S., Westergren, J., Olsson, U. (2008). Nucleation and crystal growth in supersaturated solutions of a model drug. *J. Colloid Interface Sci.*, 325, 404–413.

19. Girolami, G.S. (1994). A simple "back of the envelope" method for estimating the densities and molecular volumes of liquids and solids. *J. Chem. Educ.*, 71, 962–964.

20. Van Eerdenbrugh, B., Vermant, J., Martens, J.A., Froyen, L., Van Humbeeck, J., Van den Mooter, G., Augustijns, P. (2010). Solubility increases associated with crystalline drug nanoparticles: methodologies and significance. *Mol. Pharmaceutics*, 7, 1858–1870.

21. Good, D.J., Rodrguez-Hornedo, N. (2009). Solubility advantage of pharmaceutical cocrystals. *Cryst. Growth Des.*, 9, 2252–2264.

CHAPTER 3

THEORETICAL FRAMEWORK II: DISSOLUTION

"If you wish to make an apple pie from scratch, you must first invent the universe."
—Carl Sagan

The Noyes–Whitney equation, which describes the dissolution phenomena, was introduced more than 100 years ago [1]. Since then, the sciences of dissolution have progressed tremendously. However, there remain many unexplored areas in this field as well. Even though fluid dynamics theories are the basis of dissolution phenomena, they were merely discussed in the textbooks of pharmaceutical sciences. In this section, the sciences of dissolution are discussed using fluid dynamics theories.

Diffusion and convection govern the mass transfer phenomena. From a microscopic viewpoint, diffusion is a random walk process. For example, when a drop of ink is put into a glass of water, it gradually spreads in the water (Fig. 3.1a). After a long time, the solution becomes homogeneous. The same phenomena determines the dissolution of a drug by diffusion (Fig. 3.1b). Even though diffusion is the random walk process, there is a net movement of molecules from a high concentration region to a low concentration region. Therefore, the concentration gradient is often referred to as the *driving force of diffusion* (Fig. 2.8). The diffusion kinetics is described by Fick's laws of diffusion. On the other hand, the convection (flow) also affects the mass transfer. If we stir the water, it becomes homogeneous faster. The motion of a fluid is described by the Navier–Stokes equation.

Biopharmaceutics Modeling and Simulations: Theory, Practice, Methods, and Applications,
First Edition. Kiyohiko Sugano.
© 2012 John Wiley & Sons, Inc. Published 2012 by John Wiley & Sons, Inc.

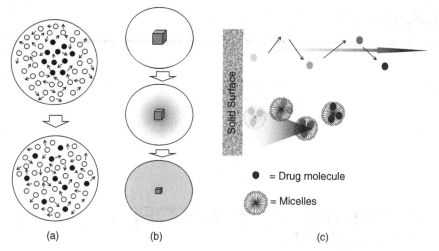

Figure 3.1 Diffusion process. (a) diffusion of a drop of ink, (b) dissolution of a drug under unstirred condition, and (c) diffusion of monomer and bile-micelle drug.

The mass transfer equation is derived from the Fick's laws of diffusion and the Navier–Stokes equation. The derivation of the mass transfer equation from these two equations is found elsewhere (Chapters 1 to 7 of the book "Mass Transfer: Basics and Application" by Kohichi Asano). In this section, we start with the obtained equation and discuss its application in biopharmaceutical modeling. Diffusion coefficient is first discussed, followed by a discussion on the convection process.

3.1 DIFFUSION COEFFICIENT

3.1.1 Monomer

A diffusion coefficient has a dimension of square length per time, for example, square centimeter per second. Several equations have been reported to calculate the diffusion coefficient of a monomer (D_{mono}) in an aqueous media. Avdeef [2] proposed the following equation to calculate the diffusion coefficient of a monomer drug molecule in water at 37 °C.

$$D_{mono}(\text{cm}^2/\text{s, } 37\,^\circ\text{C}) = 9.9 \times 10^{-5}\ \text{MW}^{-0.453} \tag{3.1}$$

For MW $= 350$ D_{mono} is calculated to be 7.3×10^{-6} cm^2/s. The average error of this equation is ca. 20%.

When a molecular volume parameter is available, various other methods can also be used, for example, Hayduk and Laudie equation,

$$D_{mono}(\text{cm}^2/\text{s, } 25\,^\circ\text{C}) = \frac{13.26 \times 10^{-5}}{\eta^{1.4} v_B^{0.589}} \tag{3.2}$$

This equation has a 13% error. By using Abraham solute descriptor,

$$\log D_{mono}(cm^2/s, 25°C) = 0.13 - 0.027\ A_H - 0.36\ V_x \tag{3.3}$$

where A_H is the hydrogen-donor strength and V_x is the McGowans molecular volume. Compared to the other drug parameters such as S_0, the estimation error of D_{mono} from the molecular structure is much smaller.

3.1.2 Bile Micelles

The diffusion coefficient of bile-micelles depends on the bile micelle concentration (Fig. 3.2). The diffusion coefficient of bile micelles is ca. 8–80 times smaller than that of a monomer molecule. In the case of taurocholic acid (TC)–egg lecithin (EL) 4:1 system, the bile-micelle diameter (d_{bm}) and diffusion coefficient of bile-micelle-bound drug (D_{bm}) can be predicted as [3, 4]

$$d_{bm}(nm) = \frac{700}{-7.90 \times C_{bile}(mM) + 37.1} \cdots C_{bile} \leq 3.98\ mM \tag{3.4}$$

$$d_{bm}(nm) = \frac{1}{0.143 \times C_{bile}(mM) - 0.562} + 5.31 \cdots C_{bile} > 3.98\ mM \tag{3.5}$$

$$D_{bm}(cm^2/s) = \frac{6.63}{d_{bm}(nm)} \times 10^{-6} \tag{3.6}$$

where C_{bile} is the concentration of TC. For example, for the fasted state simulated intestinal fluid (FaSSIF, TC = 3 mM) [5], $d_{bm} = 52$ nm and $D_{bm} = 0.13 \times 10^{-6}$ cm^2/s. It would be worth noting that D_{bm} could be different for each GI (gastrointestinal tract) position or each animal species, depending on the concentration and the composition of bile micelles. Furthermore, as a concentrated bile is diluted,

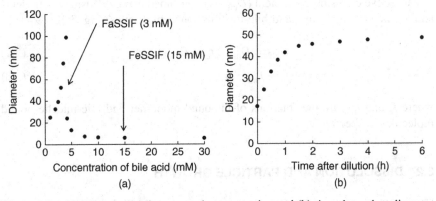

Figure 3.2 (a) Bile-micelle diameter and concentration and (b) time-dependent diameter change after dilution of concentrated FaSSIF (TC = 30 mM).

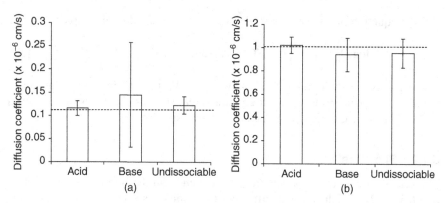

Figure 3.3 Drug inclusion and bile micelle diffusion coefficient. (a) FaSSIF and (b) FeSSIF. Acid: N = 8 drugs. Base: N = 12 drugs. Undissociable N = 23 drugs.

the bile-micelle diameter changes [4]. This dilution process might also occur in the intestine, as the bile secreted from the gall bladder is diluted in the intestine. After dilution of concentrated bile micelles, the micelles transform to liposome-like structures [6]. Okazaki et al. [7] investigated the effect of drug inclusion on the diffusion coefficient of the bile micelles (Fig. 3.3). In the case of some basic compounds, drug inclusion had a large effect on the diffusion coefficient of bile micelles, whereas undissociable and acidic compounds had little effect. Diffusion coefficient of bile micelles can be easily measured by dynamic laser scattering (Section 7.4.3).

When the bile acid concentration is less than 3 mM, the effective diffusion coefficient in the mucus layer was reported to be three times larger compared to that in water [8].

3.1.3 Effective Diffusion Coefficient

The effective diffusion coefficient (D_{eff}) is determined using diffusion coefficients and fractions of monomer and bile-micelle-bound molecules (Fig. 3.1c) [9–14]:

$$D_{eff} = D_{mono} \, f_u + D_{bm} \, f_{bm} \qquad (3.7)$$

$$f_u + f_{bm} = 1 \qquad (3.8)$$

where f_u and f_{bm} are the fractions of unbound monomer and bile-micelle-bound molecules, respectively.

3.2 DISSOLUTION AND PARTICLE GROWTH

Figure 2.8 shows the schematic representation of dissolution of a solid in a fluid. Two steps are involved in the dissolution from the solid surface. The first step is the detachment of a molecule from the solid surface. The second step is the diffusion of the detached molecule across the diffusion layer adjacent to the solid surface. In most cases, rapid equilibrium (i.e., saturation) is achieved at the solid surface. Therefore, the second step determines the dissolution rate in most cases.[1] The basic diffusion-controlled model was first described by Noyes and Whitney and later modified by Nernst and Brunner [1].

3.2.1 Mass Transfer Equations: Pharmaceutical Science Versus Fluid Dynamics

The dissolution and particle growth[2] of a drug are the mass transfer from/into the surface of a substance. The mass transfer rate is represented by the Noyes–Whitney equation as[3]

$$\frac{dX_{API}}{dt} = -SA_{API}\, k_{mass}\Delta C \tag{3.9}$$

where X_{API} is the amount of an undissolved API (active pharmaceutical ingredient), SA_{API} is the surface area of the API, k_{mass} is the mass transfer coefficient, and ΔC is the concentration gradient across the diffusion layer.

The difference between the dissolution and growth of particles depends on whether the concentration gradient around the drug particles is positive or negative. The mass transfer coefficient (k_{mass}) is defined as the ratio of diffusion coefficient (dimension: square length per time) to mass transfer resistance, which has a dimension of length.[4] The mass transfer resistance is usually scaled to the representative length (L)[5] of the substance using the Sherwood number (Sh).

$$k_{mass} = \frac{D_{eff}}{L/Sh} \tag{3.10}$$

In pharmaceutical science, the film model has been often used to express the mass transfer (Fig. 3.4) and the mass transfer resistance is represented as the thickness of the film of stagnant layer (h_{API}).

$$k_{mass} = \frac{D_{eff}}{h_{API}} \tag{3.11}$$

---

[1]This proposition may not be valid for very small particles (e.g., <100 nano scale), as the diffusion resistance (=particle radius) is very small and the diffusion mass transfer process becomes very fast.
[2]Particle growth can occur during the oral absorption process of a free base and salt.
[3]The mass transfer rate per SA is called *flux* (flux = $k_{mass}\Delta C$).
[4]The mass transfer coefficient has the same dimension with permeability (length per time). Both dissolution and passive membrane permeation are governed by the Fick's law.
[5]The representative length is the length of a substance that most largely affects the flow pattern around the substance.

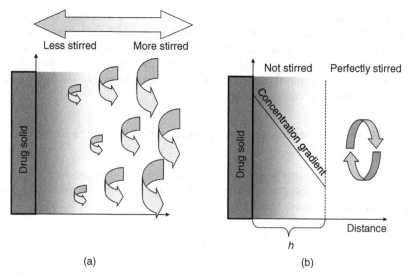

Figure 3.4 (a) Fluid dynamic and (b) pharmaceutical science views for the unstirred water layer.

By comparing Equations 3.10 and 3.11, it is trivial that

$$h_{API} = \frac{L}{Sh} \qquad (3.12)$$

This is the key equation to translate the concept of fluid dynamics to pharmaceutical science. However, as discussed later, several important factors of fluid dynamics are lost in this translation. For example, the effect of fluid viscosity, agitation strength, particle density, and particle shape on the diffusion layer thickness cannot be handled by the pharmaceutical science expression. Therefore, in this book, the fluid dynamical expression of mass transfer is mainly employed.

The mass transfer rate is expressed as

$$\frac{dX_{API}}{dt} = -SA\frac{D_{eff}}{L/Sh}\Delta C \qquad (3.13)$$

3.2.2 Dissolution Equation with a Lump Sum Dissolution Rate Coefficient (k_{diss})

Before going into the thorough discussions of mechanistic dissolution model equations, to have an overview of the dissolution models, a simple equation using a lump sum dissolution rate coefficient (k_{diss}) is first discussed.

As the SA of particles is a function of the drug amount remaining undissolved, it would be appropriate to speculate that SA is approximately in proportion to X_{API}. At the beginning of the dissolution, little amount has been dissolved from the particles and X_{API} is close to the initial dose. Therefore,

$$SA = kX_{API} = k_{Dose} \tag{3.14}$$

where k is a coefficient temporary used in this equation. At the initial time of dissolution, the concentration of the fluid is close to 0. Therefore, ΔC can be approximated as

$$\Delta C \approx S_{surface} \tag{3.15}$$

where $S_{surface}$ is the solubility of a drug at the solid surface. By using Equations 3.14 and 3.15, Equation 3.13 can be rearranged to

$$\frac{dX_{API}}{dt} = -SA_{API}\, k_{mass}\, \Delta C = -k_{Dose}\, k_{mass} S_{surface}$$

$$= -k_{Dose} \frac{D_{eff}}{h_{API}} S_{surface} = -k_{diss}\, Dose \tag{3.16}$$

The lump sum coefficient, k_{diss}, is called the *dissolution rate coefficient*. When an experimental dissolution data is available, k_{diss} can be back calculated from the initial slope of the dissolved drug concentration–time profile. In the following sections, the mechanistic model equations to estimate k_{diss} from the properties of a drug molecule and API are discussed in detail. k_{diss} is the function of solid surface solubility ($S_{surface}$), diffusion coefficient (D_{eff}), initial particle radius ($r_{p,ini}$), particle shape, and true density of the drug (ρ_p), as well as the agitation strength (ε), viscosity (μ), and density (ρ_f) of the fluid. k_{diss} can be calculated from these data (for simple cases, $k_{diss} = 3D_{eff} S_{surface}/r_{p,ini}^2 \rho_p$). However, the estimation errors of each parameter are accumulatively propagated to k_{diss}. Therefore, a direct measurement of this lump sum parameter from a dissolution test is practically useful (Section 8.5.1).

3.2.3 Particle Size and Surface Area

3.2.3.1 *Monodispersed Particles.* The SA of particles is one of the main determinants of a mass transfer rate from/into particles. We start with the calculation of the SA of a monodispersed particle. The weight of one particle is the product of the volume of one particle (V_p) and the particle density (ρ_p). The number of particles in a dose (N_p) can be calculated by dividing the weight of the dose (Dose) by the weight of one particle. In the case of spherical particles with an initial particle radius ($r_{p,ini}$), N_p can be calculated as

$$N_p = \frac{Dose}{V_p \rho_p} = \frac{Dose}{\left(\frac{4}{3}\pi r_{p,ini}^3\right)\rho_p} \tag{3.17}$$

In biopharmaceutical modeling, N_p is operationally set to be unchanged from the initial value, whereas X_{API} and r_p change with the time elapsed. A complete dissolution of a particle is represented by $r_p = 0$ or $X_{API} = 0$.

The SA of one particle (SA_p) with a particle radius (r_p) at time t is

$$SA_p = 4\pi r_p{}^2 \tag{3.18}$$

The total SA at time t is then calculated as the product of the SA of one particle and the number of the particles in the dose. Therefore,

$$SA_{API}(t) = SA_p N_p = 4\pi r_p{}^2 \frac{\text{Dose}}{\left(\dfrac{4}{3}\pi r_{p,\text{ini}}{}^3\right)\rho_p} \tag{3.19}$$

Note that r_p is not the initial particle radius, but the particle radius at time t after dissolution of the particles has occurred ($r_p < r_{p,\text{ini}}$).

Especially, at $t = 0$, this equation can be simplified as

$$SA_{API}(t = 0) = \frac{3\text{Dose}}{r_{p,\text{ini}}\,\rho_p} \tag{3.20}$$

We can see in this equation that the total SA of a dose is reciprocal to the particle size (Fig. 3.5).

Example   The number of particles in 100 mg dose with $\rho_p = 1.2$ g/cm^3, diameter (d_p) = 10 and 1 μm (assuming a spherical particle) can be calculated as follows:

$$SA = \frac{3\text{Dose}}{r_{p,\text{ini}}\,\rho_p} = \frac{3 \times 100}{0.0005 \times 1200} = 500 \text{ cm}^2$$

$$SA = \frac{3\text{Dose}}{r_{p,\text{ini}}\,\rho_p} = \frac{3 \times 100}{0.00005 \times 1200} = 5000 \text{ cm}^2$$

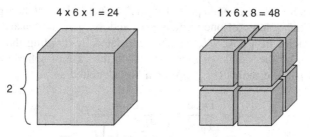

Surface area = (Area of one plate) x (Number of plate) x (Number of particle)

4 x 6 x 1 = 24   1 x 6 x 8 = 48

2

Figure 3.5   Particle size and surface area.

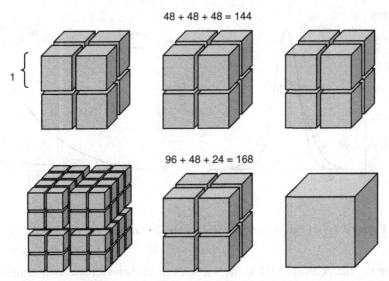

Figure 3.6 Particle size distribution and surface area.

The total SA of a dose can be very large when compared with the intestinal tube SA (the smooth tube-based SA of the entire small intestine is $2 \times 3.14 \times R_{GI}$ (1.5 cm) $\times L_{GI}$ (300 cm) = 2826 cm^2), which is important for the particle drifting effect (Section 4.7.2).

3.2.3.2 Polydispersed Particles. Particle size distribution can be expressed as the volume percentage of each particle size bin (f_{PSB}) with the particle radius ($r_{p,PSB}$)

$$N_{p,PSB} = \frac{f_{PSB} \text{Dose}}{V_p \rho_p} = f_{PSB} \frac{\text{Dose}}{\left(\frac{4}{3} \pi r_{p,ini,PSB}^3\right) \rho_p} \tag{3.21}$$

$$SA(t = 0) = \frac{3\text{Dose}}{\rho_p} \sum^{PBS} \frac{f_{PSB}}{r_{p,ini,PSB}} \tag{3.22}$$

As shown in Figure 3.6, as the particle size distribution becomes dispersed, the total SA increases. The effect of the standard deviation of particle size distribution on the SA is shown in Figure 3.7.

3.2.4 Diffusion Layer Thickness I: Fluid Dynamic Model

In this section, the diffusion layer thickness is explained based on fluid dynamics. The advantages of the fluid dynamic model are that the effects of agitation strength, fluid viscosity, and particle density are explicitly taken into

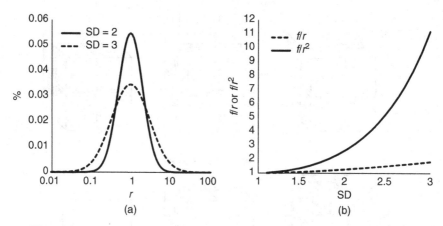

Figure 3.7 (a) Particle size distribution and (b) surface area expansion ratio.

account in the equation, and it offers a scientifically correct understanding of the mass transfer phenomena [15]. However, for most cases, the simple empirical equations, such as the Hintz–Johnson model, would offer practically appropriate accuracy (Section 3.2.5).

3.2.4.1 Reynolds and Sherwood Numbers.
The mass transfer resistance around an object has a dimension of length and is usually scaled to the representative length (L) of the object using the Sherwood number (Sh) (Fig. 3.8). The Sherwood number can be calculated from the Reynolds number (Re) and the Schmitt number (Sc) based on the Prandtl's boundary layer theory as

$$Sh \propto Re^{1/2} Sc^{1/3} \tag{3.23}$$

The Reynolds number (Re) is defined as

$$Re = \frac{U \rho_f L}{\mu} = \frac{UL}{\nu} \tag{3.24}$$

where U is the flow speed around an object, ρ_f is the density of the fluid, μ is the viscosity of the fluid, and ν is the kinematic viscosity of the fluid ($\nu = \mu/\rho_f$). The Reynolds number is often used to characterize the flow pattern of a system, namely, "laminar flow" or "turbulence." Re is the ratio of inertia of the flow (the numerator)[6] to the viscosity of the fluid (the denominator). When the viscosity surmounts the inertia ($Re < 1$), the fluid flow around the object becomes laminar, whereas when the inertia surmounts the viscosity ($Re \gg 1000$), the fluid flow becomes turbulent. As Re increases from single digit to 3–6 digit order, the flow regimen gradually changes from laminar to turbulent.

---

[6]Momentum = speed × weight (weight = density × size)

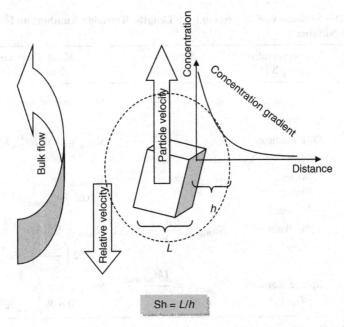

Figure 3.8 Diffusion layer thickness, representative length, and Sherwood number.

Schmidt number (*Sc*) is defined as the ratio of kinematic viscosity to the diffusion coefficient,

$$Sc = \frac{\nu}{D_{\text{eff}}} \tag{3.25}$$

For example, *Sc* of a typical drug molecule in water is ca. 1000 (MW = 400, $D_{\text{eff}} = 8 \times 10^{-6}$ cm^2/s, $\nu = 0.007$ cm^2/s in water at 37°C).

By combining Equations 3.23–3.25,

$$Sh \propto Re^{1/2}Sc^{1/3} = \left(\frac{UL}{\nu}\right)^{1/2}\left(\frac{\nu}{D_{\text{eff}}}\right)^{1/3} \tag{3.26}$$

The relationship between *Sh*, *Re*, and *Sc* for various cases are summarized in Table 3.1 and Figure 3.9.

Example The Reynolds number of a column in a water flow can be calculated as follows ($U = 1$ cm/s, $A : L = 1$ cm, $B : L = 10$ μm, $\nu = 0.007$ cm^2/s):

$$Re = \frac{UL}{\nu} = \frac{1 \text{ cm/s} \times 1 \text{ cm}}{0.007 \text{ cm}^2/\text{s}} \approx 143$$

$$Re = \frac{UL}{\nu} = \frac{1 \text{ cm/s} \times 0.001 \text{ cm}}{0.007 \text{ cm}^2/\text{s}} \approx 0.143$$

TABLE 3.1   Summary of Representative Length, Reynolds Number, and Sherwood Number

Object[a]	Representative Length (L)	Reynolds Number (Re)	Mean Sherwood Number (Sh)
Plate in a flow (A)	Plate length (l_{plate})	$Re_{plate} = \dfrac{Ul_{plate}}{\nu}$	$Sh_{plate} = 0.66\,Re_{plate}^{1/2}Sc^{1/3}$
Rotating disk (B)	Disk diameter (d_{disk})	$Re_{disk} = \dfrac{\omega d_{disk}^2}{\nu}$	$Sh_{disk} = 0.62\,Re_{disk}^{1/2}Sc^{1/3}$
Cylinder (C)	Cylinder diameter ($d_{cylinder}$)	$Re_{cylinder} = \dfrac{Ud_{cylinder}}{\nu}$	$Sh_{cylinder} = 0.66\,Re_{cylinder}^{1/2}Sc^{1/3}$
Tube flow (D)	Tube diameter (d_{tube})	$Re_{disk} = \dfrac{Ud_{tube}}{\nu}$	$Sh_{tube} = 1.52\,Gz^{1/3} = 1.52\left(\dfrac{d_{tube}}{L_{tube}}\right)^{1/3}Re_{tube}^{1/3}Sc^{1/3}$
Sphere in a flow (E)	Sphere diameter ($d_{particle}$)	$Re_{particle} = \dfrac{Ud_{particle}}{\nu}$	$Sh_{particle} = 2 + 0.6\,Re_{particle}^{1/2}Sc^{1/3}$

[a] The keys are shown in Figure 3.9.

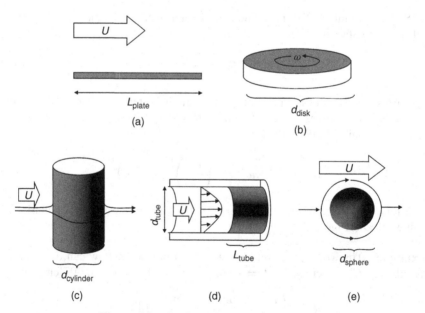

Figure 3.9   Configuration of mass transfer.

The flow pattern behind the column changes from laminar to turbulence via a periodic formation of vortices (Karman's eddy). Even though the two objects are put in the same stream, the flow pattern changes depending on the size of the object. The flow pattern behind the 100 μm object is laminar ($Re = 0.143$). However, behind the 1-cm object ($Re = 143$), periodic formation of vortices is observed. As the Re increases from several hundreds to above several thousands, this periodic vortices transit to turbulent flow.

Similarly, when the GI is considered, the Reynolds number for the drug particles (e.g., $L = r_p = 0.01$ cm) is different for tablets from that of the intestinal tube (for humans, $L = R_{GI} = 1.5$ cm).

3.2.4.2 Disk (Levich Equation). A rotating disk method is often used to measure the intrinsic dissolution rate of a drug (the dissolution rate per SA). The Sherwood number for a rotating disk (Sh_{disk}) is

$$Sh_{disk} \propto Re_{disk}^{1/2} Sc^{1/3} = \left(\frac{\pi \, \text{RPM}/60 \times d_{disk}^2}{\nu} \right)^{1/2} \left(\frac{\nu}{D_{eff}} \right)^{1/3} \tag{3.27}$$

where Re_{disk} is the Reynolds number of a disk, d_{disk} is the disk diameter, and RPM is the rotation speed. Therefore,

$$h_{API} = \frac{d_{disk}}{Sh} \propto \text{RPM}^{-1/2} \nu^{1/6} D_{eff}^{1/3} \tag{3.28}$$

This equation is called the *Levich equation*. The disk diameter does not appear in this equation, meaning that it does not affect the thickness of the diffusion layer. Therefore, the intrinsic dissolution rate becomes the same value regardless of the disk diameter. Actually, the μDISS method (3 mm diameter) gave an intrinsic dissolution rate similar to the Wood apparatus method (1 cm diameter) [16]. In the Levich equation, h_{API} is reciprocal of $\text{RPM}^{1/2}$, suggesting that the h_{API} value becomes less sensitive to rotation speed, as it is increased. Therefore, even when the mass transfer rate is not sensitive to an increase in the agitation speed, cannot be concluded that the diffusion layer is removed. This point is important when analyzing the in vitro permeability data (Section 7.9.8, Fig. 7.33).

3.2.4.3 Tube (Graetz Problem). The mass transfer in the tube with a straight laminar flow (from/into the tube wall) is referred to as the *Graetz problem* (Fig. 3.9d). In this case, the representative length is the tube diameter (d_{tube}). However, the mean Sherwood number is also affected by the tube length (l_{tube}). The Graetz number (Gz) is a dimensionless number, which characterizes the flow pattern in a tube. Equation 3.29 is called the *Leveque equation* and valid at Gz >76. Gz of approximately 1000 or less is the point at which flow would be

considered fully developed for mass transfer.

$$Sh_{\text{tube}} = 1.52 \text{Gz}^{1/3} = 1.52 \left(\frac{d_{\text{tube}}}{l_{\text{tube}}}\right)^{1/3} \left(\frac{d_{\text{tube}} U}{v}\right)^{1/3} \left(\frac{v}{D_{\text{eff}}}\right)^{1/3} \quad (3.29)$$

Graetz problem has been used to calculate the unstirred water layer thickness in the small intestine (h_{UWL}), especially for the rat in situ perfusion model [17].

3.2.4.4 Particle Fixed to Space (Ranz–Marshall Equation).

In the case of the mass transfer from/into the particles, the asymptotic diffusion often becomes significant. The asymptotic diffusion occurs as the concentration gradient is generated by spatial expansion around an object fixed in the space (Fig. 3.10a). The mass transfer by asymptotic diffusion can occur in the absence of flow. The asymptotic diffusion term in Sh for a spherical particle is 2, which can be derived from the concentration gradient around an object induced by spatial expansion (Fig. 3.10a) [detailed derivation of this term is found in Chapters 1 to 7 of the book "Mass Transfer: Basics and Application" by Kohichi Asano]. The effect of convection is then added to the asymptotic diffusion term. The Sherwood number for a spherical particle (Sh_{p}) in a laminar flow is then expressed as

$$Sh_{\text{p}} = 2 + 0.6 \, Re_{\text{p}}^{1/2} Sc^{1/3} \quad (3.30)$$

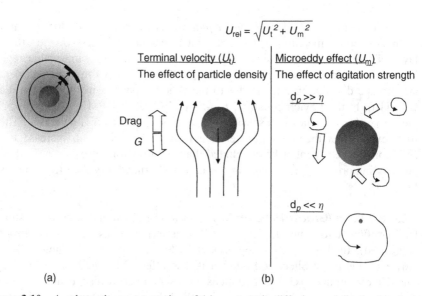

Figure 3.10   A schematic representation of (a) asymptotic diffusion and (b) the terminal sedimentation velocity and microeddy effects.

where Re_p is the Reynolds number of a sphere. This equation is called the *Ranz–Marshall equation*.

Example The Sherwood number and h_{API} of a sphere fixed in space (not freely suspended) in water can be calculated as follows ($U = 0.1$ cm/s, (a) $d_p = 1$ cm, (b) $d_p = 10$ μm, $D_{eff} = 8 \times 10^{-6}$ cm^2/s, $\nu = 0.007$ cm^2/s):
The Sherwood number for a sphere is

$$Sh_p = 2 + 0.6\,Re^{1/2}Sc^{1/3} = 2 + 0.6\left(\frac{Ud_p}{\nu}\right)^{1/2}\left(\frac{\nu}{D_{eff}}\right)^{1/3}$$

Therefore, for particle (a),

$$Sh_p = 2 + 0.6\,Re^{1/2}Sc^{1/3} = 2 + 0.6\left(\frac{1 \times 0.1}{0.007}\right)^{1/2}\left(\frac{0.007}{0.000008}\right)^{1/3} = 18.3$$

$$h_{API} = \frac{L}{Sh} = \frac{d_p}{Sh} = \frac{1}{18.3} = 0.0547 \text{ cm} = 547 \text{ μm}$$

For particle (b),

$$Sh_p = 2 + 0.6\,Re^{1/2}Sc^{1/3} = 2 + 0.6\left(\frac{0.001 \times 0.1}{0.007}\right)^{1/2}\left(\frac{0.007}{0.000008}\right)^{1/3} = 6.09$$

$$h_{API} = \frac{L}{Sh} = \frac{d_p}{Sh} = \frac{1}{6.09} = 0.000164 \text{ cm} = 1.64 \text{ μm}$$

3.2.4.5 *Floating Particle.* In the above example, the particle is fixed in a space. In this case, the absolute fluid flow equals the flow around the particle. However, in reality, the particles are suspended and float in the fluid when the fluid is agitated. The drug particles move along with the fluid flow in a synchronic manner. In this case, the relative flow velocity ($U_{rel,tot}$) can be approximated as the sum of the terminal sedimentation velocity (U_t) and the microeddy effect velocity (U_e), which is an expedient fluid velocity induced by the microeddy.

$$U_{rel,tot} = \sqrt{U_t^2 + U_e^2} \tag{3.31}$$

The terminal sedimentation velocity is determined as the balance of gravity, buoyancy, and frictional resistance. A schematic representation of the terminal sedimentation velocity is shown in Figure 3.10b. The U_t of a spherical particle can be calculated as

$$U_t = \left(\frac{4(\rho_p - \rho_f)d_p g}{3\rho_f} \times \frac{1}{C_D}\right)^{1/2} \tag{3.32}$$

where g is the gravitational acceleration constant and C_D is the resistance coefficient from the fluid.

When $Re_p < 0.3$, C_D of a spherical particle can be derived from the Navier–Stokes equation with Stokes approximation as

$$C_D = \frac{24}{Re_p} \tag{3.33}$$

$$U_t = \frac{(\rho_p - \rho_f)d_p^2 g}{18\mu} \tag{3.34}$$

When $Re_p > 0.3$, C_D can be approximated as [18]:

$$C_D = \left(\left(\frac{A}{Re_p} \right)^{1/m} + B^{1/m} \right)^m \tag{3.35}$$

$$U_t = \frac{\nu}{d_p} \left(\sqrt{\frac{1}{4}\left(\frac{A}{B}\right)^{2/m} + \left(\frac{4}{3} \times \frac{d_{p*}^3}{B}\right)^{1/m}} - \frac{1}{2}\left(\frac{A}{B}\right)^{1/m} \right)^m \tag{3.36}$$

$$d_{p*} = \left(\left(\frac{\rho_p}{\rho_f} - 1 \right) \times g \times \left(\frac{1}{\nu}\right)^2 \right)^{1/3} d_p \tag{3.37}$$

Various A, B, and m values have been reported depending on the Re_p range and particle shape. $A = 20.5$, $B = 0.310$, and $m = 2.07$ were used for spherical particles in the previous investigation [19].

The flow velocity from the microeddy effect can be calculated as [20, 21]:

$$U_e = 0.195 \times d_p^{1.1} \varepsilon^{0.525} \mu^{-0.575} \tag{3.38}$$

$$\varepsilon = \frac{P_N \rho_f \times \text{RPM}^3 \times D_{paddle}^5}{V} \tag{3.39}$$

where ε is the energy dissipation of turbulence and D_{paddle} is the paddle diameter. The microeddy effect is related to the turbulence and Kolmogorov's minimum eddy scale (η).

$$\eta = \left(\frac{\nu^3}{\varepsilon}\right)^{1/4} \tag{3.40}$$

For example, η is ca. 100 μm for the USP paddle method with 50 rpm ($\varepsilon = 0.004$ m²/s³). A schematic representation of the microeddy effect is shown in Figure 3.10b. Particles smaller than this scale are involved within this eddy (so the flow around the particle looks laminar), whereas for a particle larger than this scale, the eddies agitate the fluid near the surface.

For both terminal velocity and microeddy effects, when the particle size is small, the Reynolds number becomes small and the second term of the Ranz–Marshall equation becomes negligible (both U_t and U_e is negligible). Therefore, for the small particles ($d_p < 60$ μm), the contribution of asymptotic diffusion term becomes predominant and the Sherwood number becomes approximately 2 (for the USP paddle method with <100 rpm). Therefore, h_{API} becomes the radius of the particle ($h_{API} \approx d_p/Sh = r_p$) [19, 22]. This theoretically underwrites the well-known empirical rule in pharmaceutical sciences that h_{API} is close to the particle radius and the agitation strength has little effect on the dissolution rate of small particles. This theory of $h_{API} \approx r_p$ is validated down to 100 nm particles [23].

For coarse particles ($d_p > 60$ μm), h_{API} depends on the agitation strength and the density of particles. As the agitation strength becomes larger, the microeddy effect becomes larger, h_{API} becomes thinner, and the dissolution rate becomes faster. As the true density becomes larger, the terminal sedimentation velocity becomes larger, h_{API} becomes thinner, and the dissolution rate becomes faster. The particle size affects both U_t and U_e. Interestingly, as the result of considering these factors, h_{API} becomes relatively constant (ca. 30 μm) regardless of the particle size (Fig. 3.13).

Equations 3.31–3.40 are an open analytical solution, so that it can be used for biopharmaceutical modeling without slowing down the computational speed. However, the true density of a drug is in the 1.1–1.5 range in most cases and the agitation strength is 10–100 rpm. Therefore, a simple empirical equation with a fixed maximum $h = 30$ μm value would be appropriate for most cases (Section 3.2.5).

3.2.4.6 Nonspherical Particle.
In the case of nonspherical particles, the asymmetric term in the Ranz–Marshall equation deviates from 2. It is convenient to introduce a shape factor (Π), which has a dimension of length.

$$\Pi = Sh_{particle} \frac{SA_p}{L} \tag{3.41}$$

In Table 3.2, equations for several particle shapes are shown. However, in most cases, the particle shape is not exactly the same with those listed shapes in the table. For irregularly shaped particles, it is also convenient to use the simple approximation as

$$\Pi = 5.25 \, SA_p^{1/4} V_p^{1/6} \tag{3.42}$$

where V_p is the volume of the particle. Figure 3.11 shows the ratio of the SA and dissolution rate by asymptotic diffusion for a cylindrical particle having a volume equivalent to a sphere. As the shape of a particle deviates from the sphere, the SA and dissolution rate increases. However, the extent of increase in the dissolution

TABLE 3.2   Shape Factor for Irregular Particles

Shape of the Particle	Shape Factor $\Pi = Sh\dfrac{SA}{L}$
Sphere of diameter, d	$2\pi d$
Circular cylinder of a diameter d and length L $(0 < L/d < 8)$	$\left[8 + 4.1\left(\dfrac{2L}{d}\right)^{0.76}\right]\dfrac{d}{2}$
Cube with edge, L	$0.654(2\pi L)$
Thin rectangular plate with sides L_1 and L_2 $(L_1 > L_2)$	$\dfrac{2\pi L_1}{\ln(4L_1/L_2)}$

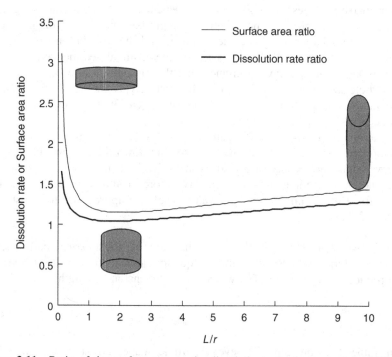

Figure 3.11   Ratio of the surface area to the dissolution rates by asymptotic diffusion for a cylindrical particle having a volume equivalent to a sphere. *Source:* Adapted from Reference 15 with permission.

rate is smaller than that in the SA. According to Equation 3.42, the dissolution rate remains within 2-fold of the spherical particle of the same volume even when the SA is increased by 16-fold. In other words, even when the particle shape deviates from spherical, the boundary layer on the particle remains (semi-) spherical and the effectiveness of SA expansion on the dissolution rate is masked

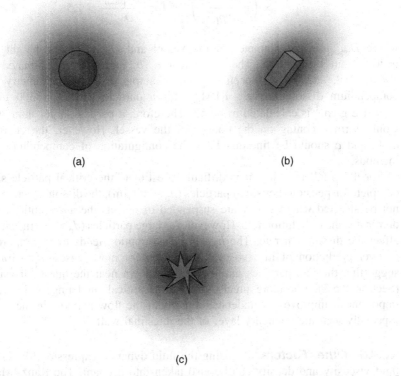

(a)

(b)

(c)

Figure 3.12 Particle shape and asymptotic diffusion. *Source:* Adapted from Reference 15 with permission.

by this semispherical diffusion layer (Fig. 3.12). This theoretically underwrites that the use of spherical approximation is appropriate for most cases.

3.2.4.7 Minimum Agitation Speed for Complete Suspension. When the terminal velocity of particles is larger than the upward flow in a system, the particles would sediment down on the bottom of a flask or the wall of the intestine. The flow around sediment particles is significantly different from that of suspended particles. In this case, estimation of the Sherwood number would be more complicated, especially when the particles are close and affect the flow pattern of each other. A simple equation for this case has not been reported yet.

For a vessel with a paddle, an equation to estimate the minimum agitation speed (RPM_{min}) for complete suspension of spherical particles was reported [24]. The general form of this equation is

$$RPM_{min} = a \left(\frac{D_{vessel}}{D_{paddle}} \right)^b \exp\left(c \frac{H_{paddle}}{D_{vessel}} \right) \frac{\left(\frac{\mu_f}{\rho_f} \right)^{0.1} d_p^{0.2}}{D_{paddle}^{0.85}}$$

$$\times \left(g \frac{\rho_p - \rho_f}{\rho_f} \right)^{0.45} \quad \text{for} \quad \frac{H_{\text{paddle}}}{D_{\text{vessel}}} > 1.5 \tag{3.43}$$

where D_{vessel} is the diameter of the vessel and H_{paddle} is the height of the paddle from the bottom. The coefficient a, b, and c were estimated to be 104.4, 1.18, and 0.41, respectively. For example, using the geometry of the compendium dissolution test, RPM_{min} for a particle with $d_p = 300$ μm and $\rho_p = 1.2$ g/cm^3 is calculated to be 53. Therefore, a particle larger than 300 μm would form a coning on the bottom of the vessel. However, the coefficients a, b, and c should be fine-tuned for the configuration of compendium paddle methods.

For the small intestine, it is difficult to estimate the critical particle size for complete suspension. For small particles ($d_p < 60$ μm), the dissolution rate would not be affected whether they are suspended or not, as the asymptotic diffusion dominates the dissolution rate. However, for large particles ($d_p > 60$ μm), it would affect the dissolution rate. The $h_{\text{API}} = r_p$ assumption tends to give appropriate or over prediction of in vivo oral absorption for many cases ($d_p > 100$ μm), suggesting that the particles may be settling down near the intestinal wall [25] (Section 8.5.2). For more precise biopharmaceutical modeling, it is critically important to improve our understanding about the flow patterns in the GI tract, especially near the boundary layer of the intestinal wall.

3.2.4.8 Other Factors. By using the fluid dynamic expression, the effect of fluid viscosity and density can be also taken into account. The Ranz–Marshall equation itself is validated in the chemical engineering area. However, literature information for a pharmaceutical application is sparse. Recently, the effect of fluid density was suggested to be important for the dissolution of lidocaine [26].

3.2.5 Diffusion Layer Thickness II: Empirical Models for Particles

Several empirical approximate equations have also been proposed to calculate the thickness of the diffusion layer on suspended particles in the USP paddle method. Hintz and Johnson [27] proposed an empirical equation (HJ model).

$$h_{\text{API}} = r_p, \quad r_p < h_{c,\text{HJ}} \tag{3.44}$$

$$h_{\text{API}} = h_{c,\text{HJ}}, \quad r_p > h_{c,\text{HJ}} \tag{3.45}$$

Wang and Flanagan [28, 29] proposed a semiempirical equation based on the film model with a spherical particle (WF model).

$$\frac{1}{h_{\text{API}}} = \frac{1}{r_p} + \frac{1}{h_{c,\text{WF}}} \tag{3.46}$$

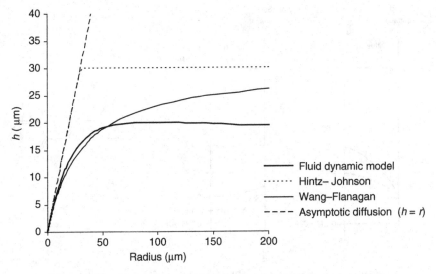

Figure 3.13   Comparison of HJ, WF, and the fluid dynamic models.

Figure 3.13 shows the comparison of HJ, WF, and the fluid dynamic models. Both $h_{c,HJ}$ and $h_{c,WF}$ are set to 30 μm, which is most often used in biopharmaceutical modeling (in the original paper, $h_{c,WF}$ was reported to be 110 μm). For the HJ model, $h_{c,HJ} = 20$ μm would result in a similar plot with the fluid dynamic model. As discussed in the previous sections, from a theoretical perspective, these simple empirical rules would have appropriate accuracy (less than twofold error) for most cases, except for a large and significantly irregular particle (aspect ratio >10) in a strong agitation condition. It should be noted that $h_{c,HJ}$ and $h_{c,WF}$ of 30 μm are for completely suspended particles but not for sediment particles.

3.2.6   Solid Surface pH and Solubility

In the case of dissociable drugs, the solid surface pH can be significantly different from the bulk fluid pH because of the buffering effect of the API. This effect can be significant especially for the dissolution of a free base in the stomach (Section 8.6) [30].

In the case of free acids or bases, chemical reactions occur within the diffusion layer. Therefore, the microclimate pH at the solid surface ($p[H^+]_0$) does not become equal to that in the bulk medium, and the solid surface solubilities ($S_{surface}$) of free acids and bases become smaller than the solubility of a drug in the bulk media ($S_{dissolv}$) (Figs. 3.14 and 3.15). The $p[H^+]_0$ can be obtained by solving the following third-degree equation (the Newton method can be used) [31, 32]:

$$pX^3 + qX^2 + rX + s = 0 \tag{3.47}$$

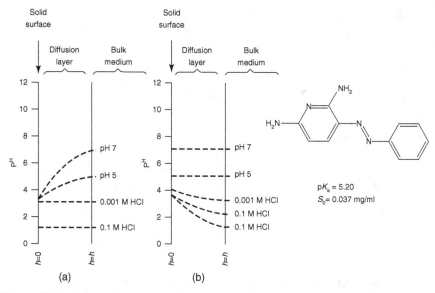

Figure 3.14 Schematic representation of the buffering effect of (a) phenazopyridine HCl and (b) phenazopyridine free base in the diffusion layers of various media. *Source:* Adapted from Reference 33 with permission.

$$p = D_w D_{buf,conj} K_{a,buf}^{-I} \sqrt{K_w^{1-I}} \qquad (3.48)$$

$$q = D_w D_{buf,unconj} \sqrt{K_w^{1-I}} + I \times D_{buf,conj} K_{a,buf}^{-I} \left(D_{OH}[OH^-]_{bulk} \right.$$

$$\left. + D_{buf,unconj}[buf\ unconj]_{bulk} - D_H[H^+]_{bulk} \right) \qquad (3.49)$$

$$r = I \times D_{buf,unconj} K_{a,buf}^{-I} \left(D_{OH}[OH^-]_{bulk} \right.$$

$$\left. - D_{buf,conj}[buf\ conj]_{bulk} - D_H[H^+]_{bulk} \right)$$

$$- I \times D_{drug} D_{buf,conj} S_0 \left(\frac{K_{a,drug}}{K_{a,buf}} \right)^{-I}$$

$$- D_{w'} D_{buf,conj} K_{a,buf}^{-I} \sqrt{K_w^{1-I}} \qquad (3.50)$$

$$r = -D_{w'} D_{buf,unconj} \sqrt{K_w^{1-I}} - I \times D_{drug} D_{buf,unconj} S_0 K_{a,drug}^I \qquad (3.51)$$

$$I = 1, X = [H^+]_0, \ W = H, W' = OH \quad \text{for free acid}$$

$$I = -1, X = [H^+]_0^{-1}, W = OH, W' = H \quad \text{for free base} \qquad (3.52)$$

where D_N is the diffusion coefficient of species, N. $[N]_{bulk}$ can be calculated from the pH of the bulk and the concentration of the buffer species (e.g., in the

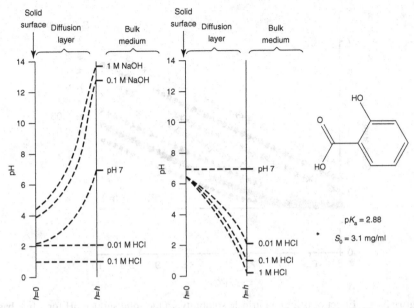

Figure 3.15 Schematic representation of the buffering effect of (a) salicylic acid and (b) sodium salicylate in the diffusion layers of various media. *Source:* Adapted from Reference 34 with permission.

case of the sodium acetate buffer, acetic acid + acetate). The "buf,conj" and "buf,unconj" are the buffer species conjugated and unconjugated to the free acid or base, respectively. For example, for an acetate buffer, "buf,conj" is acetate (CH_3COO^-) and "buf,unconj" is acetic acid (CH_3COOH). For an imidazole buffer, "buf,conj" is free imidazole and "buf,unconj" is protonated imidazole. Once $[H^+]_0$ (pH at the solid surface) is obtained, $S_{surface}$ can be calculated from the theoretical pH–solubility curve as described in Section 2.3.

The pH at the solid surface is affected by the buffer concentration ($[buf,conj]_{bulk}$ and $[buf,unconj]_{bulk}$). Usually, the buffer capacity used for a dissolution test is significantly higher than that observed in the physiological condition. Therefore, the self-buffering effect by a free drug (free acid or base) at the solid surface can be underestimated in the dissolution test [35].

Figure 3.16 shows the effect of pK_a and intrinsic solubility on the solid surface pH for a base drug at pH 1.5 (representing the stomach pH).

To incorporate the solid surface solubility, the Nernst–Brunner equation can be modified as [3]:

$$\frac{dX_{API}}{dt} = -SA \times k_{mass} S_{surface} \left(1 - \frac{C_{dissolv}}{S_{dissolv}}\right) \quad (3.53)$$

This is an approximate equation to simultaneously satisfy the initial dissolution rate and maximum $C_{dissolv}$ in the GI tract.

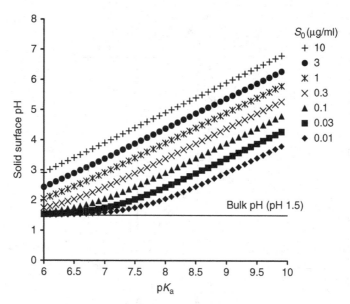

Figure 3.16   Effect of pK_a and intrinsic solubility on the solid surface pH for a free base with MW = 400 and $D_{mono} = 7 \times 10^{-6}$ cm/s at bulk pH 1.5 (with no buffer). *Source:* Calculated based on Reference 31.

3.3   NUCLEATION

In the cases the initial API form converts to another solid form during the oral absorption processes, the nucleation process of a new form has to be taken into account in biopharmaceutical modeling. The examples of API form conversions are as follows:

- salt form to free form (Fig. 3.17)[7]
- amorphous form to crystalline form
- cocrystalline form to free form
- anhydrate form to hydrate form

3.3.1   General Description of Nucleation and Precipitation Process

Figure 3.18 shows the schematic representation of a dissolution time course for a salt of a base drug (see also Figure 11.1). As the salt dissolves ①, the dissolved drug concentration increases. Even after exceeding the saturated solubility of a free base ②, the precipitation of a free base does not occur at this point because the concentration of the free base is not sufficient to induce a significant nucleation speed (in the time scale of oral absorption). As the concentration

---

[7]The solid form of a precipitant from the supersaturated solution is not necessarily crystalline but can be amorphous (cf. the Ostwald rule of stage).

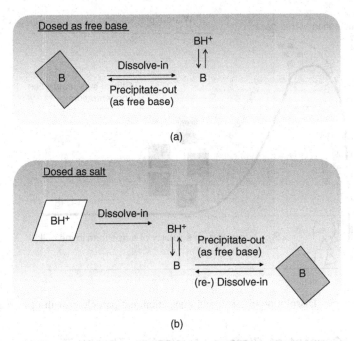

Figure 3.17   (a) Identical form precipitation and (b) different form precipitation.

of the dissolved free base increases, it then reaches the critical supersaturation concentration ③.[8] At this point, nucleation of embryo of free base particles reaches a significant speed. After nuclei are generated, the nuclei particles start to grow, bringing the dissolved free base from the solution to the free base particles ④. This particle growth is the reverse reaction of dissolution. The particle growth continues until the dissolved drug concentration reaches the equilibrium solubility of the free base ⑤.

Because the particle growth process ④ and ⑤ can be expressed by the Noyes–Whitney equation as discussed in the previous section, we focus on the mechanism of the nucleation process in this section.

3.3.2 Classical Nucleation Theory

At present, the nucleation mechanism of a drug in the GI tract are not well understood. However, as the starting point, the classical nucleation theory (CNT) can be used to simulate precipitation in biopharmaceutical modeling [3, 36]. The theory described in this section does not consider other factors such as secondary nucleation and aggregation.

---

[8]This may not occur when the dose number based on the critical supersaturation concentration is less than 1 or when the intestinal membrane permeation clearance rapidly removes the dissolved drug from the intestinal fluid.

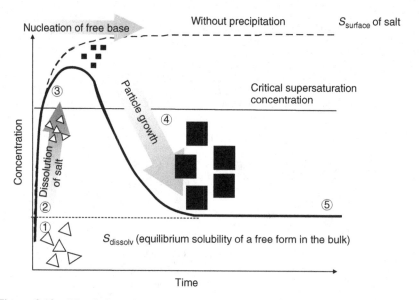

Figure 3.18   Dissolution of a salt and nucleation and particle growth of a free form.

3.3.2.1 *Concept of Classical Nucleation Theory.*

The drug molecules dissolved in a fluid can form agglomers (clusters) (Fig. 3.19). The clusters are in a dynamic equilibrium. The population of each cluster is described by the Boltzmann distribution. Even when the vast majority of the drug molecules exist as a monomer, a very small portion of the molecules can exist as clusters (cf. the Avogadro number is 6.022×10^{23} mol^{-1}). A molecule associates or dissociates to a cluster to form larger or smaller clusters. The critical cluster size at which the growth of the cluster becomes energetically favored depends on the free energy barrier to form the cluster. When the cluster size is smaller than the critical size, the increase in the interfacial energy ($\propto r^2$) by adding one molecule is larger than the decrease in the volume energy ($\propto r^3$). Therefore, in this case, the growth of the cluster is not favored and the cluster cannot grow further. Once the critical size is achieved, the growth of the cluster becomes energetically favored and the nuclei particle continues to grow.

3.3.2.2 *Mathematical Expressions.*

According to the CNT, the primary nucleation rate per volume per time (J_{nc}) can be expressed as

$$J_{nc} = \frac{dN_n}{dt}$$

$$= \text{(number of critical cluster)}$$

$$\times \text{(frequency of addition of another molecule)}$$

$$= C_{nc} \times F_{cn} \tag{3.53}$$

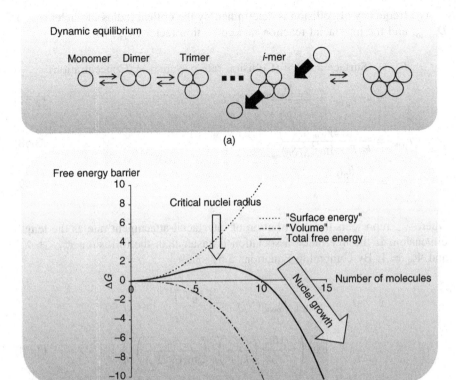

Figure 3.19 Free energy barrier for nucleation.

where N_n is the number of nuclei per volume, C_{nc} is the number of critical cluster per volume, and F_{cn} is the frequency of addition of another molecule to the critical cluster. C_{nc} is determined by the energy barrier for nucleation (ΔG_{nc}) as

$$C_{nc} = (N_A \times C_0) \exp\left(-\frac{\Delta G_{nc}}{k_B T}\right) Z_{ch} \tag{3.54}$$

where N_A is the Avogadro number, C_0 is the concentration of free monomer (mol/l), k_B is the Boltzmann constant, T is the temperature, and Z_{ch} is the Zel'dovich number. $N_A C_0$ is the concentration as the number of molecules per volume. ΔG_{cn} is expressed as (spherical nuclei assumed)

$$\Delta G_{cn} = \frac{16\pi \gamma^3 v_m{}^2}{3 \cdot (k_B T \times \ln(C_b/S_0))^2} \tag{3.55}$$

where γ is the surface energy and v_m is the molecular volume. Z_{ch} is expressed as

$$Z_{ch} = \frac{(k_B T)^{3/2}(\ln(C_0/S_0))^2}{8\pi \gamma^{3/2} v_m} \tag{3.56}$$

The frequency of collision is determined by the critical radius of nuclei ($r_{p,nc}$), D_{mono}, and the interfacial reaction rate correction factor (Ψ_{cn}) as

$$F_{cn} = \text{(Surface area)} \times \text{(Collision rate per area)} \times \text{(Concentration)}$$

$$= 4\pi r_{p,nc}{}^2 \times \frac{\varphi_{nc} D_{mono}}{r_{p,nc}} \times N_A C_0 \tag{3.57}$$

$$r_{p,nc} = \frac{2\gamma v_m}{k_B T \times \ln(C_0/S_0)} \tag{3.58}$$

$$\varphi_{nc} = \frac{h_{pUWL}}{\lambda_{nc} + h_{pUWL}} \tag{3.59}$$

where λ_{nc} represents the contribution of interfacial attachment rate as the length dimension. If the interfacial association is faster than the diffusion, $r_{p,nc} \gg \lambda_{nc}$ and $\Psi_{nc} = 1$. By combining Equations 3.52–3.59

$$J_{nc} = \varphi_{prec,k} D_{mono} (N_A C_0)^2 \left[\frac{k_B T}{\gamma}\right]^{1/2} \ln(C_0/S_0)$$

$$\exp\left(-\frac{16\pi}{3}\left(\frac{\gamma}{k_B T}\right)^3 \left(\frac{v_m}{\ln(C_0/S_0)}\right)^2\right) \tag{3.60}$$

The nucleation rate depends very steeply on C_0/S_0. C_0/S_0 represents the degree of supersaturation. The C_0/S_0 value that gives $J_{nc} \approx 1$ in the time scale of interest is defined as the *critical supersaturation ratio* (CSSR).[9] CSSR is mainly determined by γ. No nucleation occurs where $C_0/S_0 <$ CSSR in the time scale of interest. The concentration range of $S_0 < C_0 < S_0 \times$ CSSR is called the *metastable zone*.

Equation 3.60 is the theoretical equation for homogeneous precipitation. However, usually heterogeneous precipitation is more popular. In addition, γ is difficult to obtain. For heterogeneous nucleation, the lump constant (β) of the foreign particle number, sticking provability, and an apparent surface energy (γ') are introduced [37]:

$$J_{nc} = \beta D_{mono} (N_A C_0)^2 \left[\frac{k_B T}{\gamma'}\right]^{1/2} \ln(C_0/S_0)$$

$$\exp\left(-\frac{16\pi}{3}\left(\frac{\gamma'}{k_B T}\right)^3 \left(\frac{v_m}{\ln(C_0/S_0)}\right)^2\right) \tag{3.61}$$

[9]CSSR depends on the time scale. Even when the degree of supersaturation is small, after a long time elapse, nucleation occurs. This time lag is called *induction period*. This induction period is a probabilistic process that would follow the Boltzmann distribution.

where β and γ' are the drug parameters for heterogeneous nucleation. The γ' value is very difficult to measure and is usually not available during drug discovery. Therefore, it would be practical to estimate γ' from a measured CSSR value. Another unknown drug parameter, λ_{prec} can be obtained from the particle growth rate of seeded nuclei in the metastable zone [38]. The γ' and β values can be obtained by simulation fitting to in vitro precipitation experiment data, which mimics the fluid transfer from the stomach to the small intestine.

3.3.3 Application of a Nucleation Theory for Biopharmaceutical Modeling

The nucleation rate in each GI position can be calculated using a nucleation theory. Once the size and number of nuclei are calculated, a virtual particle bin can be assigned with the information of the position of the nuclei in the GI tract and the nuclei radius. The particle growth can then be calculated using the Noyes–Whitney equation with a negative concentration gradient. These mechanisms automatically give the particle size distribution of the precipitant. This particle size distribution data can then be used to calculate the redissolution of the precipitant in the GI tract.

Therefore, to represent the process of salt dissolution and free-form precipitation, we need two Noyes–Whitney equations, one for the dissolution of a salt API and the other for the particle growth and redissolution of the free base precipitant. For the dissolution of a salt, $S_{surface}$ and $S_{dissolv}$ can be set to the solubility of the salt [$= K_{sp}^{0.5}$ (common ionic effect should be considered for Cl^- and Na^+ salt cases)]. For the particle growth and redissolution of a free base precipitant, $S_{surface}$ and $S_{dissolv}$ can be set to those of the free base.

REFERENCES

1. Dokoumetzidis, A., Macheras, P. (2006). A century of dissolution research: From Noyes and Whitney to the biopharmaceutics classification system. *Int. J. Pharm.*, 321, 1–11.
2. Avdeef, A. (2010). Leakiness and size exclusion of paracellular channels in cultured epithelial cell monolayers-interlaboratory comparison. *Pharm. Res.*, 27, 480–489.
3. Sugano, K. (2009). Introduction to computational oral absorption simulation. *Expert Opin. Drug Metabol. Toxicol.*, 5, 259–293.
4. Sugano, K., Okazaki, A., Sugimoto, S., Tavornvipas, S., Omura, A., Mano, T. (2007). Solubility and dissolution profile assessment in drug discovery. *Drug Metabol. Pharmacokinet.*, 22, 225–254.
5. Galia, E., Nicolaides, E., Horter, D., Lobenberg, R., Reppas, C., Dressman, J.B. (1998). Evaluation of various dissolution media for predicting in vivo performance of class I and II drugs. *Pharm. Res.*, 15, 698–705.
6. Nawroth, T., Buch, P., Buch, K., Langguth, P., Schweins, R. (2011). Liposome Formation from bile salt-lipid micelles in the digestion and drug delivery model FaSSIF(mod) estimated by combined time-resolved neutron and dynamic light scattering. *Mol. Pharm.*, 8, 2162–2172.

7. Okazaki, A., Mano, T., Sugano, K. (2007). Theoretical dissolution model of poly disperse drug particles in biorelevant media. *J. Pharmaceut. Sci. Tech.*, Japan (meeting abstract and poster), 67.

8. Li, C.-Y., Zimmerman, C.L., Wiedmann, T.S. (1996). Diffusivity of bile salt/ phospholipid aggregates in mucin. *Pharmceut. Res.*, 13, 535–541.

9. Naylor, L.J., Bakatselou, V., Dressman, J.B. (1993). Comparison of the mechanism of dissolution of hydrocortisone in simple and mixed micelle systems. *Pharmaceut. Res.*, 10, 865–870.

10. Balakrishnan, A., Rege, B.D., Amidon, G.L., Polli, J.E. (2004). Surfactant-mediated dissolution: contributions of solubility enhancement and relatively low micelle diffusivity. *J. Pharmaceut. Sci.*, 93, 2064–2075.

11. Rao, V.M., Lin, M., Larive, C.K., Southard, M.Z. (1997). A mechanistic study of griseofulvin dissolution into surfactant solutions under laminar flow conditions. *J. Pharmaceut. Sci.*, 86, 1132–1137.

12. Granero, G.E., Ramachandran, C., Amidon, G.L. (2005). Dissolution and solubility behavior of fenofibrate in sodium lauryl sulfate solutions. *Drug Dev. Ind. Pharmaceut.*, 31, 917–922.

13. Sun, W., Larive, C.K., Southard, M.Z. (2003). A mechanistic study of danazol dissolution in ionic surfactant solutions. *J. Pharmaceut. Sci.*, 92, 424–435.

14. Okazaki, A., Mano, T., Sugano, K. (2008). Theoretical dissolution model of polydisperse drug particles in biorelevant media. *J. Pharmaceut. Sci.*, 97, 1843–1852.

15. Sugano, K. (2010). Aqueous boundary layers related to oral absorption of a drug: from dissolution of a drug to carrier mediated transport and intestinal wall metabolism. *Mol. Pharmaceut.*, 7, 1362–1373.

16. Avdeef, A., Tsinman, O. (2008). Miniaturized rotating disk intrinsic dissolution rate measurement: effects of buffer capacity in comparisons to traditional Wood's apparatus. *Pharmaceut. Res.*, 25, 2613–2627.

17. Kou, J.H., Fleisher, D., Amidon, G.L. (1991). Calculation of the aqueous diffusion layer resistance for absorption in a tube: application to intestinal membrane permeability determination. *Pharmaceut. Res.*, 8, 298–305.

18. Camenen, B. (2007). Simple and general formula for the settling velocity of particles. *J. Hydraul. Eng.*, 133, 229–233.

19. Sugano, K. (2008). Theoretical comparison of hydrodynamic diffusion layer models used for dissolution simulation in drug discovery and development. *Int. J. Pharmaceut.*, 363, 73–77.

20. Armenante, P.M., Kirwan, D.J. (1989). Mass transfer to microparticles in agitated systems. *Chem. Eng. Sci.*, 44, 2781–2796.

21. Crail, D.J., Tunis, A., Dansereau, R. (2004). Is the use of a 200ml vessel suitable for dissolution of low dose drug products? *Int. J. Pharmaceut.*, 269, 203–209.

22. Harriott, P. (1962). Mass transfer to particles: Part 1. Suspended inagitated tanks. *AICHE Journal*, 8, 93–102.

23. Galli, C. (2006). Experimental determination of the diffusion boundary layer width of micron and submicron particles. *Int. J. Pharmaceut.*, 313, 114–122.

24. Shirhatti, V., Wang, M., Williams, R., Ortega, J.R. (2007). Determination of minimum agitation speed for complete solid suspension using four electrode conductivity method. *AIP Conf. Proc.*, 914, 389–396.

25. Sugano, K. (2011). Fraction of a dose absorbed estimation for structurally diverse low solubility compounds. *Int. J. Pharmaceut.*, 405, 79–89.

26. Ostergaard, J., Ye, F., Rantanen, J., Yaghmur, A., Larsen, S.W., Larsen, C., Jensen, H. (2011). Monitoring lidocaine single-crystal dissolution by ultraviolet imaging. *J. Pharmaceut. Sci.*, 100, 3405–3410.

27. Hintz, R.J., Johnson, K.C. (1989). The effect of particle size distribution on dissolution rate and oral absorption. *Int. J. Pharmaceut.*, 51, 9–17.

28. Wang, J., Flanagan, D.R. (2002). General solution for diffusion-controlled dissolution of spherical particles. 2. Evaluation of experimental data. *J. Pharmaceut. Sci.*, 91, 534–542.

29. Wang, J., Flanagan, D.R. (1999). General solution for diffusion-controlled dissolution of spherical particles. 1. Theory. *J. Pharmaceut. Sci.*, 88, 731–738.

30. Sugano, K. (2010). Computational oral absorption simulation of free base drugs. *Int. J. Pharmaceut.*, in press.

31. Mooney, K.G., Mintun, M.A., Himmelstein, K.J., Stella, V.J. (1981). Dissolution kinetics of carboxylic acids. I: Effect of pH under unbuffered conditions. *J. Pharmaceut. Sci.*, 70, 13–22.

32. Mooney, K.G., Mintun, M.A., Himmelstein, K.J., Stella, V.J. (1981). Dissolution kinetics of carboxylic acids. II: Effects of buffers. *J. Pharmaceut. Sci.*, 70, 22–32.

33. Serajuddin, A.T.M., Jarowski, C.I. (1985). Effect of diffusion layer pH and solubility on the dissolution rate of pharmaceutical bases and their hydrochloride salts. I: Phenazopyridine. *J. Pharmaceut. Sci.*, 74, 142–147.

34. Serajuddin, A.T.M., Jarowski, C.I. (1985). Effect of diffusion layer pH and solubility on the dissolution rate of pharmaceutical acids and their sodium salts. II: Salicylic acid, theophylline, and benzoic acid. *J. Pharmaceut. Sci.*, 74, 148–154.

35. Sheng, J.J., McNamara, D.P., Amidon, G.L. (2009). Toward an in vivo dissolution methodology: a comparison of phosphate and bicarbonate buffers. *Mol. Pharmaceut.*, 6, 29–39.

36. Sugano, K. (2009). A simulation of oral absorption using classical nucleation theory. *Int. J. Pharmaceut.*, 378, 142–145.

37. Liu, X.Y. (1999). A new kinetic model for three-dimensional heterogeneous nucleation. *J. Chem. Phys.*, 111, 1628–1635.

38. Lindfors, L., Forssen, S., Westergren, J., Olsson, U. (2008). Nucleation and crystal growth in supersaturated solutions of a model drug. *J. Colloid Interface Sci.*, 325, 404–413.

CHAPTER 4

THEORETICAL FRAMEWORK III: BIOLOGICAL MEMBRANE PERMEATION

"Observations always involve theory."

—Edwin Hubble

A simple empirical linear correlation between the human intestinal membrane permeability and Caco-2 permeability of drugs (Fig. 7.27) has been used in biopharmaceutical modeling. However, there are many *in vivo* observations that cannot be simulated as far as this simple method is concerned. In the GUT framework, we dismiss this simple empirical correlation approach and introduce a mechanistic theoretical framework.

4.1 OVERALL SCHEME

The overall scheme of the intestinal membrane permeation of a drug is shown in Figure 4.1. After administering a drug, the drug molecules are dissolved in the bulk fluid of the gastrointestinal (GI) tract. The drug molecules exist in the fluid in the unbound or bile-micelle-bound state. The bulk fluid is efficiently mixed in the GI tract, and the dissolved drug molecules are conveyed close to the intestinal membrane surface by the turbulent flow or chaotic mixing. However, the unstirred water layer (UWL) exists adjacent to the intestinal

Biopharmaceutics Modeling and Simulations: Theory, Practice, Methods, and Applications,
First Edition. Kiyohiko Sugano.
© 2012 John Wiley & Sons, Inc. Published 2012 by John Wiley & Sons, Inc.

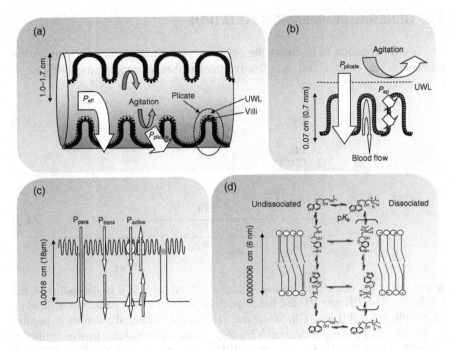

Figure 4.1 Overall scheme of intestinal membrane permeation. (a) Intestinal tube, (b) villi, (c) epithelial cell, and (d) lipid bilayer.

epithelial wall,[1] being a barrier for the transfer of drug molecules from the bulk fluid to the membrane surface. This barrier is relatively thin (ca. 300 μm) but still determines the ceiling of the effective permeability (P_{eff}) of a drug (ca. $2-8 \times 10^{-4}$ cm/s in humans). Both unbound and bile-micelle-bound drug molecules can diffuse through the UWL [1]. The unbound drug molecules then permeate the apical membrane of the epithelial cells mainly by passive diffusion, as well as by carrier-mediated transport in case of some drugs. Efflux transport from the cytosol to the apical side can occur if the drug is a substrate for an efflux transporter. Some drugs pass through the intercellular junction (the paracellular route). In the epithelial cell, a drug metabolism can occur mainly by CYP3A4 and UGTs (intestinal first-pass metabolism). After permeating the basolateral membrane, the drug molecules diffuse through the subepithelial space and then reach the villi blood flow. The villi blood flow then carries the drug molecules to the liver where the drug can be metabolized (liver first-pass metabolism).

---

[1]The *in vivo* existence of the UWL in the intestine is often argued. However, from the fluid dynamic theory, the existence of UWL is 100% sure. The question is how much diffusion resistance is maintained by the UWL. The current best guess value is 300 μm.

4.2 GENERAL PERMEATION EQUATION

The overall equation to calculate the permeation rate (dX_{perm}/dt), the permeation rate coefficient (k_{perm}), and the effective intestinal membrane permeability (P_{eff}) is expressed as[2] [2]

$$\frac{dX_{perm}}{dt} = k_{perm}X_{dissolv} = \frac{2DF}{R_{GI}}P_{eff}X_{dissolv} \tag{4.1}$$

$$P_{eff} = \frac{PE}{\dfrac{1}{P'_{ep}} + \dfrac{1}{P_{UWL}}}$$

$$= \frac{PE}{\dfrac{1}{f_u(f_0 \cdot P_{trans,0} + P_{para}) \cdot Acc \cdot VE} + \dfrac{1}{\dfrac{D_{eff}}{h_{UWL}} + P_{WC}}} \tag{4.2}$$

where DF is the degree of flatness of the intestinal tube, R_{GI} is the radius of the small intestine, PE and VE are the respective surface area expansion coefficients of the plicate (fold) and villi structures, P_{ep} is the epithelial membrane permeability ($P'_{ep} = f_u \times P_{ep} \times$ Acc $\times$ VE), Acc is the accessibility to the epithelial membrane surface [3], P_{UWL} is the UWL permeability, f_u is the free monomer fraction, f_0 is the fraction of undissociated species, $P_{trans,0}$ is the intrinsic passive transcellular permeability of undissociated species, P_{para} is the paracellular permeability (of unbound species), D_{eff} is the effective diffusion coefficient in the UWL, h_{UWL} is the effective thickness of the UWL, and P_{WC} is the permeability of the UWL by water convection. In the following sections, each component of this equation is discussed.

4.3 PERMEATION RATE CONSTANT, PERMEATION CLEARANCE, AND PERMEABILITY

The relationship between the permeation rate, the permeation rate coefficient, permeation clearance, and permeability is first discussed. Figure 4.2 shows the schematic explanation of the relationship between these parameters.

Passive membrane permeation is a mass transfer process driven by a concentration gradient across a membrane. The permeation rate is the amount of drug permeating the membrane per time (dX_{perm}/dt, dimension: amount/time). Usually, this process follows the first-order kinetics.[3]

$$\frac{dX_{perm}}{dt} = k_{perm} \cdot X_{dissolv} \tag{4.3}$$

---

[2]Equations to calculate the carrier-mediated transport are discussed later.

[3]Usually, the concentration in the GI tract is much larger than the plasma concentration. Therefore, back flux from the plasma to the GI tract is neglected in this section, unless otherwise noted.

$$\frac{\mathrm{d}X}{\mathrm{d}t} = k \cdot X \left(= \frac{\mathrm{CL} \cdot X}{V} \right) = \mathrm{CL} \cdot C = \mathrm{SA} \cdot P \cdot C$$

$$= \frac{\mathrm{SA} \cdot P \cdot X}{V} = \frac{2}{R} \cdot \mathrm{DF} \cdot P \cdot X$$

Figure 4.2 The mathematical conversions between k_{perm}, $\mathrm{CL}_{\mathrm{perm}}$, and P_{eff}.

where k_{perm} is the permeation rate coefficient (dimension: time^{-1}).[4] The permeation clearance ($\mathrm{CL}_{\mathrm{perm}}$, dimension: volume/time = length^3/time) is defined as

$$k_{\mathrm{perm}} = \frac{\mathrm{CL}_{\mathrm{perm}}}{V_{\mathrm{GI}}} \tag{4.4}$$

where V_{GI} is the fluid volume in the GI tract. By inserting Equations 4.3 and 4.4 (cf. $C_{\mathrm{dissolv}} = X_{\mathrm{dissolv}}/V_{\mathrm{GI}}$), the permeation rate is expressed as

$$\frac{\mathrm{d}X_{\mathrm{perm}}}{\mathrm{d}t} = \frac{\mathrm{CL}_{\mathrm{perm}}}{V_{\mathrm{GI}}} \cdot X_{\mathrm{dissolv}} = \mathrm{CL}_{\mathrm{perm}} \cdot C_{\mathrm{dissolv}} \tag{4.5}$$

The effective permeability (P_{eff}, dimension: length/time) is defined as the clearance per surface area (based on smooth intestinal surface) ($\mathrm{SA}_{\mathrm{GI}}$, dimension: length^2).

$$\mathrm{CL}_{\mathrm{perm}} = \mathrm{SA}_{\mathrm{GI}} \cdot P_{\mathrm{eff}} \tag{4.6}$$

where $\mathrm{SA}_{\mathrm{GI}}$ is the intestinal smooth surface area (fold and villi structure is *not* taken into account). By inserting Equations 4.5 and 4.6, the permeation rate is expressed as

$$\frac{\mathrm{d}X_{\mathrm{perm}}}{\mathrm{d}t} = k_{\mathrm{perm}} \cdot X_{\mathrm{dissolv}} = \mathrm{SA}_{\mathrm{GI}} \cdot P_{\mathrm{eff}} \cdot C_{\mathrm{dissolv}}, \qquad k_{\mathrm{perm}} = \frac{\mathrm{SA}_{\mathrm{GI}}}{V_{\mathrm{GI}}} P_{\mathrm{eff}} \tag{4.7}$$

The permeation flux (J_{perm}) is the amount of drug permeating the membrane per area per time (flux, dimension: amount/length^2/time; cf. concentration = amount/length^3).

$$J_{\mathrm{perm}} = P_{\mathrm{eff}} C_{\mathrm{dissolv}} \tag{4.8}$$

---

[4] In the case of passive diffusion, the permeation rate coefficient and permeabilities become constant. However, when a carrier-mediated transport is involved, these coefficients become concentration dependent.

These are the general expressions for membrane permeation and can be applied for any other permeation processes.

Example In an *in vitro* permeation assay, 0.1 mg dose of a drug was dissolved in the donor chamber with a volume of 1 ml. After 120 min, 0.001 mg (1%) of the dose was found in the acceptor chamber. The membrane surface area is 0.5 cm². In this case, k_{perm}, CL_{perm}, and P_{app} can be calculated as follows.

As only 1% of the drug permeated after 120 min, $X_{dissolv}$ in the donor chamber can be approximated to be constant. By integrating Equation 4.7,

$$X_{perm} = k_{perm} \cdot X_{dissolv} \cdot t$$

Therefore,

$$k_{perm} = \frac{X_{perm}}{X_{dissolv} \cdot t} = \frac{0.001}{0.1 \times 120} = 0.000083 \text{ min}^{-1}$$

$$CL_{perm} = k_{perm} \cdot V = 0.000083 \times 1 = 0.000083 \text{ ml/min}$$

$$P_{app} = \frac{CL_{perm}}{SA} = \frac{0.000083}{0.5} = 0.00017 \text{ cm/min} = 2.7 \times 10^{-6} \text{ cm/s}$$

When the donor volume was changed from 1 to 0.1 ml. The permeated percentage after 120 min can be calculated as follows:

$$k_{perm} = \frac{CL_{perm}}{V_{GI}} = 0.00083 \text{ min}^{-1}$$

$$\frac{X_{perm}}{X_{dissolv}} = k_{perm} \cdot t = 0.00083 \times 120 = 0.1 = 10\%$$

When the fluid volume is smaller, the permeation rate and permeated fraction become larger, whereas the permeability and permeation clearance remain the same. This is the same situation with the relationship between k_{el}, CL, and Vd ($k_{el} = $ CL/Vd) in pharmacokinetics.

4.4 INTESTINAL TUBE FLATNESS AND PERMEATION PARAMETERS

In Equation 4.7, P_{eff} is related to k_{perm} by the surface area/volume ratio (SA_{GI}/V_{GI}). Theoretically, SA_{GI} is a function of V_{GI} and the degree of flatness (DF).

$$SA_{GI} = f(V_{GI}, DF) \tag{4.9}$$

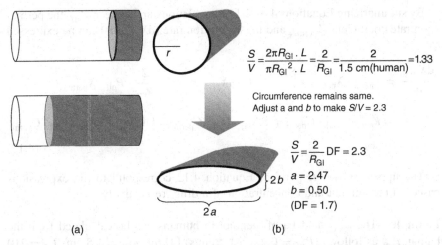

$$\frac{S}{V} = \frac{2\pi R_{GI} \cdot L}{\pi R_{GI}^2 \cdot L} = \frac{2}{R_{GI}} = \frac{2}{1.5 \text{ cm(human)}} = 1.33$$

Circumference remains same.
Adjust a and b to make $S/V = 2.3$

$$\frac{S}{V} = \frac{2}{R_{GI}} DF = 2.3$$

$a = 2.47$
$b = 0.50$
(DF $= 1.7$)

(a)   (b)

Figure 4.3 Relationship between the fluid volume and available surface area for a tube shape. (a) Fluid volume and surface area and (b) Tube shape and surface area/volume ratio.

DF can be also a function of V_{GI}.[5]

$$DF = f(V_{GI}) \tag{4.10}$$

In the case of a tube shape,[6] this ratio can be represented by the radius and degree of flatness of the tube.

$$\frac{SA_{GI}}{V_{GI}} = \frac{2\pi R_{GI} \cdot L_{GI}}{\pi R_{GI}^2 \cdot L_{GI}} DF = \frac{2}{R_{GI}} DF \tag{4.11}$$

where L_{GI} is the length of the GI tract. Because the small intestine is a tube, the surface area and fluid volume become proportional (Fig. 4.3a). For cylindrical shape, DF $= 1$. However, the shape of the intestine would be like a deflated fire hose and DF should be larger than 1. As discussed later, DF was estimated to be 1.7 (Fig. 4.3b; Section 8.4.1).

---

[5]As the membrane shape can be deformed by the fluid volume.
[6]In general, when the two objects are similar in shape, the surface area/volume ratio decreases as the volume increases,

$$\frac{SA}{V} \propto \frac{L^2}{L^3} = \frac{1}{L}$$

Therefore, the mass (and heat) transfer via the surface becomes inefficient as the volume increases. To compensate this, the surface of the object can be expanded by making folds, protuberances (villi), etc. (Section 6.1).

By summarizing Equations 4.3–4.11, the relationship between P_{eff}, the permeation rate coefficient (k_{perm}), and the absorption rate (dX_{perm}/dt) can be expressed as

$$\frac{dX_{perm}}{dt} = k_{perm} \cdot X_{perm} = \frac{SA_{GI}}{V_{GI}} \cdot P_{eff} \cdot X_{perm} = DF \cdot \frac{2}{R_{GI}} \cdot P_{eff} \cdot X_{perm}$$

$$= k_{perm} \cdot V_{GI} \cdot C_{perm} = SA_{GI} \cdot P_{eff} \cdot C_{perm} = DF \cdot \frac{2}{R_{GI}} \cdot P_{eff} \cdot V_{GI} \cdot C_{perm}$$

$$(4.12)$$

The upper and lower parts of Equation 4.12 correspond to the expressions based on the amount and concentration of a drug, respectively.

Example The k_{perm} and Fa of atenolol in humans can be calculated from the human P_{eff} as follows ($P_{eff} = 0.2 \times 10^{-4}$ cm/s) [4] (cf. $R_{GI} = 1.5$ cm, $T_{si} = 210$ min, Fa $= 1 - \exp(-k_{perm}T_{si})$):

$$k_{perm} = DF \frac{2}{R_{GI}} P_{eff} = 1.7 \times \frac{2}{1.5} \times 0.00002 = 0.000045 \text{ s}^{-1} = 0.0027 \text{min}^{-1}$$

$$Fa = 1 - \exp\left(-k_{perm}T_{si}\right) = 1 - \exp\left(-0.0027 \times 210\right) = 0.43$$

4.5 EFFECTIVE CONCENTRATION FOR INTESTINAL MEMBRANE PERMEABILITY

4.5.1 Effective Concentration for Unstirred Water Layer Permeation

In the GUT framework, the effective intestinal membrane permeability (P_{eff}) is defined based on the sum of the concentrations of molecular states being able to permeate the first permeation barrier, the UWL. Free monomers and bile-micelle-bound molecules are considered to diffuse through the UWL [1]. Therefore, P_{eff} is defined based on $C_{dissolv}$. This is the unified definition of effective concentration for both permeation and dissolution.

$$X_{dissolv} = X_{mono} + X_{bm} = f_{mono}X_{dissolv} + (1 - f_{mono})X_{dissolv} \qquad (4.13)$$

$$C_{dissolv} = \frac{X_{dissolv}}{V_{GI}} \qquad (4.14)$$

4.5.2 Effective Concentration for Epithelial Membrane Permeation: the Free Fraction Theory

In most cases, it would be appropriate to assume that only free monomers can permeate the epithetical membrane. There are many experimental data showing that bile-micelle binding reduces apparent permeability (P_{app}) *in vitro, in situ,* and *in vivo* (P_{app} is usually calculated based on $C_{dissolv}$) [5–11].[7] Bile-micelle binding is thought to be one of the main reasons for the negative food effect (Section 12).

The effective epithelial membrane permeability (P'_{ep}), which is defined based on the total dissolved drug concentration, is expressed as

$$P'_{ep} = f_u \cdot P_{ep} \tag{4.15}$$

If the UWL permeability is negligible, P_{eff} is expressed as

$$P_{eff} = f_u \cdot P_{ep} \cdot PE \cdot VE \tag{4.16}$$

This is similar to the hepatic clearance calculation, in which the intrinsic hepatic clearance ($CL_{h,int}$) and unbound fraction in the plasma (f_{up}) are related to the hepatic clearance (CL_h) as $CL_h = f_{up} CL_{h,int}$ (when $Q_h > f_{up} CL_{h,int}$; Section 4.11).

4.6 SURFACE AREA EXPANSION BY PLICATE AND VILLI

P_{eff} value is usually calculated assuming that the small intestine is a smooth tube. However, the small intestinal has a plicate and villi structure. The UWL is adjacent to the top of the villi. Therefore, P_{eff} can be expressed as

$$P_{eff} = P_{plicate} \cdot PE \tag{4.17}$$

where $P_{plicate}$ is the plicate surface permeability and PE represents the surface area expansion by the plicate structure. The plicate surface permeation is a sequence of UWL and epithelial membrane permeations.

$$P_{plicate} = \cfrac{1}{\cfrac{1}{P_{UWL}} + \cfrac{1}{f_u \cdot P_{ep} \cdot Acc \cdot VE}} \tag{4.18}$$

where P_{UWL} is the UWL permeability, Acc is the accessibility to the villi surface, and VE is the villi expansion. Acc depends on the diffusion coefficient and the epithelial membrane permeability of a drug. In the case of a drug with high permeability, drug molecules are absorbed from the top of the villi before they diffuse to the crypt of the villi (Fig. 4.4), whereas in the case of a drug with low

---

[7]Usually an *in vitro* permeability assay (e.g., Caco-2) is performed without adding bile micelles to the donor chamber. Therefore, before using an *in vitro* data for biopharmaceutical modeling, the permeability should be corrected for bile micelle binding by multiplying with f_u.

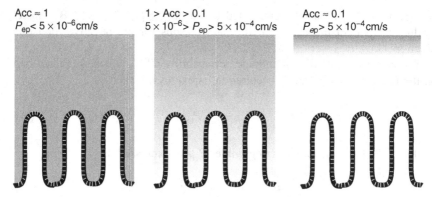

Acc $\approx$ 1
$P_{ep} < 5 \times 10^{-6}$ cm/s

$1 > $ Acc > 0.1
$5 \times 10^{-6} > P_{ep} > 5 \times 10^{-4}$ cm/s

Acc ≈ 0.1
$P_{ep} > 5 \times 10^{-4}$ cm/s

Figure 4.4   Villi available surface area for different P_{ep} drugs.

permeability, the entire surface is utilized for membrane permeation. Acc can be calculated as follows [3]:

$$q = \frac{1}{2}\left[(\beta^2 + 4)^2 + \beta\right], \quad r = \frac{1}{2}\left[(\beta^2 + 4)^2 - \beta\right] \tag{4.19}$$

$$\gamma = \left(\frac{f_u P_{ep} H_{villi}^2}{D_{eff} W_{channel}}\right)^{1/2}, \quad \beta = \left(\frac{P_{WC}^2 W_{channel}}{f_u P_{ep} D_{eff}}\right)^{1/2} \tag{4.20}$$

$$AA = \frac{\frac{1}{\gamma}\left\{\left(\frac{r}{q}\right)\exp(-r\gamma)[1 - \exp(-q\gamma)] - \left(\frac{q}{r}\right)\left[\exp(-r\gamma) - 1\right]\right\}}{q + r\exp\left[-\gamma(r + q)\right]} \tag{4.21}$$

$$BB = \frac{\left[\frac{W_{channel}}{H_{villi}}(r + q)\exp(-r\gamma)\right]}{q + r\exp[-\gamma(r + q)]} \tag{4.22}$$

$$Acc = \frac{\left(AA + BB + \frac{W_{villi}}{H_{villi}}\right)}{\left(1 + \frac{W_{channel}}{H_{villi}} + \frac{W_{villi}}{H_{villi}}\right)} \tag{4.23}$$

where P_{WC} is permeation by water conveyance, W_{villi} is the width of villi, $W_{channel}$ is the width of the channel between villi, and H_{viili} is the height of villi. Figure 4.5 shows the effect of Acc on P_{eff} calculation. In the case of low P_{ep} drugs (ca. $P_{ep} < 5 \times 10^{-6}$ cm/s at pH 6.5), P_{eff} is predominantly determined by epithelial membrane permeation and Acc has little effect. For high P_{ep} drugs (ca. $P_{ep} > 500 \times 10^{-6}$ cm/s at pH 6.5), P_{eff} is predominantly determined by the UWL and Acc has little effect. Acc has the largest effect (1.7-fold) when the UWL permeability and epithelial membrane permeability are in the same order of magnitude (ca. $P_{ep} = 5 - 500 \times 10^{-5}$ cm/s at pH 6.5, $0 < \log D_{oct} < 2$ at

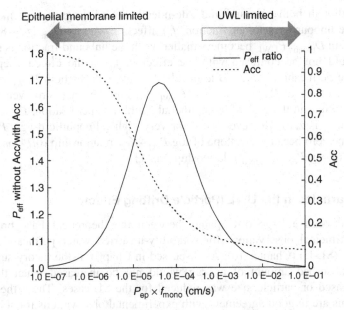

Figure 4.5   Effect of Acc on P_{eff} estimation.

pH 6.5). The maximum error by ignoring the Acc (i.e., assuming Acc = 1) is ca. 1.7-fold in P_{eff} prediction (Fig. 4.5). However, in this range, the oral absorption of a drug usually becomes rapid and complete (unless otherwise Do >1[8]). Therefore, in cases where Fa% <90%, the Acc has little effect on Fa% prediction accuracy (hence, Acc = 1 assumption is appropriate for Fa% prediction).

4.7 UNSTIRRED WATER LAYER PERMEABILITY

4.7.1 Basic Case

Both free monomers and bile-micelle-bound molecules can pass through the UWL, which partly superimposes to the mucous layer. In addition to diffusion, water conveyance would also affect UWL permeation [12, 12]. P_{UWL} can be expressed as

$$P_{UWL} = \frac{D_{eff}}{h_{UWL}} + P_{WC} = \frac{f_{mono}D_{mono} + (1 - f_{mono})D'_{bm}}{h_{UWL}} + P_{WC} \qquad (4.24)$$

D'_{bm} is the diffusion coefficient of bile-micelle-bound drug in the UWL. When the bile acid concentration is <3 mM, the effective diffusion coefficient in the mucous layer was reported to be three times higher compared to that in water [14].

---

[8]However, this case is rare (only for a compound with very high melting point (Section 2.3.7)).

Even though both unbound and bile-micelle-bound drugs can permeate the UWL, the unbound monomer fraction (f_u) affects P_{UWL}, as D_{bm} is 8–80 times smaller than D_{mono}. P_{UWL} becomes smaller when the unbound fraction is smaller. This should not be confused with the effect of f_u on the effective epithelial membrane permeability (P'_{ep}). Bile-micelle binding reduces both P_{UWL} and P'_{ep}. In the case of the UWL permeability, P_{UWL} does not become zero even when f_u is zero, whereas in the case of the epithelial membrane permeation, P'_{ep} becomes zero when f_u is zero. However, even for very highly lipophilic drugs, P'_{ep} does not become zero because the slope of log P_{oct}–K_{bm} relationship (0.74) is smaller than that of log P_{oct}–$P_{trans,0}$ relationship (ca. 1).

4.7.2 Particles in the UWL (Particle Drifting Effect)

There had been a large discrepancy between the theoretical Fa% prediction and experimental observations for solubility-unstirred water permeability limited cases (SL-U) (Chapter 10). As discussed in Chapter 1, the theory suggested that the absorbed amount of a drug would not be increased when the dose was increased or particle size was reduced for the SL cases. These theoretical suggestions are in good agreement with experimental observations for solubility-epithelial membrane permeability limited cases (SL-E) and SL-U cases with moderate particle size and dose (>5 µm and <5 mg/kg), but not for the SL-U cases with small particle size and/or large dose (<5 µm and/or >5 mg/kg) (Chapters 8 and 10; Fig. 10.2).

The particle drifting effect (PDE) was recently proposed [15] as a possible explanation for this discrepancy. The absorbed amount of a drug in solubility-permeability limited cases is determined by the solubility and permeability of the drug (but not the dissolution rate). However, the solubility of a drug is independent of the dose and particle size.[9] Therefore, even though it might be counter-intuitive, the permeability of a drug should have changed depending on the dose and particle size.

Many reports showed that a significant portion of microscale particles can drift into the UWL [16–20]. The structure of the mucous layer (i.e., micrometer-scale mesh size; Chapter 6; Fig. 6.7) also supports this experimental observation.

When the drug particles exist within the UWL, the distance from the particle to the epithelial cell surface becomes shorter. This reduction in diffusion length should be taken into account in biopharmaceutical modeling. This effect would be proportional to the drug particle surface area (i.e., dose and the inverse of particle size) in the UWL and would be significant when the surface area of the drug particles is in the same order of magnitude as the intestinal membrane surface (Section 3.2.3). These drug particles in the UWL could be the reservoir of a drug in the UWL.

In conscious humans, the total thickness of the UWL (h_{totUWL}) is reported to be ca. 0.03 cm (a plicate-surface-based value; it is 0.01 cm when based

---

[9]Unless otherwise the particle size is ≪100 nm (Sections 2.3.9 and 7.6.3.4).

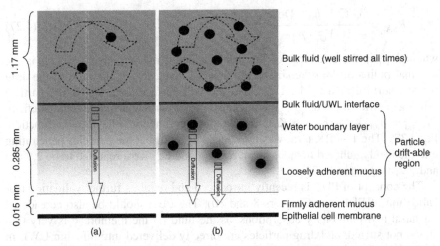

Figure 4.6 Particle drifting effect. (a) Low dose: drug molecules are supplied only from the bulk fluid/UWL interface. (b) High dose: drug molecules are supplied from both the particle surface in the UWL and the bulk fluid/UWL interface. *Source:* Adapted from Reference 15 with permission.

on a smooth surface) (Section 6.2.3.3). The UWL consists of the mucous and aqueous boundary layers (the latter is called the *Prandtl's boundary layer*, which is maintained solely by the viscosity of water; Fig. 4.6). The mucous layer is divided into two regions: the firmly adhered and loosely bound regions [21, 22]. The loosely bound mucous region can be renewed by a fluid flow.

Since the self-diffusion of micrometer-scale particles is negligibly small, the drug particles may be drifted into the UWL by the fluctuating fluid flow and/or the sedimentation by gravity (nanoscale particles may self-diffuse by Brownian motion). Fluctuation of intestinal fluid flow by the peristaltic moves of the intestinal wall is a well-known phenomenon. The loosely adhered mucus is easily removed by a flow [21, 22]. Therefore, the UWL would not be a completely static water layer. The fluid in the UWL can be renewed by an occasional strong flow and drug particles can be carried into the UWL (such as snow drifting on the hedge or sand drifting on the seacoast). However, the average flow in the UWL is weak, and the UWL becomes a barrier against self-diffusion majority of the time.

As the drug particles drift into the UWL, the effective thickness of the UWL looks reduced (Fig. 4.6). Considering the PDE, h_{UWL} is calculated as

$$h_{\text{UWL}} = h_{\text{fam}}\left[1 - \text{RK}\left(\frac{r_{\text{p,mean}}}{R_{\text{mucous}}}\right)\right] + h_{\text{pd}} - \frac{1}{2}h_{\text{pd}} \cdot R_{\text{SA}} \quad R_{\text{SA}} \leq 1 \quad (4.25)$$

$$h_{\text{UWL}} = h_{\text{fam}}\left[1 - \text{RK}\left(\frac{r_{\text{p,mean}}}{R_{\text{mucous}}}\right)\right] + \frac{1}{2} \cdot \frac{h_{\text{pd}}}{R_{\text{SA}}} \quad R_{\text{SA}} > 1 \quad (4.26)$$

$$R_{SA} = \frac{3 \cdot C_{pd} \cdot h_{pd} \cdot \text{Dose}}{V_{GI} \cdot \rho} \sum_i \frac{f_i}{r_{p,i}} \tag{4.27}$$

where h_{fam} is the thickness of the firmly adhered mucous layer, R_{mucous} is the nominal radius of the pore size of the mucous layer, R_{SA} is the ratio of the drug particle surface area in the UWL and the villi surface area, C_{pd} is the particle drifting coefficient, and h_{pd} is the thickness of the particle driftable region defined as $h_{pd} = h_{tot,UWL} - h_{fam}$. RK is a size sieving function (the Renkin function, Eq. 4.37). The $1 - $ RK term was introduced to represent the particles penetrating into the firmly adhered mucous layer. R_{mucous} and C_{pd} were reported to be 2.9 μm and 2.2, respectively [23].

The concept of PDE is recently introduced and requires further validation (for validation of PDE, see Chapters 8 and 10). The PDE should be also considered for nasal and pulmonary absorptions, as the fluid on the membrane is very thin and is not stirred, and drug particles are directly delivered into this thin UWL in these administration sites.

4.8   EPITHELIAL MEMBRANE PERMEABILITY (PASSIVE PROCESSES)

The epithelial membrane permeability (P_{ep}) can be further deduced to passive transcellular (P_{trans}) and paracellular (P_{para}) permeabilities (carrier-mediated transport is discussed later).

$$P_{ep} = P_{trans} + P_{para} \tag{4.28}$$

4.8.1   Passive Transcellular Membrane Permeability: pH Partition Theory

The cellular membrane is a lipid bilayer mainly consisting of phospholipids and cholesterol (Fig. 6.4). The lipophilic core of a lipid bilayer becomes the permeation barrier for hydrophilic molecules. In the case of dissociable drugs, P_{trans} can be represented as the weighted sum of the permeability of each species.

$$P_{trans} = f_0 \cdot P_{trans,0} + f_+ \cdot P_{trans,+} + f_- \cdot P_{trans,-} + f_{++} \cdot P_{trans,++} + \cdots \tag{4.29}$$

$$f_0 + f_+ + f_- + f_{++} + \cdots = 1 \tag{4.30}$$

where $P_{trans,0}$ is the intrinsic permeability of the undissociated species, $P_{trans,+}$ is that of $+1$ charged species, etc. The fraction of each species (f) depends on the pH near the epithelial membrane surface (microclimate pH, 5.5–6.5) and the $pK_a(s)$ of a drug (Section 6.1). Usually, the uncharged species is much more permeable

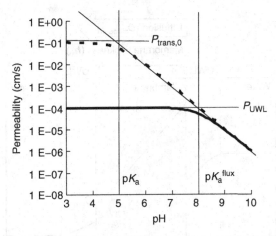

Figure 4.7   pH–permeability curve for an acidic drug.

than the charged species. Therefore, according to the pH partition theory,[10,11]

$$P_{trans} \approx f_0 \cdot P_{trans,0} \tag{4.31}$$

A typical pH–permeability curve is shown in Figure 4.7. The slope of the logarithmic plot is 1. In this slope region, one unit difference of pH or pK_a (a logarithmic scale) corresponds to a 10-fold change in permeability on a normal scale. Therefore, when a nonphysiological pH is used in an *in vitro* membrane assay for a dissociable drug, the effect of pH should be corrected before using the permeability value for biopharmaceutical modeling.[12] When the effect of the UWL is negligible, the horizontal line corresponds to $P_{trans,0}$. The crossover point of the slope line and the horizontal line is the pK_a the drug. However, when the UWL limits the permeability, the horizontal line becomes lower than $P_{trans,0}$, and the crossover point (pK_a flux) is not the same as the pK_a of the drug [26].

4.8.2 Intrinsic Passive Transcellular Permeability

4.8.2.1 Solubility–Diffusion Model. $P_{trans,0}$ can be further deduced from the interactions between a drug and the lipid bilayer. The simplest way to calculate the membrane permeability from the molecular properties of a drug and the membrane constituents is to treat the lipid bilayer as a homogeneous organic solvent membrane and apply Fick's law (Fig. 4.8) [27]. The passive permeation

---

[10]This relationship is similar to that of octanol–water partition coefficient (P_{oct}) and octanol–water distribution coefficient (D_{oct}), as $D_{oct} = f_0 P_{oct}$ (Section 7.2).

[11]Recently, it was suggested that ionized molecular species can also passively permeate the lipid bilayer (however, much slower than the neutral species) [24, 24].

[12]A pH of 7.4 is often used in an *in vitro* assay, although it is ca. 1 pH unit higher than the microclimate pH.

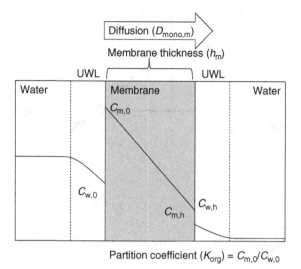

Figure 4.8 Homogeneous membrane model.

across a membrane is a diffusion process, the driving force of which is the concentration gradient across the membrane (i.e., Fick's law). If the interfacial resistance at the lipid–water interface is assumed negligible, flux (J) can be expressed as

$$J = \frac{D_m(C_{m,0} - C_{m,h})}{h_m} = \frac{D_m K_{org}(C_{W,0} - C_{W,h})}{h_m} = P_0(C_{W,0} - C_{W,h}) \quad (4.32)$$

where $D_{mono,m}$ is the diffusion coefficient of a drug in the membrane, h_m is the thickness of the membrane, and $C_{m,0}$ and $C_{m,h}$ are the concentrations of a drug at positions 0 and h in the membrane, respectively. $C_{m,0}$ and $C_{m,h}$ can be expressed by the partition coefficient between the water and the organic solvent (K_{org}) and the concentration in the water phases of the donor and acceptor sides ($C_{W,0}$ and $C_{W,h}$, respectively). Considering the sink condition, $C_{W,h}$ is approximated to be zero. Equation 4.32 indicates that the permeability is determined by the partition (a static parameter) and diffusion coefficients (a kinetic parameter) and the thickness of the membrane.[13]

The solubility–diffusion model can be extrapolated to the inhomogeneous membrane model [28]. The permeability coefficient is the reciprocal of the permeation resistance, and the total permeation resistance connected in series is the sum of each resistance (same as Ohm's law).

$$\frac{1}{P_{trans,0}} = \int_0^h \frac{1}{D_m(x)K_{org}(x)}dx \quad (4.33)$$

---

[13]This is similar to the Nernst–Brunner equation, in which the intrinsic dissolution rate is defined by the diffusion coefficient, thickness of the UWL on the particle, and solubility at the solid surface.

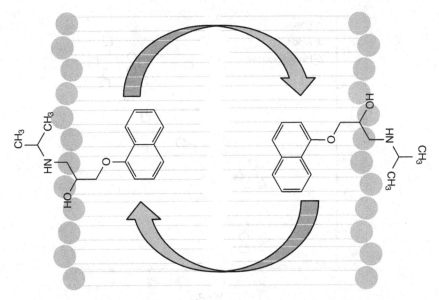

Figure 4.9   Flip-flop membrane permeation.

where $D_m(x)$ is the local diffusion coefficient at position x and $K_{org}(x)$ is the local partition coefficient between water and position x. According to Equation 4.33, the lowest permeability region (barrier domain) limits the total permeability. Therefore, Equation 4.33 can be simplified to Equation 4.32. K_{org} is the partition coefficient of a solute from water (not from the polar head group interface) to the barrier domain. The diffusion coefficient in the membrane is suggested to be lower than that in a nonpolar solvent such as hexadecane. The ordered region of the hydrophobic core (high density tail region in Figure 6.4) is suggested to behave like a soft polymer, leading to a reduction in the diffusion coefficient of this region.

According to the solubility–diffusion model, the membrane permeability coefficient can be related to the partition coefficient between water and the barrier region. If a suitable organic solvent that resembles the rate-limiting barrier is chosen, the membrane permeability coefficient can be calculated from the partition coefficient between water and the organic solvent, the diffusion coefficient, and the thickness of the barrier. In the case of a lipid bilayer mainly composed of phospholipids, simple alkanes or alkenes were suggested to reflect the rate-limiting permeation barrier for hydrophilic molecules [28–31]. Octanol was suggested to be less suitable, although it is the most often used organic solvent for QSAR (quantitative structure–activity relationship). However, the solubility diffusion theory has been investigated mainly for small molecules (MW < 100), and its applicability to druglike molecules is not known.

4.8.2.2   *Flip-Flop Model.* The flip-flop mechanism has also been investigated as the membrane permeation mechanism [32–34]. Figure 4.9 shows the concept

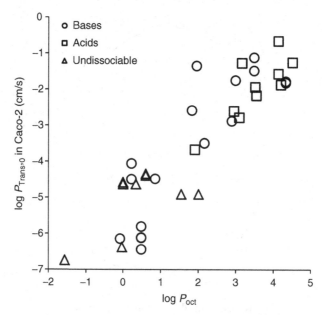

Figure 4.10   Relationship between $\log P_{oct}$ and $\log P_{trans,0}$ in Caco-2 for nontransporter substrates.

of the flip-flop mechanism. The flip-flop model has been proposed to describe the transmembrane movement of large amphiphilic molecules or peptide mimetic molecules (e.g., doxorubicin). The transmembrane movement can be described as (i) incorporation of a compound into one membrane leaflet and (ii) transfer (flip-flop) across the lipid core. In the case of fatty acids, it was found that the first step was much faster than the second flip-flop step, and the flip-flop rate decreased as the chain length increased [35, 36].

4.8.2.3 Relationship between $P_{trans,0}$ and $\log P_{oct}$.

The octanol–water partition coefficient is most often used as the surrogate of K_{org}. $P_{trans,0}$ and P_{oct} show broad but linear relationship over the range of $-2 < \log P_{oct} < 4$ and $0.0000001 < P_{trans,0} < 0.1$ cm/s.[14][15] Previously, the following equation was proposed to roughly estimate $P_{trans,0}$ in the Caco-2 assay [2, 2].

$$\log P_{trans,0}(\text{cm/s}) = 1.1 \log P_{oct} - 5.6 \qquad (4.34)$$

This equation is derived using experimental P_{oct} values. $P_{trans,0}$ is calculated from Caco-2 apparent permeability data (cf. Section 7.9.5) [37–39]. Figures 4.10

---

[14]Note that the order is not 10^{-6}. The high end value of 0.1 cm/s ($100{,}000 \times 10^{-6}$ cm/s) might look odd, as the highest apparent permeability (P_{app}) experimentally observed is usually 50×10^{-6} cm/s. However, this upper limit in P_{app} is due to the thick UWL in a standard *in vitro* setting. Once the UWL effect is corrected, $P_{trans,0}$ can reach up to 0.1 cm/s.

[15]This does not mean that octanol and lipid bilayer have exactly the same selectivity for drug permeation. The standard deviation of this relationship is ca. 1 log unit.

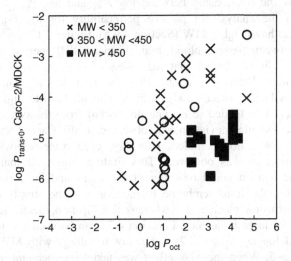

Figure 4.11 Relationship between log P_{oct} and log $P_{trans,0}$ for P-gp substrates in Caco-2 and MDCK cells under P-gp inhibition.

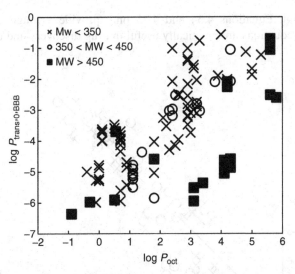

Figure 4.12 Relationship between log P_{oct} and the intrinsic blood–brain barrier permeability ($P_{trans,0,BBB}$) measured by brain perfusion experiments in P-gp knockout mice (or non-P-gp substrates). *Source:* Plotted based on References 40 and 41.

and 4.11 show the relationship between $\log P_{oct}$ and $\log P_{trans,0}$. Figure 4.11 was based on the analysis of passive permeability for the P-gp substrates, which tended to have higher MW (Section 4.9.5). Figure 4.12 shows the similar relationship between passive blood–brain barrier (BBB) permeability and log P_{oct} [40, 41]. It is interesting that regardless of the cell types (i.e., Caco-2, MDCK, and mice BBB), the relationships between $\log P_{oct}$ and $\log P_{trans,0}$ were similar. A large molecule (MW > 500) with medium to high lipophilicity ($\log D_{oct,\ pH6.5} > 1.5$) tended to deviate downward from the central correlation line. Previously, similar deviation was observed in the Caco-2 study [42], but the P-gp effect was not excluded. However, even after removing the P-gp effect, this deviation was observed. This finding suggested that the passive permeation mechanism could be different for small and large molecules. For small molecules, the transmembrane permeation may be simply described by the partition-diffusion mechanism, whereas the flip-flop mechanism would be more suitable for large molecules. Equation 4.34 can be used for the drugs with MW<500 and $\log D_{oct,\ pH6.5} = 2-5$, but not for drugs with MW > 500 and $\log D_{oct,pH\ 6.5} > 5$. When the MW effect was taken into account, the following empirical equation was obtained (Fig. 4.13).

$$\log P_{trans,0}(cm/s) = 0.89 \log P_{oct} - \frac{MW^{0.6}}{8.2} - 1.2 \qquad (4.35)$$

Even though Equations 4.34 and 4.35 only provide a rough estimation of $P_{trans,0}$, these equations are practically useful in drug discovery and development,

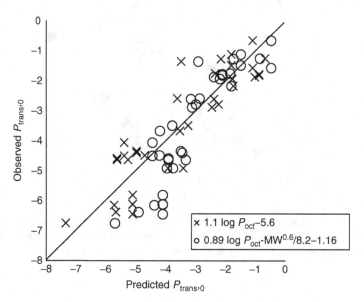

Figure 4.13 Estimated and observed $P_{trans,0}$ for nontransporter substrates.

especially for lipophilic drugs (log $D_{oct,pH\ 6.5} > 2$). Owing to the artifacts in an *in vitro* assay (Section 7.9.8), there is an inherent risk of underestimation of P_{app} for drugs with high lipophilicity (log $D_{oct,pH6.5} > 1.5$). On the other hand, experimental log $D_{oct,pH\ 6.5}$ is relatively reliable up to 4. In addition, at log $D_{oct,pH\ 6.5} > 2$, P_{eff} is governed by the UWL in most cases (except where MW > 500), and therefore, accurate estimation of P_{ep} is not required. Equations 4.34 and 4.35 should not be used if $P_{trans,0} > 0.1$ cm/s, as these equations were not validated in this range. There should be a theoretical upper limit for $P_{trans,0}$ controlled by diffusion process in the cytosol.

Example The P_{trans} of ketoprofen at pH 6.5 can be estimated from its log P_{oct} (3.2) and pK_a (4.0) as follows.[16]

$$\log P_{trans,0}(\text{cm/s}) = 1.1 \times 3.2 - 5.6 = -2.1$$

$$f_0 = \frac{1}{1 + \dfrac{10^{-4.0}}{10^{-6.5}}} = 0.0030$$

$$P_{trans} = 0.0030 \times 10^{-2.1} = 24 \times 10^{-6}\text{cm/s}$$

4.8.3 Paracellular Pathway

Small molecules can permeate the tight junction between the epithelial cells. The tight junction is maintained by the cell adhesion molecules and is negatively charged. Cationic small molecules (MW $< 200 - 400$ for humans) tend to be able to permeate the paracellular pathway, whereas large and/or negatively charged molecules cannot. Drug permeation through the paracellular pathway has been successfully modeled using a negative-charge tube model [43–50].

$$P_{para} = f_0 \cdot P_{para,0} + f_+ \cdot P_{para,+} + f_- \cdot P_{para,-} + f_{++} \cdot P_{para,++} + \cdots$$

$$= A'' \cdot \frac{1}{MW^{1/3}} \cdot RK\left(\frac{MW^{1/3}}{R_{MW}}\right)\left(f_0 + \sum^{z\,(z \neq 0)} f_z \cdot E(z)\right) \quad (4.36)$$

$$RK(R_{ratio}) = (1 - R_{ratio})^2[1 - 2.104 \cdot R_{ratio} + 2.09(R_{ratio})^3 - 0.95(R_{ratio})^5] \quad (4.37)$$

$$E(z) = \frac{Z_{para} \cdot z}{1 - \exp(-Z_{para} \cdot z)} \quad (4.38)$$

---

[16]The following misunderstanding is frequently cited in the literature of transporters: "A dissociable drug with a pK_a of 8.5 (base) or pK_a 4.5 (acid) is 99% ionized at a neutral pH and cannot permeate the lipid bilayer membrane by passive diffusion." (often followed by "Therefore, the majority of the ionizable drugs are absorbed via a transporter."). This misunderstanding might come from overlooking the point that $P_{trans,0}$ can be at least as high as $100,000 \times 10^{-6}$ cm/s.

where f_z is the fraction of each charged species (z, charge number) calculated from pK_a(s) of a drug, R_{ratio} is the ratio of the apparent pore radius of the paracellular pathway based on MW selectivity (R_{MW} (8.46 for humans)) and the molecular radius of a permeant (r_{mono}) ($R_{ratio} = MW^{1/3}/R_{MW}$), and A'' is a lump constant of the paracellular pathway population, etc. ($A'' = 3.9 \times 10^{-4}$, P_{para} in cm/s). Z_{para} corresponds to the apparent electric potential of the paracellular pathway (for the intestine, -18 to -80 mV). Owing to this negative charge, the paracellular pathway is cation selective [44, 51]. RK is a molecular sieving function (Renkin function) [52]. RK decreases as the molecular radius of a permeant increases. Even though the paracellular pathway model equation was a first approximation, it appropriately modeled the contribution of the paracellular pathway (Section 8.4.4). In addition to MW and z, the substrate's lipophilicity was also suggested to affect the paracellular pathway permeability [53, 54]. The molecular shape of a drug was suggested to affect P_{app} for specific cases such as PEGs [55].

The effective width of the paracellular pathway is different between animals and humans. The paracellular pathway is significantly leakier in dogs than in rats and humans [56] (Section 13.5.1). Caco-2 cells tend to have tighter tight junctions than the human small intestine [57]. Therefore, the paracellular pathway should be taken into account when we investigate species differences and *in vitro–in vivo* correlation.

Figure 4.14 shows the prediction of Fa% via P_{para} calculated using Equations 4.36–4.39. The paracellular pathway is often mentioned as a minor pathway when compared to passive transcellular permeation. However, many hydrophilic basic drugs ($pK_a >$ ca. 6.5) are suggested to permeate the paracellular pathway; for example, atenolol (MW = 266), metformin (MW = 129), and ranitidine (MW = 314). As P_{para} can be estimated from MW and pK_a with reasonable accuracy, the benefit/cost ratio of P_{para} calculation is appropriate.

4.8.4 Relationship between log D_{oct}, MW, and Fa%

Figure 4.15 shows the relationship between log D_{oct} (pH 6.5), MW, and Fa% calculated using Equations 4.35–4.38. The theoretical calculation is in good agreement with the experimental observation shown in Figure 8.8.

4.9 ENTERIC CELL MODEL

Figure 4.16 is the schematic presentation of an epithelial cell. To appropriately simulate the biological processes in the cytosol, the effective concentration of a drug in the cytosol should be defined as the unbound drug concentration ($f_{u1}C_1$).[17] $f_{u1}C_1$ could be significantly different from the drug concentration in the apical side. Full numerical integration of the processes in Figure 4.16 has been extensively used to investigate the pharmacokinetics in the enteric cells [58–65].

---

[17]The definitions of parameters shown in Figure 4.16 are used in this section.

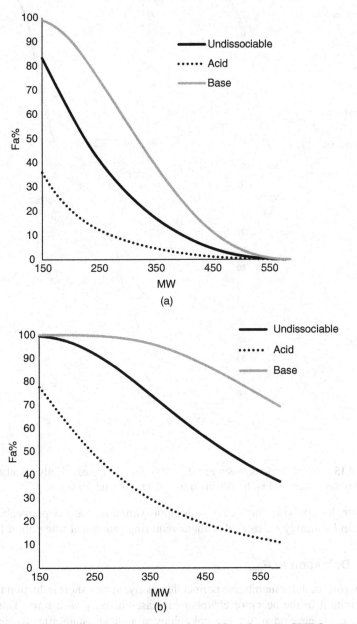

Figure 4.14 Fa% via paracellular pathway estimated based on the GUT framework. (a) Humans and (b) dogs.

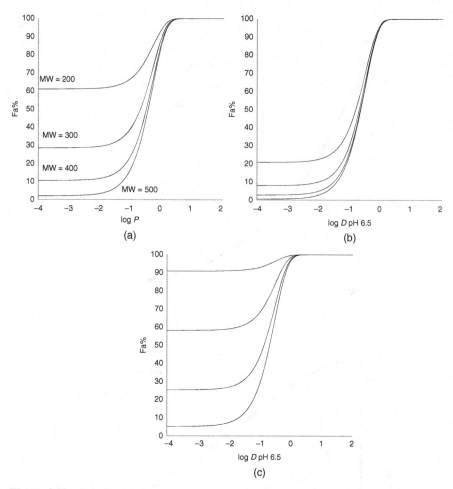

Figure 4.15 Relationship between log D_{oct}, MW, and Fa% theoretically calculated using Equations 4.35–4.39: (a) undissociable drugs, (b) acids, and (c) bases.

However, by applying the steady-state approximation, the net permeability and $f_{u1} C_1$ can be simply calculated without requiring numerical integration [66].

4.9.1 Definition of P_{app}

In an *in vitro* cellular membrane permeation assay, after a short induction time, the concentration in the acceptor chamber increases linearly with time. This means that the concentration in the cytosol achieved a steady state after the induction time. The apparent permeability (P_{app}) is calculated from this linear region as

$$P_{app} = \frac{1}{A_{well} \cdot C_{donor}} \frac{dX_{acceptor}}{dt} \tag{4.39}$$

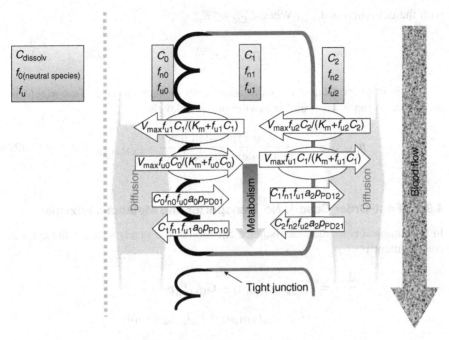

Figure 4.16 Epithelial cells' configuration.

where C_{donor} is the dissolved drug concentration in the donor well, A_{well} is the surface area of the well, and X_{acceptor} is the drug amount in the acceptor well.

In most cases, the steady-state approximation is appropriate mainly because the fluid volume in the cytosol is much smaller than the intestinal fluid.[18] In the following section, the theoretical details of the explicit cell model are discussed based on the steady-state approximation.

4.9.2 Enzymatic Reaction: Michaelis–Menten Equation

Usually, drug permeation by carrier-mediated transport is saturable, is substrate specific, and can be inhibited [67]. Intrinsic carrier-mediated permeability can be expressed as

$$p_{\text{CM}} = \frac{J_{\text{max}}}{K_{\text{m}} + C_{\text{CM}}} \tag{4.40}$$

where J_{max} is the maximum flux, K_{m} is the Michaelis–Menten constant, and C_{CM} is the effective concentration at the site of a transporter. K_{m} should be aligned

---

[18]The steady-state approximation is valid when a steady state is rapidly established in the cytosol compared to the timescale of concentration change in the donor side. Even when the C_{dissolv} changes over time, the steady-state approximation is applicable for each time point. At steady state, the ratio of the concentrations in the donor and cytosol compartments can be approximated to be constant.

with the definition of C_{CM}. When $C_{CM} \ll K_m$,

$$p_{CM} = \frac{J_{max}}{K_m} \tag{4.41}$$

J_{max} is in proportion to the expression level of each enzyme. To correct the difference in the *in vitro* and *in vivo* expression levels,

$$p_{CM,in\ vivo} = \frac{in\ vivo\ \text{expression level}}{in\ vitro\ \text{expression level}} \times p_{CM,in\ vitro} \tag{4.42}$$

4.9.3 First-Order Case 1: No Transporter and Metabolic Enzymes

In this simplest case, the mass balance equation at the steady state for the cytosol compartment is

$$\frac{dX_1}{dt} = C_0 f_{u0} f_{n0} p_{PD01} a_0 - C_1 f_{u1} f_{n1} p_{PD10} a_0$$

$$- C_1 f_{u1} f_{n1} p_{PD12} a_2 + C_2 f_{u2} f_{n2} p_{PD21} a_2 = 0 \tag{4.43}$$

where

f_n = the fraction of undissociated (uncharged) species;
f_u = the fraction of unbound species;
p = ideal permeability;
C = total dissolved drug concentration in each compartment;
a = absolute surface area;
X = compound amount in each compartment;
PD = passive diffusion;
0, 1, and 2 = compartments in Figure 4.16.

This equation is based on two assumptions:

1. Only the unbound fraction can permeate the membrane (free fraction theory).
2. Only the undissociated molecule can passively permeate the membrane (pH partition theory).

At steady state, the net mass balance in the cytosol can be approximated to be zero at each time point. The drug concentration in the basal side (C_2) is much smaller than that in the apical side and is considered to be negligible ($C_2 = 0$). By rearranging Equation 4.43 for $C_1 f_{u1}$, we obtain,

$$C_1 f_{u1} = C_0 f_{u0} \frac{f_{n0}}{f_{n1}} \frac{p_{PD01} a_0}{p_{10PD} a_0 + p_{12PD} a_2} \tag{4.44}$$

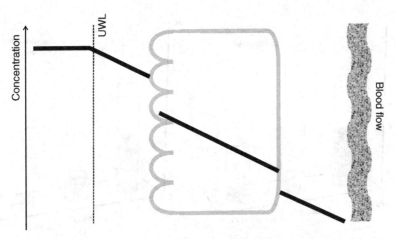

Figure 4.17   Schematic presentation of concentration gradient across the epithelial membrane. The bold line indicates the concentration gradient across the intestinal wall.

This equation can be interpreted as the unbound drug concentration in the cytosol ($C_1 f_{u1}$) is determined by the ratio of undissociated fraction in the apical and cytosol compartments (f_{n0}/f_{n1}), intrinsic passive permeability, unbound fraction in the apical site (f_{u0}), and surface area ($p_{PD01} a_0/(p_{PD10} a_0 + p_{PD12} a_2)$). f_{n0}/f_{n1} can be calculated from the pK_a of a drug and the pH of the apical and the cytosol compartments. Therefore, the information about the bound fraction of a drug in the cytosol (f_{u1}) is not required for calculation of the unbound drug concentration in the cytosol at the steady state.[19] In other words, the concentration gradient of the unbound undissociated species solely determines the passive permeation process. Figure 4.17 shows a schematic presentation of a concentration gradient across the intestinal wall. Figure 4.18 shows the concentration profile of undissociated and dissociated species.

When the passive permeability is symmetric in the influx and efflux directions and is equal in the apical and basal sides (i.e., $p_{PD01} = p_{PD10} = p_{PD12} = p_{PD21} = p_{PD}$),[20] and as the surface area ratio is 1:3 in the epithelial cells [68], Equation 4.44 becomes

$$C_1 f_{u1} = C_0 f_{u0} \frac{f_{n0}}{f_{n1}} \frac{a_0}{a_0 + a_2} = C_0 f_{u0} \frac{1}{4} \frac{f_{n0}}{f_{n1}} \tag{4.45}$$

Therefore, when the pH of the apical and cytosol compartments are equal (e.g., pH 7.4) or a drug is not dissociable, the unbound drug concentration in the cytosol

---

[19]This situation is the similar in the PK–PD theory, so the cytosol concentration in a target organ can be calculated from the plasma concentration and plasma unbound fraction (when no carrier-mediated transport is involved).

[20]This assumption is supported by the fact that passive A to B and B to A permeability values become the same at iso-pH.

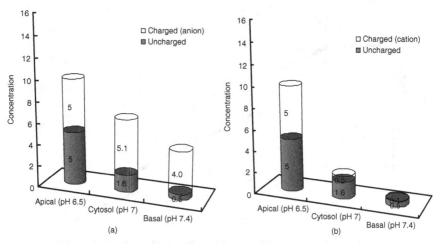

Figure 4.18 The concentration of undissociated and charged species in the epithelial cells. The concentration gradient of unbound undissociated species (gray bar) solely determines the passive permeation processes. (a) Acid and (b) base. (Both have pK_a of 6.5). Concentration gradient of unbound unionized drug molecules determines the passive permeability.

$(C_1 f_{u1})$ is one-fourth of that in the apical side $(C_0 f_{u0})$. When the pH is different (e.g., pH 6.0–6.5 in the apical side (acid microclimate pH) and 7.0–7.4 in the cytosol) and a drug is dissociable, the difference in the undissociated fraction should be taken into account. This point is especially important for prediction of drug–drug interaction in the enterocytes (Section 14.2).

Example The unbound drug concentration ratio of cimetidine (cytosol/apical) can be calculated as follows ($pK_a = 6.9$; pH of the apical and cytosol sites = 6.5 and 7.0, respectively; and no bile-micelle binding in the apical side):

$$f_{n0} = \frac{1}{1 + \dfrac{10^{-6.5}}{10^{-6.9}}} = 0.28, \quad f_{n1} = \frac{1}{1 + \dfrac{10^{-7.0}}{10^{-6.9}}} = 0.56$$

$$\frac{C_1 f_{u1}}{C_0 f_{u0}} = \frac{1}{4} \times \frac{0.28}{0.56} = 0.13$$

Using this cytosol concentration, the net permeability can be calculated as follows. At steady state, the flux across the apical membrane becomes equal to the net flux from the apical to basal side.

$$C_0 P_{app} A_{well} = C_0 f_{u0} f_{n0} P_{PD} a_0 - C_1 f_{u1} f_{n1} P_{PD} a_0 \qquad (4.46)$$

The LHS of the equation is the macroscopic net flux from the apical side to the basal side (cf. the apparent permeability (P_{app}) is defined based on the flat surface area of a cell culture well (A_{well}) and the dissolved drug concentration at the apical membrane surface (C_0)). The RHS is the microscopic net flux at the apical membrane. By substituting Equation 4.44 in Equation 4.46, we obtain

$$P_{app} = f_{n0}f_{u0}P_{PD} \frac{1}{A_{well}} \left(\frac{a_0 a_2}{a_0 + a_2} \right) \tag{4.47}$$

This equation can be interpreted as P_{app} is affected by the uncharged and unbound fractions in the apical side (f_{n0} and f_{u0}, respectively), but not by those in the cytosol (f_{n1} and f_{u1} do not appear in this equation).[21] As shown in Figure 4.18, the passive flux is determined only by the concentration gradient of unbound undissociated species [38, 69].[22,23]

4.9.4 First-Order Case 2: Efflux Transporter in Apical Membrane

When $C_1 f_{u1} \ll K_m$, the efflux transport can be treated as the first-order kinetics. For A to B direction, the mass balance in the cytosol at steady state is

$$C_0 f_{u0} f_{n0} P_{PD01} a_0 - C_1 f_{u1} f_{n1} P_{PD10} a_0 - C_1 f_{u1} f_{n1} P_{PD12} a_2 - C_1 f_{u1} P_{efflux} a_0 = 0 \tag{4.48}$$

By rearranging this equation, we obtain

$$C_1 f_{u1} = C_0 f_{u0} \frac{f_{n0}}{f_{n1}} \frac{P_{PD01} a_0}{P_{PD10} a_0 + P_{PD12} a_2 + \dfrac{P_{efflux} a_0}{f_{n1}}} \tag{4.49}$$

On the other hand, from the definition of apparent permeability and flux across the basolateral membrane at steady state, we obtain

$$C_0 P_{app,A-B} A_{well} = C_1 f_{u1} f_{n1} P_{PD12} a_2 - C_2 f_{u2} f_{n2} P_{PD21} a_2 \tag{4.50}$$

In this equation, the flux across the basolateral membrane at steady state (RHS) is equal to the total flux defined as the donor concentration and apparent permeability (LHS). Usually, P_{app} is calculated at the time point where $C_2 \approx 0$

[21] It is often argued that the pH partition theory should be incorrect because the pH in the cytosol is maintained constant (at pH 7.4) regardless of the apical pH and the basolateral permeation of a drug will be the rate-limiting step (main permeation barrier) for an acid (unless otherwise the apical intrinsic passive clearance ($a_0 P_{01}$) is significantly smaller than the basal one ($a_1 P_{12}$)). According to Equation 4.47, pH and unbound fraction in the cytosol does not affect P_{app}, and therefore, regardless of $a_0 P_{01}$ and $a_1 P_{12}$ values, the pH-partition theory is valid. It has been widely experimentally confirmed in the literature that dissociable compounds follow the pH partition theory [38, 39].
[22] Concentration and fraction should not be confused.
[23] In an *in situ* assay and *ex vivo* assay, the pH-dependent permeability of a drug is often not well observed because of the existence of microclimate pH, which is well maintained and little affected by the bulk fluid pH.

and the second term is negligible. By substituting Equation 4.49 in Equation 4.50, we obtain

$$
P_{\text{app},A-B} = \frac{C_1 f_{u1} f_{n1} P_{\text{PD}12} a_2}{C_0 A_{\text{well}}} = \frac{f_{n1} P_{\text{PD}12} a_2}{C_0 A_{\text{well}}} C_0 f_{u0} \frac{f_{n0}}{f_{n1}} \frac{P_{\text{PD}01} a_0}{P_{\text{PD}10} a_0 + P_{\text{PD}12} a_2 + \dfrac{P_{\text{efflux}} a_0}{f_{n1}}}
$$

$$
= f_{u0} f_{n0} \frac{1}{A_{\text{well}}} \frac{P_{\text{PD}01} a_0 P_{\text{PD}12} a_2}{P_{\text{PD}10} a_0 + P_{\text{PD}12} a_2 + \dfrac{P_{\text{efflux}} a_0}{f_{n1}}} \tag{4.51}
$$

In a similar way, for B to A direction,

$$
C_2 f_{u2} f_{n2} P_{\text{PD}21} a_2 - C_1 f_{u1} f_{n1} P_{\text{PD}12} a_2 - C_1 f_{u1} f_{n1} P_{\text{PD}10} a_0
$$
$$
- C_1 f_{u1} P_{\text{efflux}} a_0 = 0 \tag{4.52}
$$

$$
C_1 f_{u1} = C_2 f_{u2} \frac{f_{n2}}{f_{n1}} \frac{P_{\text{PD}21} a_2}{P_{\text{PD}12} a_2 + P_{\text{PD}10} a_0 + \dfrac{P_{\text{efflux}} a_0}{f_{n1}}} \tag{4.53}
$$

$$
C_2 P_{\text{app},B-A} A = C_2 f_{u2} f_{n2} P_{\text{PD}21} a_2 - C_1 f_{u1} f_{n1} P_{\text{PD}12} a_2 \tag{4.54}
$$

Therefore,

$$
P_{\text{app},B-A} = \frac{C_2 f_{u2} f_{n2} P_{\text{PD}21} a_2 - C_1 f_{u1} f_{n1} P_{\text{PD}12} a_2}{C_2 f_{u2} A_{\text{well}}}
$$

$$
= f_{n2} f_{u2} \frac{1}{A_{\text{well}}} \left(P_{\text{PD}21} a_2 - \frac{P_{\text{PD}12} a_2 P_{\text{PD}21} a_2}{P_{\text{PD}12} a_2 + P_{\text{PD}10} a_0 + P_{\text{efflux}} a_0 / f_{n1}} \right) \tag{4.55}
$$

When $f_{n0} = f_{n2}$ (the iso-pH condition), $f_{u0} = f_{u2}$, and $P_{\text{PD}01} = P_{\text{PD}10} = P_{\text{PD}12} = P_{\text{PD}21} = P_{\text{PD}}$, the efflux ratio (ER) becomes

$$
\text{ER} = \frac{P_{\text{app},BA}}{P_{\text{app},AB}} = 1 + \frac{P_{\text{efflux}}}{f_{n1} P_{\text{PD}}} \tag{4.56}
$$

This equation is particularly important, as it clearly shows the relationship between ER, passive diffusion, and active efflux transport. By substituting this equation in Equation 4.49, we obtain

$$
C_1 f_{u1} = C_0 f_{u0} \frac{f_{n0}}{f_{n1}} \frac{P_{01} a_0}{P_{10} a_0 + P_{12} a_2 + a_0 P_{01} (\text{ER} - 1)}
$$

$$
= C_0 f_{u0} \frac{f_{n0}}{f_{n1}} \frac{1}{1 + a_2 / a_0 + (\text{ER} - 1)} \tag{4.57}
$$

This equation collapses to Equation 4.44 when ER $= 1$. As the surface area ratio is 1:3 in the epithelial cells [68],

$$C_1 f_{u1} = C_0 f_{u0} \frac{f_{n0}}{f_{n1}} \frac{1}{4 + (\text{ER} - 1)} \tag{4.58}$$

Therefore, the unbound drug concentration in the cytosol under the effect of efflux transporter can be estimated once we have ER data.

An inhibition study is often performed to estimate the effect of an efflux transporter on oral absorption of its substrate. In this case,

$$\frac{P_{\text{app,PD}}}{P_{\text{app},A-B}} = 1 + \frac{1}{4}(\text{ER} - 1) \tag{4.59}$$

This equation suggests that an AUC change by inhibiting an apical efflux transporter is much smaller than ER. For example, when ER $= 2$, the AUC increase by inhibiting the apical efflux transporter will be 1.25.[24] Another merit of this equation is that ER can be estimated from $P_{\text{app,PD}}/P_{\text{app},A-B}$ ratio. In many cases of lipophilic P-gp substrates, the $P_{\text{app},B-A}$ exceeds the *in vitro* UWL limitation (Section 7.9.8), while $P_{\text{app},A-B}$ and $P_{\text{app,PD}}$ remain within it. In this case, Equation 4.59 can be used to calculate ER unaffected by the UWL. In addition, if $P_{\text{app,PD}}$ is not available, it can be estimated from $P_{\text{app},A-B}$ and ER (when $P_{\text{app},B-A} \ll \textit{in vitro} P_{\text{UWL}}$).

From Equation 4.59,

$$P_{\text{efflux}} = f_{n1} P_{\text{PD}} \, (\text{ER} - 1) \tag{4.60}$$

$$A_{\text{well}} \cdot p_{\text{efflux}} \equiv P_{\text{efflux}} = \frac{J_{\text{max}}}{K_m} = A f_{n1} P_{\text{PD}} (\text{ER} - 1)$$

$$\equiv P_{\text{app,PD}} \left(\frac{a_0 a_2}{a_0 + a_2} \right) (\text{ER} - 1) \tag{4.61}$$

Using Equations 4.59 and 4.61, we can estimate K_m/J_{max} both *in vitro* and *in vivo*. It would be appropriate to assume that K_m is similar *in vivo* and *in vitro*. Therefore, the difference in the expression levels can be estimated by comparing *in vitro* and *in vivo* J_{max} values. This enables mechanistic *in vitro–in vivo* extrapolation.

In Figure 4.19, *in vitro* p_{efflux} was plotted against $f_{n1} \times p_{\text{PD}}$ for structurally diverse drugs. P_{app} data were collected from the literature [70–73]. The following methods were used to estimate p_{efflux}: (i) when $P_{\text{app,PD}}$, $P_{\text{app},A-B}$, and $P_{\text{app},B-A}$ are all available and below the UWL limitation, they are used to calculate $f_{n1} \times p_{\text{PD}}$ and p_{efflux}; (ii) when $P_{\text{app},B-A}$ exceeded the UWL limitation, while $P_{\text{app,PD}}$ and $P_{\text{app},A-B}$ did not, Equation 4.59 was used to calculate ER; and (iii) when $P_{\text{app,PD}}$

---

[24]Therefore, when considering the bioequivalence (0.8–1.25 AUC and C_{max}) of oral absorption with and without inhibition, ER $= 2$ would be a good criteria.

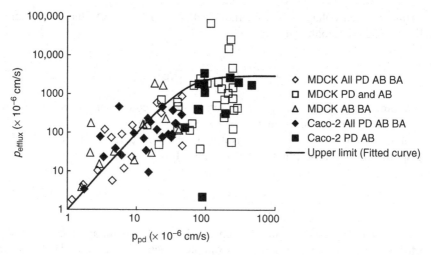

Figure 4.19 $p_{\text{efflux}} - p_{\text{PD}}$ relationship.

is not available but $P_{\text{app},A-B}$ and $P_{\text{app},B-A}$ are both below the UWL limitation, $P_{\text{app,PD}}$ is calculated from $P_{\text{app},A-B}$ and ER using Equation 4.59. The half of the highest permeability observed in the system was used as the UWL limiting criteria. All experiments were performed at pH 7.4 in both apical and basal sides (hence, $f_{n0} = f_{n1} = f_{n2}$) without any solubilizers ($f_{u0} = f_{u2} = 1$).

As shown in Figure 4.19, a correlation was observed between p_{efflux} and $f_{n1} \times p_{\text{PD}}$. This is in good agreement with the suggested mechanism of P-gp that the efflux transport is the sequence of the passive membrane partitioning step and active transmembrane transport step (Fig. 4.20) [74]. The trend line in Figure 4.19 is

$$p_{\text{efflux}} \leq \left[\frac{0.2}{\left(f_{n1} \times p_{\text{PD}}\right)^2} + \frac{1}{500} \right]^{-1} \tag{4.62}$$

where the unit of both p_{efflux} and $f_{n1} \times p_{\text{PD}}$ is 10^{-6} cm/s. Using this trend line, the maximum effect of P-gp on $P_{\text{ep}}, P_{\text{eff}}$, and Fa% can be calculated. Figure 4.21b shows the maximum increase of $P_{\text{ep}}, P_{\text{eff}}$, and Fa% by P-gp inhibition for undissociable drugs. Equations 4.35 and 4.62 were used to calculate $P_{\text{trans,0}}$ and maximum p_{efflux}, respectively. It was suggested that maximum ratio of P_{ep} would be ca. 7 (inhibition/no inhibition) for moderately lipophilic indissociable drugs, whereas when passive P_{ep} is higher than 3×10^{-3} cm/s (log D_{oct} of ca. 2.5), the P-gp effect on net P_{ep} should be minimum. Furthermore, at passive $P_{\text{ep}} > 2 \times 10^{-4}$ cm/s (log D_{oct} of ca. 1.25), the minimum value of net P_{ep} becomes ca. 50×10^{-6} cm/s and the UWL would become the limiting step, hence P-gp inhibition would have little effect on total P_{eff} and complete oral absorption is anticipated even when the drug is a P-gp substrate. These theoretical suggestions are in good agreement with the

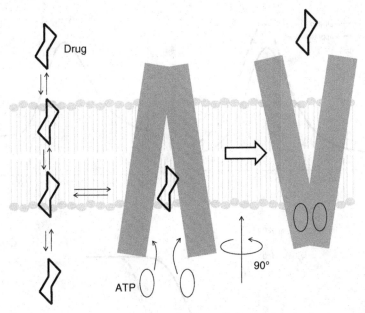

Figure 4.20 Model of substrate transport by P-gp [74]. A substrate drug partitions into the bilayer and enters the internal drug-binding pocket through an open portal. ATP binding induces a large conformational change, opening the drug-binding site to the extracellular space.

experimental observations that when the passive P_{ep} is high, P-gp has little or no effect on the *in vitro* ER [75] and *in vivo* total absorption (Section 14.4.2).

In addition, the P-gp effect would be larger for basic drugs compared to indissociable and acid drugs in *in vivo* situation (Fig. 4.22). This is due to the difference in the apical and cytosol pH. When the apical pH is changed from 7.4 to 6.5, the passive influx of a basic drug becomes ca. 10-fold smaller while P-gp efflux remains the same (as the cytosol pH remains the same). Maximum P-gp inhibition effect on Fa% (ca. sevenfold) would be observed for a basic drug with moderate permeability.

4.9.5 Apical Efflux Transporter with K_m and V_{max}

To calculate the nonlinear effect of efflux transporter, the Michaelis–Menten equation can be incorporated into the explicit cell model. In this case, the mass balance in the cell compartment can be written as

$$\frac{dM_1}{dt} = C_0 f_{n0} f_{u0} a_0 P_{PD01} - C_1 f_{n1} f_{u1} a_0 P_{PD10} - C_1 f_{n1} f_{u1} a_2 P_{PD12}$$

$$+ C_2 f_{n2} f_{u2} a_2 P_{PD21} - \frac{V_{max\,10} C_1 f_{u1}}{K_{m10} + C_1 f_{u1}} = 0 \qquad (4.63)$$

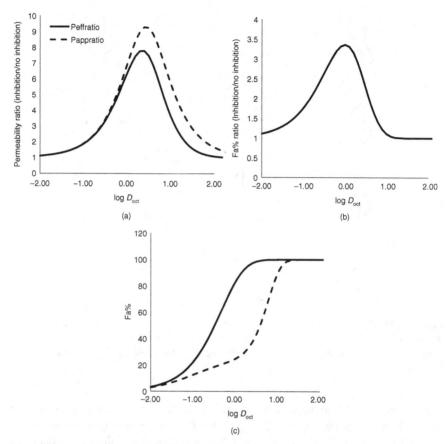

Figure 4.21 Maximum effect of P-gp inhibition on P_{eff} and Fa% (without low solubility and dissolution rate limitation, paracellular permeation, and bile-micelle binding ($f_u = 1$)). (a) P_{eff} ratio, (b) Fa% ratio, and (c) Fa%. PE = 3, VE = 10, $h_{UWL} = 0.03$ cm, $D_{mono} = 7 \times 10^{-6}$ cm/s, $H_{villi} = 0.06$ cm, $W_{channel} = 0.02$ cm, $W_{villi} = 0.05$ cm, and $P_{WC} = 0.23 \times 10^{-5}$ cm/s.

where K_{m10} is the intrinsic Michaelis constant of an efflux transporter in the apical membrane. By rearranging Equation 4.63,

$$(C_1 f_{u1})^2 (f_{n1} a_0 p_{10} + f_{n1} a_2 p_{12})$$

$$+ (C_1 f_{u1}) \left[K_{m10} (f_{n1} a_0 p_{10} + f_{n1} a_2 p_{12}) \right.$$

$$+ V_{max\,10} - (C_0 f_{n0} f_{u0} a_0 p_{01} + C_2 f_{n2} f_{u2} a_2 p_{21}) \right]$$

$$- K_{m10} (C_0 f_{n0} f_{u0} a_0 p_{01} + C_2 f_{n2} f_{u2} a_2 p_{21}) = 0 \qquad (4.64)$$

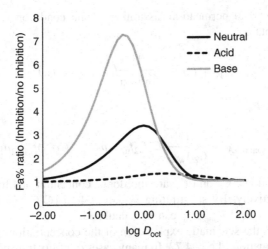

Figure 4.22 Maximum effect of P-gp inhibition on Fa% for undissociable, acid and base drugs. pK_a was set to 4 and 9 for acids and bases, respectively. Other conditions are the same with Figure 4.21.

This is a quadratic equation for $C_1 f_{u1}$. By solving Equation 4.64, $C_1 f_{u1}$ can be obtained as

$$C_1 f_{u1} = \frac{-b' + \sqrt{b'^2 - 4a'c'}}{2a'} \tag{4.65}$$

$$a' = f_{n1} a_0 p_{10} + f_{n1} a_2 p_{12} \tag{4.66}$$

$$b' = K_{m10} a' + V_{max\,10} + \frac{c'}{K_{m10}} \tag{4.67}$$

$$c' = -K_{m10}(C_0 f_{n0} f_{u0} a_0 p_{01} + C_2 f_{n2} f_{u2} a_2 p_{21}) \tag{4.68}$$

On the other hand, from the definition of $P_{app,A-B}$ (LHS of Eq. 4.69) and the mass transfer into the basal compartment (RHS of Eq. 4.69), we obtain

$$C_0 P_{app,A-B} A_{well} = C_1 f_{n1} f_{u1} a_2 p_{12} - C_2 f_{n2} f_{u2} a_2 p_{21} \tag{4.69}$$

Similarly,

$$C_2 P_{app,B-A} A_{well} = C_2 f_{n2} f_{u2} a_2 p_{21} - C_1 f_{n1} f_{u1} a_2 p_{12} \tag{4.70}$$

For apical to basal permeation, assuming a sink condition in the basal side ($C_2 = 0$), we obtain

$$P_{app,ep,A-B} = \frac{1}{C_0 A_{well}} f_{n1} a_2 p_{12} (C_1 f_{u1}) \tag{4.71}$$

Similarly, for $P_{app,B-A}$,

$$P_{app,ep,B-A} = \frac{1}{C_2 A_{well}} [C_2 f_{n2} f_{u2} a_2 p_{21} - (C_1 f_{u1}) f_{n1} a_2 p_{12}] \tag{4.72}$$

In these equations, C_0 and C_2 are the donor concentrations for $P_{app,A-B}$ and $P_{app,B-A}$, respectively. By substituting Equation 4.65 ($C_1 f_{u1}$) in Equations 4.71 and 4.72, $P_{app,A-B}$ and $P_{app,A-B}$ can be calculated.

Figure 4.23 is the schematic explanation of the concentration–P_{app} curve calculated using Equations 4.62–4.72. In many cases of efflux transporter substrates, an asymmetric concentration–P_{app} curve is observed between the A to B and B to A permeations. This asymmetry is caused by the differences in the passive clearance of the apical and basolateral membranes. Figure 4.24 shows the fitted curve for rhodamin123 and fexofenadine. In addition, the difference in expression level can change the apparent K_m value as the cytosol concentration changes depending on the P-gp expression level [64, 76, 77]. Figure 4.25 shows the fitted curve for vinblastine with a single intrinsic K_m value.

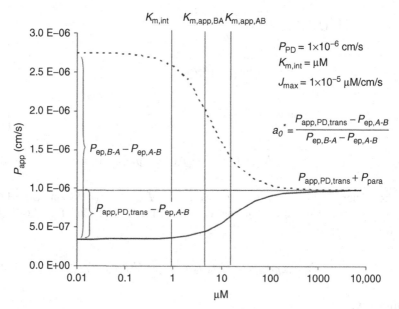

Figure 4.23 Schematic explanation of the concentration–P_{app} curve with an efflux transporter in the apical membrane. *Source:* Adapted from Reference 66 with permission.

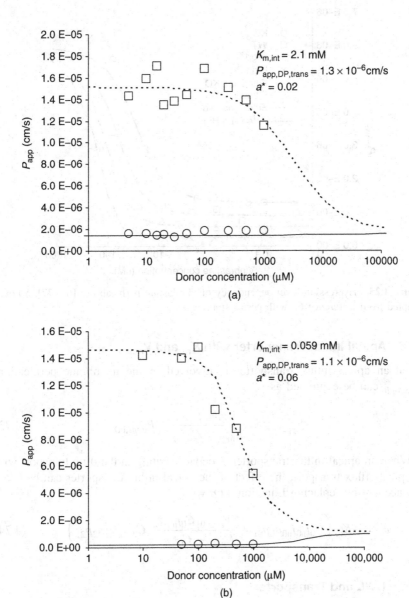

Figure 4.24 Experimental and simulated concentration–P_{app} curves of rhodamin123 and fexofenadine [66, 78, 79]. (a) Rhodamine 123 and (b) Fexofenadine. *Source:* Adapted from Reference 66 with permission.

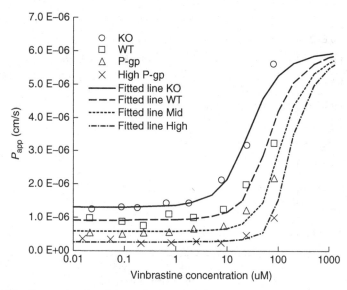

Figure 4.25 Expression-level dependency of vinblastine permeability [66, 77]. *Source:* Adapted from Reference 66 with permission.

4.9.6 Apical Influx Transporter with K_m and V_{max}

When an apical influx transporter is involved in the membrane permeation, $P_{app,A-B}$ can be expressed as

$$P_{app,A-B} = \frac{J_{max}}{K_{m01} + C_0 f_{u0}} + P_{trans,PD} \tag{4.73}$$

When an apical influx transporter is coparticipating in the drug transport with an apical efflux transport, the effect of the apical influx transporter can be taken into account by replacing Equation 4.68 with

$$c' = -K_m \left(C_0 f_{n0} f_{u0} a_0 p_{01} + \frac{V_{max01} C_0 f_{u0}}{K_{m01} + C_0 f_{u0}} + C_2 f_{n2} f_{u2} a_2 p_{21} \right) \tag{4.74}$$

4.9.7 UWL and Transporter

In the above discussions of explicit cell models, the UWL is neglected. To consider the UWL effect, the following condition can be additionally introduced:

$$(C_{dissolv} - C_0) P_{UWL} - C_0 P_{ep} = 0 \tag{4.75}$$

where C_0 is the concentration adjacent to the apical membrane in the apical chamber. This equation means that at steady state, the flux across the UWL (first term) is equal to the flux across the epithelial membrane.

4.9.7.1 No Transporter. With no transporter, by rearranging Equation 4.75, C_0/C_{dissolv} can be calculated as

$$\frac{C_0}{C_{\text{dissolv}}} = \frac{P_{\text{UWL}}}{P_{\text{UWL}} + P_{\text{ep}}} \tag{4.76}$$

When $P_{\text{UWL}} < P_{\text{ep}}$, the drug concentration at the epithelial membrane surface (C_0) is significantly smaller than C_{dissolv} because of the concentration gradient across the UWL. Furthermore, the $f_{\text{u1}}C_1$ can be 3- to 10-fold lower than $f_{\text{u0}}C_0$ for neutral and base cases (for acids, $f_{\text{u0}}C_0/f_{\text{u1}}C_1 = 2$). Therefore, to saturate or inhibit a metabolic enzyme in the cytosol, the concentration in the donor side should be significantly higher than the intrinsic K_{m} and K_{i} values. When predicting the drug–drug interaction, these concentration gradients across the UWL and the epithelial membrane should be taken into account (Section 14.2.2).

4.9.7.2 Influx Transporter and UWL. With an apical influx transporter, Equations 4.73 and 4.75 can be solved as a quaternary equation (cf. P_{ep} is a function of C_0 for nonlinear cases) [80, 81].

$$C_0 f_{\text{u0}} = \sqrt{\frac{q^2 r^2}{4} + q K_{\text{m01}} C_{\text{dissolv}} f_{\text{u0}}} - \frac{q \cdot r}{2} \tag{4.77}$$

$$P_{\text{app},A-B} = P_{\text{UWL}} \left(1 - \frac{C_0 f_{\text{u0}}}{C_{\text{dissolv}}} \right) \tag{4.78}$$

$$q = \frac{P_{\text{UWL}}}{P_{\text{UWL}} + P_{\text{trans,PD}}}, \ r = \frac{K_{\text{m01}}}{q} + \frac{J_{\text{max}}}{P_{\text{UWL}}} - C_{\text{dissolv}} f_{\text{u0}} \tag{4.79}$$

Figure 4.26 shows the concentration–$P_{\text{app},A-B}$ relationship with an apical influx transporter. If the UWL effect is neglected in the intrinsic K_{m} calculation, the intrinsic K_{m} value is overestimated (apparent $K_{\text{m}} >$ intrinsic K_{m}).

4.9.7.3 Efflux Transporter. In this case, the theoretical treatment to handle the UWL effect together with a saturable efflux transport is complicated and a simple open solution cannot be obtained. However, the following process can be used to calculate P_{app}. At steady state,

$$(C_{\text{dissolv}} - C_0)P_{\text{UWL}} - C_0 P_{\text{ep}} = 0 \tag{4.80}$$

$$P_{\text{ep}} = f(C_0) \tag{4.81}$$

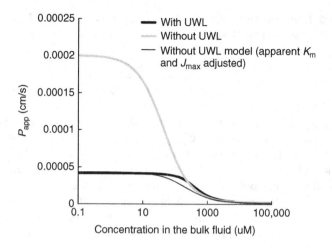

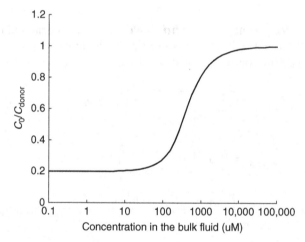

Figure 4.26   The effect of UWL on total permeability of apical influx transporter substrate. $P_{active} = 200 \times 10^{-6}$ cm/s, $K_m = 50$ μm, and $P_{UWL} = 50 \times 10^{-6}$ cm/s. No passive diffusion.

From this condition, the C_0 value satisfying Equation 4.80 can be seeked, for example, using the Newton method or the simplex method.[25] Once C_0 is obtained, P_{app} can be calculated as

$$P_{app} = \frac{C_0}{C_{dissolv}} P_{ep} \tag{4.82}$$

---

[25] *In Vivo* P_{eff} can be obtained in the same way, but surface area (fold and villi) and bile-micelle-unbound fraction should be taken into account.

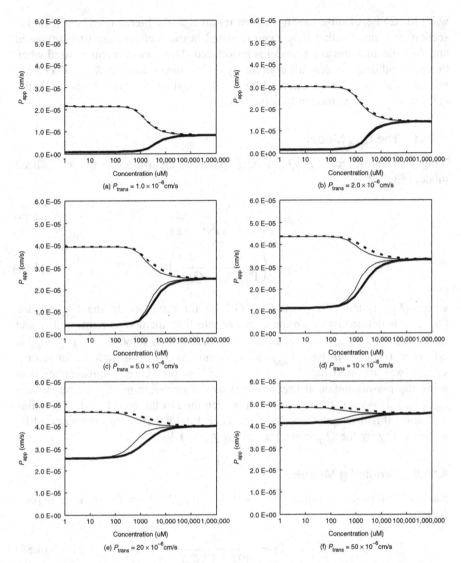

Figure 4.27 The effect of the UWL on the total permeability of an efflux transport substrate. Keys are shown in (a). $K_m = 50$ μM and $P_{UWL} = 50 \times 10^{-6}$ cm/s. Passive permeation (P_{trans}) was changed from 1 to 50×10^{-6} cm/s. p_{efflux} was calculated using Equation 4.62.

Figure 4.27 shows the effect of P_{UWL} on P_{app}.

4.10 GUT WALL METABOLISM

The gut wall metabolism could be significant especially for CYP3A4 and UGT substrates. Various methods to predict Fg (fraction not metabolized in the gut wall) for CYP3A4 substrates have been reported in the literature [82–85]. In this section, two models that have been reported in the literature are first discussed and then the anatomical Fg model is introduced. These models can be used when the unbound drug concentration in the cytosol is lower than the K_m of CYP3A4. For more advanced simulation, differential equations for an explicit epithelial cell model can be numerically solved [65].

4.10.1   The Q_{gut} Model

Yang et al. introduced the "Q_{gut} model" based on an analogy to the well-stirred model [83, 83].

$$Fg = \frac{Q_{gut}}{Q_{gut} + f_{u1}CL_{met,int}} \tag{4.83}$$

$$Q_{gut} = \left(\frac{1}{PS_{perm}} + \frac{1}{Q_{villi}} \right)^{-1} \tag{4.84}$$

where Q_{villi} is the villi blood flow (18 l/h for humans). In the Q_{gut} model, PS_{perm} was defined based on the effective intestinal membrane permeability and calculated as, PS_{perm} = intestinal smooth surface area (0.66 m^2) × P_{eff}. P_{eff} is estimated from the *in vitro* P_{app} (MDCK and Caco-2) by simple linear regression. It was reported that $f_{u1} = 1$ gave the best prediction results, rather than using the plasma unbound fraction (f_{up}) as the surrogate for f_{u1} (i.e., assuming $f_{u1} = f_{up}$). However, the reason was not identified in the report [83]. A possible reason for this discrepancy is discussed later. Figure 4.29 shows the reported Fg predictability by the Q_{gut} model assuming $f_{u1} = 1$ [83].

4.10.2   Simple Fg Models

Kato [82] proposed a simple equation to estimate Fg from the intrinsic hepatic clearance.

$$Fg = \frac{402}{402 + CL_{h,int}} \tag{4.85}$$

This equation would be valid for CYP3A substrates with high membrane permeability.

4.10.3   Theoretical Consideration on Fg

In this section, to understand the background of the Q_{gut} model and other models, a theoretical equation is derived from the anatomy of the epithelial cells and intestinal villi. As the derivation of the Q_{gut} model from the anatomical perspective was not disclosed in the original paper, we attempt to reproduce a derivation process possibly studied by the original investigator.

4.10.3.1 Derivation of the Fg Models. As shown in Figure 4.28, Fg is basically determined as the ratio of the metabolism rate ($k_{met} \times C_1 \times V_1$; V_1, fluid volume in the cell) and the escaping rate via the basolateral membrane ($k_{esc} \times C_1 \times V_1$). As the escaping rate becomes faster, the Fg becomes larger and approaches 1. This is the main concept applied in all the Fg models. Fg is interpreted as the ratio of the escaping rate in the total rate.

$$\text{Fg} = \frac{k_{esc}C_1V_1}{k_{met}C_1V_1 + k_{esc}C_1V_1} = \frac{C_1f_{u1}CL_{esc,int}}{C_1f_{u1}CL_{met,int} + C_1f_{u1}CL_{esc,int}}$$

$$= \frac{CL_{esc,int}}{CL_{met,int} + CL_{esc,int}} \tag{4.86}$$

Both metabolism and basolateral membrane permeation are driven by the unbound drug concentration. Therefore, in this equation, f_{u1} is canceled out in the numerator and dominator. The escaping process from the cytosol is the sequential process of the basolateral membrane permeation, diffusion from the basolateral membrane to the capillary vessels, and conveyance by the blood flow. One of these three steps can be the rate-limiting step.

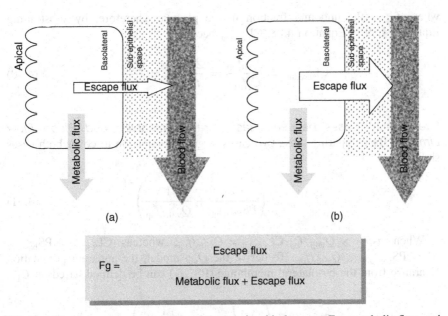

Figure 4.28 Schematic presentation of the relationship between Fg, metabolic flux, and escape flux of a drug. (a) Low Fg and (b) high Fg.

Basolateral Membrane Permeation Limited. When the permeation clearance of the basolateral membrane is much slower than the following processes,

$$\text{Fg} = \frac{\text{PS}_{\text{baso,int}}}{\text{CL}_{\text{met,int}} + \text{PS}_{\text{baso,int}}} \tag{4.87}$$

where $\text{PS}_{\text{baso,int}}$ is the basolateral permeation clearance of unbound drug molecules. For passive diffusion, $\text{PS}_{\text{baso,int}}$ can be calculated as $\text{PS}_{\text{baso,int}} = a_2 p_{\text{PD12}}$. In this case, correction for f_{u1} is not required (i.e., $f_{\text{u1}} = 1$), which in good agreement with the findings by Yang et al. [83].

Blood Flow Limited. When the basolateral membrane permeation and subepithelial diffusion are infinitely fast, the escaping rate is limited by the blood flow. The escaping rate becomes equal to the blood flow elimination rate of a drug. Therefore,

$$C_1 f_{\text{u1}} \text{CL}_{\text{esc,int}} = Q_{\text{villi}} C_{\text{p}} \tag{4.88}$$

The LHS of the equation is the escaping rate, and the RHS is the blood flow elimination rate. At this limiting condition, the unbound concentration in the cytosol and plasma becomes the same because equilibrium is rapidly established between the cytosol and plasma.

$$f_{\text{u1}} C_1 = f_{\text{up}} C_{\text{p}} \tag{4.89}$$

where f_{up} is the unbound fraction in the plasma. Therefore, by substituting Equation 4.89 in Equation 4.88, $\text{CL}_{\text{esc,int}}$ becomes

$$\text{CL}_{\text{esc,int}} = \frac{Q_{\text{villi}} C_{\text{p}}}{C_1 f_{\text{u1}}} = \frac{Q_{\text{villi}} C_{\text{p}}}{f_{\text{up}} C_{\text{p}}} = \frac{Q_{\text{villi}}}{f_{\text{up}}} \tag{4.90}$$

Intermediate Cases between Basolateral Permeability and Blood Flow Limited. By comparing these two cases, a general equation to cover both cases should be

$$\text{CL}_{\text{esc,int}} = \left(\frac{1}{\text{PS}_{\text{baso,int}}} + \frac{1}{Q_{\text{villi}}/f_{\text{up}}} \right)^{-1} \tag{4.91}$$

When $a_2 p_{12} \gg Q_{\text{villi}}/f_{\text{up}}$, $\text{CL}_{\text{esc,int}} = Q_{\text{villi}}/f_{\text{up}}$, whereas $\text{CL}_{\text{esc,int}} = \text{PS}_{\text{baso,int}}$ when $\text{PS}_{\text{baso,int}} \ll Q_{\text{villi}}/f_{\text{up}}$. To derive the Q_{gut} model, the apparent permeation clearance from the basolateral membrane (PS_{perm}) can be defined based on C_1.

$$\text{CL}_{\text{esc,int}} = \left(\frac{1}{\text{PS}_{\text{perm}}/f_{\text{u1}}} + \frac{1}{Q_{\text{villi}}/f_{\text{up}}} \right)^{-1} \tag{4.92}$$

If we assume, $f_{u1} = f_{up}$ and rearrange Equation 4.92 and substitute it in Equation 4.86, we can obtain an equation identical to the Q_{gut} model.

$$f_{u1}CL_{esc,int} = \left(\frac{1}{PS_{perm}} + \frac{1}{Q_{villi}} \right)^{-1} \equiv Q_{gut} \tag{4.93}$$

$$Fg = \frac{CL_{esc,int}}{CL_{met,int} + CL_{esc,int}} = \frac{Q_{gut/f_{u1}}}{CL_{met,int} + Q_{gut}/f_{u1}} = \frac{Q_{gut}}{f_{u1}CL_{met,int} + Q_{gut}} \tag{4.94}$$

However, the definition of PS_{perm} is ambiguous in the Q_{gut} model. Yang et al. [83] reported that $f_{u1} = 1$ gave the best prediction, whereas the assumption $f_{u1} = f_{up}$ gave poor prediction. This is in good agreement with the basolateral permeation limited cases but disagrees with the blood flow limited cases.

4.10.3.2 Derivation of the Anatomical Fg Model.
In the Q_{gut} model, the diffusion in the subepithelial space is neglected. If the subepithelial space diffusion is the rate-limiting step, based on the similar discussion with the blood flow limited case,

$$C_1 f_{u1}CL_{esc,int} = CL_{subepithelial}C_{subepithelial} \tag{4.95}$$

$$f_{u1}C_1 = f_{subepithelial}C_{subepithelial} \tag{4.96}$$

$$CL_{esc,int} = \frac{CL_{subepithelial}C_{subepithelial}}{C_1 f_{u1}} = \frac{CL_{subepithelial}}{f_{up}} \tag{4.97}$$

where $CL_{subepithelial}$ is the permeation clearance of the subepithelial space and $C_{subepithelial}$ is the concentration and unbound fraction of a drug in the subepithelial space. In this case, the fluid in the subepithelial space was assumed to be the same as the plasma ($f_{subepithelial} = f_{up}$). The diffusion clearance in the subepithelial space is

$$CL_{subepithelial} = A_{blood\ vessel} \frac{D_{mono}f_{up} + D_{albumin}(1 - f_{up})}{h_{subepithelial}} \tag{4.98}$$

where $h_{subepithelial}$ is the thickness of the subepithelial space. This clearance is based on the total concentration in the subepithelial space and the surface area of the blood vessel in the villi ($A_{blood\ vessel}$). $CL_{subepithelial}$ becomes relatively constant when $f_{up} < 0.05$ and is mainly determined by the diffusion coefficient of albumin-bound drug molecules ($D_{albumin} = 6.6 \times 10^{-7}$ cm^2/s).

When we combine the three limited cases into one general equation, it becomes

$$CL_{esc,int} = \left(\frac{1}{PS_{baso,int}} + \frac{1}{CL_{subepithelial}/f_{up}} + \frac{1}{Q_{villi}/f_{up}} \right)^{-1} \tag{4.99}$$

This is called the *anatomical Fg model* in this book. The next step is to assess which process tends to become the rate-limiting step, the subepithelial diffusion or the blood flow. Considering the villi structure (Fig. 6.2), the $h_{subepithelial}$ would be approximately 50 μm and $A_{blood\ vessel}$ is approximately 100 cm^2 in humans. In this case, $CL_{subepithelial}$ is likely to be smaller than Q_{villi}. $CL_{subepithelial}$ value becomes relatively constant, ca. 2–4 ml/min/kg at $f_{u1} < 0.05$ ($h_{subepithelial} = 50$ μm and $A_{blood\ vessel} = 88.4$ cm^2 (12.6 cm^2/ kg)). This $CL_{subepithelial}$ value becomes coincidentally close to Q_{villi}, but it is significantly smaller than Q_{villi}/f_{u1}. This could be a possible reason why $f_{u1} = 1$ operationally resulted in a better prediction in the Q_{gut} model (as PS_{baso} limited drugs are minor in the validation data set).

Another discrepancy in the Q_{gut} model is that it suggests the existence of positive food effects via Fg increase. The Q_{gut} model suggests that the Fg would be affected by the change of Q_{villi}. Food intake increases the enteric blood flow by 100% (Fig. 6.23). Therefore, if the Q_{gut} model is correct, a positive food effect is anticipated for lipophilic drugs with high Fg. However, this contradicts the experimental observations (Section 12.2.2.2). These two contradictions in the Q_{gut} model can be solved by the anatomical Fg model. As $CL_{subepithelial}$ is close to Q_{villi} for $f_{up} \ll 0.05$, the Q_{gut} model (with $f_{u1} = 1$) and the anatomical model give similar Fg value. In addition, because CYP3A4 substrate tends to have low f_{up} and high permeability, the anatomical Fg model can be simplified to the Kato Fg model, which uses a constant $CL_{esc,int}$ value (5.7 ml/min/kg for humans).

The key difference between the Q_{gut} model and the anatomical Fg model is the method to calculate $CL_{esc,int}$. To directly compare the Q_{gut} and anatomical models with the experimental $CL_{esc,int}$, the Fg was converted to $CL_{esc,int}$ as

$$CL_{esc,int} = \frac{Fg \cdot CL_{met,int}}{1 - Fg} \qquad (4.100)$$

$CL_{met,int}$ was obtained from the *in vitro* human intestinal microsome assay. Because this data is collected from various literature, it was normalized to that of midazolam (6.2 ml/min/kg) (Table 4.1). Figure 4.29 shows the comparison between the Q_{gut} and anatomical models for $CL_{esc,int}$ prediction. Even though $f_{up} = f_{u1}$ was suggested to be theoretically more appropriate, if $f_{up} = f_{u1}$ is used, the Q_{gut} model largely overestimated $CL_{esc,int}$, whereas the operational assumption $f_{u1} = 1$ gave better prediction. This is in good agreement with the previous findings by Yang et al. By the Q_{gut} ($f_{u1} = 1$) model, $CL_{esc,int}$ of many lipophilic drugs becomes a constant value ($= Q_{villi}$) value so that it becomes close to Kato's simple model. The anatomical Fg model can capture the f_{up} dependency of $CL_{esc,int}$ (Fig. 4.29c).

4.10.4 Interplay between CYP3A4 and P-gp

Recently, an interplay between CYP3A4 and P-gp has been proposed [87, 88]. This point is interesting because these enzymes have overlapping

TABLE 4.1 Clinical Fg, $CL_{int,met}$, and Predicted $CL_{esc,int}$

Drug	MW	log P_{oct}	pK_a	Acid/Base	f_{up}	$CL_{int,met}$ (In Vitro)	Fg (obs.)	$CL_{esc,int}$ (obs.)	Predicted (ml/min/kg) Q_{gut} ($f_{u1}=f_{up}$)	Q_{gut} ($f_{u1}=f_{up}$)	$CL_{esc,int}$ Anatomical Model	Predicted Fg Q_{gut} ($f_{u1}=f_{up}$)	Q_{gut} ($f_{u1}=f_{up}$)	Anatomical Model	References Fg	$CL_{int,met}$
Alfentanil	417	2.4	6.3	B	0.093	0.87	0.61	1.33	2.7	29	1.7	0.76	0.97	0.66	97	86
Alprazolam	308	4.9	2.6	B	0.300	0.00	0.92	—	4.2	14	1.4	1.00	1.00	1.00	97	85
Amlodipine	408	3.7	8.9	B	0.005	0.50	0.88	3.71	2.3	452	4.0	0.82	1.00	0.89	85	85
Atorvastatin	558	4.4	4.2	A	0.005	0.25	0.40	0.17	0.0	8	0.0	0.14	0.97	0.14	97	86
Buspirone	386	2.5	7.6	B	0.050	2.96 (1.98–3.95)	0.16	0.56	2.5	50	2.1	0.46	0.94	0.42	97	86, 98
Carbamazepine	236	0.8	—	—	0.250	<0.55	1.00	—	3.8	15	1.6	0.88	0.97	0.75	98	98
Cisapride	465	3.3	7.8	B	0.020	2.59 (2.50–2.67)	0.55	3.16	2.6	130	3.3	0.50	0.98	0.56	97	86, 98
Clonazepam	315	2.5	—	—	0.150	0.00	0.93	—	3.9	26	1.8	1.00	1.00	1.00	85	85
Cyclosporine	1203	3.5	—	—	0.068	1.14 (0.36–1.91)	0.55	1.36	0.0	0	0.0	0.01	0.24	0.01	97	86, 98
Diazepam	285	2.9	3.4	B	0.023	<0.55	1.00	—	4.1	179	5.8	0.88	1.00	0.91	98	98
Diltiazem	415	3.2	8.0	B	0.180	0.73	0.91	7.38	2.8	15	1.3	0.79	0.95	0.64	98	98
Felodipine	383	4.5	—	—	0.004	23.90 (21.34–26.47)	0.49	22.97	4.2	1162	30.6	0.15	0.98	0.56	97	86, 98
Lovastatin	404	4.5	—	—	0.050	54.81 (44.49–65.13)	0.07	4.13	4.2	84	3.2	0.07	0.60	0.05	97	86, 98
Methadone	309	4.2	9.0	B	0.210	0.07	0.82	0.29	3.8	18	1.6	0.98	1.00	0.96	97	86
Midazolam	325	3.2	5.9	B	0.035	6.20	0.54	7.13	4.1	117	4.2	0.40	0.95	0.40	97	85, 86, 98
Nicardipine	479	4.3	7.1	B	0.005	53.31 (44.76–61.85)	0.64	94.77	4.1	810	19.1	0.07	0.94	0.26	98	85
Nifedipine	346	4.5	—	—	0.050	2.44 (1.73–3.60)	0.70	5.70	4.2	84	3.3	0.63	0.97	0.57	97	85, 86, 98
Nimodipine	418	2.7	—	—	0.016	15.77	0.64	28.04	3.3	204	5.1	0.17	0.93	0.24	98	98

(*Continued*)

TABLE 4.1 *(Continued)*

Drug	MW	log P_{oct}	pK_a	Acid/Base	f_{up}	$CL_{int,met}$ (In Vitro)	Fg (obs.)	$CL_{esc,int}$ (obs.)	Predicted (ml/min/kg) Q_{gut} ($f_{ul} = f_{up}$)	Q_{gut} ($f_{ul} = f_{up}$)	$CL_{esc,int}$ Anatomical Model	Predicted Fg Q_{gut} ($f_{ul} = f_{up}$)	Q_{gut} ($f_{ul} = f_{up}$)	Anatomical Model	References Fg	$CL_{int,met}$
Nisoldipine	388	3.1	—	—	0.003	69.93	0.28	26.53	3.9	1296	21.9	0.05	0.95	0.24	97	86
Nitrendipine	360	4.5	—	B	0.020	6.72	0.44	5.28	4.2	209	6.5	0.38	0.97	0.49	98	98
Quinidine	324	2.9	8.6	B	0.260	<0.27 (0.00–0.55)	0.91	—	2.5	10	1.2	0.90	0.97	0.81	97	85, 98
Repaglinide	452	5.9	3.9	A	0.015	0.43	0.89	3.48	1.3	89	1.6	0.76	1.00	0.79	97	86
Rifabutin	846	3.2	6.5	B	0.070	0.47	0.21	0.13	0.1	2	0.1	0.23	0.81	0.22	97	86
Sildenafil	474	4.5	9.2	B	0.040	1.02	0.68	2.17	2.1	52	1.9	0.67	0.98	0.65	97	86
Simvastatin	418	4.7	—	—	0.020	59.98 (56.50–63.46)	0.14	9.76	4.2	209	6.4	0.07	0.78	0.10	97	85, 86, 98
Tacrolimus	803	3.3	—	—	0.010	15.60 (12.04–19.16)	0.14	2.54	0.3	21	0.3	0.02	0.58	0.02	97	85, 86
Terfenadine	472	5.6	9.9	B	0.003	30.09	0.40	20.06	2.8	945	7.1	0.09	0.97	0.19	97	86
Trazodone	372	3.5	7.5	B	0.070	0.22	0.83	1.05	4.0	57	2.5	0.95	1.00	0.92	97	86
Triazolam	342	5.5	—	—	0.150	<0.55	0.70	—	4.2	28	1.8	0.88	0.98	0.77	97	98
Verapamil	455	4.2	9.1	B	0.093	4.01 (2.15–6.23)	0.65	7.45	2.0	22	1.4	0.33	0.84	0.25	97	85, 86, 98
Zolpidem	307	2.5	6.4	B	0.050	0.02	0.79	0.08	3.9	78	3.1	0.99	1.00	0.99	97	86

Indinavir and saquinavir were excluded from the analysis, as they have low K_m for CP3A4 (<1 µM) and saturation of CYP3A4 was suggested [65].

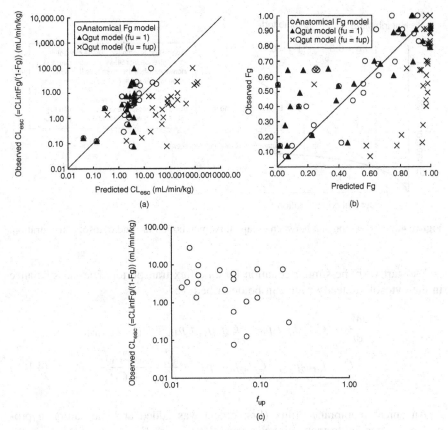

Figure 4.29 Comparison of (a) $CL_{esc,int}$ and (b) Fg predictability of the Q_{gut} and anatomical models. The relationship between $CL_{esc,int}$ and f_{up} is shown in (c). $Q_{villi} = 4.2$ ml/min/kg, $h_{subepithelial} = 0.0005$ cm, $A_{villi} = 126$ cm^2/ kg, $A_{vein} = 1.43$ cm^2/ kg, $D_{albumin} = 0.66 \times 10^{-6}$ cm^2/s, and $PS_{baso,int} = f_{n1} \times P_{trans,0} \times (a_0 a_2/(a_0 + a_2))/A_{well} \times a_2 \times A_{villi}$. $P_{trans,0}$ was calculated from experimental log P_{oct} and MW using Equation 4.35.

substrates. However, the definition of "interplay" has not been explicitly defined and there are controversies in the interpretation of experimental data. Recently, Fan and coworkers [89] performed a fully numerical simulation using a three-compartment model to solve the controversy. Here, we discuss this point using the steady-state solutions. The results from the full numerical simulation and the steady-state analytical solution are essentially the same, but the latter would be easier for interpretation and suitable for a book like this.

As discussed above, Fg is determined as the ratio of metabolic clearance and escaping clearance (Fig. 4.28). Therefore, if both processes are concentration-linear, P-gp in the apical membrane does not affect Fg and there is no interplay between P-gp and CYP3A4 on Fg. However, it is not the case when the metabolic clearance is saturable.

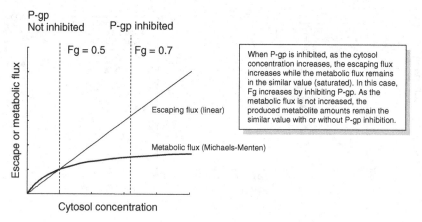

Figure 4.30 Relationship between escape flux, metabolic flux, and cytosol concentration.

We start with the similar equation for an efflux transporter. The mass balance in the cytosol at steady state can be described as:

$$\frac{dM_1}{dt} = C_0 f_{n0} f_{u0} a_0 p_{01} - C_1 f_{n1} f_{u1} a_0 p_{10} - C_1 f_{u1} a_0 p_{efflux}$$

$$- C_1 f_{n1} f_{u1} a_2 p_{12} + C_2 f_{n2} f_{u2} a_2 p_{21} - \frac{V_{max,met} C_1 f_{u1}}{K_{m,met} + C_1 f_{u1}} \quad (4.101)$$

An apical membrane efflux (first order) was added and the saturable process was amended to metabolic clearance ($CL_{met,int} = V_{max,met}/(C_1 f_{u1} + K_{m,met})$). This equation can be solved for $C_1 f_{n1}$ as a quadratic equation and substituted in Equation 4.69.

$$P_{app,ep,A-B} = \frac{1}{C_0 A_{well}}[a_0 p_{01} f_{n0} C_0 - (C_1 f_{u1})(a_0 p_{10} f_{n1} - a_0 p_{efflux} f_{n1})] \quad (4.102)$$

Figure 4.30 shows the cytosol concentration dependency of escape and metabolic flux. When an apical efflux transporter is inhibited, the cytosol concentration increases and the escape flux[26] increases proportionally (as it follows the first-order kinetics). When $f_{u1} C_0 \ll K_{m,met}$, the metabolic flux also increases proportionally (hence, Fg remains constant). However, for a nonlinear case ($f_{u1} C_0 \approx K_{m,met}$ or above), metabolic flux increases subproportionally. Therefore, Fg is increased.

The effect of an efflux transporter on Fg might be observed even when a reduction of Fa by the efflux transporter was not significant. In Figure 4.31, $P_{ep} > 10 \times 10^{-6}$ cm/s and Fa% is > 99% across the concentration range.

---

[26]Should not be confused with clearance.

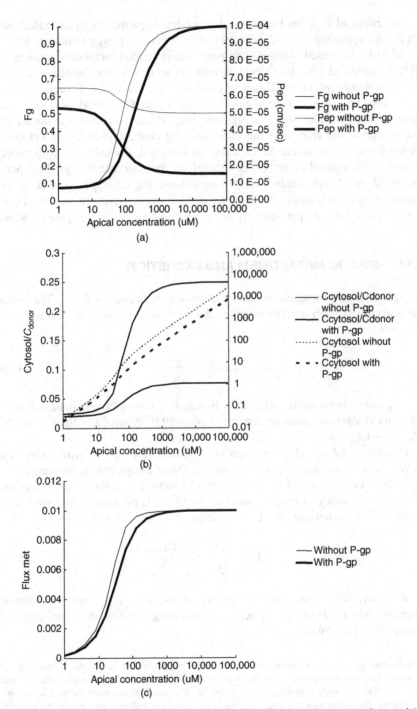

Figure 4.31   Concentration dependency of (a) Fg, P_{ep}; (b) cytosol concentration; and (c) metabolic flux. $P_{trans} = 5 \times 10^{-5}$ cm/s, $p_{efflux} = p_{PD} \times 10$, and $K_{m,met} = 1$ μM.

The effect of P-gp on the metabolic rate has been mainly investigated using CYP3A4-expressing Caco-2 cells [90–92]. When P-gp was inhibited, Fg was found to be increased. At the same time, the generated metabolite amount was slightly increased (due to a slight increase in metabolic flux by the increase in the cytosol concentration). This is in good agreement with the theoretical results.

Interestingly, it was theoretically suggested that P_{ep} would also show concentration dependency, even though the P-gp efflux was assumed linear. This occurs due to the change in the unbound drug concentration in the cytosol by metabolism. As the metabolic clearance is saturated, the unbound drug concentration in the cytosol increases, and therefore, the concentration gradient across the apical membrane is reduced, resulting in lower P_{ep} (cf. P_{ep} is the macroscopic permeability corresponding to the concentration reduction rate in the apical side[27] but not to the intrinsic permeability of each membrane (p_{01} and p_{10} are constant)).

4.11 HEPATIC METABOLISM AND EXCRETION

Hepatic first-pass metabolism often has significant impact on BA%. The following equation is often used to calculate the fraction of a drug that passes through the liver.

$$Fh = 1 - \frac{CL_h}{Q_h} \qquad (4.103)$$

CL_h can be obtained from i.v. data. Figure 4.32 shows the relationship between CL_h and BA% in humans for marketed drugs [93]. When $Fa = Fg = 1, BA\% = Fh = 1 - CL_h/Q_h$.

Hepatic metabolic clearance can be predicted from the *in vitro* assays such as S9, microsome, and hepatocyte assays. These assays can be performed with or without coexistence of plasma protein. In many cases, the intrinsic clearance (clearance of unbound drug) is used for *in vivo* CL prediction. The well-stirred model is most often used for CL prediction from *in vitro* data.

$$CL_h = \frac{Q_h \cdot f_{up} \cdot CL_{int}}{Q_h + f_{up} \cdot CL_{int}} \qquad (4.104)$$

Recently, there have been extensive investigations for more mechanistic approaches to predict CL_h, explicitly incorporating the canalicular and sinusoidal transporters [94–96].

---

[27]In *in vitro* assays, P_{app} is usually calculated from the appearance rate in the acceptor chamber assuming that appearance rate equals the concentration reduction rate in the apical side. But this is not valid when the metabolic degradation occurs in the cytosol. If extensive metabolism occurs in the cytosol, the appearance rate could be small even when the disappearance rate in the apical side is fast. Fa corresponds to the appearance rate in the cytosol (before metabolism) and is equal to the disappearance rate.

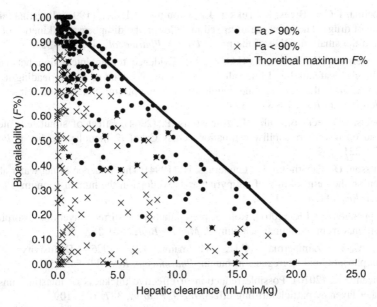

Figure 4.32   Bioavailability and CL_h in humans. *Source:* Replotted from Reference 93.

REFERENCES

1. Amidon, G.E., Higuchi, W.I., Ho, N.F.H. (1982). Theoretical and experimental studies of transport of micelle-solubilized solutes. *J. Pharmaceut. Sci.*, 71, 77–84.

2. Sugano, K. (2009). Estimation of effective intestinal membrane permeability considering bile-micelle solubilisation. *Int. J. Pharm.*, 368, 116–122.

3. Oliver, R.E., Jones, A.F., Rowland, M. (1998). What surface of the intestinal epithelium is effectively available to permeating drugs? *J. Pharmaceut. Sci.*, 87, 634–639.

4. Lennernaes, H. (2007). Intestinal permeability and its relevance for absorption and elimination. *Xenobiotica*, 37, 1015–1051.

5. Yamaguchi, T., Ikeda, C., Sekine, Y. (1986). Intestinal absorption of a b-adrenergic blocking agent nadolol. I. Comparison of absorption behavior of nadolol with those of other b-blocking agents in rats. *Chem. Pharmaceut. Bull.*, 34, 3362–3369.

6. Yamaguchi, T., Ikeda, C., Sekine, Y. (1986). Intestinal absorption of a b-adrenergic blocking agent nadolol. II. Mechanism of the inhibitory effect on the intestinal absorption of nadolol by sodium cholate in rats. *Chem. Pharmaceut. Bull.*, 34, 3836–3843.

7. Yamaguchi, T., Oida, T., Ikeda, C., Sekine, Y. (1986). Intestinal absorption of a b-adrenergic blocking agent nadolol. III. Nuclear magnetic resonance spectroscopic study on nadolol-sodium cholate micellar complex and intestinal absorption of nadolol derivatives in rats. *Chem. Pharmaceut. Bull.*, 34, 4259–4264.

8. Poelma, F.G.J., Breaes, R., Tukker, J.J. (1990). Intestinal absorption of drugs. III. The influence of taurocholate on the disappearance kinetics of hydrophilic and lipophilic drugs from the small intestine of the rat. *Pharmaceut. Res.*, 7, 392–397.

9. Poelma, F.G.J., Breas, R., Tukker, J.J., Crommelin, D.J.A. (1991). Intestinal absorption of drugs. The influence of mixed micelles on the disappearance kinetics of drugs from the small intestine of the rat. *J. Pharm. Pharmacol.*, 43, 317–324.

10. Lennernaes, H., Regaardh, C.G. (1993). Evidence for an interaction between the b-blocker pafenolol and bile salts in the intestinal lumen of the rat leading to dose-dependent oral absorption and double peaks in the plasma concentration-time profile. *Pharmaceut. Res.*, 10, 879–883.

11. Ingels, F., Beck, B., Oth, M., Augustijns, P. (2004). Effect of simulated intestinal fluid on drug permeability estimation across Caco{-}2 monolayers. *Int. J. Pharm.*, 274, 221–232.

12. Nilsson, D., Fagerholm, U., Lennernas, H. (1994). The influence of net water absorption on the permeability of antipyrine and levodopa in the human jejunum. *Pharmaceut. Res.*, 11, 1540–1544.

13. Pappenheimer, J.R. (2001). Role of pre-epithelial "unstirred" layers in absorption of nutrients from the human jejunum. *J. Membr. Biol.*, 179, 185–204.

14. Li, C.-Y., Zimmerman, C.L., Wiedmann, T.S. (1996). Diffusivity of bile salt/phospholipid aggregates in mucin. *Pharmaceut. Res.*, 13, 535–541.

15. Sugano, K. (2010). Possible reduction of effective thickness of intestinal unstirred water layer by particle drifting effect. *Int. J. Pharm.*, 387, 103–109.

16. Doyle-McCullough, M., Smyth, S.H., Moyes, S.M., Carr, K.E. (2007). Factors influencing intestinal microparticle uptake *in vivo*. *Int. J. Pharm.*, 335, 79–89.

17. Hodges, G.M., Carr, E.A., Hazzard, R.A., Carr, K.E. (1995). Uptake and translocation of microparticles in small intestine. Morphology and quantification of particle distribution. *Dig. Dis. Sci.*, 40, 967–975.

18. Limpanussorn, J., Simon, L., Dayan, A.D. (1998). Transepithelial transport of large particles in rat: a new model for the quantitative study of particle uptake. *J. Pharm. Pharmacol.*, 50, 753–760.

19. Norris, D.A., Puri, N., Sinko, P.J. (1998). The effect of physical barriers and properties on the oral absorption of particulates. *Adv. Drug Delivery Rev.*, 34, 135–154.

20. Smyth, S.H., Feldhaus, S., Schumacher, U., Carr, K.E. (2008). Uptake of inert microparticles in normal and immune deficient mice. *Int. J. Pharm.*, 346, 109–118.

21. Allen, A., Flemstroem, G. (2005). Gastroduodenal mucus bicarbonate barrier: Protection against acid and pepsin. *Am. J. Physiol.*, 288, C1–C19.

22. Atuma, C., Strugala, V., Allen, A., Holm, L. (2001). The adherent gastrointestinal mucus gel layer: thickness and physical state *in vivo*. *Am. J. Physiol.*, 280, G922–G929.

23. Sugano, K. (2011). Fraction of a dose absorbed estimation for structurally diverse low solubility compounds. *Int. J. Pharm.*, 405, 79–89.

24. Sugano, K., Nabuchi, Y., Machida, M., Asoh, Y. (2004). Permeation characteristics of a hydrophilic basic compound across a bio-mimetic artificial membrane. *Int. J. Pharm.*, 275, 271–278.

25. Fischer, H., Kansy, M., Avdeef, A., Senner, F. (2007). Permeation of permanently positive charged molecules through artificial membranes influence of physico-chemical properties. *Eur. J. Pharmaceut. Sci.*, 31, 32–42.

26. Walter, A., Gutknecht, J. (1984). Monocarboxylic acid permeation through lipid bilayer membranes. *J. Membr. Biol.*, 77, 255–264.

27. Diamond, J.M., Katz, Y. (1974). Interpretation of nonelectrolyte partition coefficients between dimyristoyl lecithin and water. *J. Membr. Biol.*, 17, 121–154.

28. Xiang, T., Xu, Y., Anderson, B.D. (1998). The barrier domain for solute permeation varies with lipid bilayer phase structure. *J. Membr. Biol.*, 165, 77–90.

29. Mayer, P.T., Xiang, T.X., Anderson, B.D. (2000). Independence of substituent contributions to the transport of small molecule permeants in lipid bilayers. *AAPS PharmSci [Electronic Resource]*, 2, E14.

30. Mayer, P.T., Anderson, B.D. (2002). Transport across 1,9-decadiene precisely mimics the chemical selectivity of the barrier domain in egg lecithin bilayers. *J. Pharmaceut. Sci.*, 91, 640.

31. Walter, A., Gutknecht, J. (1986). Permeability of small nonelectrolytes through lipid bilayer membranes. *J. Membr. Biol.*, 90, 207–217.

32. Burton, P. S., Conradi, R.A., Hilgers, A.R. (1991). Mechanisms of peptide and protein absorption. (2). Transcellular mechanism of peptide and protein absorption: passive aspects. *Adv. Drug Deliv. Rev.*, 7, 365–386.

33. Eytan, G.D., Kuchel, P.W. (1999). Mechanism of action of P-glycoprotein in relation to passive membrane permeation. *Int. Rev. Cytol.*, 190, 175–250.

34. Regev, R., Eytan, G.D. (1997). Flip-flop of doxorubicin across erythrocyte and lipid membranes. *Biochem. Pharmacol.*, 54, 1151–1158.

35. Kamp, F., Zakim, D., Zhang, F., Noy, N., Hamilton, J.A. (1995). Fatty acid flip-flop in phospholipid bilayers is extremely fast. *Biochemistry*, 34, 11928–11937.

36. Kleinfeld, A.M., Chu, P., Storch, J. (1997). Flip-flop is slow and rate limiting for the movement of long chain anthroyloxy fatty acids across lipid vesicles. *Biochemistry*, 36, 5702–5711.

37. Avdeef, A., Artursson, P., Neuhoff, S., Lazorova, L., Grasjo, J., Tavelin, S. (2005). Caco{-}2 permeability of weakly basic drugs predicted with the double-sink PAMPA pKa(flux) method. *Eur. J. Pharmaceut. Sci.*, 24, 333–349.

38. Yamashita, S., Furubayashi, T., Kataoka, M., Sakane, T., Sezaki, H., Tokuda, H. (2000). Optimized conditions for prediction of intestinal drug permeability using Caco{-}2 cells. *Eur. J. Pharmaceut. Sci.*, 10, 195–204.

39. Lee, K.J., Johnson, N., Castelo, J., Sinko, P.J., Grass, G., Holme, K., Lee, Y.H. (2005). Effect of experimental pH on the *in vitro* permeability in intact rabbit intestines and Caco{-}2 monolayer. *Eur. J. Pharmaceut. Sci.*, 25, 193–200.

40. Avdeef, A. (2011). How well can *in vitro* brain microcapillary endothelial cell models predict rodent *in vivo* blood-brain barrier permeability? *Eur. J. Pharmaceut. Sci.*, 43, 109–124.

41. Dagenais, C., Avdeef, A., Tsinman, O., Dudley, A., Beliveau, R. (2009). P-glycoprotein deficient mouse *in situ* blood-brain barrier permeability and its prediction using an in combo PAMPA model. *Eur. J. Pharmaceut. Sci.*, 38, 121–137.

42. Camenisch, G., Alsenz, J., van de Waterbeemd, H., Folkers, G. (1998). Estimation of permeability by passive diffusion through Caco{-}2 cell monolayers using the drugs' lipophilicity and molecular weight. *Eur. J. Pharmaceut. Sci.*, 6, 313–319.

43. Adson, A., Burton, P.S., Ruab, T.J., Barsuhn, C.L., Audus, L., Ho, N.F.H. (1995). Passive diffusion of weak organic electrolytes across Caco{-}2 cell monolayers: Uncoupling the contributions of hydrodynamic, transcellular and paracellular barriers. *Pharmaceut. Res.*, 84, 1197–1203.

44. Adson, A., Ruab, T.J., Burton, P.S., Barsuhn, C.L., Hilgers, A.R., Audus, K.L., Ho, N.F.H. (1994). Quantitative approaches to delineate paracellular diffusion in cultured epithelial cell monolayers. *J. Pharmaceut. Sci.*, 83, 1529–1530.

45. Sugano, K., Nabuchi, Y., Machida, M., Aso, Y. (2003). Prediction of human intestinal permeability using artificial membrane permeability. *Int. J. Pharm.*, 257, 245–251.

46. Sugano, K., Takata, N., Machida, M., Saitoh, K., Terada, K. (2002). Prediction of passive intestinal absorption using bio-mimetic artificial membrane permeation assay and the paracellular pathway model. *Int. J. Pharm.*, 241, 241–251.

47. Sugano, K., Obata, K., Saitoh, R., Higashida, A., Hamada, H., Processing of Bio-pharmaceutical Profiling Data in Drug Discovery, in: B. Testa, S. Krämer, H. Wunderli-Allenspach, G. Folkers (Eds.) Pharmacokinetic Profiling in Drug Research, Wiley-VCH, Zurich, 2006, pp. 441–458.

48. Obata, K., Sugano, K., Saitoh, R., Higashida, A., Nabuchi, Y., Machida, M., Aso, Y. (2005). Prediction of oral drug absorption in humans by theoretical passive absorption model. *Int. J. Pharm.*, 293, 183–192.

49. Avdeef, A. (2010). Leakiness and size exclusion of paracellular channels in cultured epithelial cell monolayers-interlaboratory comparison. *Pharmaceut. Res.*, 27, 480–489.

50. Reynolds, D.P., Lanevskij, K., Japertas, P., Didziapetris, R., Petrauskas, A. (2009). Ionization-specific analysis of human intestinal absorption. *J. Pharmaceut. Sci.*, 98, 4039–4054.

51. Karlsson, J., Ungell, A.l., Grasjo, J., Artursson, P. (1999). Paracellular drug transport across intestinal epithelia: influence of charge and induced water flux. *Eur. J. Pharmaceut. Sci.*, 9, 47–56.

52. Deen, W.M. (1987). Hindered transport of large molecules in liquid-filled pores. *AIChE Journal*, 33, 1409–1425.

53. Sugano, K., Yoshida, S., Takaku, M., Haramura, M., Saitoh, R., Nabuchi, Y., Ushio, H. (2000). Quantitative structure-intestinal permeability relationship of benzamidine analogue thrombin inhibitor. *Bioorg. Med. Chem. Lett.*, 10, 1939–1942.

54. Kristl, A., Tukker, J.J. (1998). Negative correlation of n-octanol/water partition coefficient and transport of some guanine derivatives through rat jejunum *in vitro*. *Pharmaceut. Res.*, 15, 499–501.

55. Avdeef, A., Tam, K.Y. (2010). How well can the caco{-}2/madin-darby canine kidney models predict effective human jejunal permeability? *J. Med. Chem.*, 53, 3566–3584.

56. He, Y., Murby, S., Warhurst, G., Gifford, L., Walker, D., Ayrton, J., Eastmond, R., Rowland, M. (1998). Species differences in size discrimination in the paracellular pathway refracted by oral bioavailability of poly(ethylene glycol) and D-peptides. *J. Pharmaceut. Sci.*, 87, 626–633.

57. Knipp, T.G., Ho, N.F.H., Barsuhn, C.L., Borchardt, R.T. (1997). Paracellular diffusion in Caco{-}2 cell monolayers: effect of perturbation on the transport of hydrophilic compounds that vary in size and charge. *J. Pharmaceut. Sci.*, 86, 1105–1110.

58. Garmire, L.X., Hunt, C.A. (2008). In silico methods for unraveling the mechanistic complexities of intestinal absorption: metabolism-efflux transport interactions. *Drug Metabol. Dispos.*, 36, 1414–1424.

59. Garmire, L.X., Garmire, D.G., Hunt, C.A. (2007). An in silico transwell device for the study of drug transport and drug-drug interactions. *Pharmaceut. Res.*, 24, 2171–2186.

60. Grant, M.R., Hunt, C.A. An in silico analogue of *in vitro* systems used to study epithelial cell morphogenesis, Computational Methods in Systems Biology, Springer, Berlin, Heidelberg, 2006, 285–297.

61. Liu, Y., Hunt, C.A. (2006). Mechanistic study of the cellular interplay of transport and metabolism using the synthetic modeling method. *Pharmaceut. Res.*, 23, 493–505.

62. Liu, Y., Hunt, C.A. (2005). Studies of intestinal drug transport using an in silico epithelio-mimetic device. *BioSystems*, 82, 154–167.

63. Heikkinen, A.T., Moenkkoenen, J., Korjamo, T. (2010). Determination of permeation resistance distribution in *in vitro* cell monolayer permeation experiments. *Eur. J. Pharmaceut. Sci.*, 40, 132–142.

64. Korjamo, T., Kemilainen, H., Heikkinen, A.T., Monkkonen, J. (2007). Decrease in intracellular concentration causes the shift in K_m value of efflux pump substrates. *Drug Metabol. Dispos.*, 35, 1574–1579.

65. Gertz, M., Houston, J.B., Galetin, A. (2011). Physiologically based pharmacokinetic modeling of intestinal first-pass metabolism of CYP3A substrates with high intestinal extraction. *Drug Metabol. Dispos.: the biological fate of chemicals*, 39, 1633–1642.

66. Sugano, K., Shirasaka, Y., Yamashita, S., Velicky, M., Bradley, D.F., Tam, K.Y., Dryfe, R.A. (2011). Estimation of Michaelis-Menten constant of efflux transporter considering asymmetric permeability Fraction of a dose absorbed estimation for structurally diverse low solubility compounds *In Situ* artificial membrane permeation assay under hydrodynamic control: permeability-pH profiles of warfarin and verapamil. *Int. J. Pharm.*, 8, 8.

67. Sugano, K., Kansy, M., Artursson, P., Avdeef, A., Bendels, S., Di, L., Ecker, G.F., Faller, B., Fischer, H., Gerebtzoff, G., Lennernaes, H., Senner, F. (2010). Coexistence of passive and carrier-mediated processes in drug transport. *Nat. Rev. Drug Discov.*, 9, 597–614.

68. Trotter, P.J., Storch, J. (1991). Fatty acid uptake and metabolism in a human intestinal cell line (Caco{-}2): comparison of apical and basolateral incubation. *J. Lipid Res.*, 32, 293–304.

69. Neuhoff, S., Ungell, A.L., Zamora, I., Artursson, P. (2005). pH-Dependent passive and active transport of acidic drugs across Caco{-}2 cell monolayers. *Eur. J. Pharmaceut. Sci.*, 25, 211–220.

70. Troutman, M.D., Thakker, D.R. (2003). Novel experimental parameters to quantify the modulation of absorptive and secretory transport of compounds by p-glycoprotein in cell culture models of intestinal epithelium. *Pharmaceut. Res.*, 20, 1210–1224.

71. Dahan, A., Amidon, G.L. (2009). Segmental dependent transport of low permeability compounds along the small intestine due to P-glycoprotein: the role of efflux transport in the oral absorption of BCS class III drugs. *Mol. Pharm.*, 6, 19–28.

72. Collett, A., Tanianis-Hughes, J., Hallifax, D., Warhurst, G. (2004). Predicting P-glycoprotein effects on oral absorption: Correlation of transport in Caco{-}2 with drug pharmacokinetics in wild-type and mdr1a(-/-) mice *in vivo*. *Pharmaceut. Res.*, 21, 819–826.

73. Varma, M. V., Sateesh, K., Panchagnula, R. (2005). Functional role of P-glycoprotein in limiting intestinal absorption of drugs: contribution of passive permeability to P-glycoprotein mediated efflux transport. *Mol. Pharm.*, 2, 12–21.

74. Aller, S. G., Yu, J., Ward, A., Weng, Y., Chittaboina, S., Zhuo, R., Harrell, P.M., Trinh, Y.T., Zhang, Q., Urbatsch, I.L., Chang, G. (2009). Structure of P-glycoprotein reveals a molecular basis for poly-specific drug binding. *Science (Washington, DC, U. S.)*, 323, 1718–1722.

75. Varma, M.V., Panchagnula, R. (2005). Prediction of *in vivo* intestinal absorption enhancement on P-glycoprotein inhibition, from rat *in situ* permeability. *J. Pharmaceut. Sci.*, 94, 1694–1704.

76. Horie, K., Tang, F., Borchardt, R.T. (2003). Isolation and characterization of caco{-}2 subclones expressing high levels of multidrug resistance protein efflux transporter. *Pharmaceut. Res.*, 20, 161–168.

77. Shirasaka, Y., Sakane, T., Yamashita, S. (2008). Effect of P-glycoprotein expression levels on the concentration-dependent permeability of drugs to the cell membrane. *J. Pharmaceut. Sci.*, 97, 553–565.

78. Petri, N., Tannergren, C., Rungstad, D., Lennernaes, H. (2004). Transport characteristics of fexofenadine in the caco{-}2 cell model. *Pharmaceut. Res.*, 21, 1398–1404.

79. Troutman, M.D., Thakker, D.R. (2003). Efflux ratio cannot assess P-glycoprotein-mediated attenuation of absorptive transport: Asymmetric effect of P-glycoprotein on absorptive and secretory transport across Caco{-}2 cell monolayers. *Pharmaceut. Res.*, 20, 1200–1209.

80. Balakrishnan, A., Hussainzada, N., Gonzalez, P., Bermejo, M., Swaan, P.W., Polli, J.E. (2007). Bias in estimation of transporter kinetic parameters from overexpression systems: Interplay of transporter expression level and substrate affinity. *J. Pharmacol. Exp. Ther.*, 320, 133–144.

81. Winne, D. (1973). Unstirred layer, source of biased Michaelis constant in membrane transport. *Biochim. Biophys. Acta.*, 298, 27–31.

82. Kato, M. (2008). Intestinal first-pass metabolism of CYP3A4 substrates. *Drug Metab. Pharmacokinet.*, 23, 87–94.

83. Yang, J., Jamei, M., Yeo, K.R., Tucker, G.T., Rostami-Hodjegan, A. (2007). Prediction of intestinal first-pass drug metabolism. *Curr. Drug Metabol.*, 8, 676–684.

84. Fagerholm, U. (2008). Prediction of human pharmacokinetics-gut-wall metabolism. *J. Pharm. Pharmacol.*, 59, 1335–1343.

85. Kadono, K., Akabane, T., Tabata, K., Gato, K., Terashita, S., Teramura, T. (2010). Quantitative prediction of intestinal metabolism in humans from a simplified intestinal availability model and empirical scaling factor. *Drug Metabol. Dispos.: the biological fate of chemicals*, 38, 1230–1237.

86. Gertz, M., Harrison, A., Houston, J.B., Galetin, A. (2010). Prediction of human intestinal first-pass metabolism of 25 CYP3A substrates from *in vitro* clearance and permeability data. *Drug Metabol. Dispos.: the biological fate of chemicals*, 38, 1147–1158.

87. Cummins, C.L., Jacobsen, W., Benet, L. Z. (2002). Unmasking the dynamic interplay between intestinal P-glycoprotein and CYP3A4. *J. Pharmacol. Exp. Ther.*, 300, 1036–1045.

88. Benet, L. Z., Cummins, C.L., Wu, C.Y. (2004). Unmasking the dynamic interplay between efflux transporters and metabolic enzymes. *Int. J. Pharm.*, 277, 3–9.

89. Fan, J., Maeng, H.J., Pang, K.S. (2010). Interplay of transporters and enzymes in the Caco{-}2 cell monolayer: I. effect of altered apical secretion. *Biopharm. Drug Dispos.*, 31, 215–227.

90. Fisher, J.M., Wrighton, S.A., Watkins, P.B., Schmiedlin-Ren, P., Calamia, J.C., Shen, D.D., Kunze, K.L., Thummel, K.E. (1999). First-pass midazolam metabolism catalyzed by 1alpha,25-dihydroxy vitamin D3-modified Caco{-}2 cell monolayers. *J. Pharmacol. Exp. Ther.*, 289, 1134–1142.

91. Hochman, J.H., Chiba, M., Nishime, J., Yamazaki, M., Lin, J.H. (2000). Influence of P-glycoprotein on the transport and metabolism of indinavir in Caco{-}2 cells expressing cytochrome P{-}450 3A4. *J. Pharmacol. Exp. Ther.*, 292, 310–318.

92. Raeissi, S.D., Hidalgo, I.J., Segura-Aguilar, J., Artursson, P. (1999). Interplay between CYP3A-mediated metabolism and polarized efflux of terfenadine and its metabolites in intestinal epithelial Caco{-}2 (TC7) cell monolayers. *Pharmaceut. Res.*, 16, 625–632.

93. Varma, M. V., Obach, R.S., Rotter, C., Miller, H.R., Chang, G., Steyn, S.J., El-Kattan, A., Troutman, M.D. (2010). Physicochemical space for optimum oral bioavailability: contribution of human intestinal absorption and first-pass elimination. *J. Med. Chem.*, 53, 1098–1108.

94. Kusuhara, H., Sugiyama, Y. (2010). Pharmacokinetic modeling of the hepatobiliary transport mediated by cooperation of uptake and efflux transporters. *Drug Metab. Rev.*, 42, 539–550.

95. Watanabe, T., Kusuhara, H., Maeda, K., Kanamaru, H., Saito, Y., Hu, Z., Sugiyama, Y. (2010). Investigation of the rate-determining process in the hepatic elimination of HMG-CoA reductase inhibitors in rats and humans. *Drug Metabol. Dispos.: the biological fate of chemicals*, 38, 215–222.

96. Watanabe, T., Kusuhara, H., Sugiyama, Y. (2010). Application of physiologically based pharmacokinetic modeling and clearance concept to drugs showing transporter-mediated distribution and clearance in humans. *J. Pharmacokinet. Pharmacodyn.*, 37, 575–590.

97. Galetin, A., Gertz, M., Houston, J.B. (2010). Contribution of intestinal cytochrome p450-mediated metabolism to drug-drug inhibition and induction interactions. *Drug Metabol. Pharmacokinet.*, 25, 28–47.

98. Nishimuta, H., Sato, K., Mizuki, Y., Yabuki, M., Komuro, S. (2010). Prediction of the intestinal first-pass metabolism of CYP3A substrates in humans using cynomolgus monkeys. *Drug Metabol. Dispos.: the biological fate of chemicals*, 38, 1967–1975.

CHAPTER 5

THEORETICAL FRAMEWORK IV: GASTROINTESTINAL TRANSIT MODELS AND INTEGRATION

"The river's current never fails, and yet the water never stays the same."

—Chomei Kamono

5.1 GI TRANSIT MODELS

5.1.1 One-Compartment Model/Plug Flow Model

The one-compartment model is the simplest model used to represent the drug absorption process for oral and other administration routes. Even though it is simple, it is often enough to represent the key features of the drug absorption process. As the Occam's razor principle suggests,[1] when the number of the parameters in the model becomes minimum, the risk of overlearning is minimum.

In the case of oral absorption, the one-compartment model assumes that the small intestine is the main absorption site and neglects the contributions of the stomach and the colon. It was found that the one-compartment model gave satisfactory results when the effect of the stomach pH is negligible [1–6].

---

[1]The simplest model that can explain the observation is the best model. This is also related to parameter distinguishing and identifying abilities.

Biopharmaceutics Modeling and Simulations: Theory, Practice, Methods, and Applications,
First Edition. Kiyohiko Sugano.
© 2012 John Wiley & Sons, Inc. Published 2012 by John Wiley & Sons, Inc.

The following equation is often used to correlate Fa% with the permeation rate coefficient of a drug.

$$Fa = 1 - \exp(-k_{perm}T_{si}) \tag{5.1}$$

5.1.2 Plug Flow Model

Amidon and coworkers [7] used the plug flow model, in which the time parameter is replaced by the distance from the pylorus. The distance is then normalized by the total length of the small intestine as

$$L_{GI}* = \frac{t \times Q_{GI}}{L_{GI}} \tag{5.2}$$

where Q_{GI} is the flow rate along the small intestine. Using this conversion, the dissolution and permeation equations can be rewritten as the function of the normalized position of a particle in the GI tract. These equations were then solved numerically to obtain Fa%. The most significant finding by this approach is that the equations are now expressed using three dimensionless parameters, which are intrinsic to oral absorption of a drug, that is, dose number (Do), dissolution number (Dn), and absorption number (An). This finding is the basis for the bioequivalence guidelines and biopharmaceutical classification system (BCS). A simpler version to derive these parameters is discussed in Section 9.2.

The plug flow model can be regarded as a variation of the one-compartment model (Fig. 5.1a). If the physiological conditions are consistent along the GI

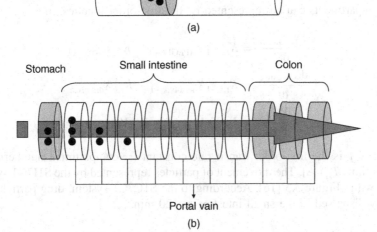

(a)

(b)

Figure 5.1 Plug flow and multiple-compartment models. (a) One-compartment model/plug flow model and (b) Multiple-compartment model (S1I7C3).

tract over time, when one plug compartment moves down the GI tract, the plug flow model becomes identical with the one-compartment model. Therefore, the analytical solution for the plug flow model and the one-compartment model becomes mathematically identical.

5.1.3 Three-Compartment Model

The GI tract should be divided into at least three compartments, the stomach, the small intestine, and the colon, to reflect the significant differences in the physiological conditions of these sections (S1I1C1 system,[2] mixed tank model). The transit kinetics could be zero order, first order, etc., to represent the observed GI transit profile. Despite of its simplicity, the predictability is appropriate for many cases and has been employed often in the literature.

5.1.4 S1I7CX (X = 1–4) Compartment Models

To represent the regional differences, the small intestine and the colon can be divided into multiple compartments. On the basis of the best fitting to the distribution of the colon exit time, when the first-order transit kinetics was applied for the transfer between the compartments, the optimal compartment number for the small intestine was found to be 7 [8, 9].

The S1I7CX $(X = 1–4)$ system is operationally convenient to represent the regional differences of the GI physiology, such as pH, bile concentration, and transporter and metabolic enzyme expression levels. Several variations of the S1I7CX system have been reported in the literature, such as the advanced compartment absorption transit (ACAT) model [10], the gastro-intestinal transit absorption (GITA) model [11–14], and the advance dissolution absorption and metabolism (ADAM) model [15] (Figs. 5.1b and 5.2).

The movement of the API particles, the dissolved drug, the GI fluid between the compartments can be represented by the first-order kinetics.

$$\frac{dN_{API,GI,k}}{dt} = K_{t,k-1}N_{API,GI,k-1} - K_{t,k}N_{API,GI,k} \tag{5.3}$$

$$\frac{dX_{dissolv,k}}{dt} = K_{t,k-1}X_{dissolv,k-1} - K_{t,k}X_{dissolv,k} \tag{5.4}$$

$$\frac{dV_{GI,k}}{dt} = K_{t,k-1}V_{GI,k-1} - K_{t,k}V_{GI,k} \tag{5.5}$$

where $K_{t,k}$ is the first-order transit rate constant ($=$ compartment number/mean transit time, T_{si}) [8]. The movement of particles represented by the S1I7C1 system is shown in Figure 5.3 [16]. According to the S1C7C1 system, drug particles are widely dispersed in the small intestine at 120 min.

---

[2]In this book, the compartment systems were expressed such as S1I1C1 in which S, I, and C corresponds to the stomach, small intestine, and colon, respectively, and the following number indicates the number of compartment.

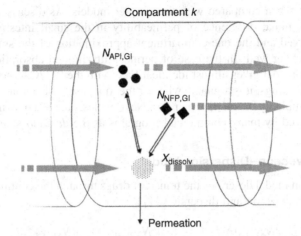

Figure 5.2 Mass balance in a compartment. N_{API} and N_{NFP} are the numbers of original API particles and newly formed precipitated particles, respectively.

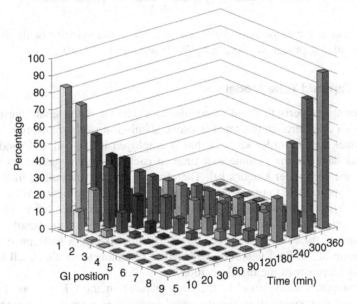

Figure 5.3 Particle distribution represented by the S1I7C1 model [16].

However, it should be stressed that the real small intestine is a continuous tube rather than a series of compartments with unlimited capacity. Therefore, this model is not a physiological model as in the same sense of the physiologically based pharmacokinetics model. In addition, when looking at the individual experimental data, the distribution of the colon exit time looks as it follows the zero-order kinetics. It is not clear how much advantage the S1I7CX systems have when compared with the simpler models. As discussed in Section 13.6.3, the regional difference of permeability in the small intestine has been merely observed and the one-compartment approximation of the small intestine has been working well. In the case of permeability-limited absorption, the one-compartment model gives almost identical Fa% with the S1I7CX model (Section 5.3.3). In most drugs, it is arguable whether the model should be made complex at the cost of simplicity or not (Chapter 16). Nevertheless, the S1I7CX model is currently employed by many commercial programs as the *de facto* standard model.

5.1.5 Convection–Dispersion Model

The dispersion model describes the transit of drugs through the continuous intestinal tube by convection and dispersion [17].

$$\frac{\partial N_{API,GI}(k,t)}{\partial t} = \text{Disp}\frac{\partial^2 N_{API,GI}}{\partial^2 k} - \text{Vc}\frac{\partial N_{API,GI}}{\partial k} \tag{5.6}$$

$$\frac{\partial X_{dissolv,GI}(k,t)}{\partial t} = \text{Disp}\frac{\partial^2 X_{dissolv,GI}}{\partial^2 k} - \text{Vc}\frac{\partial X_{dissolv,GI}}{\partial k} \tag{5.7}$$

where Disp is the dispersion coefficient and Vc is the velocity of the intestinal fluid. Similar approach was taken by Willmann et al. [18, 19].

5.1.6 Tapered Tube Model

Considering the peristaltic and mucociliary movements of the small intestine, the transit of a drug through the small intestine should follow the zero-order kinetics, rather than the first-order kinetics that is employed in the S1I7CX model. The observed data for the colonic exit time in each individual patient looks as it follows the zero-order kinetics [9]. Therefore, in biopharmaceutical modeling, it might be appropriate to treat the small intestine as a tube with a movement like a belt conveyor (Fig. 5.4). As the fluid in the stomach is excreted (cf. this is a first-order kinetic process), the fluid is pushed along the tube of the small intestine. This band of the fluid then moves down the tube like by a belt conveyor. The distribution of the fluid would be widened as the diameter of the small intestine becomes narrower in the distal position.

To computationally simulate the drug transfer in the GI tract as discussed above, it is convenient to model the small intestine as a series of compartments with a limited volume capacity. The number of the compartments should be sufficient to approximate the tapered tube shape [e.g., 100 ellipse cylinders with the length and circumference of 3 cm and 10–6 cm (proximal to distal), respectively]. The stomach can be modeled as one compartment and the stomach fluid is excreted into the small intestine following the first-order kinetics. As the fluid in the stomach is excreted into the small intestine, owing to the limited fluid capacity of each compartment, the fluid fills the compartment one after the other in the proximal small intestine. The drug particles then move down the small intestine

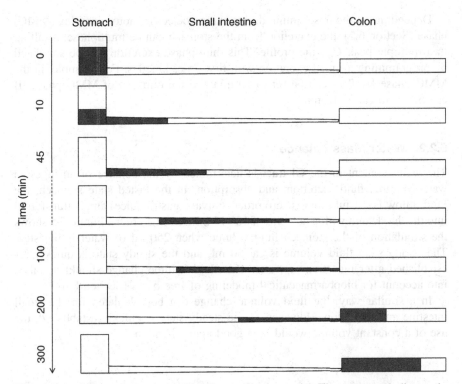

Figure 5.4 Schematic representation of tapered tube model. The gray part indicates the distribution of a drug. The stomach is modeled as one compartment. The fluid excretion from the stomach is modeled by the first-order kinetics. As the fluid in the stomach is excreted into the small intestine (0–45 min), because of the limited fluid capacity of each compartment, the fluid fills the compartment one after the other in the proximal small intestine. The drug particles then moves down the small intestine following the zero-order kinetics (like by a belt conveyor).

following the zero-order kinetics (like by a belt conveyor). The forefront of the drug particles moves to the next compartment ca. every 1 min, so that it takes ca. 100 min to exit into the colon. The zero-order flux at the small intestine–colon junction can be set to represent the colon exit time distribution with the mean exit time of 210 min and the back-end exit time to be ca. 300 min.

5.2 TIME-DEPENDENT CHANGES OF PHYSIOLOGICAL PARAMETERS

5.2.1 Gastric Emptying

Gastric empting is usually simulated as a first-order kinetic process. In the fed state, gastric emptying rate depends on the nutrition state (Sections 6.2.1.1 and 12.2.1).

Depending on the dose timing during the myoelectric motor complex (MMC) phase (Section 6.2), the excretion from the stomach can be multiphase, resulting in a multiple peak C_p time profile. This multiphase excretion can be simulated by programming a timed excretion with first-order kinetics. For example, in the MMC phase III, $T_{1/2}$ can be set to 10 min and the duration of MMC phase III can be set to ca. 2–15 min.

5.2.2 Water Mass Balance

The water content in the GI tract is determined by the balance of an ingested water volume, fluid secretion, and absorption. In the fasted state stomach, the fluid inflow is 2.1 ml/min (as zero order, saliva + gastric juice) and is transferred into the duodenum with a half-life of 10–15 min (as first order). Figure 5.5 shows the simulation of the stomach fluid volume when 250 ml of water is ingested. The steady state fluid volume is ca. 30 ml, and the steady state is quickly re-established after ingestion of water. This fluid volume change should be taken into account for biopharmaceutical modeling of free bases (Section 8.6).

In a similar way, the fluid volume change can be calculated for the small intestine and the colon. However, as the steady state is quickly established, the use of a constant volume would be a good approximation.

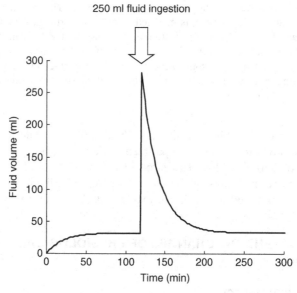

Figure 5.5 The simulated time course of the stomach volume after bonus administration of 250 ml of water. Secretion of saliva and gastric juice and gastric emptying were simulated as the zero-order (2.1 ml/min) and first-order ($T_{1/2} = 10$ min) kinetics, respectively.

Example   The steady state volume in the stomach with the secretion rate = 2.1 ml and emptying half-life = 10 min can be calculated as follows:

The mass balance at the steady state is

$$\text{Secretion per time} = \frac{\ln 2}{\text{Transfer } T_{1/2}} \cdot \text{Steady state volume}$$

By rearranging this equation and input the secretion rate and the emptying half-life,

$$\text{Steady state volume} = \text{Secretion per time} \times \frac{\text{Transfer } T_{1/2}}{\ln 2}$$

$$= 2.1 \frac{10}{0.693} = 30.3 \text{ ml}$$

5.2.3   Bile Concentration

After being secreted from the bile duct into the duodenum, the bile is diluted by the fluid coming from the stomach. As the fluid moves down the small intestine, water will be reabsorbed and the bile concentration will go up ca. twofold. At the end of the ileum, the bile acid is almost completely reabsorbed (Fig. 6.18). This dynamic change of bile concentration is suggested to be one of the reasons for the bimodal absorptions of some drugs (Section 13.6.3). The fluid composition changes more dynamically in the fed state than in the fasted state [20]. This change can be represented by assigning a different bile concentration to each small intestinal region.

5.3   INTEGRATION 1: ANALYTICAL SOLUTIONS

As the kinetic processes of oral absorption are expressed by sequential differential equations, integration of these equations is required to obtain observable values, such as the fraction of a dose absorbed (Fa) and plasma concentration (C_p) time profile. There are two methods to integrate the differential equations, analytical solution and numerical integration.

Traditionally, the quest for analytical solution(s) was the only way to apply the scientific theories for practical prediction. Some approximation is often applied to obtain an approximate analytical solution. When we obtained an analytical solution, we could say that we understood it.[3] However, analytical solution is obtainable only for very few specific cases (but these cases are often the most important and essential cases). Therefore, to solve a complex problem, computational numerical integration is required. As the computational speed increases,

---

[3]In addition, an analytical solution is less liable for calculation error. Analytical solution is often used to validate the numerical integration program.

numerical integration becomes more and more available for many scientists. Numerical integration is very powerful and enables us to have answers for many complicated cases for which analytical solution cannot be obtained.

In this book, as in the other textbooks of physics, analytical solutions for some essential cases are first discussed. Understanding of these essential cases is important for interpreting the results from numerical integration.

5.3.1 Dissolution Under Sink Condition

5.3.1.1 Monodispersed Particles. The Nernst–Brunner equation for monodispersed spherical particles with $r_{p,ini} < 30$ μm in a sink condition[4] is obtained by combining surface area per particle (SA_p), particle number (N_p), mass transfer coefficient ($D_{eff}/L/Sh$, at < 30 μm, $L/Sh = h = r_{p,ini}$), and surface solubility ($S_{surface}$)

$$\frac{dX_{API,t}}{dt} = -SA_p \times N_p \times \frac{D_{eff}}{L/Sh} \times S_{surface}$$

$$= -4\pi r_p^2 \times \frac{X_{t=0}}{\left(\frac{4}{3}\pi r_{p,ini}^3\right)\rho_p} \times \frac{D_{eff}}{r_p} \times S_{surface}$$

$$= -\frac{3D_{eff}S_{surface}}{r_{p,ini}^2\rho_p} X_{API,t=0}^{2/3} X_{API,t}^{1/3}$$

$$= -k_{diss} X_{API,t=0}^{2/3} X_{API,t}^{1/3} \tag{5.8}$$

$$\left(k_{diss} = \frac{3D_{eff}S_{surface}}{r_{p,ini}^2\rho_p}\right) \tag{5.9}$$

By rearranging Equation 5.9,

$$X_t^{-1/3}\frac{dX_t}{dt} = -k_{diss} X_{API,t=0}^{2/3} \tag{5.10}$$

By integrating this equation and rearranging, we obtain

$$\text{Dissolved } \% = 1 - \left(1 - \frac{2}{3}k_{diss}T_{si}\right)^{3/2} \qquad r_{p,t=0} < 30 \text{ μm} \tag{5.11}$$

This is the exact analytical solution of the Nernst–Brunner equation for the dissolution of monodispersed particles with $r_{p,ini} < 30$ μm in a sink condition.

---

[4]When $C_{dissolv}/S_{dissolv} < 0.3$, it is called *sink condition*.

Similarly, for > 30 μm cases, assuming that h_{API} is constant (= 30 μm), we obtain

$$k_{diss} = \frac{3D_{eff}S_{surface}}{r_{p,ini}h_{API}\rho_p} \tag{5.12}$$

$$\text{Dissolved \%} = 1 - \left(1 - \frac{1}{3}k_{diss}T_{si}\right)^3 \qquad r_{p,t=0} > 30 \text{ μm} \tag{5.13}$$

This equation is not an exact analytical solution because, as the particles dissolve, the particle radius becomes less than 30 μm and the h_{API} is no longer a constant (Fig. 5.6).

When an approximation of $X_{t=0}^{2/3} X_t^{1/3} \approx X_t$ is employed,

$$\frac{dX_{API,t}}{dt} = -k_{diss}X_t = -k_{diss}X_{API,t} \tag{5.14}$$

This is a first-order kinetic equation. Therefore, by integrating Equation 5.14, we obtain an approximate analytical solution as

$$\text{Dissolved \%} = 1 - \exp(-k_{diss}t) \tag{5.15}$$

Figure 5.6 shows the comparison between the exact and approximate analytical solutions. Considering variations of *in vivo* data and various other errors for *in vivo* predictions (Section 16.1), the first-order approximation would be reasonable for *in vivo* oral absorption prediction. In addition, when Dissolved % < 60–70%, the zero-order, first-order, and exact analytical solutions become similar.

5.3.1.2 Polydispersed Particles.

As discussed in Section 3.2.3.2, polydispersed particles can be represented as the sum of monodispersed particles. Therefore, the Noyes–Whitney equation becomes

$$\frac{dX_{API,t}}{dt} = \sum_{PSB} f_{PSB}\frac{dX_{API,PSB,t}}{dt} = \sum_{PSB} -f_{PSB}SA_{p,PSB} \times N_{p,PSB} \times \frac{D_{eff}}{L/Sh} \times S_{surface} \tag{5.16}$$

Figure 5.7 shows the comparison between the dissolution profiles of monodispersed particles and polydispersed particles under a sink condition. At the initial stage of dissolution, the dissolution rate increases as the particle becomes dispersed (cf. Fig. 3.7). However, at the final stage of dissolution, the dissolution rate becomes slower when compared to that of the monodispersed particles, as the small particles have already been vanished, whereas the large particles remain dissolved (Fig. 5.8).

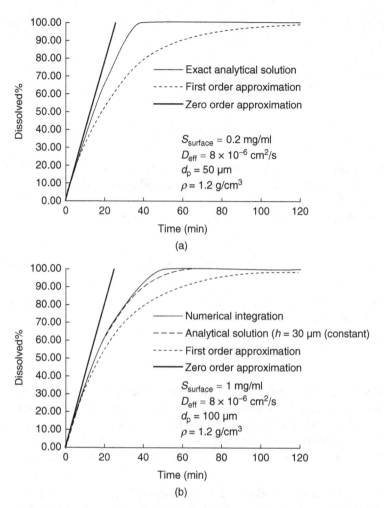

Figure 5.6 Comparison of numerical integration, analytical solution, and first-order approximation for dissolution simulation of monodispersed drug particles. (a) $d_{p,ini} < 60$ μm and (b) $d_{p,ini} > 60$ μm.

5.3.2   Fraction of a Dose Absorbed (Fa%)

The fraction of a dose absorbed (Fa%) is the ratio of the absorbed amount to the dosed amount. In this book, once drug molecules permeated the first biological barrier (e.g., apical membrane of the intestinal epithelial cells), the drug molecules were designated to be absorbed and Fa% is defined based on this definition. Usually, Fa% means the final Fa% after one dose of a drug passed through the GI tract.[5] However, Fa% is time dependent. For example, after dosing a drug,

---

[5]Similarly, the bioavailability (F or BA%) is usually the final value.

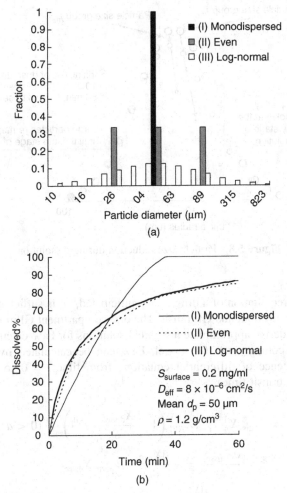

Figure 5.7 Dissolution of mono, 3 bins, and log-normal distribution particles. (a) Particle size distribution and (b) dissolution.

10% is absorbed until 1 h, 20% is absorbed until 2 h, and so on. Therefore, if the drug stays in the small intestine for infinite time, Fa% always becomes 100% regardless of the dissolution and permeation rates.

5.3.3 Approximate Fa% Analytical Solutions 1: Case-by-Case Solution

The central dogma of oral absorption consists of dissolution, nucleation, permeation, and GI transit, which are expressed as sequential differential equations. The derivations of some analytical solutions for Fa% are first discussed in this section. The numerical integration is then discussed in the next section.

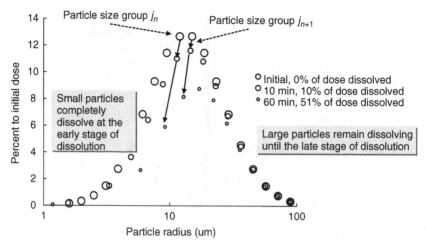

Figure 5.8 Particle size reduction during dissolution.

When the precipitation of a drug is not anticipated,[6] it is sufficient to consider dissolution, permeation, and GI transit. The one-compartment GI model (S0I1C0) can be used to derive approximate analytical solutions for Fa% calculation. When using the one-compartment GI model, Fa% can be calculated by solving the following sequence of differential equations from time $t = 0$ to $t = T_{si}$ (T_{si}: small intestine transit time).

$$\frac{dX_{API}}{dt} = -k_{diss}X_{API,t=0}^{1-a}X_{API}^{a}\left(1 - \frac{X_{dissolv}/V_{GI}}{S_{dissolv}}\right)\cdots(0 < a < 1) \quad (5.17)$$

$$\frac{dX_{dissov}}{dt} = -\frac{dX_{API}}{dt} - k_{perm}X_{dissolv} \quad (5.18)$$

$$\frac{dX_{perm}}{dt} = k_{perm}X_{dissolv} \quad (5.19)$$

As $X_{dissolv}$ appears in all equations, it is difficult to obtain an exact analytical solution for general cases.[7] First, approximate analytical solutions for three typical types of oral absorption, that is, the permeability-limited, dissolution-rate-limited, and solubility-permeability-limited cases are discussed (Section 1.2).

5.3.3.1 *Permeability-Limited Case.* When drug particles dissolve instantly and completely in the GI tract, the dissolution process becomes negligible and the

---

[6]Basically for undissociable and free acid drugs with a standard formulation.
[7]However, no existence of such an exact analytical solution has not been proved yet (so might exist but not found).

permeation process determines the Fa% of the drug. In this case, $X_{dissolv} = $ Dose at $t = 0$. Therefore, by solving Equation 5.19,

$$X_{dissolv} = \text{Dose} \cdot \exp(-k_{perm}T_{si}) \tag{5.20}$$

The fraction of the dissolved drug remaining unabsorbed at time T_{si} is then calculated as

$$\frac{X_{dissolv}}{\text{Dose}} = \exp(-k_{perm}T_{si}) \tag{5.21}$$

Considering the mass balance in the GI fluid, Fa for the permeability-limited cases (Fa_{PL}) is

$$Fa_{PL} = 1 - \frac{X_{dissolv}}{\text{Dose}} = \frac{X_{perm}}{\text{Dose}} = 1 - \exp(-k_{perm}T_{si}) = 1 - \exp(-Pn) \tag{5.22}$$

where X_{perm} is the permeated amount. As colonic absorption of drugs with low permeability is usually negligible ($< 20\%$), T_{si} can be set to the small intestine transit time. $k_{perm} \times T_{si}$ becomes a dimensionless number, the "permeation number (Pn)."[8,9] Even though this analytical solution is based on the one-compartment model, it is almost identical to the analytical solution for seven-compartment model [8] (Fig. 5.9) (Table 5.1).

$$Fa_{PL} = 1 - \exp(-k_{perm}T_{si}) \approx 1 - \left(1 + \frac{k_{perm}T_{si}}{7}\right)^{-7} \tag{5.23}$$

5.3.3.2 *Solubility-Permeability-Limited Case.* In the solubility-permeability-limited case (SL), Fa can be calculated assuming that $X_{dissolv}$ equals $S_{dissolv} \times V_{GI}$ and remains constant over time.

$$\frac{dX_{dissolv}}{dt} = -k_{perm}X_{dissolv,const} = -k_{perm}S_{dissolv}V_{GI} \tag{5.24}$$

(cf. $X_{dissolv} = C_{dissolv} \times V_{GI}$). By integrating this equation, the permeated amount until time T_{si} is calculated as

$$X_{perm} = 1 - X_{dissolv} = k_{perm}S_{dissolv}V_{GI}T_{si} \tag{5.25}$$

---

[8] As discussed later, dimensionless parameters of Do, Dn, and An ($= 1/2Pn$) were originally introduced using a plug flow model (Section 9.2). However, the derivation of these parameters using the plug flow model is difficult and its meaning is not explicitly understood from the derivation process. Therefore, in this section, the one-compartment model is used and these dimensionless parameters are discussed in a step-by-step manner.

[9] k_{perm} is basically a time-dependent value. But in most cases, k_{perm} is treated as a constant.

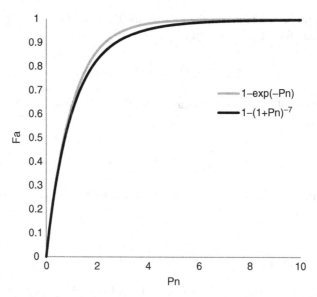

Figure 5.9 Analytical solutions for one- and seven-compartment models for a permeability-limited absorption case.

TABLE 5.1 Drug Range Used for the Investigation of Fa% Analytical Solution

Drug Parameter	Values
Dose (mg)	1, 3, 10, 30, 100, 300, 1000
$P_{\mathrm{eff}}(\times 10^{-4} \mathrm{cm/s})$	0.03, 0.1, 0.3, 1, 3, 10
$D_{\mathrm{eff}}(\times 10^{-6} \mathrm{cm}^2/\mathrm{s})$	0.1, 0.3, 1, 3, 10
S_{dissolv} (mg/ml)	0.001, 0.003, 0.01, 0.03, 0.1, 1
$d_{\mathrm{p}}(= 2r_{\mathrm{p}})$ (µm)	1, 3, 10, 30, 100, 300

Therefore, Fa is calculated as

$$\mathrm{Fa_{SL}} = \frac{X_{\mathrm{perm}}}{\mathrm{Dose}} = \frac{k_{\mathrm{perm}} S_{\mathrm{dissolv}} V_{\mathrm{GI}} T_{\mathrm{si}}}{\mathrm{Dose}} = \frac{\mathrm{Pn}}{\mathrm{Do}} (\text{if } \mathrm{Fa} > 1 \text{ then } \mathrm{Fa} = 1) \qquad (5.26)$$

$$\mathrm{Do} = \frac{\mathrm{Dose}}{S_{\mathrm{dissolv}} V_{\mathrm{GI}}} \qquad (5.27)$$

As the colonic absorption of compounds with low solubility is usually negligible, T_{si} can be set to the small intestine transit time. As it is assumed that the dissolution rate is rapid and C_{dissolv} immediately reaches S_{dissolv} in this case,

Fa_{SL} is the theoretical maximum Fa value (except for supersaturable cases). Dose $\times$ Fa_{SL} is called the *maximum absorbable dose* (MAD) [21, 22].[10]

This Fa calculation is appropriate for undissociable and free acid drugs; however, it is not appropriate for free base compounds and the salts of acid and base drugs. In the latter cases, Fa% usually becomes significantly higher than Fa_{SL}. It should be emphasized that Fa_{PL} depends on k_{perm} and $S_{dissolv}$ (so it is called *solubility–permeability* limited).

The Do, which is the ratio of the dose to the maximum dissolved amount in the fluid is introduced in the Fa_{PL} equation. The Do is the most important dimensionless number that characterizes the biopharmaceutical profile of a drug.

5.3.3.3 *Dissolution-Rate-Limited Case.*
In the case of dissolution-rate-limited (DRL) absorption, the dissolved % equals Fa%. An approximate analytical solution can be obtained, assuming $C_{dissolv}$ equals 0 (the perfect sink condition) and first-order dissolution.

$$Fa_{DRL} = 1 - \exp(-k_{diss}T_{si}) = 1 - \exp(-Dn) \tag{5.28}$$

where Dn is the dissolution number. As shown in Figure 5.6, the first-order approximation would be appropriate for many cases.

5.3.4 Approximate Fa% Analytical Solutions 2: Semi-General Equations

5.3.4.1 *Sequential First-Order Kinetics of Dissolution and Permeation.*
When Do < 1, the oral absorption of a drug can be represented as a sequential first-order process. In this case, an analytical solution for Fa (Fa_{sfo}) is

$$
\begin{aligned}
Fa_{sfo} &= 1 - \frac{k_{perm}}{k_{perm} - k_{diss}} \exp(-k_{diss}T_{si}) + \frac{k_{diss}}{k_{perm} - k_{diss}} \exp(-k_{perm}T_{si}) \\
&= 1 - \frac{Pn}{Pn - Dn} \exp(-Dn) + \frac{Dn}{Pn - Dn} \exp(-Pn) \qquad \frac{C_{dissolv}}{S_{dissolv}} < 1 \quad (5.29)
\end{aligned}
$$

Figure 5.10 shows the comparison of Fa_{sfo} and Fa numerically obtained with the S1I7C1 model (Fa_{NI}). Fa_{sfo} is only valid for Do < 1 cases. Fa_{sfo} resulted in overestimation of Fa in the case of compounds with low solubility (BCS class II and IV compounds) because of negligence of the effect of solubility limitation in the GI fluid. In the case of compounds with high solubility (BCS I and III, Do < 1), the correlation was appropriate. This is not surprising because the analytical solutions of permeation-limited cases for the S1I7C1 system are almost identical with that of the one-compartment model (Fig. 5.9). Even in the

[10]This calculation gives maximum achievable absorbed amount for undissociable compounds by increasing the dose or increasing the dissolution rate. However, for supersaturable cases such as a salt form API, supersaturated concentration could occur in the GI tract and Fa can exceed Fa_{SL}.

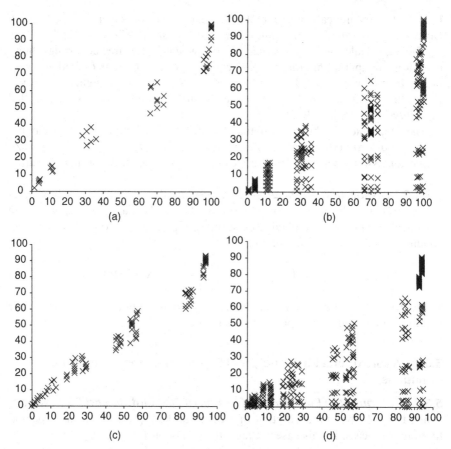

Figure 5.10   Fa calculated by sequential first-order approximation (Fa_{sfo}) versus numerical integration of the S1I7C1 system (Fa_{NI}). The ranges of the drug parameters are listed in Table 5.1. Panel a–d corresponds to BCS class I–IV, respectively.

case of BCS I, some compounds showed incomplete absorption because of a slow dissolution rate. A large particle size or a small diffusion coefficient can cause slow dissolution. As the permeabilies of BCS I drugs are high, oral absorption becomes dissolution rate limited and the first-order approximation is appropriate.

The GITA model is an extension of the sequential first-order kinetics to the seven-compartment model. Therefore, the GITA model should not be used for the solubility-permeability-limited cases.

5.3.4.2   Minimum Fa% Model.   By taking the minimum Fa value[11] among the three rate-limiting cases (Fa_{PL}, Fa_{SL}, and Fa_{DRL}), we can obtain an approximate analytical solution for Fa ($Fa_{min\,limit}$). As shown in Figure 5.11, compared to Fa_{sfo}, the $Fa_{min\,limit}$ gives much closer results to Fa_{NI}, suggesting that the simplest

---

[11]Corresponds to the rate-limiting step approximation.

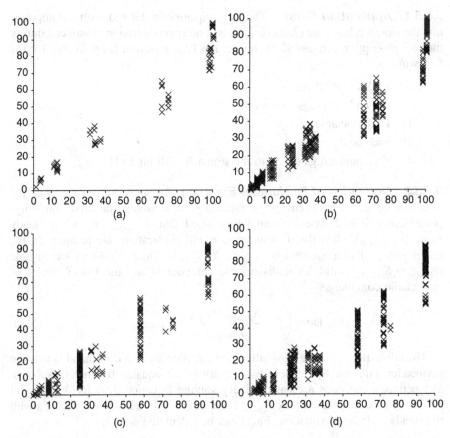

Figure 5.11 Fa calculated as the minimum value of limiting cases ($Fa_{min,limit}$) versus by numerical integration of the S1I7C1 system (Fa_{NI}). The ranges of the drug parameters are listed in Table 5.1.

Fa% calculation for each limiting case would be sufficient for most cases of drugs. However, for intermediate cases, the assumptions employed to derive the analytical solutions, that is, $X_{dissolv} = 0$ in Equation 5.29 for the dissolution-limited case or $C_{dissolv} = S_{dissolv}$ in Equation 5.26 for the solubility-permeability-limited case are not appropriate.

5.3.5 Approximate Fa% Analytical Solutions 3: Fa$_{SS}$ Equation

Recently, a general approximate Fa% analytical solution based on the steady state approximation ("Fa$_{SS}$ equation") was derived and compared with Fa_{NI} [16, 23]. The Fa$_{SS}$ equation is simple; however, it still gives Fa% values similar to Fa_{NI}. To increase the transparency of calculation, the Fa$_{SS}$ equation should be used when it is appropriate.

5.3.5.1 Application Range. The Fa_{ss} equation is derived with assumptions that the stomach has little effect on Fa% and no supersaturation is induced during the oral absorption processes. Therefore, the Fa_{ss} equation is applicable for the following:

1. All BCS I and III drugs
2. BCS II and IV drugs that are
   (a) Undissociable
   (b) Free acid
   (c) Free base drugs dosed to the stomach with high pH.

5.3.5.2 Derivation of Fa Number Equation. To appropriately calculate the intermediate cases between the permeability, dissolution rate, and solubility-permeability-limited cases, it can be assumed that $X_{dissolv}$ becomes a steady value ($X_{dissolv,ss}$) when the dissolution rate and permeation rate balance. In the initial phase of oral absorption, $X_{API} \approx X_{API,t=0}(= \text{Dose})$.[12] When we assume $S_{surface} = S_{dissolv}$ (valid for undissociable compounds and the low S_0 cases of dissociable compounds),

$$k_{diss}\text{Dose}\left(1 - \frac{X_{dissolv}/V_{GI}}{S_{dissolv}}\right) = k_{perm}X_{dissolv} \qquad (5.30)$$

The left-hand side is the dissolution rate equation and the right-hand side is the permeation rate equation. These two equations are equaled because dissolve-in and permeate-out rates are balanced. By solving Equation 5.30 for $X_{dissolv,ss}$ at the initial time, normalizing by $S_{dissolv}$, and inserting into Equation 5.28, Fa with the steady state approximation (Fa_{ss}) can be calculated as [23]

$$Fa_{ss} = 1 - \exp\left(-\frac{1}{\dfrac{1}{k_{diss}} + \dfrac{\text{Do}}{k_{perm}}} \cdot T_{si}\right)$$

$$= 1 - \exp\left(-\frac{1}{\dfrac{1}{\text{Dn}} + \dfrac{\text{Do}}{\text{Pn}}}\right) \quad \text{If Do} < 1, \text{Do} = 1. \qquad (5.31)$$

As limiting cases, Fa_{ss} smoothly connects to Fa_{PL}, Fa_{SL}, and Fa_{DRL} (cf. $x < 0.7, 1 - \exp(x) \approx x$). The initial saturation number (Sn_{ini}), which indicates the degree of sink/nonsink conditions in the intestinal fluid, can be calculated as

$$Sn_{ini} = \frac{C_{dissolv,ss}}{S_{dissolv}} = \frac{1}{1 + \dfrac{k_{perm}}{\text{Do} \cdot k_{diss}}} = \frac{1}{1 + \dfrac{\text{Pn}}{\text{Do} \cdot \text{Dn}}} \quad \text{Do} > 1 \qquad (5.32)$$

[12]More precisely, in the dissolution rate equation, the power on X_{API} is 1/3 for most cases. Therefore, we can approximate the dissolution process as zero-order kinetics (Fig. 5.6).

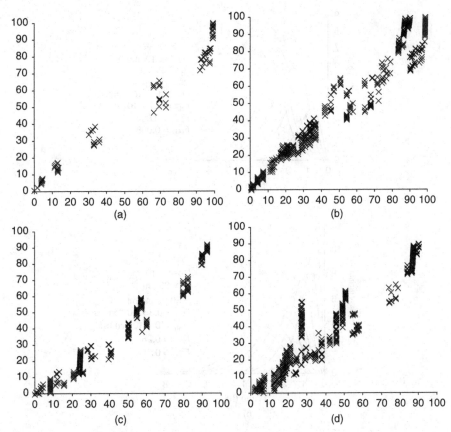

Figure 5.12   Fa calculated by the analytical solution with the steady state approximation (Fa$_{SS}$) versus by numerical integration of the S1I7C1 system (Fa$_{NI}$). The ranges of the drug parameters are listed in Table 5.1.

where $C_{dissolv,ss}$ is the steady state concentration in the intestinal fluid. When Sn$_{ini}$ is close to 1, the drug concentration in the intestinal fluid is close to the saturated solubility, whereas when Sn$_{ini}$ is close to 0, it is close to the sink condition.

As shown in Figure 5.12, even though the Fa$_{SS}$ equation is simple, it gives Fa that is almost identical to Fa$_{NI}$ that is calculated using a numerical integration of the S1I7C1 model.

5.3.5.3 *Refinement of the Fa$_{SS}$ Equation.*   Compared to Fa$_{sfo}$ and Fa$_{min\,limit}$, the Fa$_{SS}$ gives much closer results to Fa$_{NI}$. The remaining slight difference would be due to the steady state concentration assumption and the dispersion of particles along the GI tract. The following three deviation patterns were identified (Fig. 5.13):

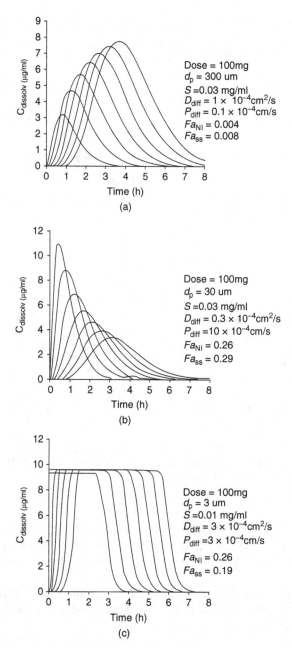

Figure 5.13 Typical case examples of deviation from the steady state approximation. (a) $C_{dissolv}$ does not reach the steady state during the GI transit, (b) the initial steady state concentration is not maintained, and (c) the steady state duration is longer than T_{si}. The drug parameters used for Fa calculation are indicated in the figures. The lines in the figure correspond to each small intestinal compartment (from the left to the right, compartment 1 to 7, proximal to distal, respectively).

(a) C_{dissolv} does not reach the steady state during the GI transit

(b) The initial steady state concentration is not maintained because of the dissolution rate being reduced (particle size reduction occurred as particles dissolve)

(c) The steady state is maintained longer than T_{si} because of the particles remaining in the GI tract after T_{si} (remaining particle effect (RPE)).

Cases (a) and (b) are due to the steady state approximation, whereas case (c) is due to negligence of the dispersion of drug particles along the GI tract.

In the case of (a), $C_{\text{dissolv}} < S_{\text{dissolv}}$. Therefore, the sequential first-order kinetic model is appropriate. Appropriate Fa can be obtained by replacing Fa_{SS} with Fa_{sfo} when $\text{Fa}_{\text{sfo}} \times 1.15 < \text{Fa}_{\text{ss}}$. The coefficient 1.15 was introduced as a margin to ensure a definite sink condition. This treatment improved the correlation at $\text{Fa} < 0.2$ range.

To correct (b) and (c), the steady state reduction correction factor (CF_{SSR}) and the extended steady state duration number (Tn_{exss}) can be introduced as

$$\text{Fa}_{\text{ss,corr}} = 1 - \exp\left(-\frac{1}{\dfrac{1}{\text{Dn}} + \dfrac{\text{Do}}{\text{Pn}}} \cdot \text{CF}_{\text{SSR}} \cdot \text{Tn}_{\text{exss}}\right) \qquad \text{If Do} < 1, \text{Do} = 1.$$

$$(5.33)$$

CF_{SSR} can be calculated considering the saturation number at time $T_{\text{si}}(\text{Sn}_{T_{\text{si}}})$. Fa is first calculated without any correction in Equation 5.31 (Fa'). Using Fa' to consider the reduction of Do and Dn during the oral absorption processes (i.e., replacing Do and Dn in Equation 5.31 with $\text{Do}(1 - \text{Fa}')$ and $\text{Dn}(1 - \text{Fa}')^{-2/3}$), and normalizing by Sn_{ini}, the steady state reduction number (SRn) can be obtained as (cf. $r_p/r_{p,t=0} \approx (1 - \text{Fa}')^{1/3}$, neglecting X_{dissolv} at time T_{si}),

$$\text{SRn} = \frac{\text{Sn}_{T_{\text{si}}}}{\text{Sn}_{\text{ini}}} = \frac{1}{\text{Sn}_{\text{ini}}\left(1 + \dfrac{\text{Pn}}{\text{Do} \cdot \text{Dn} \cdot (1 - \text{Fa}')^{1/3}}\right)} \qquad (5.34)$$

The mean and standard distribution of particle size are assumed to remain the same. CF_{SSR} is then calculated by taking the average as

$$\text{CF}_{\text{SSR}} = \frac{1}{2}(\text{Sn}_{\text{ini}} + \text{Sn}_{T_{\text{si}}}) = \frac{1}{2}\text{Sn}_{\text{ini}}(1 + \text{SRn}) \qquad (5.35)$$

The CF_{SSR} corrects the declining of drug concentration from an initial steady state concentration. CF_{SSR} was found to be in the range of 0.54–1.0.

Tn_{exss} is determined by the amount of drug particles remaining in the GI tract. The portion of a drug exited from the small intestine until time t (EXT(t)) can

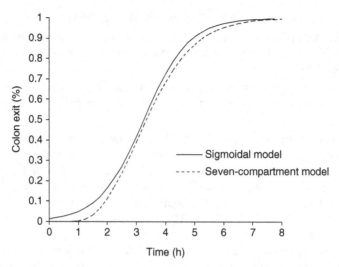

Figure 5.14   Colon exited fraction expressed by the sigmoidal curve (solid line) and the S1I7C1 system (dotted line). For the S1I7C1 system, $K_t = 7/T_{si} = 2$ (h^{-1}) and for the sigmoid curve, $k_t = 1.31$ (h^{-1}).

be expressed by the S1I7C1 model or a sigmoid curve as

$$\mathrm{EXT}(t) = 1 - \exp(-K_t \cdot t) \left(\sum_{n=1}^{7} \frac{(K_t \cdot t)^{n-1}}{(n-1)!} \right) \approx \frac{1}{1 + \exp(-k_t(t - T_{si}))} \quad (5.36)$$

Figure 5.14 shows the analytical solution of the colon exited fraction by the S1I7C1 model (Eq. 5.36, middle part) and a sigmoid curve (Eq. 5.36, right-hand side, $k_t = 1.31$ h^{-1}). Using EXT(t) and approximation of Fa $\ll$ 1, the saturation number at T_{exss} can be calculated as

$$\mathrm{Sn}_{T_{exss}} = \frac{1}{1 + \dfrac{\mathrm{Pn}}{\mathrm{Do}(1 - \mathrm{EXT}(T_{exss})) \cdot \mathrm{Dn}}} \quad (5.37)$$

Do$(1 - \mathrm{EXT}(t))$ is the Do at time t considering the colon exit of the dosed drug particles. When $\mathrm{Sn}_{T_{exss}}/\mathrm{Sn}_{ini} < 1/2$, the particle number in the small intestine cannot maintain the steady state. Using a sigmoidal curve for EXT(t), rearranging $\mathrm{Sn}_{T_{exss}}/\mathrm{Sn}_{ini} = 1/2$ and normalizing by T_{si}, we obtain the Tn_{exss}:

$$\mathrm{Tn}_{exss} = \frac{T_{exss}}{T_{si}} = 1 - \frac{1}{k_t \cdot T_{si}} \ln \left(\frac{1}{1 + \dfrac{\mathrm{Do \cdot Dn}}{\mathrm{An}}} \right) \qquad \mathrm{Do}(1 - \mathrm{EXT}(T_{exss})) > 1$$

$$(5.38)$$

The precondition of this equation is that $Do(1 - EXT(t))$ is larger than 1. The time at which the drug amount remains in the small intestine gives $Do(1 - EXT(t)) = 1(T_{Do1})$ and can be calculated by rearranging $Do(1 - EXT(T_{Do1})) = 1$ and normalizing with T_{si} as

$$Tn_{Do1} = \frac{T_{Do1}}{T_{si}} = 1 - \frac{1}{k_t \cdot T_{si}} \ln \left(\frac{1}{1 - \frac{1}{Do}} - 1 \right) \tag{5.39}$$

When $Tn_{Do1} > Tn_{exss}$, Tn_{exss} is replaced with Tn_{Do1}. Tn_{exss} was found to be in the range of 1.0–2.8.

The correlation between Fa_{SS} and Fa_{NI} was improved by applying Fa_{sfo}, CF_{SSR}, and Tn_{exss} (Fig. 5.15). The remaining deviations may be due to the approximation employed in the correction factors and the dispersion of drug

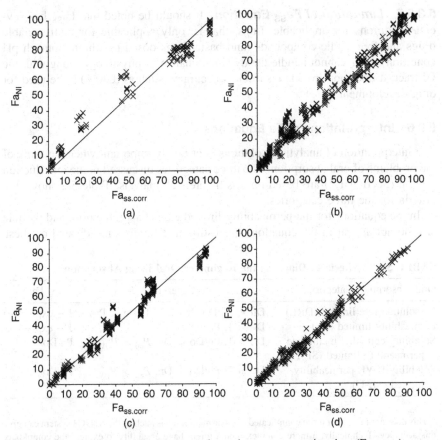

Figure 5.15 Fa calculated by corrected steady state approximation ($Fa_{SS\ corr}$) versus numerical integration of the S1I7C1 system (Fa_{NI}). (a) BCS I, (b) BCS II, (c) BCS III, and (d) BCS IV. The ranges of the drug parameters are listed in Table 5.1.

particles and dissolved drug in the small intestine, which are represented by the S1I7C1 model but not by the S0I1C0 model.

5.3.5.4 *Advantage of Fa$_{SS}$ Equation.*

Considering the convenience and clarity of the Fa$_{SS}$ equation and that many compounds with low solubility are undissociable, Fa$_{SS}$ would be beneficial for practical drug discovery uses. Figure 5.12 suggests that the difference of the GI transit models (S0I1C0 vs S1I7C1) and integration method (approximate analytical vs numerical) has little effect on Fa% prediction. Sn can be used to indicate whether the oral absorption of the drug is dissolution limited (sink condition) or solubility–permeability limited.

Fa$_{SS}$ calculation is simple, easy, and available for everybody, whereas the S1I7CX model is difficult to calculate (need programing skill). The commercial software is not available as an open source. As scientific publications should be thoroughly validated by independent readers, Fa$_{SS}$ will be important as a transparent and traceable model.

5.3.5.5 *Limitation of Fa$_{SS}$ Equation.*

It should be noted that Fa$_{SS}$ has several conditions for applicable drugs, that is, only applicable for undissociable drugs and free acidic compounds (and basic drugs dosed in a high stomach pH condition). Fa$_{SS}$ cannot handle the dynamic change of physiology along with the GI tract. It does not provide a sufficient accuracy (such as $\pm 20\%$) to be used for drug development.[13]

5.3.6 Interpretations of Fa Equations

The interpretation of analytical solutions is critically important when we think of the problems of oral absorption. The three categories discussed in the introduction section (Section 1.2) are based on this theoretical analysis. Table 5.2 shows the criteria for the three categories.

In the equations for the permeability-limited case (Fa$_{PL}$), the dose and particle size do not appear in the equation, suggesting that Fa does not depend on these

TABLE 5.2   Criteria to Diagnose the Regime of Oral Drug Absorption

Oral Absorption Category	Criteria	Fa
Dissolution rate limited (DRL)	Dn < Pn/Do (If Do < 1, Dn < Pn)	$1 - \exp(-Dn)$
Permeability limited (PL)	Do < 1, Pn < Dn	$1 - \exp(-Pn)$
Solubility-epithelial membrane permeability limited (SL-E)	Do > 1, Pn/Do < Dn, $P'_{ep} < P_{UWL}$	Pn/Do
Solubility-UWL permeability limited (SL-U)	Do > 1, Pn/Do < Dn, $P'_{ep} > P_{UWL}$	Pn/Do

[13]This does not mean that more complicated compartment models such as the S1I7C3 system can give this accuracy. Technically, a more complex model might have an ability to express the complexity of the oral absorption of a drug. However, given the uncertainty in the physiological and drug parameters, as well as the variations in the *in vivo* data, it is difficult to prove the superiority of more complicated systems over a simpler model. The Occam's razor principle should be considered.

parameters. Similarly, in the case of the dissolution-rate-limited case (Fa_{DRL}), the dose does not appear in the equation, whereas the particle size does (cf. $k_{diss} = 3D_{eff}S_{dissolv}/\rho_p r_{p,ini}^2$), suggesting that the dose strength does not affect Fa, whereas the particle size does. In the case of the solubility-permeability-limited case (Fa_{SL}), the dose and permeability appear in the equation, whereas particle size does not, suggesting that the dose and permeability[14,15] affect Fa, whereas the particle size does not.

5.3.7 Approximate Analytical Solution for Oral PK Model

The one-compartment first-order oral PK model is often used to analyze the PK profile. From Equation 5.31,

$$k_{abs} = \frac{1}{k_{diss}} + \frac{Do}{k_{perm}} \quad \text{If } Do < 1, Do = 1 \tag{5.40}$$

$$C_p(t) = \frac{Dose \cdot Fg \cdot Fh}{Vd} \cdot \frac{k_{abs}}{k_{abs} - k_{el}}(\exp(-k_{el}t) - \exp(-k_{abs}t))t < T_{si} \tag{5.41}$$

$$C_p(t) = C_p(T_{si}) \exp(-k_{el}(t - T_{si})) \qquad t > T_{si} \tag{5.42}$$

Equations 5.41 and 5.42 are different from the most often used equation, as Fg Fh is used in the pre-exponential factor instead of F (Fig. 5.16).

5.4 INTEGRATION 2: NUMERICAL INTEGRATION

As discussed earlier, the approximate analytical solution based on the one-compartment GI model is simple, easy to understand, and practically useful for many cases. However, this simple model cannot be used when the effect of the stomach and the colon is not negligible.

For appropriate biopharmaceutical modeling, the GI tract should be divided into at least three compartments, the stomach, the small intestine and the colon, to reflect the significant difference of physiological conditions in these sections. Numerical integration is required to simulate the dynamic change of $C_{dissolv}$ and the regional differences of P_{eff} and $S_{dissolv}$ in the GI tract. In this section, the mathematical treatment to perform numerical integration using multicompartment model is discussed.

---

[14]It is sometimes misunderstood that the permeability of a drug does not affect Fa% in the case of solubility-permeability-limited cases. It is obvious from the analytical solution that the permeability does affect Fa%.

[15]Except in the SL-U cases with high dose (>5 mg/kg) and small particle size (<10 μm). In these cases, the particle drifting effect may increase P_{eff}.

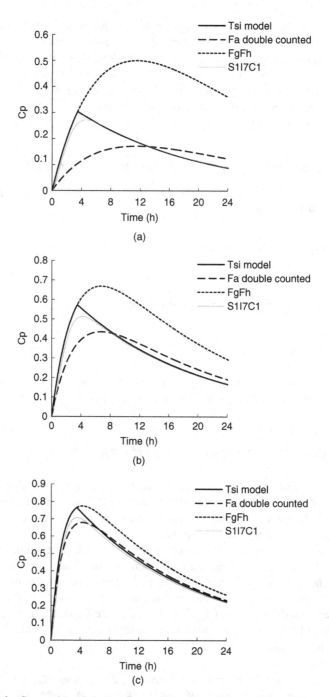

Figure 5.16 Comparison of Equations 5.41 and 5.42 (Tsi model) with the one-compartment model widely used in the literature (Fa double counted or Fa = 1 assumption (i.e., F = 1 × FgFh)), and numerical solution with the S1I7C1 model. (a) Fa = 0.34, (b) Fa = 0.65, and (c) Fa = 0.88.

5.4.1 Virtual Particle Bins

The use of virtual particle bins (VPBs) is the characteristic technical feature of computational biopharmaceutical modeling.

As discussed in Section 3.2.3, to represent the particle size distribution of API particles, a particle size bin (PSB) is assigned to each particle size. Furthermore, to represent the movement of each particle in the GI tract and the particle size reduction accompanied with dissolution, a PSB has to be further divided into VPBs. If the particle size distribution is represented by 20 PSBs and 100 VPBs are assigned to each PSB, a total of 2000 particle bins are required. As each particle group has one differential equation for dissolution, 2000 differential equations are required. However, with today's high speed computers, this number is not an issue. PSB and VPB also serves as the particle identification number.

Similarly, a PSB and a VPB can be assigned to the particles of newly formed API via nucleation (nuclei) as it is generated.

Each particle bin is associated with the data of its particle size, particle number, and the position of the particle in the GI tract (GI position: GIP). The physiological conditions that the VPB experiences, such as pH, bile-micelle concentration, and agitation strength, are used in the dissolution equation of each VPB.

$$\text{GIP(VPB)} = k, \quad k = \text{position in the GI tract} \tag{5.43}$$

$$\frac{dX_{\text{API(PSB,VPB)}}}{dt} = f\left(\text{pH}_{\text{GIP(VPB)}}, C_{\text{bile,GPI(VPB)}}, \varepsilon_{\text{GIP(VPB)}}, r_{\text{p(PSB,VPB)}},\right.$$

$$\left. N_{\text{API(PSB,VPB)}}, \text{others}\right) \tag{5.44}$$

5.4.2 The Mass Balance of Dissolved Drug Amount in Each GI Position

The mass balance of the dissolved drug in the GI fluid at a GI position (subscript k) can be expressed as

$$\frac{dX_{\text{dissolv},k}}{dt} = (K_{t,k-1} \cdot X_{\text{dissolv},k-1} - K_{t,k} \cdot X_{\text{dissolv},k})$$

$$+ \left(\sum_{\text{if GIP(PSB,VPB)}=k} \frac{dX_{\text{API(PSB,VPB)}}}{dt} + \sum_{\text{if GIP(PSB,VPB)}=k} \frac{dX_{\text{NFP(PSB,VPB)}}}{dt} \right)$$

$$- \frac{dX_{\text{perm},k}}{dt} \tag{5.45}$$

where $X_{\text{dissolv},k}$ is the dissolved drug amount at a position k (a compartment). The first parenthesis represents the flow-in of dissolved drug from the previous position and flow-out into the next position. The second parenthesis represents the dissolution and growth of both the dosed API particles (X_{API}) and the newly formed precipitant particles (X_{NFP}). The dissolved (or precipitated) amount from a VPB is added to $X_{dissolv,k}$ of the position where the particle bin is existing (i.e., GIP(VPB)). The last term represents the absorption of the dissolved drug molecules into the body. GIP represents the GI position of a particle bin at time t.

5.4.3 Controlled Release of Virtual Particle Bin

Biopharmaceutical modeling plays an important role in controlled release (CR) formulation development (Section 11.8). The development strategy of the CR formulation and the practical use of biopharmaceutical modeling are discussed in Section 11.8 in detail. Therefore, this section focuses on the computational algorithms to handle CR simulation.

CR can be categorized as prolonged release, timed release, and stimuli-triggered release. The release profile can simply be modeled by coupling a conditional binary function for each VPB with the dissolution equation.

$$CR(j) = (0 \text{ or } 1) \tag{5.46}$$

The binary function can be written by "if–then" syntax in the program. For pH triggered release,

"If pH(GIP(VPB)) < 5.5 then CR(VPB) = 1, else CR(VPB) = 0"

Similarly, for the GI position-specific release (such as colon targeting),

"If GIP(VPB) > 9 then CR(VPB) = 1, else CR(VPB) = 0"

For timed release,

"If t > 2 h then CR(VPB) = 1, else CR(VPB) = 0"

This can be expanded to any time-scheduled CR, for example, zero-order release and Weibull functional release.

Usually, the CR formulation is formulated as pellets, a tablet, or a capsule. The gastric empting patterns for these formulations are different from that of small particles (<0.5 mm) and depends on the MMC (Section 6.2). A timed gastric empting with the MMC phase III can be programmed by assigning the dosing timing during the MMC cycle (Section 5.2.1).

5.5 *IN VIVO* FA FROM PK DATA

Clinical Fa% data are required to validate biopharmaceutical modeling. However, there is no absolute method to obtain clinical Fa% from the clinical PK data. Usually, we have to put one or a few assumptions to calculate clinical Fa%. Therefore, it is preferable to compare the Fa% values if two or more methods are available.

5.5.1 Absolute Bioavailability and Fa

Absolute bioavailability (F or BA%) can be obtained from AUC ratio of i.v. and the other route (e.g., oral). Normalization by dose strength is often used assuming a linear PK profile. To avoid the effect of nonlinearity, the C_p levels from the i.v. and the other route should be set similar.

$$F = \frac{AUC_{other}/Dose_{other}}{AUC_{i.v.}/Dose_{i.v.}} \tag{5.47}$$

In the case of oral absorption, F is a composite parameter of the fraction of a dose absorbed (Fa), the fraction not metabolized in the gut wall (Fg), and the fraction not metabolized in the liver (Fh).

$$F = Fa \cdot Fg \cdot Fh \tag{5.48}$$

Therefore, to calculate Fa from F, Fh and Fg data are required. Fg can be roughly estimated from *in vitro* data or $CL_{h,int}$ (for CYP3A4 substrates) (Section 4.10). Fh can be calculated from the total clearance and urinary excretion percent (Ur%) after i.v. administration (assuming only the liver and kidney contribute the clearance).

$$Fh = 1 - \frac{CL_{tot}(1 - Ur)}{Q_h} \tag{5.49}$$

This method is often used to estimate Fa% from i.v. and p.o. data. However, this method has some deviation from the authentic Fa% data obtained using radio-labeled drug [24].

5.5.2 Relative Bioavailability Between Solid and Solution Formulations

Relative bioavailability of a solid formulation against a solution formulation can be used as a surrogate for Fa% in the case of BCS class II drugs. As a BCS class II drug has a high permeability, Fa% would be 100% after solution administration.[16] High permeability can be assessed by *in vitro* membrane permeation assays (e.g., Caco-2) or simply from log P_{oct}, MW, and pK_a. Fa% can be calculated as the ratio of AUCs from a solid dosage form to a solution dosage form ($AUC_{solid\ formulation}$ and $AUC_{solution}$, respectively).

$$Fa = \frac{AUC_{solid\ formlation}}{AUC_{solution}} \tag{5.50}$$

---

[16]Absence of precipitation should be assessed by *in vitro* experiments using a biorelevant media.

In this equation, the effect of Fg and Fh on AUC is cancelled out. Therefore, Fa% obtained by this method is free from the uncertainty in these parameters.[17]

When the Do in the fed state is less than 1 (and dissolution is rapid), the AUC in the fed state can be used as a surrogate for $AUC_{solution}$. If the food has little or no effect on the AUC of a drug from a solubility-enhancing formulation such as emulsion and solid dispersion, it is highly probable that Fa% from the formulation is nearly 100%.

5.5.3 Relative Bioavailability Between Low and High Dose

In preclinical and clinical studies, a dose escalation study is usually performed. In many cases, at lower doses, the Do is less than 1 (or dosed as a solution formulation). If we assume that clearance and volume of distribution (V_d) of the drug is concentration independent, we can use this data to calculate Fa% for high permeability cases. In many cases, it is unlikely that the V_d becomes concentration dependent (except the case there is specific systemic binding site). However, CL could be concentration dependent especially at an extremely high dose. From the elimination half-life (k_{el}), the change in clearance can be estimated. By assuming V_d being constant, Fa can be calculated as [25]

$$Fa = \frac{AUC_{high\ dose} \cdot CL_{high\ dose}}{AUC_{low\ dose} \cdot CL_{low\ dose}} \cdot \frac{Dose_{low}}{Dose_{high}} = \frac{AUC_{high\ dose} \cdot k_{el,high\ dose}}{AUC_{low} \cdot k_{el,low\ dose}} \cdot \frac{Dose_{low}}{Dose_{high}}$$

(5.51)

where the subscripts high and low indicate the parameters obtained at high and low dose strengths, respectively.

5.5.4 Convolution and Deconvolution

Deconvolution is often used to calculate F as a time course function (i.e., $F(t)$), typically from i.v. and p.o. data. Various commercial programs as well as free programs are available to perform deconvolution. The Loo–Riegelman, Nelson–Wagner, and numerical deconvolution methods are most widely used. In many textbooks, the convolution equation is given as trivial, and the deconvolution is explained via Laplace transformation. However, the concept of convolution is actually not trivial and Laplace transformation is not easy to understand. In this section, the concept of convolution and deconvolution is briefly discussed in an illustrative manner. To enhance the understanding of the concept, the mathematical expression is simplified. The readers should refer to the original publication for accurate equations [26–29].

---

[17]Assessment of high/low permeability category by Caco-2 is more reliable than Fh and Fg estimation (so it is used even for the regulatory purposes).

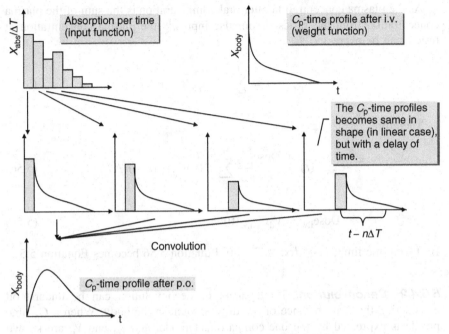

Figure 5.17   Schematic explanation of the convolution process.

5.5.4.1 *Convolution.*

When the pharmacokinetics in the body is linear, the plasma concentration at time t after oral administration ($C_{p,p.o.}(t)$) can be written as convolution of input function (F) and weight function ($C_{p,i.v.}(t)$).

$$C_{p,p.o.}(t) = \frac{\text{Dose}_{p.o.}}{\text{Dose}_{i.v.}} \int_0^t F(\tau) C_{p,i.v.}(t - \tau) \, d\tau \tag{5.52}$$

Figure 5.17 shows the schematic explanation of this convolution process. Equation 5.52 can be derived as follows. The oral absorption of a drug can be treated as the series of impulse inputs into the body. After an impulse input from the intestine, the elimination time course of the drug follows the same pattern as that of i.v. administration. The C_p time profile after ith impulse is

$$C_{p,p.o.,i}(t) V_d = \text{Dose}_{p.o.} F(i) \frac{C_{p,i.v.}(t - i\,\Delta T)}{C_{p,i.v.}(0)} \tag{5.53}$$

where $\text{Dose}_{p.o.} F(i)$ represents the fraction of a dose input to the body by the ith impulse.

By integrating this equation,

$$V_d \sum_0^i C_{p,p.o.,i}(t - i\,\Delta T) = \frac{\text{Dose}_{p.o.}}{C_{p,i.v.}(0)} \sum_0^i F(i) C_{p,i.v.}(t - i\,\Delta T) \tag{5.54}$$

As the plasma concentration after oral administration is the sum of the plasma concentration from the series of impulse inputs,[18] the plasma concentration at time t can be expressed as

$$C_{p,p.o.}(t) = \sum_{0}^{n} C_{p,p.o.,i}(t - n\Delta T) \qquad (5.55)$$

Therefore,

$$C_{p,p.o.}(t) = \frac{\text{Dose}_{p.o.}}{\text{Dose}_{i.v.}} \sum_{0}^{n} F(n) C_{p,i.v.}(t - n\Delta T) \qquad (5.56)$$

$$\text{Dose}_{i.v.} = V_d C_{p,i.v.}(0) \qquad (5.57)$$

By taking the limit, $i \to d\infty$, $\Delta T \to 0$, Equation 5.56 becomes Equation 5.52.

5.5.4.2 Deconvolution. The concept of deconvolution can be understood considering the mass balance of the drug amount in the body. When a C_p time profile is expressed by the one-compartment model and k_{el} and V_d are known from the i.v. data, the mass balance of the drug amount in the body at time t can be written as

$$V_d \frac{dC_p}{dt} = \frac{dX_{abs}}{dt} - k_{el} C_p V_d \qquad (5.58)$$

By rearranging this equation,

$$\frac{dX_{abs}}{dt} = V_d \frac{dC_p}{dt} + k_{el} C_p V_d \qquad (5.59)$$

Table 5.3 explains the stepwise deconvolution process based on this equation. In the first 1 min, the drug amount in the body (X_{body}) increased from 0 to 0.0198. At time $t = 0$ min, the elimination rate is 0. Therefore, the absorbed amount from 0 to 1 min is 0.0198. In the next 1 min, the net increase of X_{body} (left-hand side of Equation 5.58) can be calculated from the C_p time profile (In Table 5.3, it is 0.0192 (from 0.0198 to 0.0390). At time 1 min, the elimination rate is 0.0000988 ($= k_{el} \times C_p \times V_d$). Therefore, the drug amount supplied from the intestine into the plasma (dX_{abs}/t) is $0.0192 + 0.0000988$.

Another simple approach to understand the deconvolution would be reversing the convolution process by the stair case method [30]. As discussed in the convolution cases, the drug absorption from the intestine is represented as a series

---

[18]This is from the assumption of linear PK.

TABLE 5.3   Stepwise Deconvolution Process

Time, min	Observed C_p C_p (p.o.)	Deconvolution process (1) $V_d \times dC_p$	(2) $k_{el} \times V_d \times C_p$	(1) + (2)	Fa (Deconvolution)
0	0.0000 (A)	0.0198 (C) = $V_d \times ((B) - (A))$	0.0000 (D) = $V_d \times (A) \times k_{el}$	0.0198(E) = (C)+ (D)	0.0198 (F)
1	0.0198 (B)	0.0193(H) = $V_d \times ((G) - (B))$	0.0001(I) = $V_d \times (B) \times k_{el}$	0.0194(J) = (H) + (I)	0.0391(K) = (F) + (J)
2	0.0390 (G)	0.0188(M) = $V_d \times ((L) - (G))$	0.0002(N) = $V_d \times (G) \times k_{el}$	0.0190 (O) = (M) + (N)	0.0581 (P) = (K) + (O)
3	0.0578 (L)	0.0183	0.0003	0.0186	0.0767

$k_{el} = 0.005, V_d = 1.$

of impulse input. To simplify the equation, the nth pulse input ($I(n)$) and $C_{p,i.v.}$ ratio at time t against time 0 are defined as

$$A(n) \equiv \frac{C_{p,i.v.}(n\Delta T)}{C_{p,i.v.}(0)}$$

$$I(n) \equiv \text{Dose}_{p.o.}(F(n\Delta T) - F((n-1)\Delta T)) \tag{5.60}$$

The drug amount in the body at time $t = n\Delta T$ then becomes

$$X_{\text{body}}((n+1)\Delta T) = I(1)A(n+1) + I(2)A(n)$$
$$+ \cdots + I(n-1)A(1) + I(n)A(0) \tag{5.61}$$

By rearranging this equation,

$$I(n) = \frac{X_{\text{body,p.o.}}((n+1)\Delta T) - (I(1)A(n+1) + I(2)A(n-1)}{A(0)} \\ \frac{+ \cdots + I(n-2)A(2) + I(n-1)A(1))}{A(0)} \tag{5.62}$$

This is the reverse process of convolution. Starting with $n = 0$, $I(n)$ can be calculated in a step-by-step manner. In the stair case method, the i.v. pharmacokinetics is not model dependent and does not have to assume first-order kinetics. In reality, the experimental sampling time point is not equally distributed. Therefore, the time points between the experimental sampling time points have to be interpolated.

5.6 OTHER ADMINISTRATION ROUTES

5.6.1 Skin

In the case of skin permeation, the permeability coefficient can be described by the solubility–diffusion model, so that by the partition coefficient and the diffusion coefficient of a drug in the permeation barrier. Drugs permeate through the intercellular part of the stratum corneum (SC) that is mainly consist of ceramide (CER), cholesterol (CHO), and free fatty acid (FFA). These components organize a lamellar structure (cf. Fig. 6.28, the brick and mortar model). The octanol/water partition coefficient is most often used as a surrogate for the partition coefficient into the SC (K_{sc}) [31–33]. K_{sc} can be calculated as

$$\log K_{sc} = -0.024 + 0.59 \log P_{oct} \tag{5.63}$$

The regression coefficient of $\log P_{oct}$ was 0.59, indicating that the skin membrane permeation barrier is more polar than octanol or a partial desolvation of the solute caused by the water associated with the ceramide polar head group. The diffusion coefficient was found to decrease as the molecular weight and/or the hydrogen bond acidity/basicity increase. This finding is consistent with diffusion along a nonpolar pathway hindered by interaction with the immobilized polar head groups of the SC lipids.

REFERENCES

1. Takano, R., Sugano, K., Higashida, A., Hayashi, Y., Machida, M., Aso, Y., Yamashita, S. (2006). Oral absorption of poorly water-soluble drugs: computer simulation of fraction absorbed in humans from a miniscale dissolution test. *Pharm. Res.*, 23, 1144–1156.

2. Takano, R., Furumoto, K., Shiraki, K., Takata, N., Hayashi, Y., Aso, Y., Yamashita, S. (2008). Rate-limiting steps of oral absorption for poorly water-soluble drugs in dogs; prediction from a miniscale dissolution test and a physiologically-based computer simulation. *Pharm. Res.*, 25, 2334–2344.

3. Takano, R., Takata, N., Saitoh, R., Furumoto, K., Higo, S., Hayashi, Y., Machida, M., Aso, Y., Yamashita, S. (2010). Quantitative analysis of the effect of supersaturation on *in vivo* drug absorption. *Mol. Pharmaceutics*, 7, 1431–1440.

4. Sugano, K. (2011). Fraction of a dose absorbed estimation for structurally diverse low solubility compounds. *Int. J. Pharm.*, 405, 79–89.

5. Dressman, J.B., Fleisher, D. (1986). Mixing-tank model for predicting dissolution rate control or oral absorption. *J. Pharm. Sci.*, 75, 109–116.

6. Johnson, K.C. (2003). Dissolution and absorption modeling: model expansion to simulate the effects of precipitation, water absorption, longitudinally changing intestinal permeability, and controlled release on drug absorption. *Drug Dev. Ind. Pharm.*, 29, 833–842.

7. Oh, D.M., Curl, R.L., Amidon, G.L. (1993). Estimating the fraction dose absorbed from suspensions of poorly soluble compounds in humans: a mathematical model. *Pharm. Res.*, 10, 264–270.

8. Yu, L.X., Lipka, E., Crison, J.R., Amidon, G.L. (1996). Transport approaches to the biopharmaceutical design of oral drug delivery systems: prediction of intestinal absorption. *Adv. Drug Delivery Rev.*, 19, 359–376.

9. Yu, L.X., Amidon, G.L. (1998). Characterization of small intestinal transit time distribution in humans. *Int. J. Pharm.*, 171, 157–163.

10. Yu, L.X. (1999). An integrated model for determining causes of poor oral drug absorption. *Pharm. Res.*, 16, 1883–1887.

11. Sawamoto, T., Haruta, S., Kurosaki, Y., Higaki, K., Kimura, T. (1997). Prediction of the plasma concentration profiles of orally administered drugs in rats on the basis of gastrointestinal transit kinetics and absorbability. *J. Pharm. Pharmacol.*, 49, 450–457.

12. Haruta, S., Iwasaki, N., Ogawara, K.I., Higaki, K., Kimura, T. (1998). Absorption behavior of orally administered drugs in rats treated with propantheline. *J. Pharm. Sci.*, 87, 1081–1085.

13. Fujioka, Y., Kadono, K., Fujie, Y., Metsugi, Y., Ogawara, K.I., Higaki, K., Kimura, T. (2007). Prediction of oral absorption of griseofulvin, a BCS class II drug, based on GITA model: Utilization of a more suitable medium for in-vitro dissolution study. *J. Controlled Release*, 119, 222–228.

14. Fujioka, Y., Metsugi, Y., Ogawara, K.I., Higaki, K., Kimura, T. (2008). Evaluation of *in vivo* dissolution behavior and GI transit of griseofulvin, a BCS class II drug. *Int. J. Pharm.*, 352, 36–43.

15. http://www.simcyp.com.

16. Sugano, K. (2009). Introduction to computational oral absorption simulation. *Expert Opin. Drug Metab. Toxicol.*, 5, 259–293.

17. Ni, P.F., Ho, N.F.H., Fox, J.L., Leuenberger, H., Higuchi, W.I. (1980). Theoretical model studies of intestinal drug absorption. V. Non-steady-state fluid flow and absorption. *Int. J. Pharm.*, 5, 33–47.

18. Willmann, S., Schmitt, W., Keldenich, J., Dressman, J.B. (2003). A physiologic model for simulating gastrointestinal flow and drug absorption in rats. *Pharm. Res.*, 20, 1766–1771.

19. Willmann, S., Schmitt, W., Keldenich, J., Lippert, J., Dressman, J.B. (2004). A physiological model for the estimation of the fraction dose absorbed in humans. *J. Med. Chem.*, 47, 4022–4031.

20. Clarysse, S., Psachoulias, D., Brouwers, J., Tack, J., Annaert, P., Duchateau, G., Reppas, C., Augustijns, P. (2009). Postprandial changes in solubilizing capacity of human intestinal fluids for BCS class II drugs. *Pharm. Res.*, 26, 1456–1466.

21. Johnson, K.C., Swindell, A.C. (1996). Guidance in the setting of drug particle size specifications to minimize variability in absorption. *Pharm. Res.*, 13, 1795–1798.

22. Avdeef, A., High-throughput solubility, permeability, and the MAD PAMPA model, in: B. Testa, S. Krämer, H. Wunderli-Allenspach, G. Folkers (Eds.) *Pharmacokinetic Profiling in Drug Research*, Wiley-VCH, Zurich, 2006. pp. 221–241.

23. Sugano, K. (2009). Fraction of dose absorbed calculation: comparison between analytical solution based on one compartment steady state approximation and dynamic seven compartment model. *CBI J.*, 9, 75–93.

24. Nomeir, A.A., Morrison, R., Prelusky, D., Korfmacher, W., Broske, L., Hesk, D., McNamara, P., Mei, H. (2009). Estimation of the extent of oral absorption in animals from oral and intravenous pharmacokinetic data in drug discovery. *J. Pharm. Sci.*, 98, 4027–4038.

25. Wagner, J.G. (1967). Method of estimating relative absorption of a drug in a series of clinical studies in which blood levels are measured after single and/or multiple doses. *J. Pharm. Sci.*, 56, 652–653.

26. Loo, J.C., Riegelman, S. (1968). New method for calculating the intrinsic absorption rate of drugs. *J. Pharm. Sci.*, 57, 918–928.

27. Wagner, J.G. (1974). Application of the Wagner-Nelson absorption method to the two-compartment open model. *J. Pharmacokinet Biopharm*, 2, 469–486.

28. Wagner, J.G. (1975). Application of the Loo-Riegelman absorption method. *J. Pharmacokinet Biopharm*, 3, 51–67.

29. Wagner, J.G., Nelson, E. (1963). Per cent absorbed time plots derived from blood level and/or urinary excretion data. *J. Pharm. Sci.*, 52, 610–611.

30. Vaughan, D.P., Dennis, M. (1978). Mathematical basis of point-area deconvolution method for determining in vivo input functions. *J. Pharm. Sci.*, 67, 663–665.

31. Pugh, W.J., Degim, I.T., Hadgraft, J. (2000). Epidermal permeability-penetrant structure relationships: 4, QSAR of permeant diffusion across human stratum corneum

in terms of molecular weight, H-bonding and electronic charge. *Int. J. Pharm.*, 197, 203–211.

32. Pugh, W.J., Roberts, M.S., Hadgraft, J. (1996). Epidermal permeability—penetrant structure relationships: 3. The effect o f hydrogen bonding interactions and molecular size on diffusion across the stratum corneum. *Int. J. Pharm.*, 138, 149–165.

33. Potts, R.O., Guy, R.H. (1992). Predicting skin permeability. *Pharm. Res.*, 9, 663–669.

CHAPTER 6

PHYSIOLOGY OF GASTROINTESTINAL TRACT AND OTHER ADMINISTRATION SITES IN HUMANS AND ANIMALS

"Animals, whom we have made our slaves, we do not like to consider our equal."
—Charles Darwin

It is critically important to use accurate physiological data in biopharmaceutical modeling. The GI physiology has been summarized in many excellent reviews [1–10]. The data presented in this chapter is recompiled from these reviews. Therefore, particular reference is not indicated for each data unless otherwise it is quoted from a specific reference.

6.1 MORPHOLOGY OF GASTROINTESTINAL TRACT

6.1.1 Length and Tube Radius

The tube radius of the small intestine (R_{GI}) is ca. 1.5–2 cm in humans, 0.5 cm in dogs, and 0.2 cm in rats. In monkeys, the intestinal radius ranges from 0.4 cm (cynomolgus monkey) [11] to 0.8 cm (rhesus monkey). In humans, the tube radius of the small intestine decreases while descending the small intestine, from ca. 1.7 cm in the upper intestine to ca. 1.0 at the end of the small intestine.

These differences cause the differences in the surface–volume ratio (SA_{GI}/V_{GI}) (Section 4.4). The permeation rate coefficient (k_{perm}) becomes larger as the intestinal radius becomes smaller, even when the effective intestinal

Biopharmaceutics Modeling and Simulations: Theory, Practice, Methods, and Applications,
First Edition. Kiyohiko Sugano.
© 2012 John Wiley & Sons, Inc. Published 2012 by John Wiley & Sons, Inc.

membrane permeability (P_{eff}) is the same (cf. $k_{perm} = 2/R_{GI} \times DF \times P_{eff}$). This species difference in the intestinal tube radius is canceled out by the difference in P_{eff} (caused by the differences in the fold and villi structures), resulting in similar k_{perm} and Fa% values between animals and humans in case of passive transcellular and UWL-limited permeation (Section 13.5.1).

The postmortem anatomical length of the human small intestine is ca. 680 cm. The living physiological length is ca. 282 cm. The length of the duodenum, jejunum, and ileum is 21, 105, and 156 cm, respectively.

In contrast to humans, the portion of ileum in the small intestine is very small in rats and dogs, ca. 2% and 4%, respectively (Table 6.1).

6.1.2 Surface Area

6.1.2.1 Small Intestine. In humans, the surface area of the small intestine is expanded by the fold (plicae, $\times 3$), villi ($\times 10$), and microvilli ($\times 20$) (Fig. 6.1; Table 6.2). On the basis of the smooth surface geometry, the surface area of the small intestine is ca. 3000 cm^2. The surface area is expanded to 10,000, 100,000, and 2,000,000 cm^2 by the fold, villi, and microvilli structures, respectively. However, drug particles are inhomogeneously distributed along the small intestine and the intestinal surface is not fully exposed to the drug. Dogs and rats lack the fold structure.

Figure 6.2 shows the structure of villi. Rats have shorter villi length than dogs and humans. As the effective intestinal membrane permeability (P_{eff}) is defined on the basis of the smooth tube surface, the morphological differences of the fold and the villi are one of the reasons for the species differences in P_{eff}. These morphological differences decrease P_{eff} threefold in dogs (except for paracellular permeants[1]) and sixfold in rats compared to that in humans. Monkeys have plicate and villi structure; however, the surface area information is not available. In monkeys, the P_{eff} values of several UWL-limited permeation drugs are ca. threefold lower than those in humans [11], suggesting that the surface area expansion by the plicate structure might be less significant in monkeys. Caco-2 cells do not have the fold and villi structures but have a microvilli structure.

TABLE 6.1 Percentage of Length of Small Intestinal Parts[a]

	Human, %	Dog, %	Rat, %
Duodenum	4	6	8
Jejunum	38	90	90
Ileum	58	4	2

[a]Reference 3.

[1]In one commercial software (as of 2011), the P_{eff} value of any drug in dogs is assumed to be threefold larger than that in humans regardless of the permeation pathway of the drug. However, this assumption is not valid for the transcellular and UWL-controlled cases, in which, the P_{eff} in dogs is threefold lower than that in humans.

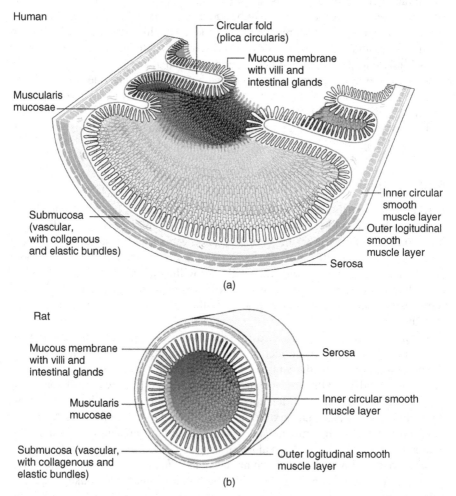

Figure 6.1 Structure of the small intestine in humans and rats. *Source:* Adapted from Reference 2 with permission.

TABLE 6.2 Surface Expansion by Plicae and Villi

	Human	Dog	Rabbit	Rat
Plicae (PE; small intestine)	3	1	1	1
Villi (VE; small intestine)	10	10	5.7	5
Microvilli (small intestine)	20	25	24	20
DF (small intestine)	1.7	—	—	—
DF (colon)	5.3	—	—	—

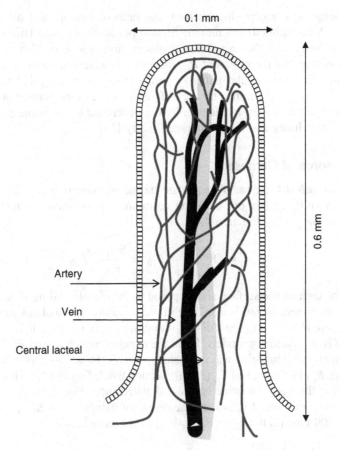

Figure 6.2   Structure of the villi [12].

Therefore, the epithelial membrane permeability (P_{app}) in the Caco-2 models is ca. 30-fold smaller than the human P_{eff} value in case of epithelial-membrane-limited permeation.[2]

6.1.2.2   Colon. The effective permeability of a drug in the colon is usually lower than that in the small intestine due to the lack of both plicate and villi structures in the colon. The ratio of the available surface area is ca. 1:30 in humans (colon/small intestine).

In rats, both the small intestine and colon lack the plicate structure. The villi expansion was ca. fivefold in the rat intestine, whereas no villi exist in the

---

[2]This cannot be applied for the UWL permeation cases. The UWL thickness of the _in vitro_ planner membrane system is 5- to 10-fold thicker than that of the _in vivo_ intestine. The apparent permeability (P_{app}) of an _in vitro_ assay, which is usually reported in the literature, is the composite parameter of the UWL permeability (P_{UWL}) and epithelial membrane permeability (P_{ep}) as $1/P_{app} = 1/P_{ep} + 1/P_{UWL}$.

colon. Using these morphological data, the ratio of colonic and intestinal P_{eff} becomes 1:5 for epithelial-membrane-limited permeation cases. This value is in good agreement with the experimental observations (Section 13.6.1). It would be worth noting that the observed P_{eff} ratio values were similar between passive transcellular and paracellular pathway permeations, suggesting that the relative P_{eff} ratio is mainly determined by the difference between the surface areas of the small intestine and colon, rather than by the difference between the pore size of paracellular pathway and the membrane fluidity [13].

6.1.3 Degree of Flatness

6.1.3.1 Small Intestine. To calculate the permeation rate coefficient (k_{perm}) of a drug from P_{eff}, either one of the two combinations of information is required, DF–R_{GI} or SA$_{GI}$–V_{GI} (Section 4.4).

$$k_{perm} = DF \cdot \frac{2}{R_{GI}} \cdot P_{eff} = \frac{SA_{GI}}{V_{GI}} \cdot P_{eff} \tag{6.1}$$

Neither the data on the surface area exposed to the dissolved drug (SA$_{GI}$) nor the direct measurement of DF is available in the literature. In this book and most of the commercial software, the DF–R_{GI} combination is used, as it is compatible with the GI compartment models. From the experimental P_{eff}, and Fa% data, DF of the human small intestine was estimated to be 1.7 (Fa = $1 - \exp(-2DF/R_{GI} \times P_{eff} \times T_{si})$, R_{GI} (1.5 cm), and T_{si} (3.5 h); Section 8.4.1; Figure 8.2). This DF value denotes that the small intestine is like a deflated tube (Fig. 4.3). From the fluid volume in the intestine (130 ml) and the degree of flatness (1.7), SA$_{GI}$ is estimated to be ca. 300 cm^2 ($2DF/R_{GI} = SA_{GI}/V_{GI}$) in the fasted state.

6.1.3.2 Colon. Owing to the substantial residence time in the ascending colon and the limited free water volume in the transverse and descending colon, the primary region of interest with regard to drug/dosage form performance in the lower gut is the ascending colon [14].

Owing to the lack of the colon P_{eff} data in humans, we were not able to obtain DF value in humans from the Fa–P_{eff} relationship. However, the DF of the human ascending colon (DF$_{AC}$)[3] can be estimated from the relative Fa% of drugs with low permeability from the small intestine and the colon, using the following equation:

$$\frac{Fa_{AC}}{Fa_{SI}} = \frac{2DF_{AC}/R_{GI,AC}}{2DF_{SI}/R_{GI,SI}} \frac{P_{eff,AC}T_{si}}{P_{eff,SI}T_{AC}} \tag{6.2}$$

Considering the lack of villi and plicae in the colon (10- and 3-fold expansion, respectively), if we assume that the difference in the P_{eff} is due to its surface

[3]The subscripts AC and SI indicate the ascending colon and the small intestine, respectively.

area,[4] $P_{eff,AC}/P_{eff,SI}$ should be 1:30 in humans in case of epithelial membrane permeability. The radius of the small intestine and colon is 1.5 and 2.5 cm and the transit times are 3.5 and 13 h, respectively. The average of the observed relative Fa (Fa_{AC}/Fa_{SI}) for BCS class III compounds ($Fa_{oral}\% < 70\%$) was 0.29 ± 0.13 ($n = 10$) (including all charges (neutral, positive, and negative) and wide MW range (217–538)) [15]. When limited to the passive transcellular permeation of neutral compounds, which would not be affected by the possible difference of the paracellular pathway and pH, the observed Fa_{AC}/Fa_{SI} was 0.24 ($n = 2$). DF_{SI} is 1.7. From these data and Equation 6.2, DF_{AC} was estimated to be 5.3.

This high DF value in the colon compared to the small intestine may be due to the small fluid volume in the colon (15 ml) spread on the colonic wall (Section 6.3.1) [14].

6.1.4 Epithelial Cells

The intestinal epithelial membrane consists of intestinal epithelial cells tightly connected each other (Fig. 4.1). The tight junction restricts the lateral diffusion of the membrane components. The apical side has a microvilli structure. However, the surface area ratio of the apical and basolateral sides was measured to be ca. 1–3 [16], probably because the tight junction exists close to the apical side and the most part of the side face of the cell contacts the basolateral space.

Drug molecules can permeate across the layer of the epithelial membrane via the cellular membrane (transcellular) and the tight junction (paracellular). Transcellular permeation of most drugs occurs mainly by passive diffusion, but some drugs permeate the membrane mediated by a carrier protein(s) (transporter). In addition, drugs can be metabolized in the enterocyte (intestinal first-pass metabolism). Transporters and metabolic enzymes in the intestinal epithelial cells are discussed in Section 6.4.

6.1.4.1 *Apical and Basolateral Lipid Bilayer Membranes.* Typical lipid components of biological membranes are shown in Figure 6.3. Phosphatidylcholine (PC) and phosphatidylethanolamine (PE) are zwitterionic phospholipids with zero net charge at neutral pH. Phosphatidylserine (PS) has two negatively charged moieties (pK_a on the membrane, carboxylate ($pK_a = 5.5$) and phosphate ($pK_a < 1$)) and one positively charged moiety (amine ($pK_a = 11.3$)), with a net charge of -1. Phosphatidylinositol (PI) and phosphatidylglycerol (PG) have one negatively charged moiety (phosphate ($pK_a = 2.7$ (PI), 2.9 (PG))). The lipid bilayer of the intestinal epithelial cells contains significant amount of anionic phospholipids (Table 6.3) [17, 18]. The distribution of negatively charged lipid is nearly symmetrical in the intestinal brush border membrane, which is in contrast to the red blood cells (Table 6.4) [19, 20].

---

[4]This assumption is validated by the $P_{eff,AC}/P_{eff,SI}$ ratio in rats, which is ca. 0.2 as this value is in good agreement with the fivefold surface expansion by villi and plicae in the small intestine in rats (Table 13.1).

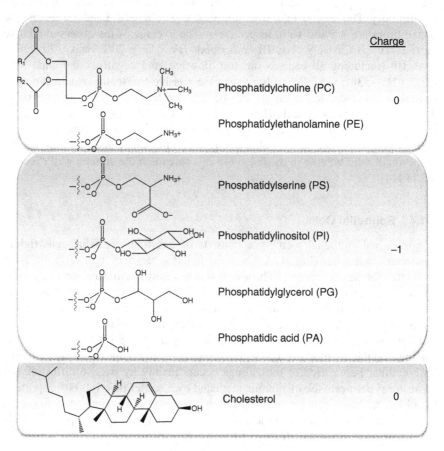

Figure 6.3 Chemical structure of lipid bilayer components.

TABLE 6.3 Lipid Bilayer Component

Lipid	Brush Border Membrane (Rat)	Caco-2	Egg Lecithin	Soybean Lecithin
PC	20	53	73	24
PE	18	19	11	18
PS	6	17	—	—
PI	7	8	1	12
Sphingomyelin	7	3	—	—
CHO	37	—	—	—
Triglyceride	—	—	13	37

TABLE 6.4 Inner and Outer Leaflet Distribution of Lipid Component

	Rabbit Intestinal Brush Border		Red Blood Cell	
Lipids	Outer Layer, %	Inner Layer, %	Outer Layer, %	Inner Layer, %
PC	32	68	76	24
PE	34	66	20	80
PS	44	56	0	100
PI	40	60	—	—
Sphingomyelin	—	—	82	18

A lipid bilayer is a heterogeneous system that can be roughly divided into four regions (Fig. 6.4), although the boundary of each region is not explicit [21, 22].

- Low Density Head Group Region. This region ranges from the point where the membrane begins to perturbate the bulk water structure to the point where the water density and head group density are comparable. This region can be large because the perturbation of water molecules can extend over a long range.
- High Density Head Group Region. This region is ca. 7.5 Å wide. In this region, bulk water structure no longer exists. It has a high dielectric constant (ε = ca. 30) and high viscosity and is abundant in hydrogen bond acceptors.
- High Density Tail Region. This region is ca. 7 Å wide. It has a low dielectric constant and high viscosity. The hydrocarbon tail has a high density and is highly ordered. The region is considered to resemble a soft polymer.
- Low Density Tail Region. This region is ca. 11 Å wide (both halves of the bilayer). It has a low dielectric constant (ε = ca. 2) and low viscosity. This region is considered to resemble a low density alkane fluid, such as dodecane or hexadecane.

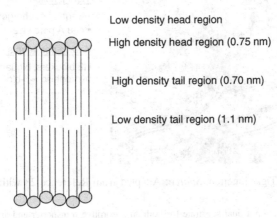

Low density head region

High density head region (0.75 nm)

High density tail region (0.70 nm)

Low density tail region (1.1 nm)

Figure 6.4 Regions of lipid bilayer.

Drug molecules diffuse through the lipid bilayer, depending on the physicochemical property of a drug, especially lipophilicity. Unlike the carrier-protein-mediated transport, passive diffusion is not structure specific. Therefore, the passive diffusion is, and will continue to be,[5] the main permeation mechanism for most drugs.

6.1.4.2 Tight Junction. The epithelial cells of the GI tract are tightly connected by cell adhesion proteins such as occludens [23]. The apparent pore radius of the tight junction is ca. 6 Å in humans and 9 Å in dogs [24–26]. The pore radius of the tight junction of Caco-2 cells has a large laboratory to laboratory variation [27], and therefore, it should be measured in each laboratory. In many cases, it is smaller than that in humans. The tight junction is negatively charged with 70 mV in humans [24] and 17 mV in Caco-2 cells (Fig. 6.5) [28, 29]. Owing to this negative charge, a positively charged molecule is more permeable than a negatively charged molecule (Fig. 4.14). Masaoka et al. [13] reported that the effective pore sizes of the paracellular pathway were similar between the small intestine and the colon.

Recent quantitative assessments suggested that paracellular permeation is more significant than it was originally thought for drug absorption [24, 30–33]. Many drugs such as H2 blockers and β-blockers permeate this pathway significantly. As shown in Figure 4.14, in the case of basic drugs of MW up to 350, this route can contribute an Fa% more than 30%, which is sufficient to launch on the market.

6.1.4.3 Mucous Layer. The mucous layer exists adjacent to the epithelial cells (Fig. 6.6). Figure 6.7 shows the structure of the mucous layer [34]. The mucous layer is thought to maintain the UWL and microclimate pH. The mucous

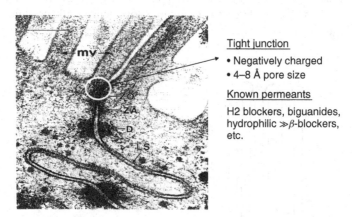

Figure 6.5 Tight junction. *Source*: Adapted from Reference 28 with permission.

[5]It is difficult to design a dual substrate for both an absorptive transporter and an pharmacological target, as the substrate specificity of the former tends to be narrow and selective.

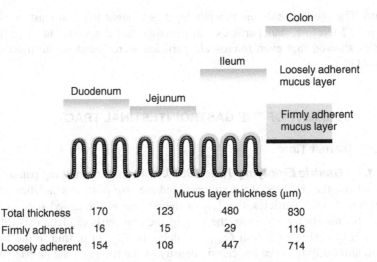

Figure 6.6 A schematic figure showing the thickness of the mucous gel layers *in vivo* [36].

		Mucus layer thickness (μm)		
Total thickness	170	123	480	830
Firmly adherent	16	15	29	116
Loosely adherent	154	108	447	714

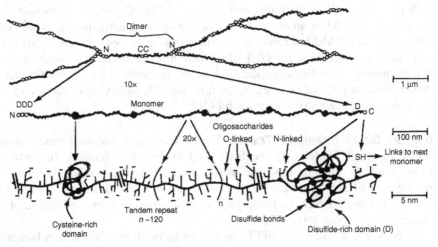

Figure 6.7 Structure of the mucous layer. *Source:* Adapted from Reference 34 with permission.

layer is divided into two regions, the firmly adhered and loosely bound regions [35, 36]. The loosely bound mucus can be wiped away by the luminal fluid flow. In places where intestinal chyme wipes away the mucous blanket, the glycocalyx (0.5 μm thick) forms the final barrier that can prevent pathogens and drug delivery particles from adhering to the epithelial cell surface. The secretion of mucus is rapid, and the mucous layer grows ca. 1 μm/s in the rat small intestine [36].

The mucin fibers that form mucous gel are long flexible strings densely coated with short glycans, most of which are functionalized with a carboxyl or sulfate group. The mesh size of the mucous layer is thought to be at least greater than 0.4 μm. Therefore, nanoparticles can penetrate to the mucous layer [34]. Many studies showed that even microscale particles were found in the mucous layer [37–41].

6.2 MOVEMENT OF THE GASTROINTESTINAL TRACT

6.2.1 Transit Time

6.2.1.1 Gastric Emptying Time (GET). The gastric emptying pattern largely depends on the contents of the stomach and the size of the formulation [42]. For liquids and small particles, the $T_{1/2}$ of the content in the fasted state in humans is ca. 10 min. In the fed state, the $T_{1/2}$ of the content is ca. 1 h. This difference causes a typical reduction in C_{max} and delay in T_{max} of a drug in the fed state. The relationship between the caloric density of the food and the gastric emptying rate is shown in Table 6.5 and Figure 6.8 [43]. Factors such as posture, pain, and disease conditions affect gastric emptying time (GET) [44].

On the other hand, the GET of solid objects larger than ca. 0.5 mm is associated with phase II or III of migrating motor complex (MMC), which is observed in the fasted state. When an object with this size range is administered in the fed state, only after MMC has resumed, gastric emptying of these objects occurs [5].

In dogs and monkeys, the GET of a solution in the fasted state is similar to that in humans [45]. However, the GET in the fed state is longer in dogs than that in humans [46]. In pigs, the mean time for 50% emptying of the liquid in the fasted state is approximately 1.4 h [42].

6.2.1.2 Small Intestinal Transit Time. The small intestinal transit time (SITT) is ca. 3.5 h for both the fasted and fed states in humans. In contrast to the stomach emptying time, the intestinal transit time is not largely affected by the size of the formulation [42]. However, it is significantly shortened to 1.7–2.4 h when a tablet is administered 45 min before food intake because of a strong housekeeping wave [47].

In dogs and monkeys, the SITT was suggested be shorter than that in humans (3.5 vs 2 h, respectively) [45].

TABLE 6.5 The Caloric Density of Food and the Gastric Emptying Rate[a]

Caloric Load, kcal	Meal Volume, ml			
	200	400	600	800
200	56	41	42	38
300	74	59	60	56
400	92	77	78	74

[a]Reference 5.

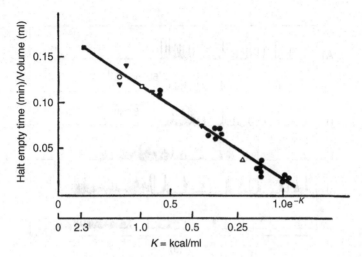

Figure 6.8 Gastric emptying time and caloric density of the food. *Source*: Adapted from Reference 43 with permission.

6.2.1.3 Colon Transit Time.

The ascending colon transit time in humans was reported to be ca. 13 h and not significantly different depending on the formulation size [48].

6.2.2 Migrating Motor Complex

In the fasted state, the MMC controls the motility pattern (Fig. 6.9) [49]. The MMC cleanses the stomach and the small intestine acting as "the housekeeper wave." The MMC consists of at least three distinct phases (Tables 6.6 and 6.7) with a combined total average duration of about 100 min:

phase I (ca. 60 min)—less than three pressure waves per 10 min;
phase II (ca. 30 min)—period of irregular contractions;
phase III (ca. 2–15 min)—regular rhythmic contractions at high frequency.

There is also a phase IV, a brief period of transitional motor activity from the intense phase III to the quiescent phase I.

The propagation velocity in the duodenum, the proximal jejunum, and the distal ileum is 10, 7, and 1 cm/min, respectively. Only half of them propagate beyond the middle jejunum, and only 10% reaches the distal ileum.

When food is taken in, the MMC activity is lost and fed state motility is reached (Fig. 6.10). The partial secretion of bile in the fasted state is related to the MMC (Section 6.6.1).

Dogs have an MMC pattern similar to that in humans. However, as the gastric emptying of food is slower than that in humans, the MMC phase III also resumes

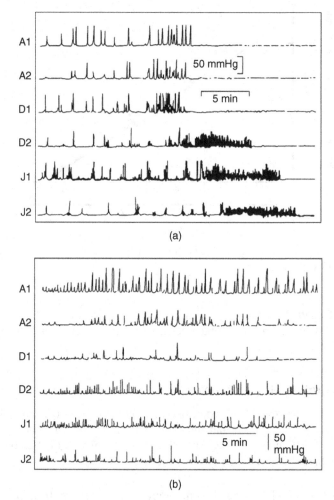

Figure 6.9 Intraluminal pressure recordings in the (a) fasted and (b) fed states of a healthy volunteer. *Source*: Adapted from Reference 49 with permission.

TABLE 6.6   Return of MMC Phase III After Meal[a]

Species		Time for MMC Phase III to Resume, min
Human	285 kcal, liquid	156 ± 54 (SD)
	500 kcal, solid	288 ± 90 (SD)
Dog	30 kcal/kg solid	324 ± 23 (SE)
	60 kcal/kg solid	561 ± 31 (SE)
	90 kcal/kg solid	799 ± 33 (SE)

[a]Reference 46.

TABLE 6.7   Mean Flow Rate in Various Intestinal Segments in Humans[a]

MMC Phase	Mean Flow Rate, ml/min, mean ± SD		
	Jejunum	Ileum	Terminal Ileum
I–II	0.58 ± 0.12	0.17 ± 0.03	0.33 ± 0.01
III	1.28 ± 0.18	0.50 ± 0.13	0.65 ± 0.01
Mean phase (I–III)	0.73 ± 0.11	0.33 ± 0.09	0.43 ± 0.06
Fed state	3.00 ± 0.67	2.35 ± 0.28	2.09 ± 0.16

[a]Reference 51.

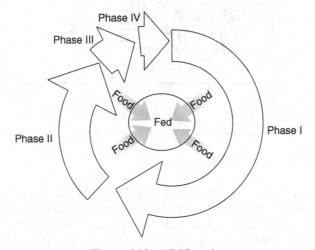

Figure 6.10   MMC cycles.

more slowly [46]. Rats have indistinct MMC pattern and shorter MMC cycle time (20–30 min) [50].

6.2.3   Agitation

6.2.3.1   *Mixing Pattern.* The mixing pattern in the stomach is not homogeneous. Using computational fluid dynamic (CFD) simulation, Pal et al. [52] investigated the role of antral contraction wave (ACW) activity of gastric fluid motions, pressure, and mixing. Gastric mixing was found to be limited to the antrum where occluding ACW generates strong gastric fluid motions (Fig. 6.11). Dillard et al. [53] investigated the mixing pattern at the pylorus and superior duodenum. It was found that the asymmetric geometry of the pyloric orifice in concert with intermittent gastric outflow and luminal constriction is likely to enhance homogenization of gastric effluent with duodenal secretion.

There are two types of large-scale intestinal wall movements in the unanesthetized state, the periodic segmental contraction and the periodic peristaltic

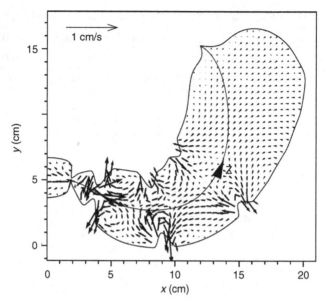

Figure 6.11   Mixing patterns in the stomach. *Source*: Adapted from Reference 52 with permission.

movement (Fig. 6.12), the former was suggested to be the main contributor for mixing, whereas the latter moves the chyme toward the distal position. The periodic segmental contraction and peristaltic movement of the intestine would knead and mix the intestinal fluid effectively in spite of the low Reynolds number in the intestine with little turbulent flow (= little eddy diffusion and dissipation). In

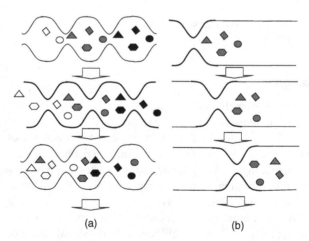

(a)   (b)

Figure 6.12   Segmental contraction and the periodic peristaltic movement. *Source*: Adapted from Reference 55 with permission.

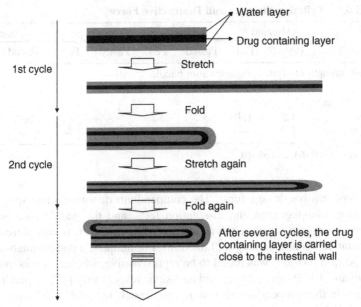

Water layer

Drug containing layer

1st cycle

Stretch

Fold

2nd cycle

Stretch again

Fold again

After several cycles, the drug
containing layer is carried
close to the intestinal wall

Figure 6.13 Baker's transformation. *Source*: Adapted from Reference 55 with permission.

other words, the fluid mixing pattern can be chaotic even without turbulence (periodic laminar mixing is also called *chaotic mixing* [54] and is related to Baker's transformation (Fig. 6.13)). This mixing pattern brings the drug and nutrient molecules close to the intestinal wall, hence reducing the UWL thickness adjacent to the intestinal membrane. Theoretical estimation of the effect of laminar mixing on the UWL thickness would be the subject of future investigation.

The villous mobility (mainly vertical shrinking) [56, 57], which is present in humans and dogs but not in rats, was suggested to be not effective to reduce the UWL thickness [58]. This is in good agreement with the Reynolds number of villi being much less than 1 (much smaller than the *Re* for the intestinal tube scale). The microfluidics induced by the villous motility would be laminar and no mixing would occur. At $Re \ll 1$, viscosity significantly surmounts the inertia of fluid velocity and the fluid is stagnant on the wall, that is, the fluid moves together with the villi wall dragged by viscosity. The vertical shrinking movement would not produce a knead-and-mix pattern.

There were several experimental attempts to characterize the flow regime of the intestine. Janssen et al. [59] reported that some elements of turbulence were observed when the intestinal fluid had a viscosity close to water, whereas it was absent when the intestinal fluid had higher viscosity such as in the fed state chyme.

6.2.3.2 Agitation Strength.
The effective agitation strength in the GI tract was assessed by comparing the *in vitro* and *in vivo* drug release profiles for a

TABLE 6.8 Agitation Strength and Destructive Force[a]

	Humans		Dogs		Monkeys		Rats	
	Fasted	Fed	Fasted	Fed	Fasted	Fed	Fasted	Fed
Agitation strength (as rpm in compendium paddle speed)								
	10	—	100	—	10–50	—	10 ~ 50	—
Destructive force, N								
Stomach	1.5	1.9	3.2	3.2	—	—	—	—
Small intestine	1.2	—	1.2	—	—	—	—	—

[a]References 45, 60–63, and 65–68.

matrix-type erosive dosage form. The compendium dissolution test was used as the *in vitro* disintegration and dissolution tests, and the paddle rotation speed that gives a release profile equivalent to *in vivo* release was considered as the representative agitation strength (Table 6.8). For humans, a paddle rotation speed of 10–30 rpm [60–63] was found to be representative, whereas it was more than 100 rpm and 10–50 rpm in dogs and monkeys, respectively [45]. A paddle speed of 50 rpm in the compendium dissolution test equals to 0.004 m^2/s^3 (energy input per time) [64].

The destruction force is not equal to the agitation strength, as the contact with the intestinal wall can influence the destruction force. In humans in the fasted state, the destruction force is 1.5 and 1.9 N in the stomach and intestine, respectively [65]. In dogs, the destruction force in the stomach is 3.2 N, which is higher than that in humans. The highest destruction force would be observed when the formulation passes through the antrum.

6.2.3.3 Unstirred Water Layer on the Intestinal Wall.

The existence of the UWL in the intestine *in vivo* is often argued. From the fluid dynamic theory, the existence of the UWL is 100% sure. When the intestinal wall moves, the fluid adjacent to the wall also moves in a synchronized manner towed by the viscosity of the fluid. In addition, the eddy of turbulence cannot reach the intestinal wall. Therefore, by the action of the viscosity of the fluid, even though the intestinal fluid is agitated by the movement of the intestinal wall, the UWL cannot be completely removed. The question is how much diffusion resistance is maintained by the UWL.[6] In this book, based on the following discussion, 300 μm is used as the best guess value for UWL thickness.

There had been a controversy in the literature about the UWL thickness (h_{UWL}) in the small intestine. Previously, the UWL thickness was estimated to be ca. 700 μm from the rat small intestinal perfusion experiments under anesthetized conditions [69]. On the other hand, in conscious humans, it was estimated to be

[6]The concept of the "thickness of UWL" is based on the film model. The h_{UWL} is an operational term because the well-mixed phase and the UWL are not well defined. Therefore, the so-called UWL thickness corresponds to the effective diffusion resistance of the boundary layer, which has the dimension of length.

30–130 µm (based on the smooth tube surface) [70, 71]. When corrected for the fold (plicae) structure (threefold), the actual thickness of the UWL was found to be 90–400 µm. This is in good agreement with the mucous layer thickness of 100–200 µm on the villi tip obtained by a direct measurement (Fig. 6.6). Recently, the UWL thickness was retrospectively estimated from human Fa% of several model drugs whose oral absorption is solubility-UWL limited [72]. To neglect the particle drifting effect, Dose <5 mg/kg and $d_p > 10$ µm were selected (cilostazol, irbesartan, phenytion, and spironolactone). The estimated UWL thickness was 332 µm. This value is very close to the experimentally estimated value by Lennernäs (384 µm based on glucose P_{eff} at the infusion rate of 1.5 ml/min (after plicae effect correction)) [71] and the computationally simulated value by Wang et al. (Fig. 6.14) [73]. The lower values reported in the literature (40 µm based on the smooth tube surface) were obtained from an infusion study with the flow rate of 7.5–20 ml/min [70]. These high perfusion rates might cause an artifactual reduction in the UWL thickness, as the normal flow rate in the proximal small intestine has been reported to be 0.6–4.2 ml/min in humans, including both fasted and fed states [74].

The UWL thickness values in rats, dogs, and monkeys are not well known. In dogs, the UWL was estimated to be 35 and 50 µm at the perfusion rates of 26 and 5 ml/min, respectively [70]. Considering the difference in the intestinal diameter, these flow rates in dogs are also very high. From the absorption flux data of glucose (threefold lower in dogs compared to humans) [75] and the difference in the fold structure (dogs do not have the fold structure), the UWL thickness of dogs is suggested to be similar to that in humans.

In rats, the UWL thickness is suggested to be similar to that in humans, based on the similar discussion for dogs [75]. In monkeys, due to the lack of information about the plicae expansion, it is difficult to estimate the UWL thickness. On the basis of the effective permeability of antipyrine and assuming that the plicae

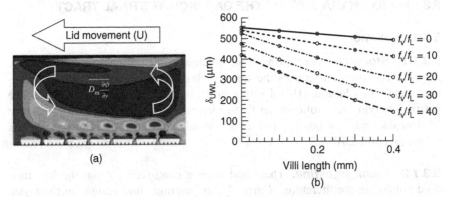

Figure 6.14 UWL simulation results. (a) Vertical diffusional mass transfer. The gray concentration corresponds to the UWL. (b) The effect of villi length and oscillation frequency on the UWL thickness. f_v/f_L is the frequency ratio of cavity eddy and the villi oscillation. *Source*: Adapted from Reference 73 with permission.

expansion was not as large as that in humans, the UWL thickness of monkeys is suggested to be similar to that in humans [11].

The thickness of the UWL is theoretically estimated to be greater than 1 cm in humans if the flow pattern is a straight laminar flow (the Graetz problem (Section 3.2.4.3)). Therefore, the *in vivo* UWL (ca. 300 μm) is very thin, suggesting that the intestinal fluid is effectively agitated. Therefore, the flow pattern should not be a straight laminar flow in the conscious human. At the same time, the Reynolds number calculated for the intestinal tube, tablet, and drug particles suggests that the flow patterns around these objects in the intestine could be only weakly turbulent. As discussed above, "periodical laminar mixing" could be an additional mechanism for the effective mixing in the GI tract (Fig. 6.12).

Figure 6.14 shows the CFD simulation results for the flow and mass transfer patterns in the small intestine reported by Wang et al. [73]. To simulate the macro- and microscale phenomena simultaneously, a two-dimensional multiscale lattice Boltzmann model was used. The flow pattern was modeled as a lid-driven cavity flow with oscillating villi at the lower surface. The cavity characteristics were set to roughly consistent with the macroscales of the human jejunum: cavity length and height $L \times H = 6\text{mm} \times 3$ mm and lid velocity $U = 2$ mm/s. Figure 6.14 shows the visual pattern of the mass transfer in the cavity. Convective flux is overall larger than diffusive flux everywhere except in the diffusion-dominated UWL adjacent to the villi surfaces. The estimated UWL thickness is in the range of 200–500 μm.

In contrast to the conscious *in vivo* situation, the UWL under anesthetized state was suggested to be much thicker [75].

In the colon, due to solidified chyme (high viscosity), significantly thick mucous layer, and lesser mobility, the UWL thickness would be significantly thicker than that in the small intestine.

6.3 FLUID CHARACTER OF THE GASTROINTESTINAL TRACT

6.3.1 Volume

6.3.1.1 Stomach. The resting fluid volume in the stomach is ca. 30 ml in humans. The stomach secretes the stomach fluid at the rate of 1.2 ml/min (zero-order rate). In addition, 0.9 ml saliva flows into the stomach per minute. The gastric emptying rate follows the first-order rate of 0.0693 min^{-1}. The balance of flow-ins and flow-out determines the steady-state resting volume to be ca. 30 ml (Section 2.10).

6.3.1.2 Small Intestine. There had been a controversy about the intestinal fluid volume in the literature.[7] Currently, the average fluid volume in the fasted

---

[7]In some reports, $V_{GI} = 600$ ml was used with the surface area of 800 cm^2, that is, $SA_{GI}/V_{GI} = 1.3$, which is equal to the cylindrical tube shape. Compared to the current most credible values of $V_{GI} = 130$ ml and $SA_{GI}/V_{GI} = 2.3$, the previous V_{GI} is larger and the previous SA_{GI}/V_{GI} is smaller. These

human small intestine is estimated to be ca. 130 ml, but it has a large variation. The following evidence support this value:

- direct measurements by MRI in conscious states (107 and 10–100 ml) [76, 77];
- direct measurement in postmortem state (207 ml) [4];
- indirect estimation from the dose–Fa% profiles of four SL-E compounds (130 ml) [72];
- indirect estimation from the intubations study of the precipitation–absorption study (130 ml) [78];
- K_i value and dose–CYP inhibition relationship of cimetidine (ca. 190 ml)[8] [79, 80].

These fluid volume values are in good agreement with the deflated tube shape and the surface–volume ratio of 2.4–2.6 (i.e., degree of flatness (DF) = 1.7).

The intestinal fluid is heterogeneously distributed across the small intestine as four to five water pockets (Fig. 6.15) [76]. Therefore, it was suggested that the dosage form is not always soaked in the intestinal fluid during the GI transit. In the fasted state, when 28 capsules were ingested by multiple human subjects, only 50% of the capsules were completely soaked in the intestinal fluid.

It is difficult to estimate the fluid volume in the fed state, as a large portion of the fluid is bound to the food and might not be available for drug dissolution. From the retrospective analysis using the fed/fasted AUC ratio of SL-E drugs, the effective fluid volume was estimated to be 1.2-fold larger than that in the fasted state [81].

The intestinal fluid volume tended to be higher in men than in women (ca. twofold) [82].

6.3.1.3 Colon. The fluid volume in the human ascending colon is ca.15 ml in both fasted and fed states [83]. Most of the cavity is filled with 200 ml of gas, which is roughly equal to the geometric capacity of the ascending colon.

6.3.2 Bulk Fluid pH and Buffer Concentration

The ranges of pH values for various animal species are shown in Table 6.9.

---

errors worked in opposite directions and were coincidently canceled out, resulting in semiquantitative Fa% prediction for solubility-permeability-limited cases. However, with $V_{GI} = 600$ ml, the inflation point in the dose–AUC curve would be upshifted (Fig. 10.1). In addition, with $SA_{GI}/V_{GI} = 1.3$, for permeability-limited cases, human Fa% is underestimated by ca. twofold from the experimental P_{eff} values in humans (Fig. 8.2).

[8]In the original paper, the fluid volume was estimated to be 1900 ml based on the assumption that the cytosol and luminal free drug concentration is equal. However, the cytosol free drug concentration should be significantly smaller. When the concentration gradient across the apical and basolateral sides is taken into account, the V_{GI} can be estimated to be 190 ml.

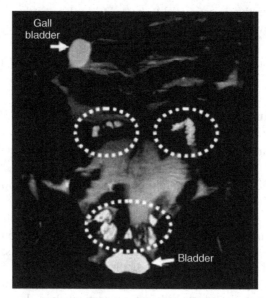

Figure 6.15 Magnetic resonance images showing the identification and segmentation of intestinal fluid pockets in the fasted state. *Source*: Adapted from Reference 76 with permission.

TABLE 6.9 Gastrointestinal Fluid pH and Bile Concentration[a]

	Humans		Dogs		Monkeys		Rats[b]	
	Fasted	Fed	Fasted	Fed	Fasted	Fed	Fasted	Fed
Fluid volume, ml								
Stomach	30	—	—	—	—	—	0.5	1.1
Small intestine	130	156	—	—	—	—	1.5	3.8
Colon	15	17	—	—	—	—	0.6	2.2
Bulk pH								
Stomach anterior	1.5–5.0	6	1.5–5.5	—	4.7–5.0	—	3.9	3.2
Stomach posterior	5.0–7.0	—	1.5–3.4	—	2.3–2.8	—	—	—
Duodenum	6.0–7.0	—	6.2	—	5.6–6.0	—	5.89	5.00
Jejunum	7.0–7.4	—	6.2–7.3	—	5.8–6.0	—	6.13	5.10
Ileum	5.7–5.9	—	7.5	—	6.0–6.7	—	5.93	5.94
Cecum	5.5–7.5	—	6.4	—	4.9–5.1	—	6.58	5.90
Colon[c]	7.8	6	6.5	—	5.0–5.9	—	5.88–6.23	5.51–5.77
Rectum/feces	—	—	6.2	—	5.5	—	—	—
Bile								
Stomach	~0	~0	—	—	—	—	—	—
Small intestine	3	15	5	—	—	—	20	—
Colon[c]	0.11	0.59	—	—	—	—	—	—

[a]References 3 and 14.
[b]Rat data from References 89 and 90.
[c]Human colon values from Reference 83.

6.3.2.1 Stomach. In humans, in the fasted state, the pH in the stomach after the administration of 250 ml of water is 1.2–7.4 (median 1.7). In the fed state, the pH in the stomach increases to about 7 and gradually decreases to the normal range within 1.5 h [46]. The concentrations of Cl^- and Na^+ ions in the stomach are 102 and 68 mM, respectively [84]. The stomach pH is slightly higher in females than in males (2.2 vs 2.8) [82].

In dogs, the gastric pH is highly variable due to lower basal secretion of HCl (0.1 mEq/h) than in humans (2–5 mEq/h). Therefore, a pretreatment to control the stomach pH is often used [85, 86]. Pentagastrin injection has been most often used to achieve a low pH. An H2 blocker is often used to keep the stomach pH neutral [87]. When a pH modulator is used, it is important to avoid drug–drug interaction in the metabolic and excretion processes. In the fed state, the pH initially increases to ca. 4; however, it immediately drops to ca. 1.2 [88].

In monkeys, the stomach pH is similar to that in humans [45]. In rats, the stomach pH is 3–5 [1].

6.3.2.2 Small Intestine. In humans in the fasted state, the pH values of the bulk fluid in the duodenum and jejunum are 6.2–7.0 and 6.8, respectively. In the fed state, the pH is slightly lower than that in the fasted state, that is, 5.9.

The buffer concentration is also an important factor that determines the solid surface pH of a drug (Section 2.3.3). The main buffer species in the intestine is sodium carbonate. The concentration of carbonate in the human intestine was reported to be 6.7 mM in the fasted state. The concentrations of Cl^- and Na^+ ions in the jejunum are 126 and 142 mM, respectively [84].

6.3.2.3 Colon. The pH in the human ascending colon is 7.8 and 6.0 in the fasted and fed states, respectively [83]. The mean buffer capacity is 21.4 and 37.7 mmol/l/ΔpH in the fasted and fed states, respectively.

6.3.3 Microclimate pH

The microclimate pH is the pH at the epithelial membrane surface. This pH is lower than that of the luminal bulk fluid. In biopharmaceutical modeling, the microclimate pH should be used when calculating the membrane permeability of a drug, whereas the bulk fluid pH should be used when calculating the solubility and dissolution rate in the bulk fluid.

6.3.3.1 Small Intestine. The acid microclimate pH exists adjacent to the epithelial membrane surface [91]. The pH is ca. 0.5 units lower than the average bulk fluid and is ca. 6.0–6.5. This microclimate pH is maintained constant by the Na^+/H^+ antiporter. A perturbation of the bulk fluid pH from 3 to 10 did not alter the microclimate pH (Fig. 6.16) [92]. The microclimate pH affects the passive diffusion of acid and base drugs as suggested by the pH partition theory. In addition, this microclimate pH is also important for PEP-T1 and OATP transporters, as the pH gradient between the microclimate pH and cytosol pH is the

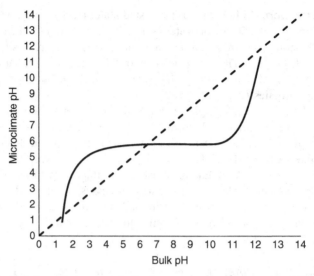

Figure 6.16 Relationship between bulk phase and microclimate pHs. Microclimate pH showed little change when the bulk pH was changed between 3.0 and 10.0. Beyond this range, there was a precipitous drop or rise in microclimate pH [92].

energy source for these transporters. Because the microclimate pH is maintained constant against pH perturbation in the bulk fluid, the membrane permeability of a drug should be insensitive to the change in the bulk pH [93, 94], for example, changes caused by food intake.

6.3.3.2 Colon. The acid microclimate pH is also maintained in the colon [95, 96]. In humans and rats, the microclimate pH was 6.4–6.7 when the luminal pH was changed from 6.1 to 7.6.

6.3.4 Bile Micelles

Bile micelles not only increase the solubility and dissolution rate of a drug but also decrease the unbound drug fraction and the effective permeability [97–103]. The concentration of bile micelles has large species differences and fed/fasted state differences. The structures of a bile acid is shown in Figure 6.17. The surface of

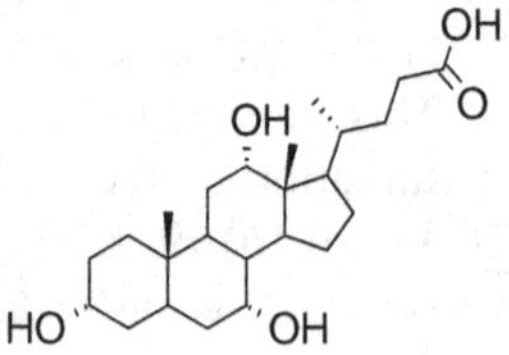

Figure 6.17 Chemical structure of bile acid.

the bile micelles is negatively charged because of the presence of sulfate (SO_3^-) or carboxylate (COO^-) group. Therefore, both lipophilicity and the charge of a drug affect bile-micelle binding. Another interesting feature of bile acids is that all hydroxyl groups are located on the same face of the cholesterol plane. This could result in a somewhat different behavior of bile acids (such as no distinct critical micelle concentration) from the regular surfactants.

6.3.4.1 Stomach. The bile concentration in the stomach is almost negligible. However, there is a small portion of surfactant that is enough to work as wetting agent [105].

6.3.4.2 Small Intestine. In humans, the average bile salt concentration in the jejunum is ca. 3 mM in the fasted state and ca. 5–15 mM in the fed state. However, the bile concentration shows a great deal of individual variation (Fig. 6.18) [104]. The bile salt/phospholipid ratio is ca. 4:1. In the fed state, the concentration and the composition of the drug-solubilizing component in the intestinal fluid changes as the digestion of food progresses. In Table 7.2, the snapshots of the intestinal fluid mimicking each digestion state are summarized. As water absorption occurs, the bile-micelles are concentrated. Therefore, the bile-micelle concentration might be slightly higher in the jejunum than in the duodenum [89, 106] (Fig. 6.19). Most of the bile acid is reabsorbed in the ileum mainly by a bile acid transporter, namely, ASBT (apical sodium-dependent bile acid transporter;

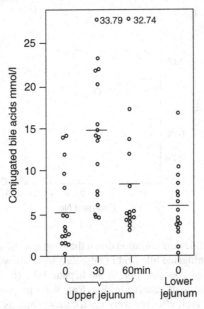

Figure 6.18 Bile concentration in humans in the fasted and fed states. *Source:* Adapted from Reference 104 with permission.

SLC10A2), which is critical for enterohepatic circulation of bile acids by mediating its absorption at the apical membranes of enterocytes [107]. This reduces the concentration of bile-micelles at the end of ileum and increases the unbound fraction of a drug, resulting in an increase in both the effective permeability in the ileum and bimodal absorption [108] (Section 13.6.3).

The bile-micelle concentration in the fed state depends on the food components [109]. The secretion of bile-micelles into the duodenum is stimulated by the lipids [110]. The long-chain triglycerides (LCTs) induce higher bile acid secretion than medium-chain triglycerides (MCTs). MCTs do not induce gallbladder contraction, whereas LCTs do [110]. On the other hand, carbohydrates do not stimulate bile secretion but increase the agitation in the GI tract [111].

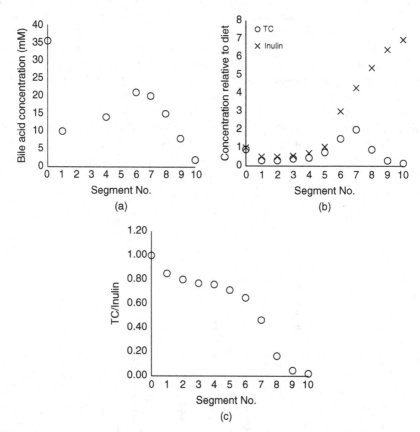

Figure 6.19 Regional bile concentration down the length of the small intestine of rats. (a) The concentration of conjugated bile acid in rats. Rats were allowed to eat ad lib. The time zero point is the bile acid concentration in the hepatic bile. (b) and (c) Taurocholic acid (TC) and inulin concentrations relative to diet. Rats were prepared surgically by ligation of the common hepatic duct; after recovery (24 h), these animals were intragastrically fed with a liquid diet containing (TC)-[14]C (10 μmol/ml) and inulin-[3]H. *Source*: Replotted from Reference 89.

In dogs, bile acid concentrations in the fasted and fed states were reported to be 4.9 (2.4–9.39 mM, $N = 3$) and 15.9 mM (12.8–18.0 mM, $N = 3$), respectively [112].

Rats lack the gallbladder and the bile continuously flows into the GI tract. The average bile salt concentration in the jejunum is ca. 15–20 mM [89].

6.3.4.3 *Colon.* As most of the bile is reabsorbed at the end of ileum, the bile concentration is very small in the colon [83]. Mean total bile acid concentration is 0.12 and 0.59 mM in the fasted and fed states, respectively.

6.3.5 Enzymes and Bacteria

Pepsin can degrade some drugs with amide and ester groups. In the fasted human stomach, the pepsin concentration ranges between 0.1 and 1.3 mg/ml. In the fed stomach, the pepsin concentration ranges from 0.26 to 1.72 mg/ml [5].

Lipase also plays important roles in the oral absorption of a drug from a lipid-based formulation (Section 11.3). Lipase activity in the fed stomach is from 11.4 to 43.9 U/ml [5]. Some drugs and formulations are degraded by the bacteria in the GI tract, for example, sulfasalazine (Table 6.10).

6.3.6 Viscosity, Osmolality, and Surface Tension

Osmolality can affect the disintegration of a formulation ([5] and references therein). Gastric osmolality in the fasted state is in the range of 29–276 mOsm/kg. After a meal, the median value in the stomach was found to be 559 mOsm/kg after 30 min and 217 mOsm/kg after 210 min. In the upper small intestine, osmolality values range from 124 to 278 mOsm/kg in the fasted state and 250 to 367 mOsm/kg in the fed state.

Viscosity of the intestinal fluid has not been reported. The viscosity of water at 37°C is 0.691 cP, while typical meals have viscosities in the range of 10 to 100,000 cP.

Surface tension of the fluid affects the wetting speed of drugs and excipients. The lower the surface tension, the higher the wetting speed. The surface tension of water is 70 mN/m at 37°C. Gastric surface tension values in the fasted and fed states range from about 41 to 46 and 30 to 31 mN/m, respectively [5]. In

TABLE 6.10 Bacterial Population in the Lower Bowel in Humans

	Distal Ileum	Cecum	Feces
Enterobacteria	3.3	6.2	7.4
Enterococci	2.2	3.6	5.6
Clostridia	<2	3.0	5.4
Lactobacilli	<2	6.4	6.5
Bacteroides	5.7	7.8	9.8
Gram-positive nonsporing anaerobes	5.8	8.4	10

the upper small intestine, surface tension values range from 28 to 46 mN/m in the fasted state and from 27 to 37 mN/m in the fed state. Surface tension in the colon is significantly lower than that of water, 39 and 43 mN/m in the fasted and fed states, respectively.

6.4 TRANSPORTERS AND DRUG-METABOLIZING ENZYMES IN THE INTESTINE

6.4.1 Absorptive Drug Transporters

6.4.1.1 PEP-T1. As an absorptive influx transporter, PEP-T1 is well known to contribute to oral absorption of some drugs, especially antibiotics.

In humans, the mRNA level of PEP-T1 is similar between the duodenum and ileum, but almost null in the colon [107, 113]. The mRNA level of PEP-T1 is similar between humans and rats [114].

6.4.1.2 OATP. OATP is an influx transporter located on the apical membrane. Fexofenadine is one of the most well-characterized OATP substrates. In humans, the mRNA level of OATP is similar in the duodenum, ileum, and colon [113].

6.4.2 Efflux Drug Transporters

6.4.2.1 P-gp. P-gp is an efflux transporter located on the apical membrane. P-gp is a 170-kd transmembrane glycosylated protein and the gene product of MDR1. P-gp has a few binding sites for substrates [115].

A proposed efflux mechanism of P-gp is shown in Figure 4.20 (the vacuum cleaner mechanism). A substrate first partitions into the lipid bilayer and then enters the cavity of the enzyme from a portal opening into the lipid bilayer.

In humans, the P-gp expression level is ca. 1.5-fold higher in the ileum than in the jejunum [116] (Fig. 6.20). This trend is also found in the functional activity level [117] and mRNA level [118]. The interindividual variation of the P-gp expression level is within twofold, which is smaller than that for CYP3A4 (>10-fold) [116].

The apparent K_m values of P-gp showed significant species differences, whereas efflux ratio has lesser species differences [119]. In addition, the degree and tendency of these species differences was different between cyclosporine and diltiazem. These results suggest that the effect of P-gp on oral absorption in humans cannot be simply quantitatively extrapolated from that in animals.

6.4.3 Drug-Metabolizing Enzymes

6.4.3.1 CYP3A4. CYP3A4 is the dominant CYP species in the intestinal wall (Fig. 6.21) [120]. The total amount of CYP3A in the intestinal wall is about 1% of that in the liver. However, intestinal CYP3A could significantly reduce the bioavailability of a drug.

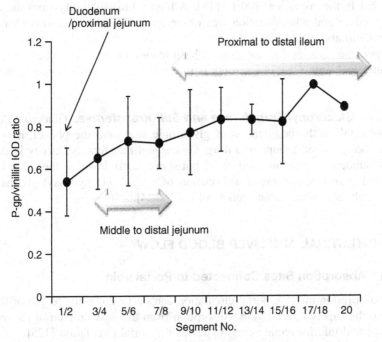

Figure 6.20 6.20 P-gp expression level along the GI tract. P-gp content (P-gp/villin integrated optical density (IOD) ratio, normalized to the maximum value) for each segment of the human small intestine are shown. Segment 1/2, duodenum/proximal jejunum; segments 3/4, 5/6, and 7/8, middle to distal jejunum; and 9/10-20, proximal to distal ileum. Segments 1/2-13/14, $n = 4$; 15/16, $n = 3$; 17/18, $n = 2$; and 20, $n = 1$. *Source*: Replotted from Reference 116.

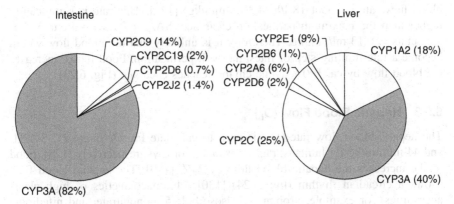

Figure 6.21 CYP in the small intestine and liver [120].

The mRNA expression level of CYP3A4 is much higher in the small intestine than that in the colon, ca. 100:1 [118]. A higher bioavailability from the colon compared to oral administration was observed for CYP3A4 substrates, such as atrovastatin and nisoldipine [15].

Significant species differences have been reported in the metabolic enzymes in the intestinal wall. CYP3A4 activity is much higher in monkeys than in humans [11].

6.4.3.2 Glucuronyl Transferase and Sulfotransferase.

Glucuronyl transferases catalyze the conjugation of glucuronic acid onto the phenol, hydroxyl, and carboxylic acid groups of a drug. Glucuronyl transferases activity is similar in the duodenum, jejunum, and ilium, but significantly lower in the colon [121]. Sulfonyl transferases catalyze sulfonation of phenol and hydroxyl groups of a drug, such as terbutaline and fenoterol [122–124].

6.5 INTESTINAL AND LIVER BLOOD FLOW

6.5.1 Absorption Sites Connected to Portal Vein

Drug absorption into the portal circulation can occur down the length of the GI tract to the superior rectal vein. Absorption from the lower region of the rectum (middle and inferior rectal veins) bypasses the portal circulation [125].

6.5.2 Villous Blood Flow (Q_{villi})

The villous blood flow (Q_{villi}) is used to calculate the extent of intestinal first-pass metabolism by the Q_{gut} model (Section 4.10). The blood supply to the small intestine is provided by the superior mesenteric artery (Fig. 6.22). The mucosal blood flow is about 80% of the total mesenteric flow of 37.2 l/h, about 60% of which then pours into the epithelial cells of the villi. Therefore, the villous blood flow rate is about 18 l/h (4.3 ml/min/kg) [127]. This rate is significantly higher than the maximum permeation clearance, $SA_{GI} \times P_{eff} = 300$ cm^2 $\times 5 \times 10^{-4}$cm/s $= 0.13$ ml/min/kg. Therefore, it is unlikely that the blood flow would become a rate-limiting step of intestinal wall permeation. Food intake increases the blood flow by ca. 100% as the chyme reaches each site (Fig. 6.23).

6.5.3 Hepatic Blood Flow (Q_h)

The hepatic blood flow rate (Q_h) is used to calculate Fh. Q_h is ca. 21, 84, 31, and 44 ml/min/kg for humans, rats, dogs, and monkeys, respectively [128]. Food intake increases the hepatic blood flow by 34% [129]. The hepatic blood flow shows a circadian rhythm (Fig. 6.24) [130]. Pharmacokinetics of high clearance drugs, for example, propranolol, isosorbide-5-mononitrate, and nifedipine [131–133], were shown to be dependent on the time of day at which they were administered.

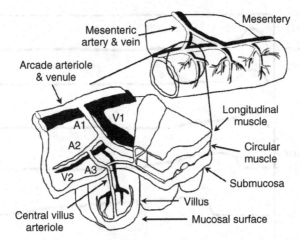

Figure 6.22 Intestinal blood flow. Outline of the intestinal microvasculature emphasizing the mucosal blood supply with the inflow (A1), transitional (A2), and premucosal (A3) arteriolar structure as well as outflow (V1) and transitional (V2) venules. *Source*: Adapted from Reference 126 with permission.

6.6 PHYSIOLOGY RELATED TO ENTEROHEPATIC RECIRCULATION

Physiology of the liver related to the enterohepatic recirculation is discussed in this section. The first-pass drug metabolism in the liver significantly affects the bioavailability of many drugs. However, it is not covered in this book, as it would be beyond the scope of this book.

6.6.1 Bile Secretion

After an overnight fast, the gallbladder volume is 17–25 ml [134]. In the fasted state, ca. 30% of the secreted bile directly excretes into the duodenum and ca. 70% accumulates in the gallbladder. The average bile secretion from the liver is 500–600 ml/d in humans [135]. The gallbladder fills to its maximum capacity (40–70 ml) in approximately 6 h [136]. More than 90% water is reabsorbed in the gallbladder.

The gallbladder is not static during the fasted state. Secretion of bile into the duodenum occurs periodically as part of the MMC. During the interdigestive period, the volume of the gallbladder decreases to up to 30–35%, starting in the first half of MMC phase II.

On the sight, smell, or ingestion of food, the bile stored in the gallbladder is released into the duodenum. Food intake causes the gallbladder to be emptied up to 75%. After ingestion of a meal, fats, and proteins, endogenous neurohormones such as cholecystokinin (CCK) and secretin are released by the endocrine cells of the small intestine. CCK, acting on the CCK-A type receptors of smooth muscle fibers, contracts the gallbladder and relaxes the sphincter of Oddi [136].

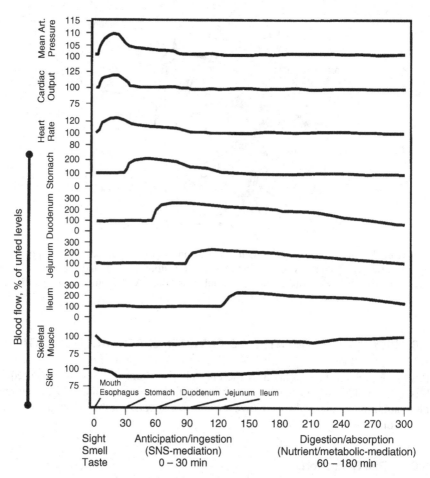

Figure 6.23 Effect of food on the gastrointestinal blood flow. Blood flow increases in specific organs as digestive chyme reaches that organ. Indications along the time axis mark the point at which the chyme reaches the stomach, duodenum, jejunum, and ileum to initiate the metabolically mediated digestion and absorption stages of postprandial hyperemia. *Source*: Adapted from Reference 126 with permission.

6.6.2 Mass Transfer into/from the Hepatocyte

6.6.2.1 *Sinusoidal Membrane (Blood to Hepatocyte)*. Mass transfer of drugs from the circulation into the hepatocyte has been intensively investigated. The majority of small lipophilic compounds enter the hepatocyte via the sinusoidal membrane by simple passive diffusion (Fig. 6.25). However, some hydrophilic drugs, such as pravastatin, can enter the hepatocyte by carrier-mediated transport across the sinusoidal membrane [125] (cf. many hydrophilic drugs are usually excreted into the urine via the kidney). The role of plasma protein binding on the uptake of highly protein-bound drugs has been

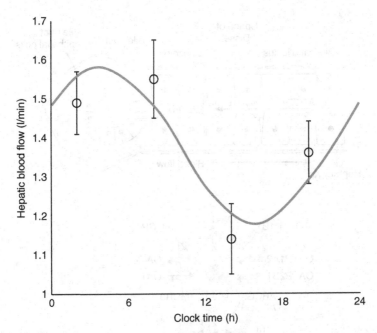

Figure 6.24 Circadian rhythm in hepatic blood flow in humans estimated from indocya-
nine green clearance. Data were fitted by a cosine function with a period of 24 h. Values
are shown as mean and SE ($n = 10$). *Source*: Replotted from Reference 130.

a controversial issue. Recent studies in this area have provided evidence that
uptake may occur from both the unbound and protein-bound fractions [125].

6.6.2.2 *Canalicular Membrane (Hepatocyte to Bile Duct).* Hepatobiliary
elimination requires active efflux transporters to move drugs from hepatocytes
into the canalicular space [137]. As the volume of biliary fluid is very small,
biliary excretion becomes significant only when the drug concentration in the
bile is higher than that in the plasma. The bile/plasma concentration ratio is most
commonly between 10 and 1000.

Biliary elimination of anionic compounds is mediated by MRP2, whereas bile
salts are excreted by a bile salt export pump (BSEP). P-glycoprotein, the multidrug resistance (MDR) gene product, is exclusively located on the canalicular
membrane of hepatocytes [125].

6.7 NASAL

The morphology of the nasal cavity has large species differences (Table 6.11;
Fig. 6.26). Rats and dogs have significantly larger surface area/body weight than
humans. Drugs applied to the mucous lining of the nasal cavity move toward
the nasopharynx, eventually entering into the GI tract. This mechanism is called

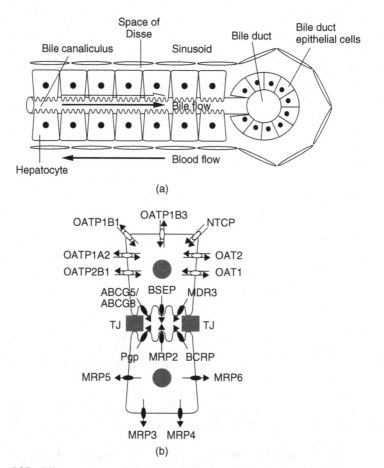

(a)

(b)

Figure 6.25 Microanatomy of the hepatobiliary tract. (a) At the cellular level, hepatocytes are organized in cords and bathed by sinusoidal blood from the basolateral side; the canalicular membranes form the bile canaliculi. Bile flows in the opposite direction to blood and drains into bile ducts and (b) Transport proteins involved in the uptake and excretion of drugs. Adjacent hepatocytes form tight junctions (TJs) to seal the canalicular domain from the basolateral domain. *Source*: Adapted from Reference 136 with permission.

TABLE 6.11 Nasal Cavity

	Body Weight, kg	Length, cm	Surface Area, cm^2	Fluid Volume, ml	MMC $T_{1/2}$, min	Surface Area/Body Weight, cm^2/ kg
Rat	0.25	2.3	10.4–14	0.013	5	49
rabbit	3	4.7	61.9	0.058	10	21
Dog (beagle)	10	10	220.7	0.207	20	22
Rhesus monkey	7	5.3	61.6	0.058	10	9
Man	70	7–8	160–181	0.15	15	2

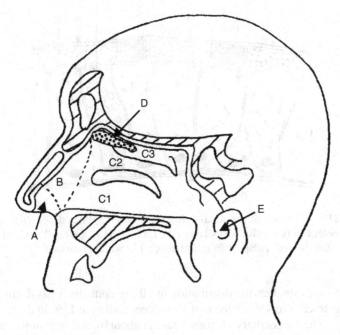

Figure 6.26 Nasal cavity. The (a) nasal vestibule; (b) atrium; (c) respiratory area: inferior turbinate (C1), middle turbinate (C2), and superior turbinate (C3); (d) the olfactory region; and (e) nasopharynx. *Source*: Adapted from Reference 139 with permission.

mucociliary clearance. Substances administered intranasally are rapidly cleared from the human nose, with a clearance half-life of approximately 21 min [138]. The mucous blanket is approximately 5 μm thick (Fig. 6.27). Together with the limited volume that can be administered, the nasal administration presents formulation challenges for poorly soluble drugs. Owing to the direct access to the circulation, the hepatic first-pass metabolism is avoided.

6.8 PULMONARY

6.8.1 Fluid in the Lung

The large absorptive surface at the air interface in the lung is covered by an extremely small volume of fluid (10–20 ml) [140]. The alveolar surface is coated with a liquid layer of 0.2 μm. This fluid is rich in surfactants, comprising approximately 90% lipids and 10% proteins. Within the lipid fraction, the most abundant component is 1,2-dipalmitoyl phosphatidylcholine (ca. 45%). The blood flow lies just beneath the absorptive surface.

6.8.2 Mucociliary Clearance

Ciliated epithelial cells cover 30–65% of the airway epithelial cells in the human respiratory tract. Each ciliated cell has about 200 cilia of 5–6 μm [141]. As the

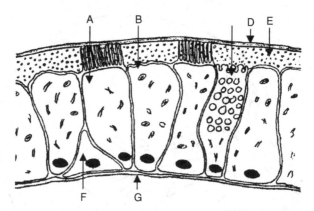

Figure 6.27   Cell types of the nasal epithelium showing ciliated cell (A), nonciliated cell (B), goblet cell (C), gel mucous layer (D), sol layer (E), basal cell (F), and basement membrane (G). *Source*: Adapted from Reference 139 with permission.

airway becomes smaller, the distribution of ciliary epithelial cells decreases from 53% in the trachea to 45% in the first airway generation to 15% in the fifth airway generation. The mucociliary clearance rate is about10 mm/min in the trachea.

6.8.3   Absorption into the Circulation

Aerosol particles in the alveolar space and terminal airway can be removed by absorptive or nonabsorptive processes [141]. Drug absorption from the lungs occurs primarily across the alveolar epithelium. The human lungs contain about 3×10^8 alveoli and have a total surface area of 130 m^2. Each alveolus contains 100 alveolar macrophages, which typically phagocytose 50–70% of particles within 2 h. As the geometric diameters of the particles increase above about 5 μm, removal by phagocytosis becomes less efficient. The adhesion of particles to alveolar macrophages is mediated through electrostatic interaction or receptor mediation, and particles are then internalized through surface cavitation or vacuole and pseudopod formation. Depending on the nature of the particles, internalization is followed by further metabolization or digestion by peptidases in the case of proteins.

6.9   SKIN

The transdermal permeation of most drugs is limited by the stratum corneum (SC) [142, 143]. The thickness of the SC is different at each body part, about 15 μm in the abdominal skin and 10 μm in the dorsal skin. The pH near the surface of the skin is about 5. The structure of the SC is represented by the brick and mortar model, in which keratin-filled cells (corneocytes, brick) are embedded within intercellular lipids (mortar) (Fig. 6.28). The intercellular lipids

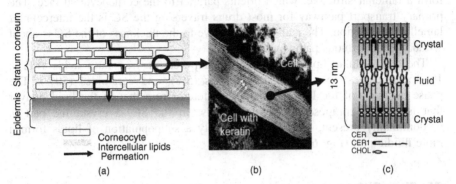

Figure 6.28 Schematic of the stratum corneum. *Source*: Adapted from Reference 142 with permission.

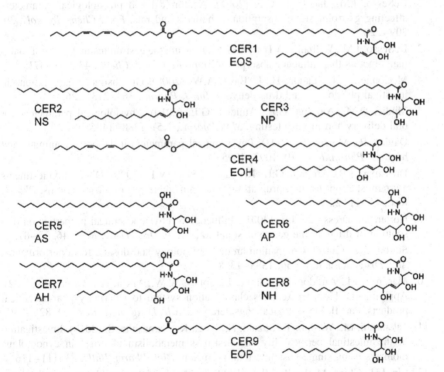

Figure 6.29 Chemical structure of the stratum corneum components. *Source:* Adapted from Reference 45 with permission.

form a lamellar structure, which orients parallel to the corneocyte surface. The primary transport pathway for most drugs traversing the SC is the intercellular lamellar lipid region. The path length relative to the thickness of the SC is about 13 due to the tortuous pathway.

The intercellular lipids are mainly composed of free fatty acids (FFAs, 10–15%), cholesterol (25%), sterol esters (5%), and ceramides (50%). The phase behavior of the lamellar lipid is different from that of the lipid bilayer that is mainly composed of phospholipids. In the SC, a crystalline part is predominantly present, while most probably a subpopulation of lipids form a more fluidic part (Fig. 6.29) [144].

REFERENCES

1. Kararli, T.T. (1995). Comparison of the gastrointestinal anatomy, physiology, and biochemistry of humans and commonly used laboratory animals. *Biopharm. Drug Dispos.*, 16, 351–380.

2. DeSesso, J.M., Jacobson, C.F. (2001). Anatomical and physiological parameters affecting gastrointestinal absorption in humans and rats. *Food Chem. Toxicol.*, 39, 209–228.

3. DeSesso, J.M., Williams, A.L. (2008). Contrasting the gastrointestinal tracts of mammals: factors that influence absorption. *Annu. Rep. Med. Chem.*, 43, 353–371.

4. McConnell, E.L., Fadda, H.M., Basit, A.W. (2008). Gut instincts: explorations in intestinal physiology and drug delivery. *Int. J. Pharm.*, 364, 213–226.

5. Mudie, D.M., Amidon, G.L., Amidon, G.E. (2010). Physiological parameters for oral delivery and in vitro testing. *Mol. Pharm.*, 7(5), 1388–1405.

6. Davies, B., Morris, T. (1993). Physiological parameters in laboratory animals and humans. *Pharm. Res.*, 10, 1093–1095.

7. Dressman, J.B., Amidon, G.L., Reppas, C., Shah, V.P. (1998). Dissolution testing as a prognostic tool for oral drug absorption: immediate release dosage forms. *Pharm. Res.*, 15, 11–22.

8. Horter, D., Dressman, J.B. (2001). Influence of physicochemical properties on dissolution of drugs in the gastrointestinal tract. *Adv. Drug Deliv. Rev.*, 46, 75–87.

9. Sutton, S.C. (2004). Companion animal physiology and dosage form performance. *Adv. Drug Deliv. Rev.*, 56, 1383–1398.

10. Martinez, M., Amidon, G., Clarke, L., Jones, W.W., Mitra, A., Riviere, J. (2002). Applying the biopharmaceutics classification system to veterinary pharmaceutical products. Part II. Physiological considerations. *Adv. Drug Deliv. Rev.*, 54, 825–850.

11. Takahashi, M., Washio, T., Suzuki, N., Igeta, K., Yamashita, S. (2010). Investigation of the intestinal permeability and first-pass metabolism of drugs in cynomolgus monkeys using single-pass intestinal perfusion. *Biol. Pharm. Bull.*, 33, 111–116.

12. Lin, J.H., Chiba, M., Baillie, T.A. (1999). Is the role of the small intestine in first-pass metabolism overemphasized? *Pharmacol. Rev.*, 51, 135–158.

13. Masaoka, Y., Tanaka, Y., Kataoka, M., Sakuma, S., Yamashita, S. (2006). Site of drug absorption after oral administration: assessment of membrane permeability and luminal concentration of drugs in each segment of gastrointestinal tract. *Eur. J. Pharm. Sci.*, 29, 240–250.

14. Diakidou, A., Vertzoni, M., Goumas, K., Soderlind, E., Abrahamsson, B., Dressman, J., Reppas, C. (2009). Characterization of the contents of ascending colon to which drugs are exposed after oral administration to healthy adults. *Pharm. Res.*, 26, 2141–2151.

15. Tannergren, C., Bergendal, A., Lennernas, H., Abrahamsson, B. (2009). Toward an increased understanding of the barriers to colonic drug absorption in humans: implications for early controlled release candidate assessment. *Mol. Pharm.*, 6, 60–73.

16. Trotter, P.J., Storch, J. (1991). Fatty acid uptake and metabolism in a human intestinal cell line (Caco-2): comparison of apical and basolateral incubation. *J. Lipid Res.*, 32, 293–304.

17. Proulx, P. (1991). Structure-function relationships in intestinal brush border membranes. *Biochim. Biophys. Acta*, 1071, 255–271.

18. Dias, V.C., Wallace, J.L., Parsons, H.G. (1992). Modulation of cellular phospholipid fatty acids and leukotriene B4 synthesis in the human intestinal cell (CaCo-2). *Gut*, 33, 622–627.

19. Lipka, G., Op den Kamp, J.A., Hauser, H. (1991). Lipid asymmetry in rabbit small intestinal brush border membrane as probed by an intrinsic phospholipid exchange protein. *Biochemistry*, 30, 11828–11836.

20. Verkleij, A.J., Zwaal, R.F., Roelofsen, B., Comfurius, P., Kastelijn, D., van Deenen, L.L. (1973). The asymmetric distribution of phospholipids in the human red cell membrane. A combined study using phospholipases and freeze-etch electron microscopy. *Biochim. Biophys. Acta*, 323, 178–193.

21. Marrink, S.J., Berendsen, H.J.C. (1996) Permeation process of small molecules across lipid membranes studied by molecular dynamics simulations. *J. Phys. Chem.*, 100, 16729–16738.

22. Marrink, S.-J., Berendsen, H.J.C. (1994). Simulation of water transport through a lipid membrane. *J. Phys. Chem.*, 98, 4155–4168.

23. Anderson, J.M. (2001). Molecular structure of tight junctions and their role in epithelial transport. *News Physiol. Sci.*, 16, 126–130.

24. Sugano, K., Takata, N., Machida, M., Saitoh, K., Terada, K. (2002). Prediction of passive intestinal absorption using bio-mimetic artificial membrane permeation assay and the paracellular pathway model. *Int. J. Pharm.*, 241, 241–251.

25. Sugano, K. (2009). Theoretical investigation of passive intestinal membrane permeability using Monte Carlo method to generate drug like molecule population. *Int. J. Pharm.*, 373, 55–61.

26. He, Y., Murby, S., Warhurst, G., Gifford, L., Walker, D., Ayrton, J., Eastmond, R., Rowland, M. (1998). Species differences in size discrimination in the paracellular pathway refrected by oral bioavailability of poly(ethylene glycol) and D-peptides. *J. Pharm. Sci.*, 87, 626–633.

27. Avdeef, A. (2010). Leakiness and size exclusion of paracellular channels in cultured epithelial cell monolayers-interlaboratory comparison. *Pharm. Res.*, 27, 480–489.

28. Adson, A., Ruab, T.J., Burton, P.S., Barsuhn, C.L., Hilgers, A.R., Audus, K.L., Ho, N.F.H. (1994). Quantitative approaches to delineate paracellular diffusion in cultured epithelial cell monolayers. *J. Pharm. Sci.*, 83, 1529–1530.

29. Adson, A., Burton, P.S., Ruab, T.J., Barsuhn, C.L., Audus, L., Ho, N.F.H. (1995). Passive diffusion of weak organic electrolytes across Caco-2 cell monolayers: uncoupling the contributions of hydrodynamic, transcellular and paracellular barriers. *Pharm. Res.*, 84, 1197–1203.

30. Pade, V., Stavchansky, S. (1997). Estimation of the relative contribution of the transcellular and paracellular pathway to the transport of passively absorbed drugs in the Caco-2 cell culture model. *Pharm. Res.*, 14, 1210–1215.

31. Sugano, K., Nabuchi, Y., Machida, M., Aso, Y. (2003). Prediction of human intestinal permeability using artificial membrane permeability. *Int. J. Pharm.*, 257, 245–251.

32. Avdeef, A., Tam, K.Y. (2010). How well can the Caco-2/Madin-darby canine kidney models predict effective human jejunal permeability? *J. Med. Chem.*, 53, 3566–3584.

33. Tam, K.Y., Avdeef, A., Tsinman, O., Sun, N. (2010). The permeation of amphoteric drugs through artificial membranes—an in combo absorption model based on paracellular and transmembrane permeability. *J. Med. Chem.*, 53, 392–401.

34. Cone, R.A. (2009). Barrier properties of mucus. *Adv. Drug Delivery Rev.*, 61, 75–85.

35. Allen, A., Flemstroem, G. (2005). Gastroduodenal mucus bicarbonate barrier: protection against acid and pepsin. *Am. J. Physiol.*, 288, C1–C19.

36. Atuma, C., Strugala, V., Allen, A., Holm, L. (2001). The adherent gastrointestinal mucus gel layer: thickness and physical state in vivo. *Am. J. Physiol.*, 280, G922–G929.

37. Doyle-McCullough, M., Smyth, S.H., Moyes, S.M., Carr, K.E. (2007). Factors influencing intestinal microparticle uptake in vivo. *Int. J. Pharm.*, 335, 79–89.

38. Hodges, G.M., Carr, E.A., Hazzard, R.A., Carr, K.E. (1995). Uptake and translocation of microparticles in small intestine. Morphology and quantification of particle distribution. *Dig. Dis. Sci.*, 40, 967–975.

39. Limpanussorn, J., Simon, L., Dayan, A.D. (1998). Transepithelial transport of large particles in rat: a new model for the quantitative study of particle uptake. *J. Pharm. Pharmacol.*, 50, 753–760.

40. Norris, D.A., Puri, N., Sinko, P.J. (1998). The effect of physical barriers and properties on the oral absorption of particulates. *Adv. Drug Delivery Rev.*, 34, 135–154.

41. Smyth, S.H., Feldhaus, S., Schumacher, U., Carr, K.E. (2008). Uptake of inert microparticles in normal and immune deficient mice. *Int. J. Pharm.*, 346, 109–118.

42. Davis, S.S., Hardy, J.G., Fara, J.W. (1986). Transit of pharmaceutical dosage forms through the small intestine. *Gut*, 27, 886–892.

43. Hunt, J.N., Stubbs, D.F. (1975). The volume and energy content of meals as determinants of gastric emptying. *J. Physiol.*, 245, 209–225.

44. Nimmo, W.S. (1976). Drugs, diseases and altered gastric emptying. *Clin. Pharmacokinet.*, 1, 189–203.

45. Ikegami, K., Tagawa, K., Narisawa, S., Osawa, T. (2003). Suitability of the cynomolgus monkey as an animal model for drug absorption studies of oral dosage forms from the viewpoint of gastrointestinal physiology. *Biol. Pharm. Bull.*, 26, 1442–1447.

46. Dressman, J. (1986). Comparison of canin and human gastrointestinal physiology. *Pharm. Res.*, 3, 123–130.

47. Fadda, H.M., McConnell, E.L., Short, M.D., Basit, A.W. (2009). Meal-Induced Acceleration of Tablet Transit Through the Human Small Intestine. *Pharm. Res.*, 26, 356–360.

48. Watts, P.J., Barrowb, L., Steedb, K.P., Wilsonb, C.G., Spillerc, R.C., Meliaa, C.D., Davies, M.C. (1992). The transit rate of different-sized model dosage forms through the human colon and the effects of a lactulose-induced catharsis. *Int. J. Pharm.*, 87, 215–221.

49. Hansen, M.B. (2002). Small intestinal manometry. *Physiol. Res.*, 51, 541–556.

50. Takahashi, T. (2007). Effects of food intake on interdigestive migrating motor complex (MMC). *Neurogastroenterology*, 10, 76–77.

51. Steffen, D., Physiological parameters relevant to dissolution testing, in: J. Dressman and J. Krämer (Eds.) Pharmaceutical Dissolution Testing, Informa Healthcare, Florida, 2005, pp. 127–191.

52. Pal, A., Indireshkumar, K., Schwizer, W., Abrahamsson, B., Fried, M., Brasseur James, G. (2004). Gastric flow and mixing studied using computer simulation. *Proc. Biol. Sci.*, 271, 2587–2594.

53. Dillard, S., Krishnan, S., Udaykumar, H.S. (2007). Mechanics of flow and mixing at antroduodenal junction. *World J. Gastroenterol.*, 13, 1365–1371.

54. Funakoshi, M. (2008). Chaotic mixing and mixing efficiency in a short time. *Fluid Dyn. Res.*, 40, 1–33.

55. Sugano, K. (2010). Aqueous boundary layers related to oral absorption of a drug: from dissolution of a drug to carrier mediated transport and intestinal wall metabolism. *Mol. Pharm.*, 7, 1362–1373.

56. Womack, W.A., Barrowman, J.A., Graham, W.H., Benoit, J.N., Kvietys, P.R., Granger, D.N. (1987). Quantitative assessment of villous motility. *Am. J. Physiol.*, 252, G250–G256.

57. Strocchi, A., Levitt, M.D. (1993). Role of villous surface area in absorption. Science versus religion. *Dig. Dis. Sci.*, 38, 385–387.

58. Mailman, D., Womack, W.A., Kvietys, P.R., Granger, D.N. (1990). Villous motility and unstirred water layers in canine intestine. *Am. J. Physiol.*, 258, G238–G246.

59. Janssen, P.W.M., Lentle, R.G., Asvarujanon, P., Chambers, P., Stafford, K.J., Hemar, Y. (2007). Characterization of flow and mixing regimes within the ileum of the brushtail possum using residence time distribution analysis with simultaneous spatiotemporal mapping. *J. Physiol.*, 582, 1239–1248.

60. Katori, N., Aoyagi, N., Terao, T. (1995). Estimation of agitation intensity in the GI tract in humans and dogs based on in vitro/in vivo correlation. *Pharm. Res.*, 12, 237–243.

61. Rostami-Hodjegan, A., Shiran, M.R., Tucker, G.T., Conway, B.R., Irwin, W.J., Shaw, L.R., Grattan, T.J. (2002). A new rapidly absorbed paracetamol tablet containing sodium bicarbonate. II. Dissolution studies and in vitro/in vivo correlation. *Drug Dev. Ind. Pharm.*, 28, 533–543.

62. Parojcic, J., Vasiljevic, D., Ibric, S., Djuric, Z. (2008). Tablet disintegration and drug dissolution in viscous media: paracetamol IR tablets. *Int. J. Pharm.*, 355, 93–99.

63. D'Arcy, D.M., Healy, A.M., Corrigan, O.I. (2009). Towards determining appropriate hydrodynamic conditions for in vitro in vivo correlations using computational fluid dynamics. *Eur. J. Pharm. Sci.*, 37, 291–299.

64. Crail, D.J., Tunis, A., Dansereau, R. (2004). Is the use of a 200ml vessel suitable for dissolution of low dose drug products? *Int. J. Pharm.*, 269, 203–209.

65. Kamba, M., Seta, Y., Kusai, A., Nishimura, K. (2002). Comparison of the mechanical destructive force in the small intestine of dog and human. *Int. J. Pharm.*, 237, 139–149.

66. Kamba, M., Seta, Y., Kusai, A., Ikeda, M., Nishimura, K. (2000). A unique dosage form to evaluate the mechanical destructive force in the gastrointestinal tract. *Int. J. Pharm.*, 208, 61–70.

67. Kamba, M., Seta, Y., Kusai, A., Nishimura, K. (2001). Evaluation of the mechanical destructive force in the stomach of dog. *Int. J. Pharm.*, 228, 209–217.

68. Kamba, M., Seta, Y., Takeda, N., Hamaura, T., Kusai, A., Nakane, H., Nishimura, K. (2003). Measurement of agitation force in dissolution test and mechanical destructive force in disintegration test. *Int. J. Pharm.*, 250, 99–109.

69. Chiou, W.L. (1994). Effect of 'unstirred' water layer in the intestine on the rate and extent of absorption after oral administration. *Biopharm. Drug Dispos.*, 15, 709–717.

70. Levitt, M.D., Furne, J.K., Strocchi, A., Anderson, B.W., Levitt, D.G. (1990). Physiological measurements of luminal stirring in the dog and human small bowel. *J. Clin. Invest.*, 86, 1540–1547.

71. Lennernäs, H. (2007). Intestinal permeability and its relevance for absorption and elimination. *Xenobiotica*, 37, 1015–1051.

72. Sugano, K. (2011). Fraction of a dose absorbed estimation for structurally diverse low solubility compounds. *Int. J. Pharm.*, 405, 79–89.

73. Wang, Y., Brasseur, J.G., Banco, G.G., Webb, A.G., Ailiani, A.C., Neuberger, T. (2010). A multiscale lattice Boltzmann model of macro- to micro-scale transport, with applications to gut function. *Philos. Trans. R. Soc. London, Ser. A*, 368, 2863–2880.

74. Knutson, T., Fridblom, P., Ahlstrom, H., Magnusson, A., Tannergren, C., Lennernas, H. (2008). Increased understanding of intestinal drug permeability determined by the LOC-I-GUT approach using multislice computed tomography. *Mol. Pharm.*, 6, 2–10.

75. Pappenheimer, J.R. (1998). Scaling of dimensions of small intestines in non-ruminant eutherian mammals and its significance for absorptive mechanisms. *Comp. Biochem. Physiol., A Mol. Integr. Physiol.*, 121, 45–58.

76. Schiller, C., Frohlich, C.P., Giessmann, T., Siegmund, W., Monnikes, H., Hosten, N., Weitschies, W. (2005). Intestinal fluid volumes and transit of dosage forms as assessed by magnetic resonance imaging. *Aliment. Pharmacol. Ther.*, 22, 971–979.

77. Marciani, L., Cox Eleanor, F., Hoad Caroline, L., Pritchard, S., Totman John, J., Foley, S., Mistry, A., Evans, S., Gowland Penny, A., Spiller Robin, C. (2010). Postprandial changes in small bowel water content in healthy subjects and patients with irritable bowel syndrome. *Gastroenterology*, 138, 469–477, e461.

78. Sutton, S.C. (2009). Role of physiological intestinal water in oral absorption. *AAPS J.*, 11, 277–285.

79. Tachibana, T., Kato, M., Watanabe, T., Mitsui, T., Sugiyama, Y. (2009). Method for predicting the risk of drug-drug interactions involving inhibition of intestinal CYP3A4 and P-glycoprotein. *Xenobiotica*, 39, 430–443.

80. Sugano, K., Shirasaka, Y., Yamashita, S., Velicky, M., Bradley, D.F., Tam, K.Y., Dryfe, R.A. (2011). Estimation of Michaelis-Menten constant of efflux transporter considering asymmetric permeability. Fraction of a dose absorbed estimation for

structurally diverse low solubility compounds. In situ artificial membrane permeation assay under hydrodynamic control: permeability-pH profiles of warfarin and verapamil. *Int. J. Pharm.*, 8, 8.

81. Sugano, K., Kataoka, M., Mathews, Cd.C., Yamashita, S. (2010). Prediction of food effect by bile micelles on oral drug absorption considering free fraction in intestinal fluid. *Eur. J. Pharm. Sci.*, 40, 118–124.

82. Freire, A.C., Basit, A.W., Choudhary, R., Piong, C.W., Merchant, H.A. (2011). Does sex matter? The influence of gender on gastrointestinal physiology and drug delivery. *Int. J. Pharm.*, 415, 15–28.

83. Diakidou, A., Vertzoni, M., Goumas, K., Soederlind, E., Abrahamsson, B., Dressman, J., Reppas, C. (2009). Characterization of the contents of ascending colon to which drugs are exposed after oral administration to healthy adults. *Pharm. Res.*, 26, 2141–2151.

84. Lindahl, A., Ungell, A.-L., Knutson, L., Lennernaes, H. (1997). Characterization of fluids from the stomach and proximal jejunum in men and women. *Pharm. Res.*, 14, 497–502.

85. Yamada, I., Goda, T., Kawata, M., Ogawa, K. (1990). Use of gastric acidity-controlled beagle dogs in bioavailability studies of cinnarizine. *Yakugaku Zasshi*, 110, 280–285.

86. Polentarutti, B., Albery, T., Dressman, J., Abrahamsson, B. (2010). Modification of gastric pH in the fasted dog. *J. Pharm. Pharmacol.*, 62, 462–469.

87. Akimoto, M., Nagahata, N., Furuya, A., Fukushima, K., Higuchi, S., Suwa, T. (2000). Gastric pH profiles of beagle dogs and their use as an alternative to human testing. *Eur. J. Pharm. Biopharm.*, 49, 99–102.

88. Sagawa, K., Li, F., Liese, R., Sutton, S.C. (2009). Fed and fasted gastric pH and gastric residence time in conscious beagle dogs. *J. Pharm. Sci.*, 98, 2494–2500.

89. Dietschy, J.M. (1968). Mechanisms for the intestinal absorption of bile acids. *J. Lipid Res.*, 9, 297–309.

90. McConnell, E.L., Basit, A.W., Murdan, S. (2008). Measurements of rat and mouse gastrointestinal pH, fluid and lymphoid tissue, and implications for in-vivo experiments. *J. Pharm. Pharmacol.*, 60, 63–70.

91. Said, H.M., Blair, J.A., Lucas, M.L., Hilburn, M.E. (1986). Intestinal surface acid microclimate in vitro and in vivo in the rat. *J. Lab. Clin. Med.*, 107, 420–424.

92. Shiau, Y.F., Fernandez, P., Jackson, M.J., McMonagle, S. (1985). Mechanisms maintaining a low-pH microclimate in the intestine. *Am. J. Physiol.*, 248, G608–G617.

93. Lee, K.J., Johnson, N., Castelo, J., Sinko, P.J., Grass, G., Holme, K., Lee, Y.H. (2005). Effect of experimental pH on the in vitro permeability in intact rabbit intestines and Caco-2 monolayer. *Eur J Pharm Sci.*, 25, 193–200.

94. Hoegerle, M.L., Winne, D. (1983). Drug absorption by the rat jejunum perfused in situ. Dissociation from the pH-partition theory and role of microclimate-pH and unstirred layer. *Naunyn Schmiedebergs Arch. Pharmacol.*, 322, 249–255.

95. McNeil, N.I., Ling, K.L., Wager, J. (1987). Mucosal surface pH of the large intestine of the rat and of normal and inflamed large intestine in man. *Gut*, 28, 707–713.

96. Genz, A.K., v Engelhardt, W., Busche, R. (1999). Maintenance and regulation of the pH microclimate at the luminal surface of the distal colon of guinea-pig. *J. Physiol.*, 517(Pt.2), 507–519.

97. Yamaguchi, T., Ikeda, C., Sekine, Y. (1986). Intestinal absorption of a b-adrenergic blocking agent nadolol. I. Comparison of absorption behavior of nadolol with those of other b-blocking agents in rats. *Chem. Pharm. Bull.*, 34, 3362–3369.

98. Yamaguchi, T., Ikeda, C., Sekine, Y. (1986). Intestinal absorption of a b-adrenergic blocking agent nadolol. II. Mechanism of the inhibitory effect on the intestinal absorption of nadolol by sodium cholate in rats. *Chem. Pharm. Bull.*, 34, 3836–3843.

99. Yamaguchi, T., Oida, T., Ikeda, C., Sekine, Y. (1986). Intestinal absorption of a b-adrenergic blocking agent nadolol. III. Nuclear magnetic resonance spectroscopic study on nadolol-sodium cholate micellar complex and intestinal absorption of nadolol derivatives in rats. *Chem. Pharm. Bull.*, 34, 4259–4264.

100. Amidon, G.E., Higuchi, W.I., Ho, N.F.H. (1982). Theoretical and experimental studies of transport of micelle-solubilized solutes. *J. Pharm. Sci.*, 71, 77–84.

101. Ingels, F., Beck, B., Oth, M., Augustijns, P. (2004). Effect of simulated intestinal fluid on drug permeability estimation across Caco-2 monolayers. *Int. J. Pharm.*, 274, 221–232.

102. Poelma, F.G.J., Breaes, R., Tukker, J.J. (1990). Intestinal absorption of drugs. III. The influence of taurocholate on the disappearance kinetics of hydrophilic and lipophilic drugs from the small intestine of the rat. *Pharm. Res.*, 7, 392–397.

103. Poelma, F.G.J., Breas, R., Tukker, J.J., Crommelin, D.J.A. (1991). Intestinal absorption of drugs. The influence of mixed micelles on the disappearance kinetics of drugs from the small intestine of the rat. *J. Pharm. Pharmacol.*, 43, 317–324.

104. Tangerman, A., van Schaik, A., van der Hoek, E.W. (1986). Analysis of conjugated and unconjugated bile acids in serum and jejunal fluid of normal subjects. *Clin. Chim. Acta*, 159, 123–132.

105. Kalantzi, L., Goumas, K., Kalioras, V., Abrahamsson, B., Dressman, J.B., Reppas, C. (2006). Characterization of the human upper gastrointestinal contents under conditions simulating bioavailability/bioequivalence studies. *Pharm. Res.*, 23, 165–176.

106. Perez de la Cruz Moreno, M., Oth, M., Deferme, S., Lammert, F., Tack, J., Dressman, J., Augustijns, P. (2006). Characterization of fasted-state human intestinal fluids collected from duodenum and jejunum. *J. Pharm. Pharmacol.*, 58, 1079–1089.

107. Meier, Y., Eloranta, J.J., Darimont, J., Ismair, M.G., Hiller, C., Fried, M., Kullak-Ublick, G.A., Vavricka, S.R. (2007). Regional distribution of solute carrier mRNA expression along the human intestinal tract. *Drug Metab. Dispos.*, 35, 590–594.

108. Lennernaes, H., Regaardh, C.G. (1993). Evidence for an interaction between the b-blocker pafenolol and bile salts in the intestinal lumen of the rat leading to dose-dependent oral absorption and double peaks in the plasma concentration-time profile. *Pharm. Res.*, 10, 879–883.

109. Ladas, S.D., Isaacs, P.E., Murphy, G.M., Sladen, G.E. (1984). Comparison of the effects of medium and long chain triglyceride containing liquid meals on gall bladder and small intestinal function in normal man. *Gut.*, 25, 405–411.

110. Hopman, W.P., Jansen, J.B., Rosenbusch, G., Lamers, C.B. (1984). Effect of equimolar amounts of long-chain triglycerides and medium-chain triglycerides on plasma cholecystokinin and gallbladder contraction. *Am. J. Clin. Nutr.*, 39, 356–359.

111. Scholz, A., Abrahamsson, B., Diebold, S.M., Kostewicz, E., Polentarutti, B.I., Ungell, A.-L., Dressman, J.B. (2002). Influence of hydrodynamics and particle size on the absorption of felodipine in labradors. *Pharm. Res.*, 19, 42–46.

112. Kalantzi, L., Persson, E., Polentarutti, B., Abrahamsson, B., Goumas, K., Dressman, J.B., Reppas, C. (2006). Canine intestinal contents vs. simulated media for the assessment of solubility of two weak bases in the human small intestinal contents. *Pharm. Res.*, 23, 1373–1381.

113. Englund, G., Rorsman, F., Roennblom, A., Karlbom, U., Lazorova, L., Grasjoe, J., Kindmark, A., Artursson, P. (2006). Regional levels of drug transporters along the human intestinal tract: co-expression of ABC and SLC transporters and comparison with Caco-2 cells. *Eur. J. Pharm. Sci.*, 29, 269–277.

114. Cao, Xea. (2006). Why is it challenging to predict intestinal drug absorption and oral bioavailability in human using rat model. *Pharm. Res.*, 23, 1675–1686.

115. Aller, S.G., Yu, J., Ward, A., Weng, Y., Chittaboina, S., Zhuo, R., Harrell, P.M., Trinh, Y.T., Zhang, Q., Urbatsch, I.L., Chang, G. (2009). Structure of P-glycoprotein reveals a molecular basis for poly-specific drug binding. *Science (Washington, DC)*, 323, 1718–1722.

116. Mouly, S., Paine, M.F. (2003). P-glycoprotein increases from proximal to distal regions of human small intestine. *Pharm. Res.*, 20, 1595–1599.

117. Makhey, V.D., Guo, A., Norris, D.A., Hu, P., Yan, J., Sinko, P.J. (1998). Characterization of the regional intestinal kinetics of drug efflux in rat and human intestine and in Caco-2 cells. *Pharm. Res.*, 15, 1160–1167.

118. Thorn, M., Finnstrom, N., Lundgren, S., Rane, A., Loof, L. (2005). Cytochromes P450 and MDR1 mRNA expression along the human gastrointestinal tract. *Br. J. Clin. Pharmacol.*, 60, 54–60.

119. Katoh, M., Suzuyama, N., Takeuchi, T., Yoshitomi, S., Asahi, S., Yokoi, T. (2006). Kinetic analyses for species differences in P-glycoprotein-mediated drug transport. *J. Pharm. Sci.*, 95, 2673–2683.

120. Paine, M.F., Hart, H.L., Ludington, S.S., Haining, R.L., Rettie, A.E., Zeldin, D.C. (2006). The human intestinal cytochrome P450 "pie". *Drug Metab. Dispos.*, 34, 880–886.

121. Beaumont, K., The importance of gut wall metabolism in determining drug bioavailability, in: H. van de Waterbeemd, H. Lennernäs, P. Artursson (Eds.) Drug Bioavailability: Estimation of Solubility, Permeability, Absorption and Bioavailability, Wiley-VCH Verlag GmbH & Co. KGaA, New York, 2003, pp. 311–328.

122. Borgstrom, L., Nyberg, L., Jonsson, S., Lindberg, C., Paulson, J. (1989). Pharmacokinetic evaluation in man of terbutaline given as separate enantiomers and as the racemate. *Br. J. Clin. Pharmacol.*, 27, 49–56.

123. Hochhaus, G., Mollmann, H. (1992). Pharmacokinetic/pharmacodynamic characteristics of the beta-2-agonists terbutaline, salbutamol and fenoterol. *Int. J. Clin. Pharmacol. Ther. Toxicol.*, 30, 342–362.

124. Mizuma, T., Kawashima, K., Sakai, S., Sakaguchi, S., Hayashi, M. (2005). Differentiation of organ availability by sequential and simultaneous analyses: intestinal conjugative metabolism impacts on intestinal availability in humans. *J. Pharm. Sci.*, 94, 571–575.

125. Roberts, M.S., Magnusson, B.M., Burczynski, F.J., Weiss, M. (2002). Enterohepatic circulation: physiological, pharmacokinetic and clinical implications. *Clin. Pharmacokinet.*, 41, 751–790.

126. Matheson, P.J., Wilson, M.A., Garrison, R.N. (2000). Regulation of intestinal blood flow. *J. Surg. Res.*, 93, 182–196.

127. Yang, J., Jamei, M., Yeo, K.R., Tucker, G.T., Rostami-Hodjegan, A. (2007). Prediction of intestinal first-pass drug metabolism. *Curr. Drug Metab.*, 8, 676–684.

128. Nomeir, A.A., Morrison, R., Prelusky, D., Korfmacher, W., Broske, L., Hesk, D., McNamara, P., Mei, H. (2009). Estimation of the extent of oral absorption in animals from oral and intravenous pharmacokinetic data in drug discovery. *J. Pharm. Sci.*, 98, 4027–4038.

129. Olanoff, L.S., Walle, T., Cowart, T.D., Walle, U.K., Oexmann, M.J., Conradi, E.C. (1986). Food effects on propranolol systemic and oral clearance: support for a blood flow hypothesis. *Clin. Pharmacol. Ther.*, 40, 408–414.

130. Lemmer, B., Nold, G. (1991). Circadian changes in estimated hepatic blood flow in healthy subjects. *Br. J. Clin. Pharmacol.*, 32, 627–629.

131. Langner, B., Lemmer, B. (1988). Circadian changes in the pharmacokinetics and cardiovascular effects of oral propranolol in healthy subjects. *Eur. J. Clin. Pharmacol.*, 33, 619–624.

132. Lemmer, B., Nold, G., Behne, S., Kaiser, R. (1991). Chronopharmacokinetics and cardiovascular effects of nifedipine. *Chronobiol. Int.*, 8, 485–494.

133. Lemmer, B., Scheidel, B., Blume, H., Becker, H.J. (1991). Clinical chronopharmacology of oral sustained-release isosorbide-5-mononitrate in healthy subjects. *Eur. J. Clin. Pharmacol.*, 40, 71–75.

134. Shaffer, E.A. (2000). Review article: control of gall-bladder motor function. *Aliment. Pharmacol. Ther.*, 14 (Suppl. 2), 2–8.

135. Merck. *Merck Manual* http://merckmanual.jp/mmpej/seco3/cho0/cho30/cho3oa. html.

136. Ghibellini, G., Leslie, E.M., Brouwer, K.L. (2006). Methods to evaluate biliary excretion of drugs in humans: an updated review. *Mol. Pharm.*, 3, 198–211.

137. Yang, X., Gandhi, Y.A., Duignan, D.B., Morris, M.E. (2009). Prediction of biliary excretion in rats and humans using molecular weight and quantitative structure-pharmacokinetic relationships. *AAPS J.*, 11, 511–525.

138. Soane, R.J., Frier, M., Perkins, A.C., Jones, N.S., Davis, S.S., Illum, L. (1999). Evaluation of the clearance characteristics of bioadhesive systems in humans. *Int. J. Pharm.*, 178, 55–65.

139. Ugwoke, M.I., Verbeke, N., Kinget, R. (2001). The biopharmaceutical aspects of nasal mucoadhesive drug delivery. *J. Pharm. Pharmacol.*, 53, 3–21.

140. Patton, J.S., Fishburn, C.S., Weers, J.G. (2004). The lungs as a portal of entry for systemic drug delivery. *Proc. Am. Thorac. Soc.*, 1, 338–344.

141. Hardy, J.G., Chadwick, T.S. (2000). Sustained release drug delivery to the lungs: an option for the future. *Clin. Pharmacokinet.*, 39, 1–4.

142. Bouwstra, J.A., Honeywell-Nguyen, P. L., Gooris, G.S., Ponec, M. (2003). Structure of the skin barrier and its modulation by vesicular formulations. *Prog. Lipid Res.*, 42, 1–36.

143. Hadgraft, J. (2004). Skin deep. *Eur. J. Pharm. Biopharm.*, 58, 291–299.

144. Talreja, P., Kleene, N.K., Pickens, W.L., Wang, T.F., Kasting, G.B. (2001). Visualization of the lipid barrier and measurement of lipid pathlength in human stratum corneum. *AAPS Pharm. Sci.*, 3, E13.

145. de Jager, M.W., Gooris, G.S., Dolbnya, I.P., Ponec, M., Bouwstra, J.A. (2004). Modelling the stratum corneum lipid organisation with synthetic lipid mixtures: the importance of synthetic ceramide composition. *Biochim. Biophys. Acta*, 1664, 132–140.

CHAPTER 7

DRUG PARAMETERS

"It is much easier to make measurements than to know exactly what you are measuring."

—J. W. N. Sullivan

It is critically important to prepare high quality input data for high quality biopharmaceutical modeling. Even though it might look easy, the experiments are actually very difficult and meticulous care is required to obtain high quality data. More than twofold error could occur easily. Considering the propagation of error, even a small error in each parameter could pile up to a significant error in the final output. It is important to understand the specification of each experiment, pros and cons of each method, and accuracy level of each data. In this section, experimental methods to obtain the drug parameters for biopharmaceutical modeling are discussed.

7.1 DISSOCIATION CONSTANT (pK_a)

The dissociation constant (K_a) of a drug is one of the most important parameter for biopharmaceutical modeling. pK_a affects solubility (Henderson–Hasselbalch equation; Section 2.3.2), the dissolution rate (solid surface pH; Section 3.2.6), and permeability (pH partition theory; Section 4.8). Even though computational prediction from the chemical structure is available, it is highly recommended

Biopharmaceutics Modeling and Simulations: Theory, Practice, Methods, and Applications,
First Edition. Kiyohiko Sugano.
© 2012 John Wiley & Sons, Inc. Published 2012 by John Wiley & Sons, Inc.

to use a measured pK_a value for biopharmaceutical modeling. Computational prediction often has circa 1 pK_a unit error (10-fold error as K_a) [1, 2]. The pH titration, pH–UV shift, and capillary electrophoresis methods are most often used in drug discovery and development. In the case of compounds with low solubility, pK_a should also be obtained from the pH–solubility profile and compared with the values from other methods.

7.1.1 pH Titration

The pH titration method is one of the authentic methods to obtain pK_a values [3]. When the solution containing a drug is titrated by an acid or an alkali such as HCl or KOH solution, the pH change becomes less sensitive to the titrated amount around the pK_a of a drug because of the buffering effect of the drug molecules. The advantage of this method is that the pK_a of a dissociable group, which is not near the chromosphere, can be measured. The disadvantage is that this method requires 5–10 mg sample. For drugs with low solubility, an organic solvent can be added to the test solution and the pK_a values at each percentage of organic solvent are extrapolated to 0%. Automated instruments are commercially available.

7.1.2 pH–UV Shift

When a dissociable group is within or close to the chromophore of a drug, the UV spectrum changes when pH is shifted [4]. The advantages of this method are that this method requires less than 1 mg sample and a DMSO sample stock solution can be used. The disadvantage of this method is that the pK_a of a dissociable group not near the chromosphere cannot be measured. Automated instruments are commercially available. Impurities in a sample can affect the result when it has a strong chromophore.

Similar concept can be used with NMR spectroscopy, but the pK_a of a dissociable group not near the chromophore can also be measured.

7.1.3 Capillary Electrophoresis

The capillary electrophoresis method is becoming more popular recently [5–7]. When a charged molecule is put in an electric field, it migrates toward the electrode of the opposite charge. The migration index at each pH depends on f_z and z. From the pH migration index relationship (usually 10–20 pH points between pH 2–11), the pK_a value of a drug can be obtained. The advantages of this method are that this method requires less than 0.1 mg sample, a DMSO sample stock solution can be used, and this method is suitable for less pure samples. The pK_a of samples with low solubility can be measured as far as it is detectable. The 96-well format and the pressure-supported method have been implemented to increase the throughput of this method [5, 8–11].

7.1.4 pH–Solubility Profile

The pK_a of a drug can be calculated from the pH–solubility profile (Fig. 2.11) [12]. For a drug with low solubility, this method is very useful. Usually, the pH–solubility profile data becomes available at the late discovery stage [13, 14]. Because the other method can have an error in pK_a for a drug with low solubility, this method should always be applied when the pH–solubility profile is available.

7.1.5 Calculation from Chemical Structure

Even though calculation from the chemical structure is still not accurate enough to be an alternative to experimental measurements, it can support pK_a assignment. Assignment of pK_a to a functional group is often not obvious for heterocyclic drugs and other structurally complex drugs. The most often encountered misunderstandings are "nitrogen is always a base," "$pK_a > 7$ always denoted basicity," "$pK_a < 7$ always denoted acidity," etc. Some programs predict both macro- and micro-pK_as for multivalent drugs.

7.1.6 Recommendation

The pK_a data is the most crucial data for biopharmaceutical modeling. It affects solubility, dissolution rate, permeability, cytosol concentration, etc. Therefore, pK_a should be obtained with good precision (<0.1 log unit error is preferable). To increase the robustness, two or more methods can be used and the pK_a values can be compared. In real drug discovery, it is often the case that a discrepancy between the methods is observed, especially for drugs with low solubility.

7.2 OCTANOL–WATER PARTITION COEFFICIENT

The octanol–water partition coefficient of a drug is one of the most reliably obtainable data in drug discovery and should be experimentally measured before starting biopharmaceutical modeling. The importance of log P_{oct} is often underestimated. This is the key parameter not only for biopharmaceutical modeling but also for understanding the pharmacokinetics of a drug, for example, distribution to each organ (including CNS and liver) [15–17] and renal reabsorption. Furthermore, log P_{oct} is often related to the toxicity of a drug, for example, phospholipidosis [18]. In biopharmaceutical modeling, log P_{oct} is used for estimating $P_{trans,0}$, intrinsic solubility, K_{bm}, etc. log P_{oct} value is the most consistent data obtained from laboratories. log P_{oct} is a common language among many disciplines in drug discovery and development. We have a huge wealth of knowledge about log P_{oct}. Therefore, as the *de facto* standard lipophilicity parameter, log P_{oct} has an irreplaceable value in drug discovery.

Even though there are many *in silico* log P_{oct} prediction programs, the prediction accuracy for a newly synthesized compound is usually not sufficient

Figure 7.1 log P_{oct} and log D_{oct}.

(on average, circa 10-fold error) [19, 20]. Therefore, it is highly recommended to use an experimental log P_{oct} data for biopharmaceutical modeling.

Figure 7.1 explains the difference between log P_{oct} and log D_{oct}. log P_{oct} is the logarithm of the partition coefficient of undissociated (unionized) drug molecules between octanol and water, whereas log D_{oct} is the logarithm of the distribution coefficient as the sum of undissociated and ionized species at a pH.

To measure log P_{oct}, a pH in which the drug does not dissociate is used. log P_{oct} can be also back-calculated from log D_{oct}, pK_a, and pH (cf. $D_{\text{oct}} = f_0 P_{\text{oct}}$). When using the latter method, the ion pair partitioning of the dissociated species should be kept at a minimum [21].

For zwitterions, it is impossible to separately measure the concentration of neutral and zwitterionic species. Therefore, log D_{oct} should be measured at a physiological pH of interest [22]. The lipophilicity of zwitterion species is usually higher than that of the monoanionic and monocationic species and the pH–lipophilicity profile becomes bell shaped. Even when the zwitterionic species is predominant at a physiological pH, many zwitterionic drugs have good membrane permeability, for example, fluoroquinolones [23]. It should be noted that some software calculate log P_{oct} as of the undissociated species ([AH-B] in Figure 2.5), while the others calculate it as of the total of neutral species ([AHB] + [A-BH$^+$]).

7.2.1 Shake Flask Method

The shake flask (SF) method is the gold standard method to experimentally determine log P_{oct} and log D_{oct}. With a standard SF method, log D_{oct} can be reliably measured within $-2 < \log D_{\text{oct}} < 4$ range ($0.01 < D_{\text{oct}} < 10,000$). This dynamic range is significantly wider than that of an *in vitro* membrane permeability assay such as Caco-2 (0.1–20×10^{-6} cm/s for P_{ep} measurement). However, when log $D_{\text{oct}} > 4$, standard experimental methods could have significant artifact as a result of the contamination of octanol and water phases. An improved method to avoid the octanol-phase contamination has been reported [24, 25].

7.2.2 HPLC Method

HPLC-based methods have been extensively investigated [26–28]. The retention time of reverse phase HPLC correlates with the lipophilicity of a drug. However, the chemical selectivity largely depends on the characteristics of the stationary and mobile phases. Therefore, the stationary and mobile phases have to be carefully selected so that the chemical selectivity of an HPLC method becomes similar to that of real octanol–water partitioning. The advantage of this method is that it can be applied for high log P_{oct} range. The disadvantage of this method is that the chemical selectivity is not perfectly identical to octanol–water partitioning, especially for acidic compounds. Micelle capillary electrophoresis has also been used to estimate log P_{oct} [29–32].

7.2.3 Two-Phase Titration Method

The pH titration curve shifts with and without the coexistence of organic phase [33, 34]. The two-phase titration method can be used to obtain the partition coefficient of both unionized and ionized species.

7.2.4 PAMPA-Based Method

Recently, a PAMPA (parallel artificial membrane permeation assay)-based method was reported (Section 7.9.4). The PAMPA setup enables HTS (high throughput screening) measurement. To measure log P_{oct} by PAMPA [35], octanol is impregnated into the filter membrane for permeability measurement. The permeability value is then converted to the partition coefficient.

7.2.5 *In Silico* Method

Various algorithms have been investigated to calculate the octanol–water partition coefficient from the chemical structure. However, the prediction accuracy is still often more than 10-fold (>1 log unit) for a newly synthesized compound [19]. If two or more software are available, it would be a good practice to compare the results. If the prediction values from different algorithms converge to a similar value, the estimated value would be more reliable. This consensus-based approach was found to predict the log P_{oct} value more accurately compared to the sole use of a software [19].

7.2.6 Recommendation

As an authentic method, the SF method is recommended as the first choice. This data is often used for regulatory submission. An *in silico* method can be helpful for experimental design and sanity check of the experiment. For the drugs with log $D_{oct} > 4$, the standard SF method cannot be applied. On the other hand, *in silico* prediction tends to be more reliable for compounds with high lipophilicity, as they have less intramolecular hydrogen bonds [19]. Therefore, for the drugs with log $D_{oct} > 4$, *in silico* log P_{oct} prediction could be more reliable than the experimental ones unless otherwise a specialized experimental method is used. In biopharmaceutical modeling, when log $D_{oct} > 3$, the prediction error of log D_{oct} has little impact on P_{eff} prediction.

7.3 BILE-MICELLE PARTITION COEFFICIENT (K_{BM})

Bile-micelles affect not only the solubility and dissolution rate but also the effective permeability of a drug. Without considering bile-micelle binding, P_{eff} cannot be appropriately estimated. The bile-micelle binding is especially important to estimate the food effect (both positive and negative food effects). Owing to the amphiphilic nature of bile micelles, even a hydrophilic drug such as nadolol can bind to bile micelles.

Prediction of K_{bm} from log P_{oct} is discussed in Section 2.2.5. In this section, experimental methods are discussed. As the bile micelles do not have a distinct critical micelle concentration and as a dynamic equilibrium exist between monomer, aggregates, and micelles, equilibrium dialysis and ultrafiltration are not suitable to separate free monomer molecules from bile-micelle-bound molecules.

7.3.1 Calculation from Solubility in Biorelevant Media

K_{bm} can be calculated from the experimental solubility data in a biorelevant media and a simple buffer [36, 37]. This method is useful for compounds with low solubility. For dissociable compounds, $K_{bm,z}$ of cation and anion species can be estimated as one-tenth and one-hundredth of $K_{bm,0}$, respectively [38, 39].

Example The $K_{bm,0}$ for a base with $pK_a = 7$ from the solubility in 3 mM bile-micelle media $S_{dissolv} = 40$ µg/ml and $S_0 = 2.4$ µg/ml can be calculated as follows. By assuming K_{bm+} is one-tenth of the K_{bm0}, Equation 2.27 can be rearranged to

$$K_{bm,0} = \left[\frac{S_{dissolv}}{S_0} - \left(1 + \frac{[H^+]}{K_a} \right) \right] \left(\frac{\text{Water}}{\text{Bile acid}} \right) \left(1 + \frac{[H^+]}{K_a} \frac{1}{10} \right)^{-1}$$

$$= \left[\frac{40}{2.4} - \left(1 + \frac{10^{-6.5}}{10^{-7}} \right) \right] \frac{55600}{3} \left(1 + \frac{10^{-6.5}}{10^{-7}} \frac{1}{10} \right)^{-1} = 1.8 \times 10^5$$

7.3.2 Spectroscopic Method

The UV and fluorescent spectroscopies can be used to obtain K_{bm} [40]. When a chromophore is put in different environments, such as water and bile micelles, its spectrum changes. Therefore, like the pH–UV titration method for pK_a measurement, a bile micelle titration curve can be obtained. This method is useful for compounds with high solubility. Even though it is often neglected in the literature, many hydrophilic bases such as nadolol and atenolol can bind to bile micelles, resulting in reduction of the effective permeability [41–43].

7.3.3 Recommendations

For drugs with low solubility, the solubility method is most appropriate. The solubility data in the blank media and biorelevant media such as the fasted state simulated intestinal fluid (FaSSIF) is usually readily available in drug discovery and development. For drugs with high solubility, the solubility method might not be suitable. In this case, the spectroscopic method would be suitable.

7.4 PARTICLE SIZE AND SHAPE

Particle size is one of the most important information for biopharmaceutical modeling. There are several methods to define the size of a particle (Fig. 7.2).

In biopharmaceutical modeling, weight-based particle size distribution is used, as it is straightforward to apply for the dissolution equations. D50 is the accumulative value at which it becomes 50% of the weight. D50 and D90 are often used to characterize the particle size distribution. D[4, 3] is also used as a representative diameter. The definitions of these parameters are illustrated in Figure 7.3 and Table 7.1.

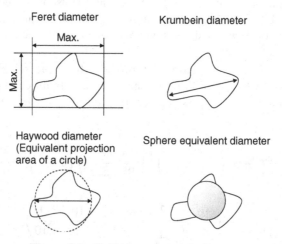

Figure 7.2   Definition of particle diameter.

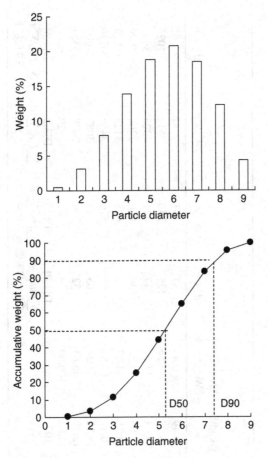

Figure 7.3 Definition of D50 and D90.

Aerodynamic diameter (d_{AD}) is also used to characterize an inhalation formulation.

$$d_{AD} = d\frac{\rho}{\rho_0} \quad (\rho_0 = 1\text{g/ml}) \tag{7.1}$$

7.4.1 Microscope

Even though it is the most classical method, microscopic observation is of great importance. A small amount of sample (<0.1 mg) is required for microscopic analysis. To increase the visibility of the sample, the drug powder is often mixed with an inert oil such as silicon oil. The particle size can be easily calculated using graphical analysis software.

The flow particle image analyzer (FPIA) is an application of this method. A dilute suspension of particles is passed through a measurement cell where

TABLE 7.1 Example of D[4,3] Calculation

Diameter of Particle Bin, $d (= 2r)$	Particle Number in Each Bin, n	Volume per Particle, $v_p = 4/3\pi r^3 n$	Weight in Particle Size Bin, $v_p \times \rho$	Weight, %	Accumulative Weight, %	$d \times n$	$d^2 \times n$	$d^3 \times n$	$d^4 \times n$
1	81	0.523	42	0.49	0.49	81	81	81	81
2	64	4.187	268	3.07	3.56	128	256	512	1024
3	49	14.130	692	7.94	11.50	147	441	1323	3969
4	36	33.493	1206	13.83	25.32	144	576	2304	9216
5	25	65.417	1635	18.75	44.07	125	625	3125	15625
6	16	113.040	1809	20.74	64.81	96	576	3456	20736
7	9	179.503	1616	18.52	83.34	63	441	3087	21609
8	4	267.947	1072	12.29	95.63	32	256	2048	16384
9	1	381.510	382	4.37	100.00	9	81	729	6561
Total —	285	—	8721	100	—	D[1,0] $\sum dn / \sum n$ 2.894737	D[2,1] $\sum d^2 n / \sum dn$ 4.04	D[3,2] $\sum d^3 n / \sum d^2 n$ 5	D[4,3] $\sum d^4 n / \sum d^3 n$ 5.712871

214

images of each particle are captured using stroboscopic illumination and a CCD camera.

7.4.2   Laser Diffraction

The laser diffraction method is widely used in drug discovery and development as a convenient and robust method. This method is suitable for one to several hundred micrometer range, covering most of the API particle size. This method assumes a spherical particle shape.

7.4.3   Dynamic Laser Scattering (DLS)

Dynamic laser scattering (DLS) is used to measure the particle size less than the micrometer range, such as nanomilled particle, emulsions, and micelles. The measurement is very simple and easy, and it is routinely used in formulation investigations. Figure 7.4 shows the size of bile micelles measured by DLS. This method can be combined with the zeta potential (surface charge) measurement.

7.4.4   Recommendations

Microscopic observation should be performed every time a new batch of API is synthesized. The particle size can change during formulation preparation. Therefore, the particle size should be monitored before and after the formulation process.

7.5   SOLID FORM

Even though the information about the solid form of a drug is not directly used in biopharmaceutical modeling, this information is critically important to interpret the results of biopharmaceutical modeling. Different solid forms show different apparent solubility and dissolution profiles. The information about the solid form must be presented together with the results of biopharmaceutical modeling. Therefore, this subject is briefly discussed in this section to cover the minimum knowledge required for biopharmaceutical modeling. This knowledge would also enhance the communication among the biopharmaceutical scientists, solid state chemists, and formulation scientists.

7.5.1   Nomenclature

7.5.1.1   Crystalline and Amorphous. Figure 7.5 illustrates the difference between amorphous and crystalline forms. In crystalline forms, the atoms of a drug have defined positions in a crystal lattice. On the other hand, the amorphous form has little regularity in the arrangement of the atoms. The solid form is diagnosed as crystalline by (i) sharp peaks of powder X-ray diffraction (PXRD), (ii) defined melting point, (iii) sharply defined particle shape, and (iv) birefringence under polarized light microscopy (PLM). An amorphous form does not have

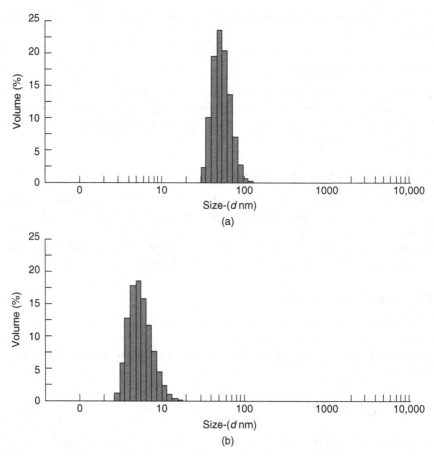

Figure 7.4 DLS data of (a) fasted and (b) fed state simulated intestinal fluids (FaSSIF and FeSSIF).

these characteristics. Even though an amorphous form shows no sharply defined melting point, it has a glass-transition temperature (T_g). Below T_g, the amorphous form has certain properties of a crystalline solid, such as plastic deformation, and is referred to as *glassy*, whereas above T_g, it has certain properties of a liquid, such as molecular mobility, and is referred to as *rubbery* [44].

7.5.1.2 *Salts, Cocrystals, and Solvates.*

Salts, cocrystals, and solvates are binary- or multiple-component systems. The difference between a salt and cocrystal is the nature of the chemical bond. In the salt form, the chemical bond between the drug and the cofactor is an ionic bond, whereas in cocrystals, it is the hydrogen bond and other intermolecular interactions. When the countercomponent of a cocrystal is a solvent, it is referred to as a *solvate*. Except ethanolate and hydrate, no solvate has been marketed.

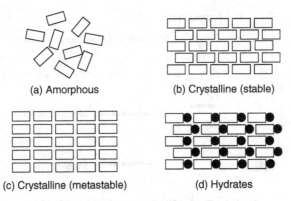

(a) Amorphous   (b) Crystalline (stable)

(c) Crystalline (metastable)   (d) Hydrates

Figure 7.5 Crystalline and amorphous forms.

7.5.1.3 Hydrate. Hydrate is a kind of solvate. Many of the marketed drugs are manufactured as hydrates. In water, a hydrate has lower solubility than an anhydrate [45]. To find a hydrate, the drug is suspended as a slurry in various solvents with different water activity and the conversion of the solid form is monitored. Dynamic vapor sorption (DVS) data is also useful to identify and characterize a hydrate form. To measure the critical relative humidity, long-term sample weight monitoring would be suitable. The samples are stored in humidity-controlled chambers and the sample weight and solid form are monitored. The use of saturated salt solution is a convenient and inexpensive method to control the humidity in a chamber.

In a suspension formulation, an anhydrate can transform into a hydrate during formulation preparation and storage. Therefore, when using a suspension formulation for preclinical and clinical PK studies, the solid form of API particles in the suspension formulation should be confirmed.

7.5.2 Crystal Polymorph

7.5.2.1 True Polymorph and Pseudopolymorph. When solid forms of a drug have the same molecular component but different stacking patterns, the relationship between these solids is "true polymorph" (Fig. 7.5b and c). On the other hand, when the solids have the additional molecular component, the relationship between these solids is "pseudopolymorph" (Fig. 7.5d), for example, hydrates and cocrystalline forms.

7.5.2.2 Kinetic Resolution versus Stable Form. When solid forms of a drug show multiple polymorphs, the most stable form is usually selected for drug development to mitigate the risks of polymorph change during the manufacture processes and long-term storage. When discussing the thermodynamic stability of solid forms, the following two perspectives should be kept in mind: kinetic resolution and enantiotropy.

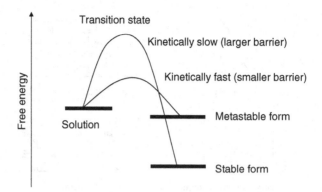

Figure 7.6 Kinetic resolution and stable form.

When various solvents are used for recrystallization, different solids form can be recrystallized from different solvents. However, the most stable form is basically always the same even in different solvents and atmosphere (except pseudopolymorphs).[1] The reason for having different polymorphs from recrystallization with different solvents is that the free energy barrier at the transition state of crystallization is different from that at equilibrium (Fig. 7.6). A metastable form can precipitate out faster than a more stable form via a kinetically favored route (with lower free energy barrier). The Ostwald rule of stage suggests that a less stable form tends to precipitate out faster [46]. The less stable form first generated in a recrystallization process would then eventually become a more stable form, leading to the most stable form if we wait for infinite time.

7.5.2.3 *Dissolution Profile Advantages of Less Stable Forms.* A less stable form of a drug can induce a supersaturated dissolved drug concentration in the GI tract, which eventually settles down to the equilibrium solubility of more stable forms. An amorphous form can induce a significantly higher dissolved drug concentration compared to a crystal form [47]. Therefore, a less stable form is advantageous compared to a more stable form for oral absorption. However, it is disadvantageous for manufacturing and long-term storage.

The difference in solubility between amorphous and crystalline forms could reach 10,000-fold [47]. On the other hand, the difference between polymorphs is less than fourfold in more than 80% cases [45].

7.5.2.4 *Enantiotropy.* In the case of enantiotropic polymorphs, the rank order of the stability of each solid form switches as temperature changes. The more stable form can be different at room temperature and a higher temperature (e.g., at a melting point; Fig. 7.7). Therefore, a polymorph with the highest melting point is not always the most stable form at room temperature. To compare the stability of polymorphs at room temperature, two polymorphs are put together

[1]So the solvent slurry method can be used to identify a more stable form in the air atmosphere.

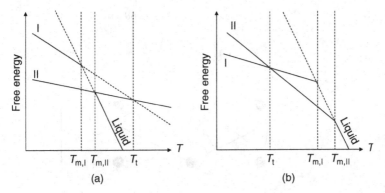

Figure 7.7 Free energy relationships of (a) monotropic and (b) enantiotropic crystalline forms.

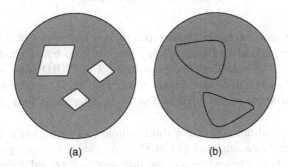

Figure 7.8 PLM image of (a) crystalline and (b) amorphous forms.

in a solvent as a slurry [48]. A less stable form eventually converts to a more stable form at room temperature.

7.5.3 Solid Form Characterization

7.5.3.1 Polarized Light Microscopy (PLM). The first step to characterize the solid form of a drug would be PLM (Fig. 7.8). Under the cross-polarized light, the crystalline forms look bright, whereas amorphous forms look dark. Crystalline/amorphous form can be also judged from the sharpness of the edge of particles. Owing to its convenience and small sample requirement, PLM is usually used as the first measure to diagnose crystalline/amorphous form.

7.5.3.2 Powder X-Ray Diffraction (PXRD). PXRD is most often used as a definitive method to identify a solid form. When the difference between the path length ($d \sin\theta$, where d is the spacing between the plains of crystal lattice and θ is the incident angle) and the wavelength of the X-ray (λ) satisfy the Bragg equation, $2d \sin\theta = n\lambda$, interference of the X-ray occurs (Fig. 7.9).

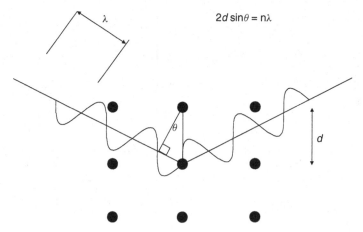

$$2d\sin\theta = n\lambda$$

Figure 7.9   Bragg's equation.

The PXRD chart of an API is interpreted as a fingerprint of polymorphs (an example can be found in Figure 11.4). The position, but not the intensity, of the peak is used to identify the crystal form. The PXRD pattern can be used to diagnose the crystalline/amorphous form. The PXRD spectrum of a crystal shows multiple sharp peaks, whereas that of an amorphous form shows a broad halo spectrum.

Usually, a small amount of the solid sample (>1–5 mg) is put on a sample plate. The inlet beam angle of (2θ in $5° \sim 35°$ range) is usually used for solid form identification. Depending on the difference in crystal habit and sample orientation, the relative intensity of each peak can be changed (even a peak can appear or disappear). The amorphous content can be semiquantitatively estimated from the PXRD data, for example, by the Ruland method [49].

7.5.3.3 *Differential Scanning Calorimeter (DSC) and Thermal Gravity (TG).* Differential scanning calorimeter (DSC) and thermal gravity (TG) are used to characterize the thermal behavior of a solid form. The DSC methods are further categorized as power compensation DSC and heat flow DSC. TG is often coupled with differential thermal analysis (TG/DTA).

The analytical principles of heat flow DSC and DTA are the same, but the former is designed to enhance quantitative analysis. Figure 7.10 is the schematic of a DSC instrument. The reference material and the analytical sample ($\sim$5 mg) are put in the heater chamber. The chamber is then heated gradually (e.g., 10°C/min). The temperature of the sample and the reference is recorded. When the sample melts, the temperature of the sample becomes lower than that of the reference. In the case of power compensation DSC, as a temperature difference between the sample and the reference is detected, the sample is heated to maintain identical temperatures (Fig. 7.11).

From the DSC data, the melting point (T_m) and heat of fusion (ΔH_m, the area of the peak) can be obtained. As the free energy (G) of the solid and melt

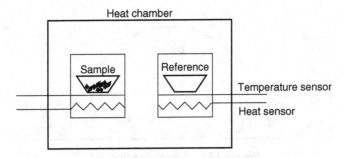

Figure 7.10 Differential scanning calorimeter.

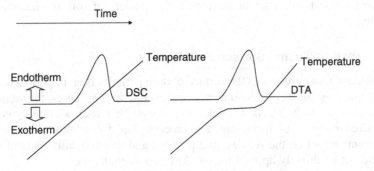

Figure 7.11 DSC and DTA charts.

material becomes the same at the melting point temperature (i.e., $\Delta G = 0$),[2] the entropy of melting (ΔS_m) can be calculated as

$$\Delta S_m = \frac{\Delta H_m}{T_m} \qquad (\text{cf.} \Delta G = T_m \Delta S_m - \Delta H_m) \qquad (7.2)$$

ΔS_m is used to estimate the difference in solubility between crystalline and amorphous forms (Section 2.3.8).

From the TG data, information about solvates (e.g., hydrates) can be obtained. In addition, decomposition of a drug by heating is often observed as an exothermic event.

7.5.3.4 High Throughput Solid Form Screening.
It is preferable to find the most stable form at ambient temperatures. However, it is challenging to arrive at a concrete conclusion about the possibility of finding a new and more stable form. Structure-based computational approach and high throughput solid form screening would be helpful to increase the success rate in finding the most stable form. Recent advances in laboratory automation enabled fast screening of a vast number of crystallization conditions [50–52]. To maximize the chance of finding

[2]In other words, the solid and liquid states are in equilibrium at the melting point temperature.

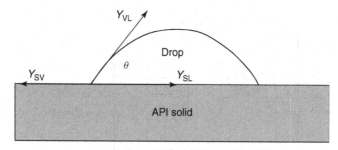

Figure 7.12   Sessile drop method.

the most stable form, a set of solvents with a variety of solvent characters can be selected.

7.5.4   Wettability and Surface Free Energy

The initial wetting process of the surface of drug particles is an important determinant of the dissolution profile in an aqueous media. In most cases, the wettability issue can be fixed during the formulation process. Therefore, wettability is rarely considered in the API form selection process. The formulation process has a significant impact on the API wetting process, and the wettability data of a pure API cannot be directly applied for the API in a formulation.

The sessile drop method (Fig. 7.12) is most often used, although it is not a robust and convenient method. The surface energy between (i) solid and liquid (γ_{SL}), (ii) solid and vapor (γ_{SV}), and (iii) liquid and vapor (γ_{LV}) and the contact angle (θ) are related by the Young equation.

$$\gamma_{SV} = \gamma_{SL} + \gamma_{LV} \cos \theta \qquad (7.3)$$

7.5.5   True Density

The true density of an API is used to calculate the dissolution rate in biopharmaceutical modeling. It affects the surface area per weight of drug particles (Section 3.2.3). In addition, true density affects the sedimentation terminal velocity of API particles and hence the UWL thickness on API particles (Section 3.2.4).

The true density[3] of drugs (ρ_p) is in the 1.1–1.5 g/cm^3 range in most cases, and 1.2 g/cm^3 is often used as the average value. Girolami developed a simple "back of the envelope" method to calculate true density from a chemical formula [53, 54].

$$\rho_p(g/cm^3) = \frac{MW}{v_m} \qquad (7.4)$$

where v_m is the molecular volume (Section 2.3.9).

---

[3]This should not be confused with bulk density and tap density, which are usually less than 1 g/cm^3.

7.6 SOLUBILITY

Solubility of a drug plays one of the central roles in biopharmaceutical modeling. In this section, we start with the terminology of solubility and then move toward the experimental methods. The definition of "solution" or "dissolved state" is discussed in Section 2.1.

7.6.1 Terminology

Most scientists are familiar with the word "solubility," and it is often used carelessly, leading to various misconceptions. These misconceptions may be caused by unclear terminology.

7.6.1.1 Definition of Solubility. Solubility is an equilibrium value per se. However, to avoid confusion, in this book, the term *equilibrium solubility* is used when needed. Equilibrium solubility is defined as the concentration of a compound in a solution that is in contact with an excess amount of the solid compound (equilibrium maker) when the concentration and the solid form do not change over time (i.e., the system is at equilibrium). A time course measurement is essential to confirm that the system reached equilibrium.

7.6.1.2 Intrinsic Solubility. In the literature, the term *intrinsic solubility* implicitly refers to the equilibrium solubility of a free form. Therefore, strictly speaking, it should be referred to as *intrinsic solubility of a free form*. The same definition is used in this book unless otherwise noted. The intrinsic solubility of a stable free form can be measured at a pH at which the drug does not dissociate (Fig. 2.9).

As discussed in Chapter 2, the intrinsic solubilities of a salt, a cocrystal, a metastable form, an anhydrate, and an amorphous form can be "theoretically" defined. In this book, these are referred as the intrinsic solubility of the form, for example, "the *intrinsic solubility of HCl salt*".

7.6.1.3 Solubility in Media. The solubility of a drug in a medium, such as a phosphate buffer and FaSSIF, is also defined as an equilibrium value. However, in this case, the solid form can convert to a different form that is more stable in the media. For example, in the pH-controlled region, a salt form dissociates to a free form. Therefore, the *equilibrium solubility* in the pH-controlled region becomes identical regardless of the starting material being a salt or a free form.[4] Therefore, when we measure the solubility of a drug, the final solid form should always be checked and this information should always be associated with the solubility value when interpreting the data (Section 16.3).

---

[4]One of the most often observed mistakes in biopharmaceutical modeling is that a salt form and a free form are considered to have different equilibrium solubility at a pH in a buffer.

7.6.1.4   Initial pH and Final pH. When measuring the equilibrium solubility of a drug, an excess amount of the drug is added to the media. In the case of a dissociable drug, the pH can be shifted from the initial pH by the dissolving drug, especially when a buffer with weak buffer capacity is used.[5] In this book, the pH after achieving equilibrium (i.e., the final pH) is used unless otherwise noted.

7.6.1.5   Supersaturable API. In this book, salts, cocrystals, anhydrates, amorphous forms, and other metastable forms are called *supersaturable API*. As discussed above, regardless of the starting material being a salt or a free form, in the pH-controlled region (as final pH), the "experimental" equilibrium solubility of a drug usually becomes the same (strictly speaking, after infinite time, but usually within 24 h). In other words, salt formation does not increase the equilibrium solubility of a drug in the pH-controlled region. The reason a salt form increases the oral absorption of a drug is that (i) it increases the dissolution rate and (ii) it can induce the supersaturated drug concentration.[6] This point is discussed in detail in Section 11.1.

7.6.1.6   Critical Supersaturation Concentration and Induction Time. The degree of supersaturation can be defined as the drug concentration over the equilibrium solubility of a solid form ($C_{dissolv}/S_{dissolv}$). Critical supersaturation concentration (CSSC) is the dissolved drug concentration where nucleation of the solid form (or liquid droplet) occurs during the timescale of interest, which is several hours in biopharmaceutical modeling. Usually, the nucleation rate is steeply dependent on the degree of supersaturation (Section 3.3). Therefore, the CSSC of a drug can be defined as a characteristic value for the timescale of interest.[7]

In the literature, the term *kinetic solubility* is often used. However, literally speaking, the terms *kinetic* and *solubility* are contradictory concepts, as solubility is an equilibrium value per se. In most cases,[8] the kinetic solubility of a drug refers to the transient concentration of dissolved drug molecules immediately after the addition of a concentrated sample solution (e.g., in DMSO) to an aqueous media (typically within the timescale of several minutes to 1–2 h) [55–58]. Therefore, kinetic solubility represents the precipitation tendency in a short period of time [59]. To avoid confusion, "kinetic solubility" is not used in this book. Instead, we use "critical supersaturation concentration."

[5]In a transporter inhibition study, this point should be remembered. The concentration of inhibitor is often higher than the buffer capacity of incubation media such as Hank's balanced solution. This can result in an artifact reduction of the permeability of a dissociable drug.
[6]The experimental equilibrium solubility of a salt (which is usually the same as that of the free form) is often used in biopharmaceutical modeling for a salt. This can result in underestimation of oral absorption.
[7]Even when the degree of supersaturation is very small, after a very long time (e.g., several hundred million years), nucleation occurs at some time point and the dissolved drug concentration settles down to the equilibrium solubility. Therefore, if the timescale of interest is longer, CSSR becomes lower (Figure 11.1).
[8]Interestingly, some people use this term as "dissolution rate."

7.6.1.7 Dissolution Rate and Dissolution Profile. The dissolution rate is the rate of a drug dissolving into a media and is measured in units of amount/time (this is different from the dissolution rate coefficient (k_{diss})). In this book, the term *dissolution profile* is used as a comprehensive term, which includes equilibrium solubility, dissolution rate, supersaturation, etc.

7.6.2 Media

As the real human intestinal fluid is difficult to obtain, an artificial fluid is usually used in solubility measurements.

7.6.2.1 Artificial Stomach Fluids. As an artificial fluid for the stomach, simple HCl solutions at pH 1.2–2 are often used. More advanced media has been proposed [60].

7.6.2.2 Artificial Small Intestinal Fluids. The FaSSIF and FeSSIF (fed state simulated intestinal fluid) have been most widely used as a surrogate for the real human intestinal fluid [61, 62]. The composition of FaSSIF and FeSSIF is shown in Table 7.2. These simulated fluids contain phosphatidylcholine (PC) and taurocholic acid (TC) to mimic the bile micelles in the small intestine. When PC purified from a natural source is used, it could cause a laboratory to laboratory variation. In addition, the preparation method has a significant effect on the solubility of a drug in these media. During the preparation of FaSSIF, after dissolving PC and TC powders in a buffer, the obtained media often becomes slightly turbid. To avoid this, a concentrated FaSSIF (e.g., 30–300 mM) can be first prepared. This solution usually becomes transparent. This solution is then diluted with a blank buffer to prepare FaSSIF. After dilution, the diameter of bile micelles grows to an equilibrium value in a few hours (Fig. 3.2) [63]. This preparation process mimics the dilution of bile juice secreted from the gall bladder into the small intestine.

As a variation of FaSSIF, the bile concentration can be increased to 5 mM for dogs [64].

7.6.3 Solubility Measurement

7.6.3.1 Standard Shake Flask Method. To measure the solubility of a drug, an excess amount of the drug that would exceed the solubilization capacity (solubility × fluid volume) is added to the medium [12, 65–67]. The fluid and the undissolved solid drug are then separated by filtration (< 0.45 μm mesh size) or sedimentation.[9] When using sedimentation (usually with centrifuge), contamination of floating particles should be avoided. The first supernatant can be recentrifuged to avoid contamination (double centrifuge method).

Filter binding is often observed especially when the drug concentration is less than 10 μg/ml, resulting in an artifact low solubility. The first portion of the filtrate

---

[9]These methods cannot be used for nanoparticles.

TABLE 7.2 Artificial Intestinal Fluids

	Fasted State		Fed State (Snapshot Media for Fed State)				
	FaSSIF	FaSSIF-V2	Early	Middle	Late	FeSSIF	FeSSIF-V2
Sodium taurocholate, mM	3	3	10	7.5	4.5	15	10
Lecithin, mM	0.75	0.2	3	2	0.5	3	2
Glyceryl monooleate, mM	0	0	6.5	5	1	0	5
Sodium oleate, mM	0	0	40	30	0.8	0	0.8
Buffer, mM	28[a]	19.12[b]	28.6[b]	44[b]	58.09[b]	144[c]	55.02[b]
Sodium chloride, mM	—	68.62	145.2	122.8	51	—	125.5
pH	6.5	6.5	6.5	5.8	5.4	5.0	5.8
Osmolality, mOsm/kg	270	180 ± 10	400 ± 10	390 ± 10	240 ± 10	635	390 ± 10
Buffer capacity, mM/ΔpH	—	10	25	25	15	—	25

[a] Phosphate.
[b] Maleic acid.
[c] Acetate.

226

should be discarded to ensure that the filter binding is saturated. In the case of compounds with very low solubility (typically <1 µg/ml), the compound could bind to the test tube, pipette, etc. A recovery process with an organic solvent can be used to avoid the artifacts of these nonspecific bindings.

The dissolved drug concentration is then measured by the UV, HPLC, or LC-MS method. Usually, the detection limit of LC-MS or HPLC (<0.05 µg/ml for many cases) does not become an issue because a solubility value less than 0.1 µg/ml is practically not reliable due to significant experimental artifacts.

It is critically important to assure that the system reached equilibrium. A time course measurement is preferable to confirm equilibrium. After adding an aqueous media to a drug powder sample, it should be strongly agitated for more than 24 h. The final pH and the solid form of the undissolved drug at equilibrium must be recorded [68].

7.6.3.2 Measurement from DMSO Sample Stock Solution. It is preferable to use a solid drug material (preferably crystalline) as starting material. However, a sample stock solution is often used in early drug discovery due to its availability and ease of handling.

A sample stock solution in a rich solvent such as DMSO (>10 mM) is mixed with aqueous media. The precipitant is then separated by filtration or centrifuge. In the turbidity detection method, the stock solution is titrated into an aqueous media and the concentration at which turbidity is first observed is recorded as the solubility of the drug. A long incubation time, for example, more than 24 h, is highly recommended.

The solubility measured using a sample stock solution could be significantly higher than that measured from a solid crystalline material [69]. Three reasons have been suggested for this discrepancy: (i) the solubilization effect of DMSO, (ii) the short incubation time, and (iii) the effect of the solid state. Sugaya et al. [70] suggested that the discrepancy might be due to the difference in the solid form.

If 30 mM stock solution is available, 2 µl DMSO stock solution +200 µl aqueous media would give an upper limit of 300 µM (for MW = 400, 120 µg/ml). When a dilute DMSO stock solution is used, it can be concentrated using a centrifuge vacuum evaporator. This process might also stimulate the nucleation and increase the portion of the crystalline precipitant.

PLM analysis can be combined with this assay to obtain crystalline/amorphous information of precipitants [69]. PLM gives rapid and reasonably accurate crystalline/amorphous information. Using reversed microscope with an automatic stage, the microscopic pictures of precipitants can be taken automatically. It can be further combined with automatic graphical analysis. A disposable 96-well glass bottom plate is commercially available (<$10 per plate). On the basis of our experience, during the drug discovery stage, the drug precipitants become crystalline in about 36% cases.

7.6.3.3 Solid Surface Solubility. The surface solubility ($S_{surface}$) of a drug determines the dissolution rate of the drug. In the case of dissociable drugs, because of the buffering effect of drug molecules dissolving from the solid surface, the pH near the solid surface deviates from the bulk fluid solubility during the dissolution process. $S_{surface}$ can be lower (for free base and acid) or higher (for salts) than the equilibrium bulk solubility of the drug at a pH.

The slurry pH method can be used to estimate the solid surface solubility [71–73]. The pH values of the concentrated drug slurry in water (20–40% w/w) represent the solid surface pH.

7.6.3.4 Method for Nanoparticles. The baseline conclusion is that standard nanomization (>100 nm) does not increase the solubility of a drug.[10] The Ostwald–Freundlich equation predicts that a particle size of much less than 100 nm is required to increase the solubility of a drug (Section 2.3.9). This theoretical prediction was recently confirmed by carefully designed experiments for drugs [74]. In a standard solubility measurement method, the use of filtration and centrifuge can cause an artifactual increase in solubility by nanomization, as they cannot completely separate nanoparticles from a fluid.

The solid drug titration method would be suitable for solubility measurements of nanoparticles [74]. In this method, a suspension of nanoparticles is gradually titrated into an aqueous media and the DLS signals or turbidity signals are monitored. When the added drug amount is smaller than the solubilization capacity (solubility × volume), the drug particles completely dissolve and there is no increase in the signals. As the added amount increases, it exceeds the solubilization capacity and the signals increase. The point at which the signal starts to appear is the solubility of a drug. Using this method, it was found that by nanomizing, the increase in solubility of typical low solubility drugs[11] is only 15%, which is in good agreement with the Ostwald–Freundlich equation (Section 2.3.9). Even if we assume a very high interfacial tension of 50 mN/m, the solubility increase would be up to 20% in the greater than 100 nm range. As it is practically difficult to reduce the particle size to less than 100 nm, the effect of nanomizing on the solubility of a drug would be basically negligibly small.

7.6.4 Recommendation

The quality of solubility data is one of the key factors that affects the accuracy of biopharmaceutical modeling. When considering the cost-effectiveness, the following method would be recommended for use in drug discovery and development. Currently, computational prediction from the chemical

---

[10] A mechanism that explains why nanomilling increases the oral absorption of solubility-permeability limited cases is discussed in Section 4.7.2.

[11] Itraconazole (interfacial tension (mN/m) = 20, hereinafter the same), loviride (27.5), phenytoin (24.4), and naproxen (23.6).

structure has significant error and cannot be used for biopharmaceutical modeling [75].

7.6.4.1 Early Drug Discovery Stage (HTS to Early Lead Optimization).
Considering the throughput required at this stage, the DMSO sample stock solution would be the starting material. The 96-well format is usually used at this stage. Even in this format, PLM, PXRD, and Raman spectroscopy can be used to determine the solid forms of precipitants with a practical throughput. Owing to the quality of the data, simple classification or mapping of drugs would be the practical use of the data at this stage. When the precipitant is crystalline, the solubility of a drug will not drop dramatically (within fourfold in 80% cases [45]) even if a more stable form appears in the later stages of drug discovery. Without the information whether the precipitant is crystalline/amorphous, a structure–solubility relationship study will be meaningless.

7.6.4.2 Late Lead Optimization Stage.
At the stage before one candidate compound is selected, medium throughput/medium contents screening would be preferable. At this stage, compounds are synthesized in a singleton manner rather than combinatorially. The solubility data is used for structure design as well as to interpret the *in vivo* data. At this stage, a preclinical PK study is often performed in animals.

Considering the above situations, a miniaturized SF method would be appropriate for this stage. When more than 5 mg is available, the powder sample can be weighed into a small test tube. Simulated gastric and intestinal fluids can be used as the media. The solid state of samples should be confirmed before and after incubation. Cross-validation with the Yalkowsky equation would be useful if the melting point of a drug is available (Section 2.3.7).

These data can be used to perform biopharmaceutical modeling. As both the solid form and the dose strength for drug development are not yet known at this stage, Fa% prediction using the approximate analytical Fa% equation would be sufficient (Section 5.3.3). This would give us the minimum absorbable dose with a standard formation effort.

7.6.4.3 Transition Stage between Discovery and Development.
After one or a few candidate compounds are selected, a detailed solubility profiling should be performed. Usually, detailed solid form information becomes available at this stage. A few hundred milligrams to a few grams of drug material become available for solubility measurements and the other pharmaceutical profiling (often called *preformulation*).

The pH–solubility profile (pH 1–11) with the solid form characterization should be performed at this stage [13, 14]. The pK_a and S_0 values of a drug can be estimated from this data. In addition, the solubility in FaSSIF and FeSSIF should be measured. The K_{bm} value of a drug can be estimated from this data. The pH–solubility profile data is also useful for parenteral formulation development and the other purposes in drug development.

7.7   DISSOLUTION RATE/RELEASE RATE

7.7.1   Intrinsic Dissolution Rate

The intrinsic dissolution rate (IDR) of an API is the dissolution rate per surface area per time (unit: amount/surface area/time). To measure IDR, an API powder is filled into a hole with a defined opening area and compressed to make a flat surface. The Wood apparatus has been used to measure the IDR. Recently, a miniaturized apparatus is available, such as µDISS (Fig. 7.13) [76]. It is sometimes difficult to compress the pure API into a tablet in a hole. The wetting process of the drug surface can cause a lag time.

The IDR data can be useful to differentiate between the dissolution rates of API polymorphs and salts. During the IDR experiments, conversion of the solid form is sometimes observed on the disk surface. In this case, the dissolution rate changes during the experiment.

7.7.2   Paddle Method

The paddle method is most often used as a dissolution test. Comparing the paddle apparatus with the real GI tract for their shapes, the agitation patterns, and the dynamic changes of chemical environments, it is rather fair to admit that

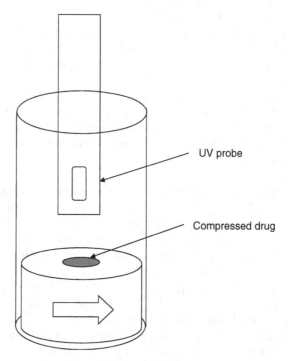

UV probe

Compressed drug

Figure 7.13   µDISS apparatus.

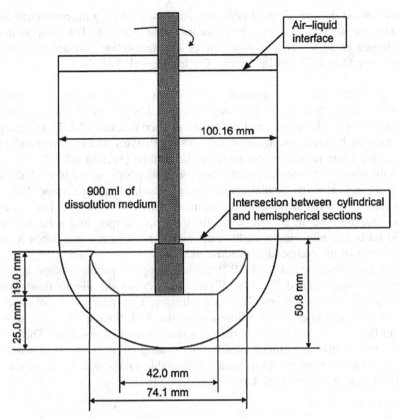

Figure 7.14 Basic geometry of USP Dissolution Testing Apparatus II. *Source:* Adapted from Reference 77 with permission.

quantitative *in vitro–in vivo* correlation is unlikely to be attainable per se using the paddle method. This notion has led to investigations for more physiological dissolution tests. However, the paddle apparatus is well standardized and the interexperimental variation is usually very small. Therefore, this method is currently used as the de facto standard method for quality control purposes.

7.7.2.1 Apparatus. The bottom of the flask is usually round, and the paddle is a semicircular plane (Fig. 7.14). In most pharmacopeias, circa 1-l flask is used for the paddle method. A miniscale paddle method (50–200 ml scale) can be used to measure the dissolution rate of API particle in drug discovery and early development.

7.7.2.2 Fluid Condition. A compendium dissolution test is usually performed under a sink condition (<30% of the saturated solubility). About 900 ml of a buffer with pH 1–7.4 is most often used. In the case of compounds with low solubility, SDS is often used to enhance the dissolution profile (up to 9% found in the FDA dissolution database). High salt concentration is not compatible with SDS, as it forms insoluble material. The temperature is maintained at 37°C. The monographs of the dissolution test are available at http://www.fda.gov/Drugs/InformationOnDrugs/ucm135742.htm.

7.7.2.3 *Agitation.* The agitation strength is of great importance for the disintegration of a formulation and the dissolution of a large particle (D50 > 50 μm). The paddle speed for a compendium paddle method is usually 50, 75, or 100 rpm. However, in humans, the agitation strength is relatively weak, corresponding to less than 50 rpm in the compendium paddle method (Section 6.2.3.2).

In the minipaddle method, even when the same paddle speed is used, the agitation strength is much smaller compared to a standard paddle method. Equation 3.39 can be used to calculate the agitation strength in each system. For example, with a paddle size of 2.5 cm, a paddle speed of 50 rpm, and a fluid volume of 50 ml in the minipaddle method, the agitation strength corresponds to circa 10–25 rpm in the compendium paddle method.

The fluid dynamics in the USP (US Pharmacopeia) paddle method has been extensively investigated [77–80]. Figure 7.15 shows the distribution of fluid velocity at the flask bottom. The shear stress is high near the paddle and the flask wall. There is an upward flow around the flask bottom; however, there is a dead-flow region where the coning phenomenon is often observed. The coning results in a slower dissolution profile. The coning effect is observed when the dosage form contains a high amount of insoluble excipients. To avoid coning, usage of a peak bottom flask has been reported [81].

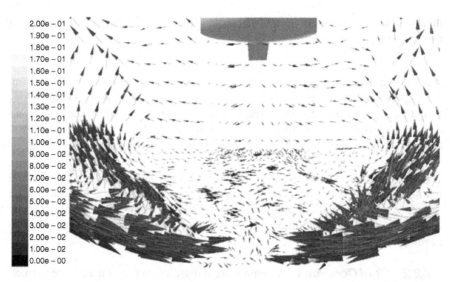

Figure 7.15 Distribution of fluid velocity in the USP paddle method. Numerically predicted velocity vectors (m/s) on the plane perpendicular to the impeller plane at the vessel bottom. *Source:* Adapted from Reference 77 with permission.

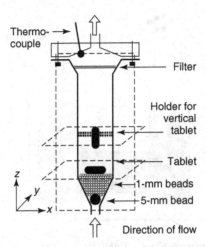

Figure 7.16 Geometry of the USP 4 flow-through method. *Source:* Adapted from Reference 82 with permission.

7.7.3 Flow-Through Method

Figure 7.16 shows the flow-through dissolution test apparatus [82]. The advantage of the flow-through method is that the dissolution media can be changed continuously, for example, from pH 1.2 to 6.8. In addition, a sink condition can be consistently maintained. Therefore, the flow-through method is suitable especially for controlled-release formulations and drugs with poor solubility (dissolution rate limited cases).

7.7.4 Multicompartment Dissolution System

Several multicompartment dissolution systems have been developed to represent the effect of gastric pH on the oral absorption of a drug. In these systems, a gastric compartment was sequentially connected to an intestinal compartment [83–86]. Furthermore, a membrane can be attached to the intestinal compartment [87]. These systems are especially useful for investigating the oral absorption of poorly soluble free bases, for example, ketoconazole, albendazole, cinnarizine, and dipyridamole. The bioavailability of these drugs was largely affected by the gastric pH (Table 12.4).

7.7.5 Dissolution Permeation System

Simultaneous assessment of dissolution and permeation is required to evaluate the performance of special formulations such as solid dispersion and self-emulsifying drug delivery systems (SEDDS), since the molecular state of a drug released from these formulations has not been well characterized. Therefore, the concentration of a drug available for permeation cannot be well defined for biopharmaceutical modeling (Section 4.4).

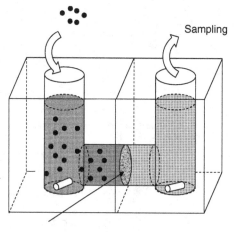

Membrane (Caco-2/PAMPA)
- Drug particles or formulations

Dissolved drug

Dissolution media (FaSSIF,FeSSIF, etc.)(8 ml)

Acceptor media (4% BSA, pH 7.4) (5 ml)

Figure 7.17 The D/P system.

Several types of *in vitro* systems in which the dissolution and permeation processes were combined were reported [87–89]. Kataoka et al.
developed a dissolution/permeation (D/P) system (Fig. 7.17). The D/P system
can evaluate the food effect and has the potential to be applied for the evaluation
of prototype formulations as well [90].

The D/P system consists of two half-chambers and a Caco-2 monolayer
(1.77 cm^2) mounted between them. Both sides of the monolayer are filled with
transport media (apical side, pH 6.5, 8 ml (circa 6% of the intestinal fluid
volume) and basal side, pH 7.4, 5 ml) and are constantly mixed by magnetic
stirrers. Compounds are applied to the apical side as a solid, suspension, or
solution. One-hundredth of the clinical dose is applied to the system. Compared
to the *in vivo* situation, due to its small surface area/volume ratio (0.22 in the
D/P system vs circa 2.3 in humans), the permeation clearance provided by the
Caco-2 membrane is quite low. However, the fluid volume/dose ratio is sixfold
higher in the D/P system than that *in vivo*. This excess fluid volume provides
an additional clearance of a drug equivalent to Pn = 6.

By the D/P system, the food effect was correctly evaluated. The modified
FaSSIF and FeSSIF with isotonic osmolality were used as the apical side fluid
[88]. The applicability for lipid-based formulation was confirmed by albendazole
and danazol formulations [89]. The D/P system was also found to be useful
to evaluate various formulations [90, 91], including nanoparticles [92]. PAMPA
membrane can be used as an alternative to Caco-2 membrane [93].

Sugano and Sakai [94] suggested the possibility of constructing a D/P system in a 96-well format. Their method is an application of the PAMPA (Section 7.9.4). One disadvantage of PAMPA for the formulation study is the lack of the mucous layer. Without the mucous layer, the formulations (particles, micelles, etc.) can directly interact with the membrane. To attach the mucous layer onto the artificial lipid membrane, the hot molten agarose/mucin gel (1% (w/v)) was impregnated into the hydrophilic fiber scaffold, which is physically attached on the membrane. The hydrophilic scaffold enables the formation of a thin mucous layer. Without the hydrophilic scaffold, the agarose/mucin mixture makes a droplet on the hydrophobic PAMPA membrane and does not form a uniform thin layer. They demonstrated that the food effect can be adequately assessed by the mucous-layer-adhered PAMPA.

7.7.6 Recommendation

There is no versatile technology for all stages in drug discovery. The minipaddle method is suitable for the early stages of drug discovery and development. μDISS can be also used in these stages. The USP method is most often used in the late stages of drug development. The main purpose of a dissolution test is to measure the dissolution rate of a drug rather than the saturated solubility. In most cases, a sink condition is used. The dissolution rate is then used in biopharmaceutical modeling (Section 8.5.1). The biopharmaceutical modeling can be modified to emulate the D/P system. As the D/P system can experimentally evaluate the effective concentration of a drug for membrane permeation, it can be used to validate a modeling hypothesis for the absorption mechanism of a special formulation such as solid dispersion.

7.8 PRECIPITATION

Development of an *in vitro* method, which correctly reflects an *in vivo* supersaturation profile, has not been successful so far. In most cases, an *in vitro* method underestimates the supersaturation of a drug *in vivo*, probably because of the difference in the chemical composition of the fluids, the containers (glass vs mucus), the pH neutralization processes, the agitation methods (stirring bar/paddle vs wall movement), etc. Therefore, the methods introduced here should be understood as a qualitative measure of supersaturation profiles.

7.8.1 Kinetic pH Titration Method

A kinetic pH titration method can be used to assess the ability of a drug to supersaturate in an aqueous solution [95]. A drug is first dissolved at a pH where it is dissolved predominantly in its ionized form, and then the pH is changed by titrating HCl or KOH. As pH shifts to the range close to the pK_a of a drug, the portion of undissociated form (f_0) increases. In the case when a drug is supersaturable

(Fig. 7.18b),[12] the dissolved drug concentration of the undissociated form in the solution ($C_{\text{dissolv},0}$) transiently exceeds the intrinsic solubility (S_0). Once $C_{\text{dissolv},0}$ hits the critical supersaturation ratio ($C_{\text{dissolv},0}/S_0 > \text{CSSR}$),[13] nucleation occurs. Subsequently, the rate of pH change by precipitation or dissolution of the drug is monitored. In the case when a drug is not supersaturable (Fig. 7.18a), the pH titration curve simply follows that of the pH–equilibrium solubility profile.

7.8.2 Serial Dilution Method

When a series of concentrated stock solutions of a drug in a rich solvent (such as DMSO or DMA (dimethylacetamide)) was diluted with an aqueous buffer, precipitation of the drug is observed when the dissolved drug concentration exceeds the CSSC (Fig. 7.19). Figure 7.20 shows the plot of dissolved drug concentration against the initially added drug amount [96].

7.8.3 Two-Chamber Transfer System

A two-chamber transfer system was used to investigate the precipitation of a base [83]. A base drug was first completely dissolved in a HCl solution and then infused into a neutral pH solution with sufficient buffer capacity to maintain the neutral pH. a paddle apparatus was used as the neutral pH chamber. Figures 7.21 and 7.22 show the dissolved drug concentration–time profile of dipyridamole and AZ0865, respectively.

However, this *in vitro* method was found to overestimate the precipitation *in vivo* (underestimate supersaturation) (Fig. 7.23) [97]. Figure 7.24 shows the dissolved drug concentration (C_{dissolv}) of AZ0865 in the small intestine after oral solution administration simulated by the S1I7C1 model. It was suggested that C_{dissolv} exceeded the critical supersaturated concentration in the *in vitro* method (Figs. 7.22 and 7.23). However, precipitation was not observed in clinical trials. The discrepancy was much smaller when a paddle stirrer was used compared to a magnetic stirrer.

7.8.4 Nonsink Dissolution Test

A nonsink dissolution test may be able to discriminate the effects of formulation components on the supersaturation and precipitation rate of a drug. Gu et al. showed that the use of appropriate dose/volume ratio is critical to evaluate the supersaturation and precipitation of a drug [98].

---

[12]As supersaturable compounds chase the equilibrium, it is called *chaser* by the investigators.

[13]CSSR can change depending on the titration speed. In addition, the local pH near the dispenser tip can be different from the bulk pH. Furthermore, mechanical stirring can stimulate nucleation. Therefore, the CSSR observed in this method does not necessarily quantitatively correlate with the *in vivo* supersaturation profile.

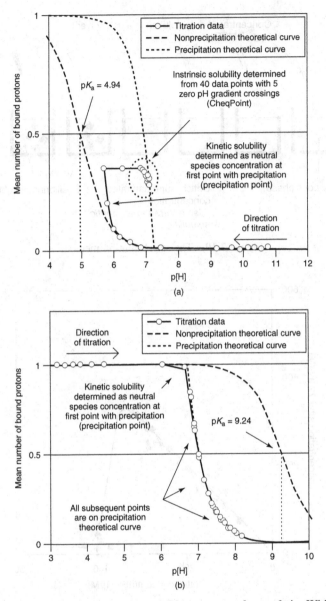

Figure 7.18 pH-supersaturation profile. (a) Bjerrum curve for warfarin. While the sample is fully dissolved, the experimental data fit well with the nonprecipitation theoretical curve. After precipitation, the points lie close to the precipitation theoretical curve at the CheqPoint. The precipitation point, when precipitation was first observed, lies a long way from the CheqPoint. The fact that the precipitation point does not lie on the precipitation theoretical curve indicates that the solution was supersaturated at the moment the sample first precipitated. (b) Bjerrum curve for chlorpromazine. As soon as the saturation level is reached, the sample precipitates, and points follow the precipitation theoretical curve. The precipitation point also lies on the precipitation theoretical curve, indicating no supersaturation. *Source:* Adapted from Reference 95 with permission.

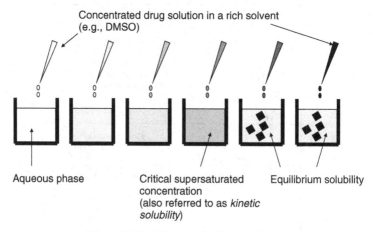

Figure 7.19   The serial dilution method.

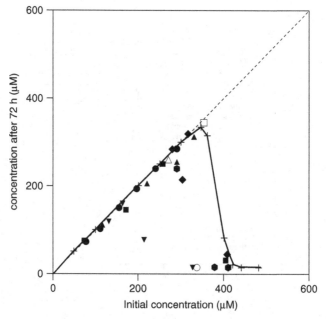

Figure 7.20   Result of the serial dilution method. Bicalutamide was used as a model drug. The solubility of crystalline material is 14.5 μM. The different symbols indicate that experiments have been performed at different occasions. The solid line with crosses represents calculated results for the bulk concentration after 72 h incubation versus initial concentration for different supersaturation ratio. In the calculations, $\lambda = 6.5$ μm and a crystal-water interfacial tension $\gamma_{SL} = 22.1$ mN/m were used together with experimental data for other parameters in the theory. *Source:* Adapted from Reference 96 with permission.

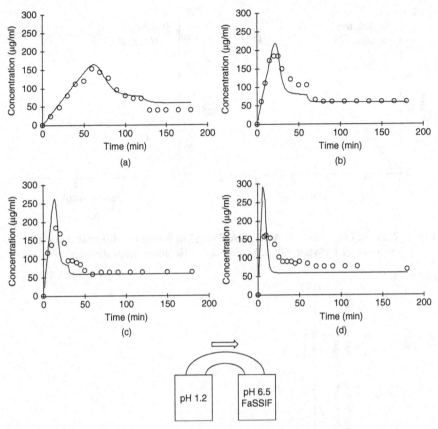

Figure 7.21 Two-chamber transfer method. (a) 0.5 ml/min, (b) 2 ml/min, (c) 4 ml/min, and (d) 9 ml/min.

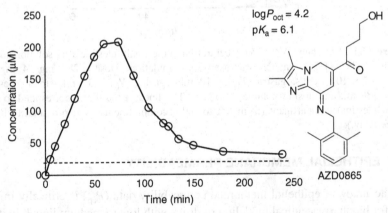

Figure 7.22 Mean ($\pm$SD) concentration of AZD0865 dissolved in FaSSIF over time from supersaturated solution using the two-chamber transfer method ($n = 3$). Dotted line represents the equilibrium solubility in FaSSIF. *Source:* Replotted from Reference 97.

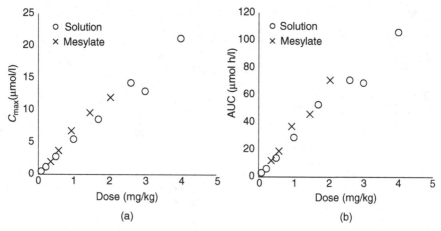

Figure 7.23 (a) C_{max} and (b) AUC of AZD0865 in humans at different doses administered as solution or mesylate salt (tablet). *Source:* Replotted from Reference 97.

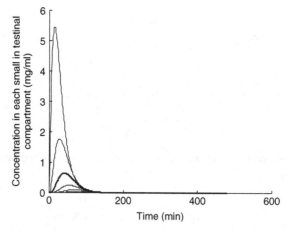

Figure 7.24 Simulated AZ0865 concentration in the small intestine after solution administration. The S1I7C3 model was used for simulation. Dose = 280 mg (4 mg/kg), $P_{eff} = 3.2 \times 10^{-4}$ cm/s, gastric $T_{1/2} = 10$ min, gastric $V_{GI} = 30$ ml, small intestinal $V_{GI} = 130$ ml, and dosing volume = 250 ml. The lines in the figure correspond to each small intestinal compartment (from left to right, compartments 1–7, proximal to distal, respectively.)

7.9 EPITHELIAL MEMBRANE PERMEABILITY

The accuracy of epithelial membrane permeability data (P_{ep}) is critically important for biopharmaceutical modeling of drugs with low to medium lipophilicity.[14]

---

[14]But it is not critically important for compounds with high lipophilicity (log $D_{oct,pH6.5}$ > circa 2) because the UWL resistance dominates P_{eff}.

To ensure the reliability of P_{ep} data, it is preferable to compare P_{ep} values obtained from two or three different methods.

7.9.1   Back-Estimation from Fa%

When Fa% of a drug administered as a solution is less than 75%[15] (i.e., low permeability), P_{ep} values can be back-estimated from the Fa% as

$$P_{ep} = \frac{R_{GI}}{2DF \cdot PE \cdot VE \cdot f_{mono}} \frac{1}{T_{si}} \cdot \ln(1 - Fa)$$

This method is practically useful in drug discovery, as Fa% in rats is usually routinely measured. A drug with low permeability tends to be less liable to the gut wall metabolism (i.e., Fg $\approx$ 1) and Fh can be calculated from i.v. data. Therefore, the equation $F = FaFgFh$ can be used to calculate Fa from F. The UWL effect and colonic absorption are negligible for drugs with low permeability (Section 11.8.5.2). The Acc of a drug with low permeability is circa 1 (Section 4.6). Data obtained from dogs should not be used for this method as the paracellular pathway in dogs is larger than that in humans. This method cannot be used for Fa% > 75% cases, as $\ln(1 - Fa)$ becomes sensitive to a small error in Fa%.

Example P_{ep} of a drug can be estimated from Fa% in rats after solution administration (without precipitation in the GI tract). For example, when Fa% = 50%,

$$P_{ep} = \frac{0.2}{2 \times 1.7 \times 1 \times 5 \times 1} \frac{1}{2 \times 60 \times 60} \cdot \ln(1 - 0.5) = 1.1 \times 10^{-6} \text{cm/s}$$

And then, P_{eff} and Fa% in humans can be estimated by assuming that P_{ep} is identical in both species (in this case, f_{mono} of this drug is assumed to be 1 in both species).

$$P_{eff,human} = PE \cdot VE \cdot f_{mono} \cdot P_{ep} = 3 \times 10 \times 1 \times 1.1 \times 10^{-6} \text{ cm/s}$$

$$= 0.33 \times 10^{-4} \text{ cm/s}$$

$$Fa_{human} = 1 - \exp\left(-\frac{2DF}{R_{GI}} P_{eff} T_{si}\right)$$

$$= 1 - \exp\left(-\frac{2 \times 1.7}{1.5} 0.33 \times 10^{-4} \times 3.5 \times 60 \times 60\right) = 61\%$$

7.9.2   *In Situ* Single-Pass Intestinal Perfusion

The Loc-I-Gut system has been used to measure the effective permeability values in humans [99]. This permeability value is considered as the authentic P_{eff} value

---

[15]Without precipitation in the GI tract.

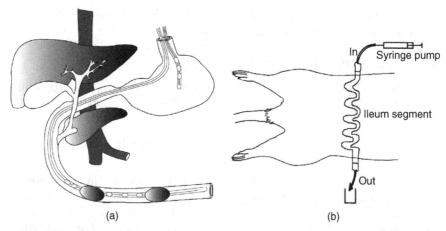

(a)   (b)

Figure 7.25   (a) Luc-I-Gut and (b) rat *in situ* perfusion methods. Loc-I-Gut is a perfusion technique for the proximal region of the human jejunum. The multichannel tube is 175 cm long and is made of polyvinyl chloride, with an external diameter of 5.3 mm. It contains six channels and is provided distally with two 40-mm-long, elongated latex balloons, placed 10 cm apart and each separately connected to one of the smaller channels. The two wider channels in the center of the tube are for infusion and aspiration of the perfusate. The two remaining peripheral smaller channels are used for administration of marker substances and/or for drainage. A tungsten weight is attached to the distal end of the tube to facilitate passage of the tube into the jejunum. The balloons are filled with air when the proximal balloon has passed the ligament of Treitz. *Source:* Adapted from References 99 and 100 with permission.

in the literature. Figure 7.25a shows the Loc-I-Gut system. Two balloons are inflated in the human intestine and drug solution is perfused. As the human subject is maintained conscious during the experiment, the GI mobility is kept intact. However, this experiment is expensive and not suitable for drug discovery and development.

Rat single-pass intestinal perfusion (SPIP) has been widely used to investigate the intestinal membrane permeability in drug discovery (Fig. 7.25b) [100]. The advantage of this method is that the physiological characteristics of the small intestine, such as paracellular pathway and carrier-mediated transport, are maintained intact (except the GI mobility). The disadvantages of this method are (i) the variation in data could be large when not performed carefully and (ii) the experiment is labor intensive. This method is not suitable for drugs with high lipophilicity, as the UWL of an anesthetized intestine is significantly larger than that of a nonanesthetized intestine.

P_{eff} can be calculated by the well-stirred model [101] as

$$P_{\text{eff}} = \frac{Q_{\text{in}}\left(\dfrac{C_{\text{in}}}{C_{\text{out}}} - 1\right)}{2\pi R_{\text{GI}}L} \tag{7.5}$$

or by the parallel tube model (for open or semiopen SPIP models in humans) as

$$P_{eff} = \frac{-Q_{in} \ln (C_{out}/C_{in})}{2\pi R_{GI} L} \qquad (7.6)$$

In both the models, the tube shape does not affect the P_{eff} value of a drug. The transit time of a drug from the inlet to the outlet is determined by V_{GI} and the infusion rate (Q_{in}) as V_{GI}/Q_{in}. A decrease in the V_{GI} of the tube fastens the transit of a solution, whereas it increases k_{perm} (cf. CL_{perm}/V_{GI}), canceling out to give a same P_{eff}).

7.9.3 Cultured Cell Lines (Caco-2, MDCK, etc.)

The Caco-2 cell model is most often used as an *in vitro* cell model [102–104]. The Caco-2 cells originated from human colon cancer and represent many common features with the small intestine. When cultured on an adhesive filter support, the Caco-2 cells form a planner membrane with a tight junction. Many transporters such as P-gp, BCRP, and PEP-T1 are expressed in the apical membrane. However, the expression level of these transporters could have significant laboratory to laboratory variations [105].

The MDCK cell model is also often used in drug discovery and development. The MDCK cells originated from the dog kidney and represent some common features with the small intestine. However, transporter expression in the MDCK cells is very different from that in the human small intestine. As for the passive diffusion, Caco-2 and MDCK give similar values (Fig. 7.26) [106]. However, these cells give different values for PEP-T1 transport [107]. The MDCK cells transfected with the P-gp gene (MDCK-MDR1) are also often used in drug discovery [108].

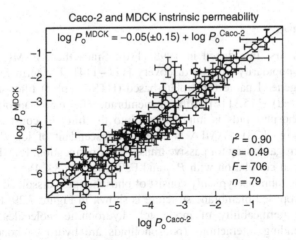

Figure 7.26 Correlation between $P_{trans,0}$ of Caco-2 and MDCK cells. *Source:* Adapted from Reference 106 with permission.

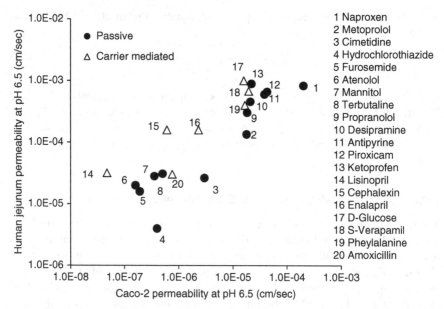

Figure 7.27 Correlation between human jejunum (*in vivo* perfusion) and Caco-2 mono-layers (*in vitro*) permeability data for 20 compounds. *Source:* Adapted from Reference 99 with permission.

Figure 7.27 shows the correlation between P_{eff} and P_{app} [109]. This type of empirical relationship has been widely used for biopharmaceutical modeling. However, there are a few cautions for this empirical correlation: (i) this relationship is validated for compounds with low to moderate lipophilicity but not for drugs with high lipophilicity, (ii) the effect of bile-micelle binding is not taken into account, and (iii) the error is greater than 0.5 log unit.

7.9.4 PAMPA

PAMPA was first introduced in 1998 [110]. Since then, PAMPA has rapidly gained wide popularity in drug discovery [111–114]. The term *PAMPA* is now used as the general name for a plate-based (HTS enabled) filter-supported (filter immobilized) [115, 116] artificial membrane. Typically, an organic solvent containing phospholipids is impregnated into the filter to construct a PAMPA membrane (Fig. 7.28). PAMPA is a refined descendant of log P_{oct} and is an improved surrogate assay for passive transcellular permeation. PAMPA was found to show a good correlation with P_{eff} and Fa% (Section 8.4.4).

PAMPA membranes typically consist of phospholipids dissolved in an organic solvent. A proposed membrane structure is shown in Figure 7.29. Phospholipids facilitate the permeability of moderately hydrophilic molecules by ionic or hydrogen bonding interactions (phospholipids are hydrogen bond acceptors). This enables appropriate assessment of permeability for moderately lipophilic

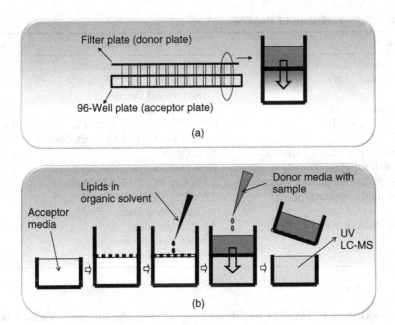

Figure 7.28 Experimental procedure of PAMPA. (a) 96-Well configuration and (b) Experimental procedure (top to bottom permeation).

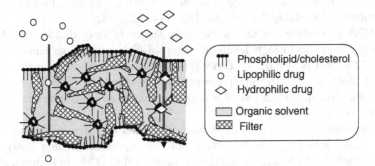

Figure 7.29 Proposed structure of PAMPA membrane.

compounds [117]. Recently, it was shown that anionic phospholipid(s) increases the permeation of basic compounds by ion pair mechanism [118–120]. In many PAMPA variations (and other artificial membrane tools), anionic phospholipid(s) is added to the membrane to increase the predictability for *in vivo* absorption. However, even though the phospholipids may add some similarity to the biological membrane, the organic solvent remaining in the membrane could have a large impact on the permeability. The solubility diffusion theory (Section 4.8.2.1) would support the use of an alkane or alkylidene as an organic solvent in PAMPA [121].

TABLE 7.3   Variations of PAMPA

Name	Composition	References
Original	10% Egg lecithin/n-dodecane	110
Double sink (DS)	20% Phospholipid mixture/n-dodecane	132
n-Hexadecane (HM)	100% n-Hexadecane	112
Biomimetic (BM)	0.8% PC, 0.8% PE, 0.2% PS, 0.2% PI, 1% CHO/1,7-octadiene	111
Lipid/oil/lipid trilayer membrane	Neat DOPC	131
Immobilized phospholipids vesicles	Neat phospholipids vesicles	133
Lipid/cholesterol/octanol mixture	1.7% Egg PC, 2.1% CHO/octanol	129
Three lipid-component model	2.6% PS18:1, 0.9% PC18:1, 1.5% CHO/n-dodecane	119
Blood–brain barrier (BBB)	2% Porcine brain extract/n-dodecane	113
Skin	70% silicone-30% IPM	134

Composition of PAMPA membranes reported in the literature varies from a pure organic solvent to a pure phospholipid. At the first international conference of PAMPA in 2002 (http://www.pampa2002.com/), it was agreed that these variations would be notated as initials or as a short adjective on the head of PAMPA, for example, BM-PAMPA for the biomimetic PAMPA. The variations of PAMPA are summarized in Table 7.3 [35, 94, 110–114, 122–131].

PAMPA is suitable for use at the early stages of drug discovery. PAMPA membrane is stable to high levels of water-miscible organic solvents (e.g., up to 10–30%, AcCN, EtOH, or DMSO) [135]. Unlike cell monolayer systems, PAMPA does not require any preincubation. A simple UV detection method can be used for quantification of a drug because there is no interference from biological contaminants.

Other artificial membrane assays have also been extensively investigated in the last two decades, such as surface plasmon liposome binding assay [136, 137], immobilized artificial membrane column HPLC [138–144], immobilized liposome chromatography [145–148], and solid-supported lipid membrane [149, 150].

7.9.5   Estimation of $P_{trans,0}$ from Experimental Apparent Membrane Permeability

To use the *in vitro* P_{app} value in a mechanistic model, it must be first converted to $P_{trans,0}$. P_{trans0} can be estimated from P_{app} as

$$P_{trans,0} = \frac{1}{f_0} \left(\frac{1}{\frac{1}{P_{app}} - \frac{h_{UWLvitro}}{D_{mono}}} - P_{para,vitro} \right)$$

where $h_{UWLvitro}$ is the UWL thickness in an *in vitro* permeability assay. It is preferable to use more than two P_{app} values at different pH points. This calculation becomes unstable when a P_{app} value is close to the UWL permeability (circa $20-50 \times 10^{-6}$ cm/s). $P_{para,vitro}$ is the paracellular permeability in the *in vitro* cellular system. To calculate $P_{para,vitro}$, the mesh size and electric potential of the paracellular pathway must be characterized at each laboratory, as these values are known to have large laboratory to laboratory variations [151]. These values can be calculated using the permeability values of model paracellular permeants such as mannitol, urea, atenolol, and nadolol. $h_{UWLvitro}$ can be estimated by various methods (Section 7.9.8.1). $P_{trans,0}$ is then converted to *in vivo* P_{eff}, considering the pH, P_{para}, P_{UWL}, the unbound fraction, the surface area expansion by the fold and villi structures, etc. (Chapter 4). A simple empirical correlation such as Figure 7.27 cannot consider these factors. It would be noteworthy that for structure–permeability relationship analysis, the use of $P_{trans,0}$ is more straightforward than using P_{app}, as a linear free energy relationship can be obtained for $P_{trans,0}$ [125].

7.9.6 Estimation of $P_{trans,0}$ from Experimental log P_{oct}

The correlation between $P_{trans,0}$ and P_{oct} is discussed in Section 4.8.2.3. It is highly recommended to use experimental log P_{oct} value rather than the *in silico* prediction.

7.9.7 Mechanistic Investigation

It is of great importance to understand what process is involved in membrane permeation of a drug. By comparing artificial membrane and Caco-2 permeabilities, the contribution of transporters can be identified (Fig. 7.30) [124].

Comparison of permeabilities in apical-to-basal (A to B) and B to A directions is often used to identify the contribution of transporters. An iso-pH condition (e.g., 7.4/7.4) must be used in this experiment [152]. An inhibition study is often used to identify the contribution of a transporter. A high inhibitor concentration (>1 mM) is often used. In this case, the dissolved inhibitor can change the pH. Therefore, pH should be readjusted after dissolving the inhibitor.

The Michaelis–Menten equation can be used to analyze the concentration dependency of permeation flux (Fig. 7.31). Using the Michaelis–Menten equation, the saturable and nonsaturable components can be separated. The nonsaturable component is usually regarded to undergo passive diffusion because it is nonsaturable and usually identical to the permeability under inhibition and/or in the mock cells.

7.9.8 Limitation of Membrane Permeation Assays

It is important to understand the limitations of each method. Owing to the following reasons, an *in vitro* method may have only a little value for drugs with high lipophilicity or could even give an erroneous low P_{ep} value.

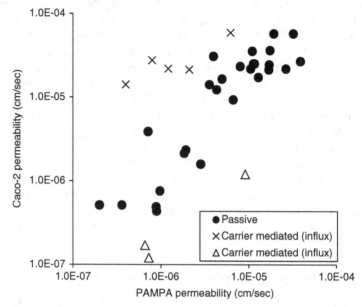

Figure 7.30 Comparison of PAMPA and Caco-2 to study the participation of carrier-mediated transport. •, passive diffusion substrates; ▲, efflux transporter substrates; and ♦, influx transporter substrates. *Source:* Adapted from Reference 124 with permission.

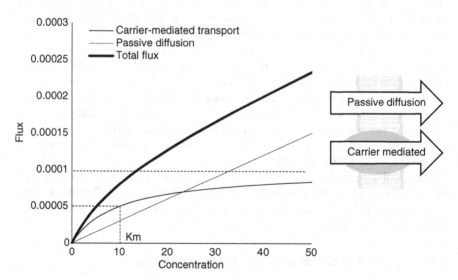

Figure 7.31 Michaelis–Menten equation and passive permeation.

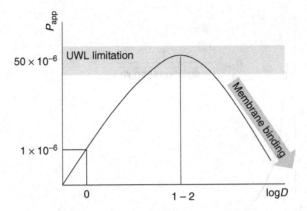

Figure 7.32   Typical lipophilicity–permeability profile.

7.9.8.1   *UWL Adjacent to the Membrane.*   The UWL is only circa 300 μm in the GI tract (Section 6.2.3.3). However, in an *in vitro* permeability assay (planar membrane),[16] the UWL adjacent to the membrane can be up to 1500–4000 μm thick.

When using a planar membrane system, the plate can be shaken to minimize the effects of the UWL. In an *in situ* perfusion study, the flow rate can be increased. A bubbling method can be used to agitate the fluid in the Ussing chamber method. However, an orbital shaker is often not effective, especially for a small-well plate such as the 96-well plate. The agitation effectiveness can be improved by adding beads in the wells. Without strong stirring, the UWL dominates the apparent permeability at $P_{app} >$ ca 30×10^{-6} cm/s. Recently, it has been clearly demonstrated that the quantitative structure–activity relationship was interfered if the effect of the UWL was not removed [20, 125].

The thickness of the UWL in an *in vitro* model ($h_{UWLvitro}$) can be estimated from the pH–permeability profile of a drug, such as ketoprofen. Figure 4.7 shows a typical pH–permeability profile. The merit of using an acidic compound is that the contribution of paracellular pathway can be less significant. Another method to estimate $h_{UWLvitro}$ is to use the P_{app}–lipophilicity profile. Figure 7.32 shows the typical relationship between log D_{oct} and P_{app}. $h_{UWLvitro}$ can be calculated from the P_{app} of compounds in the ceiling region of this profile.

Theoretically, the thickness of the UWL depends on the square or cube root of the flow speed (e.g., the infusion speed (U) for the perfusion model or the rotation speed of the plate) (Section 3.2.4).

$$h_{UWL} = \frac{L}{Sh} \propto Re^{-1/2 \text{ or } 1/3} Sc^{-1/3} = \left(\frac{UL}{\nu}\right)^{-1/2 \text{ or } 1/3} \left(\frac{\nu}{D}\right)^{-1/3} \qquad (7.7)$$

---

[16]The thickness of the UWL in the suspended cells or liposomes would be the same as the radius of the cells (Section 3.2.4.5).

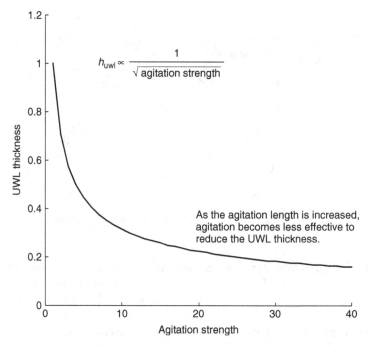

As the agitation length is increased, agitation becomes less effective to reduce the UWL thickness.

$$h_{uwl} \propto \frac{1}{\sqrt{\text{agitation strength}}}$$

Figure 7.33 Agitation strength versus unstirred water layer thickness.

This equation suggests that, as the agitation strength becomes higher, the UWL thickness becomes insensitive to the increase in the agitation strength (Fig. 7.33) [153]. Therefore, insensitiveness of apparent permeability to the agitation increment cannot be the proof for the permeability being dominated by P_{ep}. Even when a strong agitation is used, the UWL still exists and can become a permeation barrier for drugs with high lipophilicity.

7.9.8.2 Membrane Binding. Membrane binding can also retard the permeability of lipophilic drugs, resulting in artifactual low permeability [154, 155]. As a rule of thumb, when log D_{oct} (at assay pH) is greater than 1.5, the membrane binding could become an issue [155]. This experimental artifact may be mitigated by adding BSA in the acceptor fluid [155–161]. *In vivo*, the blood flow removes the compound from the basolateral side [162].

7.9.8.3 Low Solubility. The solubility of a drug in an assay media should be checked before running the assay. The concentration of a drug in the assay media should be set below the solubility of the drug. When a solubilizing agent is used, the free fraction and activity of a drug would be reduced, resulting in artifactual low permeability (cf., P_{app} is usually calculated based on the total dissolved drug concentration). In addition, the cells could be damaged when a solubilizer is used at high concentration [163, 164]. Generally, only low levels of solubilizing solvents, for example, less than 1% DMSO, can be used to avoid toxicity issues.

7.9.8.4 *Differences in Paracellular Pathway.* PAMPA does not have aqueous pores and is therefore not suitable for examining the paracellular transport of a drug. Some cell models, for example, Caco-2 and MDCK, have a narrower tight junction compared to the *in vivo* human intestine and may underestimate the paracellular transport. The paracellular permeability of a drug in dogs is significantly larger than that in humans. However, contribution of the paracellular pathway can be corrected using an *in silico* approach (Section 4.8.3).

7.9.8.5 *Laboratory to Laboratory Variation.* In cell-based assays, significant laboratory to laboratory variations have been observed [105]. Permeability differences can be attributed to a number of factors, e.g., heterogeneity of cell line, passage number, culture conditions, characteristics of the filter membrane, age of monolayers, level of differentiation, and experimental methodologies [165]. Paracellular and carrier-mediated transports tend to show larger laboratory to laboratory variations compared to passive transcellular permeation [105, 151].

7.9.8.6 *Experimental Artifacts in Carrier-Mediated Membrane Transport.* To obtain K_m and V_{max} values for transporters, P_{app} data at a wide range of concentration is required. It is sometimes difficult to achieve a high concentration. P-gp substrates often have low solubility. Both A to B and B to A permeation data should be obtained with an isotropic pH condition (usually pH 7.4 for both sides) [152]. To obtain K_m accurately, the effect of the UWL should be minimized by efficient stirring [166]. Especially for moderately lipophilic efflux transporter substrates, $P_{app,B-A}$ tends to exceed the UWL permeability (Fig. 4.27). As the unbound drug concentration in the cytosol is lower than that in the donor fluid, the intrinsic K_m value should be obtained by the equations introduced in Section 4.9. The contribution of a carrier-mediated transport *in vivo* is often overestimated by an *in vitro* experiment. This point is discussed in detail in Section 14.4.

7.9.9 Recommendation for P_{ep} and P_{eff} Estimation

Cross-validation of P_{ep} data using multiple methods would increase the reliability of the data. Usually, as the project moves from early discovery to late development, the number of available P_{ep} estimation methods increases. It should be remembered that even though the Caco-2 assay is often refereed to as the golden standard, it has various limitations as discussed above.

7.9.9.1 *Hydrophilic Drugs.* Hydrophilic drugs (log $D_{oct,pH6.5} < 0.5$) are usually free from experimental artifacts associated with *in vitro* membrane permeability assays. Thus, Caco-2, MDCK, and other *in vitro* data can be used as a reliable data source. However, the paracellular pathway and transporter expressions of these cell lines could be significantly different from that *in vivo* [167]. Fa% and SPIP data in rats can be used to estimate P_{ep} in humans.

7.9.9.2 Lipophilic Drugs. For a lipophilic drug (log $D_{\text{oct,pH6.5}} > 2$), estimation of P_{ep} from experimental log P_{oct} would be more reliable than that from *in vitro* permeability assays because an *in vitro* membrane permeation assay could underestimate P_{ep} due to the experimental artifacts. After all, the *in vivo* P_{eff} of these compounds is usually determined by the UWL, and therefore, the accuracy of P_{ep} estimation has little effect on P_{eff} prediction.

7.9.9.3 Drugs with Medium Lipophilicity. The estimation of P_{ep} is most difficult for drugs of $0.5 < \log D_{\text{oct,pH6.5}} < 2$. Fortunately, the drugs in this lipophilicity range usually have sufficient solubility and permeability to show good Fa%. However, for appropriate calculation of Fg, P_{ep} should be obtained with sufficient accuracy (Section 4.10).

When not stirred vigorously, because of the very thick UWL *in vitro*, P_{app} becomes significantly smaller than P_{ep}. Drugs with high lipophilicity and MW > 500 also often show moderate passive permeability. When Do < 1, the estimation error of P_{eff} has little effect on Fa%. However, when Do > 1, it would affect Fa% prediction. In the case of dissociable drugs, the pH of the *in vitro* cellular assay can be changed to give a P_{app} value at which the UWL has little effect ($<10 \times 10^{-6}$ cm/s) and then converted to P_{ep} and P_{eff} at a physiological pH.

7.10 *IN VIVO* EXPERIMENTS

In vivo PK data is often used to check the appropriateness of biopharmaceutical modeling (Chapter 15). In drug discovery and development, *in vivo* plasma concentration (C_p)–time profile data is usually available. However, the focus of an *in vivo* PK study in drug discovery tends to be drug disposition and it is often the case that little attention is paid to formulation. As the formulation of a drug has a significant impact on *in vivo* oral absorption, the formulation preparation and characterization for an *in vivo* study are discussed in this section.

7.10.1 P.O

To assess the effect of solubility and the dissolution rate of a drug on *in vivo* oral absorption, the formulation must be carefully prepared before performing *in vivo* experiments. As the reference data, it is preferable to have the PK data from the most stable form. In addition, it is preferable to have the PK data from a solution formulation as the best possible formulation. Precipitation from solution formulation can be tested by an *in vitro* test before the *in vivo* study [168].

In preclinical animal studies, a test compound is often administered as suspensions in vehicles. In this case, it is important to evaluate the crystal form and particle size of a drug in the vehicle. A suspension vehicle is most often composed of an inactive polymer (e.g., methylcellulose) and a small amount of wetting agent (e.g., Tween 80 (<0.1%)). A conventional preparation method to prepare a drug suspension is to use a mortar and pestle. During this preparation process, an API is subjected to destructive forces by sliding, crushing, and/or compression, which may change the characteristics of the API, such as particle size. In addition, the solid form of an API can change to another form when it is dispersed in an aqueous media (e.g., an anhydrate to a hydrate, a salt to a free form). Therefore, the particle size and solid form of an API should be checked before and after formulation preparation. PXRD, DSC, TG/DTA, PLM, and laser diffraction can be used to characterize the API form and the particle size (Sections 7.4 and 7.5). In addition, the above characteristics might change during storage so that it is preferable to confirm the stability of the formulation during the study period. Preferably, the homogeneity of the suspension should be also confirmed. If a formulation is not homogeneous, the dose amount will vary among individual animals, resulting in larger variations of the PK profiles.

7.10.2 I.V

The PK data after i.v. administration is required to calculate the bioavailability of a drug. In the case of a compound with low solubility, a solubilizer is often used to enable i.v. formulation [169, 170]. However, high concentration of the solubilizer can cause hemolysis. When using a solubilizer, hemolysis should be checked by mixing the formulation with blood. In addition, precipitation at the administered site could also be a problem.

7.10.3 Animal Species

Selection of animal species is important for biopharmaceutical investigations. The difference in physiology between animals and humans should be taken into consideration (Chapter 6).

Dogs are preferentially used to assess the performance of a formulation. Working on gastric-acidity-controlled dogs may reveal the effect of stomach pH on oral absorption [171–173]. A pentagastrin or acidic buffer treatment can be used to consistently lower the stomach pH. A dosing volume of 30–50 ml would be representative for humans (and for dogs with 10 kg body weight). Dogs are also suitable to investigate the food effects [174, 175]. The amount of food should be scaled down for dogs. However, for low permeability drugs, an oral absorption study should not be performed in dogs, as the pore size of the paracellular pathway in dogs is larger than that in humans. For evaluation of the controlled-release formulation, the short GI transit time and the strong mechanical stress in dogs should be carefully considered. The intestinal transit time in dogs can be prolonged to approximate that in humans by coadministration of atropine [176–178]. This dog model was used to evaluate the sustained release and pulsate formulations.

For drugs with low permeability, rats would be more appropriate [179]. A dose volume of 1 ml corresponds to circa 250 ml in humans. It is technically difficult to administer a capsule or a tablet to rats (a special capsule for rats is commercially available if necessary). In rats, the bile is continuously secreted into the duodenum and the bile-micelle concentration is significantly higher than that in humans.

Little is known about the agitation strength in the rat intestine. Owing to these reasons, rats are not suitable to assess the oral absorption of drugs with low solubility.

7.10.4 Analysis

Deconvolution is often used to analyze oral PK data. The blood sampling time schedule should be set to provide sufficient data points in the absorption phase.

The *in vivo* animal PK data is often used to adjust a model parameter before predicting the oral absorption of a drug in humans. However, this model optimization should be performed very carefully. Rather, it should be avoided in many cases because it is difficult to surely identify the parameter truly responsible for the discrepancy between simulated and observed PK profiles. If a significant discrepancy is observed, the reason for the discrepancy should be identified by an independent mechanistic investigation. This point is further discussed in Section 16.2.

REFERENCES

1. Lee, P.H., Ayyampalayam, S.N., Carreira, L.A., Shalaeva, M., Bhattachar, S., Coselmon, R., Poole, S., Gifford, E., Lombardo, F. (2007). In silico prediction of ionization constants of drugs. *Mol. Pharm.*, 4, 498–512.

2. Manchester, J., Walkup, G., Rivin, O., You, Z. (2010). Evaluation of pKa estimation methods on 211 druglike compounds. *J. Chem. Inf. Model.*, 50, 565–571.

3. Comer, J., Ionization constant and ionization profile, in: B. Testa, H. van de Waterbeemd (Eds.) Comprehensive medicinal chemistry II Volume 5 ADME-Tox approach, Elsevier, Oxford, 2007, pp. 357–397.

4. Box, K., Bevan, C., Comer, J., Hill, A., Allen, R., Reynolds, D. (2003). High-throughput measurement of pKa values in a mixed-buffer linear pH gradient system. *Anal. Chem.*, 75, 883–892.

5. Ishihama, Y., Nakamura, M., Miwa, T., Kajima, T., Asakawa, N. (2002). A rapid method for pK(a) determination of drugs using pressure-assisted capillary electrophoresis with photodiode array detection in drug discovery. *J. Pharm. Sci.*, 91, 933–942.

6. Poole, S., Patel, S., Dehring, K., Workman, H., Poole, C. (2004). Determination of acid dissociation constants by capillary electrophoresis. *J. Chromatogr., A*, 1037, 445–454.

7. Shalaeva, M., Kenseth, J., Lombardo, F., Bastin, A. (2008). Measurement of dissociation constants (pKa values) of organic compounds by multiplexed capillary electrophoresis using aqueous and cosolvent buffers. *J. Pharm. Sci.*, 97, 2581–2606.

8. Jia, Z., Ramstad, T., Zhong, M. (2001). Medium-throughput pKa screening pharmaceuticals by pressure-assisted capillary electrophoresis. *Electrophoresis*, 22, 1112–1118.

9. Wan, H., Holmen, A., Nagard, M., Lindberg, W. (2002). Rapid screening of pKa values of pharmaceuticals by pressure-assisted capillary electrophoresis combined with short-end injection. *J. Chromatogr., A*, 979, 369–377.

10. Wan, H., Holmen, A.G., Wang, Y., Lindberg, W., Englund, M., Nagard, M.B., Thompson, R.A. (2003). High-throughput screening of pKa values of pharmaceuticals by pressure-assisted capillary electrophoresis and mass spectrometry. *Rapid Commun. Mass Spectrom.*, 17, 2639–2648.

11. Zhou, C., Jin, Y., Kenseth, J.R., Stella, M., Wehmeyer, K.R., Heineman, W.R. (2005). Rapid pKa estimation using vacuum-assisted multiplexed capillary electrophoresis (VAMCE) with ultraviolet detection. *J. Pharm. Sci.*, 94, 576–589.

12. Volgyi, G., Baka, E., Box, K.J., Comer, J.E., Takacs-Novak, K. (2010). Study of pH-dependent solubility of organic bases. Revisit of Henderson-Hasselbalch relationship. *Anal. Chim. Acta.*, 673, 40–46.

13. Fiese, E.F. (2003). General pharmaceutics-the new physical pharmacy. *J. Pharm. Sci.*, 92, 1331–1342.

14. Balbach, S., Korn, C. (2004). Pharmaceutical evaluation of early development candidates "the 100mg-approach". *Int. J. Pharm.*, 275, 1–12.

15. Poulin, P., Theil, F.-P. (2000). A priori prediction of tissue:plasma partition coefficients of drugs to facilitate the use of physiologically-based pharmacokinetic models in drug discovery. *J. Pharm. Sci.*, 89, 16–35.

16. Rodgers, T., Rowland, M. (2006). Physiologically based pharmacokinetic modelling 2: predicting the tissue distribution of acids, very weak bases, neutrals and zwitterions. *J. Pharm. Sci.*, 95, 1238–1257.

17. Rodgers, T., Rowland, M. (2007). Mechanistic approaches to volume of distribution predictions: understanding the processes. *Pharm. Res.*, 24, 918–933.

18. Tomizawa, K., Sugano, K., Yamada, H., Horii, I. (2006). Physicochemical and cell-based approach for early screening of phospholipidosis-inducing potential. *J. Toxicol. Sci.*, 31, 315–324.

19. Mannhold, R., Poda, G.I., Ostermann, C., Tetko, I.V. (2009). Calculation of molecular lipophilicity: state-of-the-art and comparison of log P methods on more than 96,000 compounds. *J. Pharm. Sci.*, 98, 861–893.

20. Avdeef, A., Bendels, S., Di, L., Faller, B., Kansy, M., Sugano, K., Yamauchi, Y. (2007). Parallel artificial membrane permeability assay (PAMPA)-critical factors for better predictions of absorption. *J. Pharm. Sci.*, 96, 2893–2909.

21. Wenlock, M.C., Barton, P., Luker, T. (2011). Lipophilicity of acidic compounds: impact of ion pair partitioning on drug design. *Bioorg. Med. Chem. Lett.*, 21, 3550–3556.

22. Pagliara, A., Carrupt, P.A., Caron, G., Gaillard, P., Testa, B. (1997). Lipophilicity profiles of ampholytes. *Chem. Rev.*, 97, 3385–3400.

23. Bermejo, M., Avdeef, A., Ruiz, A., Nalda, R., Ruell, J.A., Tsinman, O., Gonzalez, I., Fernandez, C., Sanchez, G., Garrigues, T.M., Merino, V. (2004). PAMPA–a drug absorption model*1: 7. Comparing rat, Caco-2, and PAMPA permeability of fluoroquinolones. *Eur. J. Pharm. Sci.*, 21, 429.

24. Nishimura, I., Hirano, A., Yamashita, T., Fukami, T. (2009). Improvement of the high-speed logD assay using an injection marker for the water plug aspiration/injection method. *J. Chromatogr., A*, 1216, 2984–2988.

25. Dohta, Y., Yamashita, T., Horiike, S., Nakamura, T., Fukami, T. (2007). A system for LogD screening of 96-well plates using a water-plug aspiration/injection method combined with high-performance liquid chromatography-mass spectrometry. *Anal. Chem.*, 79, 8312–8315.

26. Lombardo, F., Shalaeva, M.Y., Tupper, K.A., Gao, F., Abraham, M.H. (2000). Elog-Poct: a tool for lipophilicity determination in drug discovery. *J. Med. Chem.*, 43, 2922–2928.

27. Lombardo, F., Shalaeva, M.Y., Tupper, K.A., Gao, F. (2001). ElogD(oct): a tool for lipophilicity determination in drug discovery. 2. Basic and neutral compounds. *J. Med. Chem.*, 44, 2490–2497.

28. Yamagami, C., Kawase, K., Iwaki, K. (2002). Hydrophobicity parameters determined by reversed-phase liquid chromatography. XV: optimal conditions for prediction of log P(oct) by using RP-HPLC procedures. *Chem. Pharm. Bull. (Tokyo)*, 50, 1578–1583.

29. Herbert, B.J., Dorsey, J.G. (1995). n-octanol-water partition coefficient estimation by micellar electrokinetic capillary chromatography. *Anal. Chem.*, 67, 744–749.

30. Poole, S.K., Patel, S., Dehring, K., Workman, H., Dong, J. (2003). Estimation of octanol-water partition coefficients for neutral and weakly acidic compounds by microemulsion electrokinetic chromatography using dynamically coated capillary columns. *J. Chromatogr., B Analyt. Technol. Biomed. Life Sci.*, 793, 265–274.

31. Razak, J.L., Cutak, B.J., Larive, C.K., Lunte, C.E. (2001). Correlation of the capacity factor in vesicular electrokinetic chromatography with the octanol:water partition coefficient for charged and neutral analytes. *Pharm. Res.*, 18, 104–111.

32. Poole, S.K., Durham, D., Kibbey, C. (2000). Rapid method for estimating the octanol–water partition coefficient (log P ow) by microemulsion electrokinetic chromatography. *J. Chromatogr., B Biomed. Sci. Appl.*, 745, 117–126.

33. Avdeef, A. (1993). pH-metric log P. II: refinement of partition coefficients and ionization constants of multiprotic substances. *J. Pharm. Sci.*, 82, 183.

34. Slater, B., McCormack, A., Avdeef, A., Comer, J.E. (1994). pH-metric log P. 4. Comparison of partition coefficients determined by HPLC and potentiometric methods to literature values. *J. Pharm. Sci.*, 83, 1280.

35. Faller, B., Grimm, H.P., Loeuillet-Ritzler, F., Arnold, S., Briand, X. (2005). High-throughput lipophilicity measurement with immobilized artificial membranes. *J. Med. Chem.*, 48, 2571–2576.

36. Glomme, A., März, J., Dressman, J., Predicting the intestinal solubility of poorly soluble drugs, in: B. Testa, S. Krämer, H. Wunderli-Allenspach, G. Folkers (Eds.) Pharmacokinetic Profiling in Drug Research, Wiley-VCH, Zurich, 2006, pp. 259–280.

37. Wiedmann, T.S., Kamel, L. (2002). Examination of the solubilization of drugs by bile salt micelles. *J. Pharm. Sci.*, 91, 1743–1764.

38. Avdeef, A., Box, K.J., Comer, J.E., Hibbert, C., Tam, K.Y. (1998). pH-metric logP 10. Determination of liposomal membrane-water partition coefficients of ionizable drugs. *Pharm. Res.*, 15, 209–215.

39. Miyazaki, J., Hideg, K., Marsh, D. (1992). Interfacial ionization and partitioning of membrane-bound local anesthetics. *Biochim. Biophys. Acta*, 1103, 62–68.

40. de Castro, B., Gameiro, P., Guimaraes, C., Lima, J.L., Reis, S. (2001). Partition coefficients of beta-blockers in bile salt/lecithin micelles as a tool to assess the role of mixed micelles in gastrointestinal absorption. *Biophys. Chem.*, 90, 31–43.

41. Yamaguchi, T., Ikeda, C., Sekine, Y. (1986). Intestinal absorption of a b-adrenergic blocking agent nadolol. I. Comparison of absorption behavior of nadolol with those of other b-blocking agents in rats. *Chem. Pharm. Bull.*, 34, 3362–3369.

42. Yamaguchi, T., Ikeda, C., Sekine, Y. (1986). Intestinal absorption of a b-adrenergic blocking agent nadolol. II. Mechanism of the inhibitory effect on the intestinal absorption of nadolol by sodium cholate in rats. *Chem. Pharm. Bull.*, 34, 3836–3843.

43. Yamaguchi, T., Oida, T., Ikeda, C., Sekine, Y. (1986). Intestinal absorption of a b-adrenergic blocking agent nadolol. III. Nuclear magnetic resonance spectroscopic study on nadolol-sodium cholate micellar complex and intestinal absorption of nadolol derivatives in rats. *Chem. Pharm. Bull.*, 34, 4259–4264.

44. Giron, D., Testa, B., van de Waterbeemd, H. (Eds.), Artificial membrane technologies to assess transfer and permeation of drugs in drug discovery, in Comprehensive Medicinal Chemistry II Volume 5 ADME-Tox Approach, Elsevier, Oxford, 2007, pp. 509–530.

45. Pudipeddi, M., Serajuddin, A.T.M. (2005). Trends in solubility of polymorphs. *J. Pharm. Sci.*, 94, 929–939.

46. Threlfall, T. (2003). Structural and thermodynamic explanations of Ostwald's rule. *Org. Process Res. Dev.*, 7, 1017–1027.

47. Hancock, B.C., Parks, M. (2000). What is the true solubility advantage for amorphous pharmaceuticals? *Pharm. Res.*, 17, 397–404.

48. Miller, J.M., Collman, B.M., Greene, L.R., Grant, D.J.W., Blackburn, A.C. (2005). Identifying the stable polymorph early in the drug discovery-development process. *Pharm. Dev. Technol.*, 10, 291–297.

49. Ruland, W. (1961). X-ray determination of crystallinity and diffuse disorder scattering. *Acta Crystallogr.*, 14, 1180–1185.

50. Gardner, C.R., Walsh, C.T., Almarsson, O. (2004). Drugs as materials: valuing physical form in drug discovery. *Nat. Rev. Drug Discov.*, 3, 926–934.

51. Morissette, S.L., Almarsson, O., Peterson, M.L., Remenar, J.F., Read, M.J., Lemmo, A.V., Ellis, S., Cima, M.J., Gardner, C.R. (2004). High-throughput crystallization: polymorphs, salts, co-crystals and solvates of pharmaceutical solids. *Adv. Drug Delivery Rev.*, 56, 275–300.

52. Kojima, T., Onoue, S., Murase, N., Katoh, F., Mano, T., Matsuda, Y. (2006). Crystalline form information from multiwell plate salt screening by use of raman microscopy. *Pharm. Res.*, 23, 806–812.

53. Girolami, G.S. (1994). A simple "back of the envelope" method for estimating the densities and molecular volumes of liquids and solids. *J. Chem. Educ.*, 71, 962–964.

54. Cao, X., Leyva, N., Anderson, S.R., Hancock, B.C. (2008). Use of prediction methods to estimate true density of active pharmaceutical ingredients. *Int. J. Pharm.*, 355, 231–237.

55. Lipinski, C.A., Lombardo, F., Dominy, B.W., Feeney, P.J. (1997). Experimental and computational approaches to estimate solubility and permeability in drug discovery and development settings. *Adv. Drug Delivery Rev.*, 23, 3–25.

56. Dehring, K.A., Workman, H.L., Miller, K.D., Mandagere, A., Poole, S.K. (2004). Automated robotic liquid handling/laser-based nephelometry system for high throughput measurement of kinetic aqueous solubility. *J. Pharm. Biomed. Anal.*, 36, 447–456.

57. Chen, T.-M., Shen, H., Zhu, C. (2002). Evaluation of a method for high throughput solubility determination using a multi-wavelength UV plate reader. *Comb. Chem. High Throughput Screen.*, 5, 575–581.

58. Pitt, A. (2005). High-throughput screening to determine aqueous drug solubility. *Pharm. Discov.*, 5, 46–49.

59. Bhattachar, S.N., Deschenes, L.A., Wesley, J.A. (2006). Solubility: it's not just for physical chemists. *Drug Discov. Today*, 11, 1012–1018.

60. Vertzoni, M., Dressman, J., Butler, J., Hempenstall, J., Reppas, C. (2005). Simulation of fasting gastric conditions and its importance for the dissolution of lipophilic compounds. *Eur. J. Pharm. Biopharm.*, 60, 413–417.

61. Galia, E., Nicolaides, E., Horter, D., Lobenberg, R., Reppas, C., Dressman, J.B. (1998). Evaluation of various dissolution media for predicting performance of class I and II drugs. *Pharm. Res.*, 15, 698–705.

62. Jantratid, E., Janssen, N., Reppas, C., Dressman, J.B. (2008). Dissolution media simulating conditions in the proximal human gastrointestinal tract: an update. *Pharm. Res.*, 25, 1663–1676.

63. Sugano, K., Okazaki, A., Sugimoto, S., Tavornvipas, S., Omura, A., Mano, T. (2007). Solubility and dissolution profile assessment in drug discovery. *Drug Metab. Pharmacokinet.*, 22, 225–254.

64. Scholz, A., Kostewicz, E., Abrahamsson, B., Dressman, J.B. (2003). Can the USP paddle method be used to represent in-vivo hydrodynamics? *J. Pharm. Pharmacol.*, 55, 443–451.

65. Baka, E., Comer, J.E., Takacs-Novak, K. (2008). Study of equilibrium solubility measurement by saturation shake-flask method using hydrochlorothiazide as model compound. *J. Pharm. Biomed. Anal.*, 46, 335–341.

66. Volgyi, G., Baka, E., Kovacs, M., Takacsne, N.K. (2011). Good laboratory practice of equilibrium solubility measurement II. Study of pH-dependent solubility of ionizable compounds. *Acta Pharm. Hung.*, 81, 87–95.

67. Baka, E. (2011). Good laboratory practice of equilibrium solubility measurement. *Acta Pharm. Hung.*, 81, 18–28.

68. Seadeek, C., Ando, H., Bhattachar, S.N., Heimbach, T., Sonnenberg, J.L., Blackburn, A.C. (2007). Automated approach to couple solubility with final pH and crystallinity for pharmaceutical discovery compounds. *J. Pharm. Biomed. Anal.*, 43, 1660–1666.

69. Sugano, K., Kato, T., Suzuki, K., Keiko, K., Sujaku, T., Mano, T. (2006). High throughput solubility measurement with automated polarized light microscopy analysis. *J. Pharm. Sci.*, 95, 2115–2122.

70. Sugaya, Y., Yoshiba, T., Kajima, T., Ishihama, Y. (2002). Development of solubility screening methods in drug discovery. *Yakugaku Zasshi*, 122, 237–246.

71. Pudipeddi, M., Zannou, E.A., Vasanthavada, M., Dontabhaktuni, A., Royce, A.E., Joshi, Y.M., Serajuddin, A.T.M. (2008). Measurement of surface pH of pharmaceutical solids: a critical evaluation of indicator dye-sorption method and its comparison with slurry pH method. *J. Pharm. Sci.*, 97, 1831–1842.

72. Serajuddin, A.T.M., Jarowski, C.I. (1985). Effect of diffusion layer pH and solubility on the dissolution rate of pharmaceutical acids and their sodium salts. II: salicylic acid, theophylline, and benzoic acid. *J. Pharm. Sci.*, 74, 148–154.

73. Serajuddin, A.T.M., Jarowski, C.I. (1985). Effect of diffusion layer pH and solubility on the dissolution rate of pharmaceutical bases and their hydrochloride salts. I: phenazopyridine. *J. Pharm. Sci.*, 74, 142–147.

74. Van Eerdenbrugh, B., Vermant, J., Martens, J.A., Froyen, L., Van Humbeeck, J., Van den Mooter, G., Augustijns, P. (2010). Solubility increases associated with crystalline drug nanoparticles: methodologies and significance. *Mol. Pharm.*, 7, 1858–1870.

75. Llinas, A., Glen, R.C., Goodman, J.M. (2008). Solubility challenge: can you predict solubilities of 32 molecules using a database of 100 reliable measurements? *J. Chem. Inf. Model.*, 48, 1289–1303.

76. Avdeef, A., Tsinman, K., Tsinman, O., Sun, N., Voloboy, D. (2009). Miniaturization of powder dissolution measurement and estimation of particle size. *Chem. Biodivers.*, 6, 1796–1811.

77. Bai, G., Armenante, P.M. (2008). Velocity distribution and shear rate variability resulting from changes in the impeller location in the USP dissolution testing apparatus II. *Pharm. Res.*, 25, 320–336.

78. Bai, G., Armenante, P.M. (2009). Hydrodynamic, mass transfer, and dissolution effects induced by tablet location during dissolution testing. *J. Pharm. Sci.*, 98, 1511–1531.

79. Bai, G., Armenante, P.M., Plank, R.V. (2007). Experimental and computational determination of blend time in USP dissolution testing apparatus II. *J. Pharm. Sci.*, 96, 3072–3086.

80. Bai, G., Armenante, P.M., Plank, R.V., Gentzler, M., Ford, K., Harmon, P. (2007). Hydrodynamic investigation of USP dissolution test apparatus II. *J. Pharm. Sci.*, 96, 2327–2349.

81. Mirza, T., Joshi, Y., Liu, Q., Vivilecchia, R. (2005). Evaluation of dissolution hydrodynamics in the USP, Peakand flat-bottom vessels using different solubility drugs. *Dissolut. Technol.*, 12, 11–16.

82. Shiko, G., Gladden, L.F., Sederman, A.J., Connolly, P.C., Butler, J.M. (2011). MRI studies of the hydrodynamics in a USP 4 dissolution testing cell. *J. Pharm. Sci.*, 100, 976–991.

83. Kostewicz, E.S., Wunderlich, M., Brauns, U., Becker, R., Bock, T., Dressman, J.B. (2004). Predicting the precipitation of poorly soluble weak bases upon entry in the small intestine. *J. Pharm. Pharmacol.*, 56, 43–51.

84. Carino, S.R., Sperry, D.C., Hawley, M. (2010). Relative bioavailability of three different solid forms of PNU-141659 as determined with the artificial stomach-duodenum model. *J. Pharm. Sci.*, 99, 3923–3930.

85. Carino, S.R., Sperry, D.C., Hawley, M. (2005). Relative bioavailability estimation of carbamazepine crystal forms using an artificial stomach-duodenum model. *J. Pharm. Sci.*, 95, 116–125.

86. Gu, C.-H., Rao, D., Gandhi, R.B., Hilden, J., Raghavan, K. (2005). Using a novel multicompartment dissolution system to predict the effect of gastric pH on the oral absorption of weak bases with poor intrinsic solubility. *J. Pharm. Sci.*, 94, 199–208.

87. Sugawara, M., Kadomura, S., He, X., Takekuma, Y., Kohri, N., Miyazaki, K. (2005). The use of an dissolution and absorption system to evaluate oral absorption of two weak bases in pH-independent controlled-release formulations. *Eur. J. Pharm. Sci.*, 26, 1–8.

88. Kataoka, M., Masaoka, Y., Sakuma, S., Yamashita, S. (2006). Effect of food intake on the oral absorption of poorly water-soluble drugs: assessment of drug dissolution and permeation assay system. *J. Pharm. Sci.*, 95, 2051–2061.

89. Kataoka, M., Masaoka, Y., Yamazaki, Y., Sakane, T., Sezaki, H., Yamashita, S. (2003). system to evaluate oral absorption of poorly water-soluble drugs: simultaneous analysis on dissolution and permeation of drugs. *Pharm. Res.*, 20, 1674–1680.

90. Buch, P., Langguth, P., Kataoka, M., Yamashita, S. (2009). IVIVC in oral absorption for fenofibrate immediate release tablets using a dissolution/permeation system. *J. Pharm. Sci.*, 98, 2001–2009.

91. Kataoka, M., Sugano, K., da Costa Mathews, C., Wong, J.W., Jones, K.L., Masaoka, Y., Sakuma, S., Yamashita, S. (2011). Application of dissolution/permeation system for evaluation of formulation effect on oral absorption of poorly water-soluble drugs in drug development. *Pharm. Res*. DOI: 10.1007/s11095-011-0623-2.

92. Tavornvipas, S., Sugimoto, S., Sugano, K., Hashimoto, N., Mano, T., Yamashita, S. (2007). Application of dissolution-permeation system PAMPA system for predicttion of oral drug absorption of nanoparticle. *J. Pharm. Sci. Tech. Jpn.*, 67, 381.

93. Takada, K., Masaoka, Y., Kataoka, M., Sakuma, S., Takano, R., Hayashi, Y., Asoh, Y., Yamashita, S. (2005). assessment of oral absorption of poorly-soluble drugs: use of artificial lipid membrane in dissolution/permeation system. *Drug Metab. Rev.*, 288.

94. Sugano, K., Sakai, K., Mucopolysaccharide-layered lipid membrane, membrane permeability-measuring filter/apparatus/kit, membrane permeability evaluation method, and test substance-screening method, in, JP, 2005, p. 13.

95. Box, K.J., Volgyi, G., Baka, E., Stuart, M., Takacs-Novak, K., Comer, J.E.A. (2006). Equilibrium versus kinetic measurements of aqueous solubility, and the ability of compounds to supersaturate in solution-a validation study. *J. Pharm. Sci.*, 95, 1298–1307.

96. Lindfors, L., Forssen, S., Westergren, J., Olsson, U. (2008). Nucleation and crystal growth in supersaturated solutions of a model drug. *J. Colloid Interface Sci.*, 325, 404–413.

97. Carlert, S., Palsson, A., Hanisch, G., von Corswant, C., Nilsson, C., Lindfors, L., Lennernas, H., Abrahamsson, B. (2010). Predicting intestinal precipitation–a case example for a basic BCS class II drug. *Pharm. Res.*, 27, 2119–2130.

98. Gu, C.H., Gandhi, R.B., Tay, L.K., Zhou, S., Raghavan, K. (2004). Importance of using physiologically relevant volume of dissolution medium to correlate the oral exposure of formulations of BMS-480188 mesylate. *Int. J. Pharm.*, 269, 195–202.

99. Lennernaes, H. (2007). Animal data: the contributions of the Ussing Chamber and perfusion systems to predicting human oral drug delivery. *Adv. Drug Delivery Rev.*, 59, 1103–1120.

100. Salphati, L., Childers, K., Pan, L., Tsutsui, K., Takahashi, L. (2001). Evaluation of a single-pass intestinal-perfusion method in rat for the prediction of absorption in man. *J. Pharm. Pharmacol.*, 53, 1007–1013.

101. Lennernaes, H. (2007). Intestinal permeability and its relevance for absorption and elimination. *Xenobiotica*, 37, 1015–1051.

102. Hidalgo, I.J., Raub, T.J., Borchardt, R.T. (1989). Characterization of the human colon carcinoma cell line (Caco-2) as a model system for intestinal epithelial permeability. *Gastroenterology*, 96, 736–749.

103. Artursson, P., Karlsson, J. (1991). Correlation between oral absorption in humans and apparent drug permeability coefficients in human intestinal epithelial Caco2 cells. *Biochem. Biophys. Res. Commun.*, 175, 880–885.

104. Artursson, P., Matsson, P., Cell culture absorption models-state of the art, in: B. Testa, S. Krämer, H. Wunderli-Allenspach, G. Folkers (Eds.) Pharmacokinetic Profiling Drug Research, Wiley-VCH, Zurich, 2006, pp. 71–78.

105. Hayeshi, R., Hilgendorf, C., Artursson, P., Augustijns, P., Brodin, B., Dehertogh, P., Fisher, K., Fossati, L., Hovenkamp, E., Korjamo, T., Masungi, C., Maubon, N., Mols, R., Mullertz, A., Monkkonen, J., O'Driscoll, C., Oppers-Tiemissen, H.M., Ragnarsson, E.G., Rooseboom, M., Ungell, A.L. (2008). Comparison of drug transporter gene expression and functionality in Caco-2 cells from 10 different laboratories. *Eur. J. Pharm. Sci.*, 35, 383–396.

106. Avdeef, A., Tam, K.Y. (2010). How well can the Caco-2/Madin-darby canine kidney models predict effective human jejunal permeability? *J. Med. Chem.*, 53, 3566–3584.

107. Putnam, W.S., Pan, L., Tsutsui, K., Takahashi, L., Benet, L.Z. (2002). Comparison of bidirectional cephalexin transport across MDCK and caco-2 cell monolayers: interactions with peptide transporters. *Pharm. Res.*, 19, 27–33.

108. Thiel-Demby, V.E., Humphreys, J.E., St. John Williams, L.A., Ellens, H.M., Shah, N., Ayrton, A.D., Polli, J.W. (2009). Biopharmaceutics classification system: validation and learnings of an permeability assay. *Mol. Pharm.*, 6, 11–18.

109. Lennernäs, H. (2007). Animal data: the contributions of the Ussing Chamber and perfusion systems to predicting human oral drug delivery. *Adv. Drug Delivery Rev.*, 59, 1103–1120.

110. Kansy, M., Senner, F., Gubernator, K. (1998). Physicochemical high throughput screening: parallel artificial membrane permeation assay in the description of passive absorption processes. *J. Med. Chem.*, 41, 1007–1010.

111. Sugano, K., Hamada, H., Machida, M., Ushio, H. (2001). High throuput prediction of oral absorption: Improvement of the composition of the lipid solution used in parallel artificial membrane permeation assay. *J. Biomol. Screen.*, 6, 189–196.

112. Wohnsland, F., Faller, B. (2001). High-throughput permeability pH profile and high-throughput alkane/water log P with artificial membranes. *J. Med. Chem.*, 44, 923–930.

113. Di, L., Kerns, E.H., Fan, K., McConnell, O.J., Carter, G.T. (2003). High throughput artificial membrane permeability assay for blood-brain barrier. *Eur. J. Med. Chem.*, 38, 223–232.

114. Avdeef, A., Strafford, M., Block, E., Balogh, M.P., Chambliss, W., Khan, I. (2001). Drug absorption model: filter-immobilized artificial membranes; 2. Studies of the permeability properties of lactones in Piper methysticum Forst. *Eur. J. Pharm. Sci.*, 14, 271–280.

115. Tanaka, M., Fukuda, H., Nagai, T. (1978). Permeation of a drug through a model membrane consisting of millipore filter with oil. *Chem. Pharm. Bull.*, 26, 9–13.

116. Camenisch, G., Folkers, G., van de Waterbeemd, H. (1997). Comparison of passive drug transport through Caco-2 cells and artificial membranes. *Int. J. Pharm.*, 147, 61–70.

117. Avdeef, A., Absorption and Drug Development, Wiley-Interscience, NJ, Hoboken, 2003.

118. Sugano, K., Nabuchi, Y., Machida, M., Asoh, Y. (2004). Permeation characteristics of a hydrophilic basic compound across a bio-mimetic artificial membrane. *Int. J. Pharm.*, 275, 271–278.

119. Seo, P.R., Teksin, Z.S., Kao, J.P.Y., Polli, J.E. (2006). Lipid composition effect on permeability across PAMPA. *Eur. J. Pharm. Sci.*, 29, 259–268.

120. Teksin, Z.S., Hom, K., Balakrishnan, A., Polli, J.E. (2006). Ion pair-mediated transport of metoprolol across a three lipid-component PAMPA system. *J. Controlled Release*, 116, 50–57.

121. Xiang, T., Xu, Y., Anderson, B.D. (1998). The barrier domain for solute permeation varies with lipid bilayer phase structure. *J. Membr. Biol.*, 165, 77–90.

122. Kansy, M., Avdeef, A., Fischer, H. (2004). Advances in screening for membrane permeability: high-resolution PAMPA for medicinal chemists. *Drug Discove. Today: Technol.*, 1, 349–355.

123. Ano, R., Kimura, Y., Shima, M., Matsuno, R., Ueno, T., Akamatsu, M. (2004). Relationships between structure and high-throughput screening permeability of peptide derivatives and related compounds with artificial membranes: application to prediction of Caco-2 cell permeability. *Bioorg. Med. Chem.*, 12, 257.

124. Fujikawa, M., Ano, R., Nakao, K., Shimizu, R., Akamatsu, M. (2005). Relationships between structure and high-throughput screening permeability of diverse drugs with artificial membranes: application to prediction of Caco-2 cell permeability. *Bioorg. Med. Chem.*, 13, 4721–4732.

125. Fujikawa, M., Nakao, K., Shimizu, R., Akamatsu, M. (2007). QSAR study on permeability of hydrophobic compounds with artificial membranes. *Bioorg. Med. Chem.*, 15, 3756–3767.

126. Flaten, G.E., Bunjes, H., Luthman, K., Brandl, M. (2006). Drug permeability across a phospholipid vesicle-based barrier: 2. Characterization of barrier structure, storage stability and stability towards pH changes. *Eur. J. Pharm. Sci.*, 28, 336–343.

127. Flaten, G.E., Dhanikula, A.B., Luthman, K., Brandl, M. (2006). Drug permeability across a phospholipid vesicle based barrier: a novel approach for studying passive diffusion. *Eur. J. Pharm. Sci.*, 27, 80–90.

128. Flaten, G.E., Skar, M., Luthman, K., Brandl, M. (2007). Drug permeability across a phospholipid vesicle based barrier: 3. Characterization of drug-membrane interactions and the effect of agitation on the barrier integrity and on the permeability. *Eur. J. Pharm. Sci.*, 30, 324–332.

129. Corti, G., Maestrelli, F., Cirri, M., Furlanetto, S., Mura, P. (2006). Development and evaluation of an method for prediction of human drug absorption I. Assessment of artificial membrane composition. *Eur. J. Pharm. Sci.*, 27, 346–353.

130. Corti, G., Maestrelli, F., Cirri, M., Zerrouk, N., Mura, P. (2006). Development and evaluation of an method for prediction of human drug absorption. *Eur. J. Pharm. Sci.*, 27, 354–362.

131. Chen, X., Murawski, A., Patel, K., Crespi, C.L., Balimane, P.V. (2008). A novel design of artificial membrane for improving the parallel artificial membrane permeability assay model. *Pharm. Res.*, 25, 1511–1520.

132. Avdeef, A. (2007). Solubility of sparingly-soluble ionizable drugs. *Adv. Drug Delivery Rev.*, 59, 568–590.

133. Flaten, G.E., Bunjes, H., Luthman, K., Brandl, M. (2006). Drug permeability across a phospholipid vesicle-based barrier. *Eur. J. Pharm. Sci.*, 28, 336–343.

134. Ottaviani, G., Martel, S., Carrupt, P.-A. (2006). Parallel artificial membrane permeability assay: a new membrane for the fast prediction of passive uman skin permeability. *J. Med. Chem.*, 49, 3948–3954.

135. Sugano, K., Hamada, H., Machida, M., Ushio, H., Saitoh, K., Terada, K. (2001). Optimized conditions of bio-mimetic artificial membrane permeation assay. *Int. J. Pharm.*, 228, 181–188.

136. Danelian, E., Karlen, A., Karlsson, R., Winiwarter, S., Hansson, A., Lofas, S., Lennernas, H., Hamalainen, M.D. (2000). SPR biosensor studies of the direct interaction between 27 drugs and a liposome surface: correlation with fraction absorbed in humans. *J. Med. Chem.*, 43, 2083–2086.

137. Frostell-Karlsson, A., Widegren, H., Green, C.E., Hamalainen, M.D., Westerlund, L., Karlsson, R., Fenner, K., van de Waterbeemd, H. (2005). Biosensor analysis of the interaction between drug compounds and liposomes of different properties; a two-dimensional characterization tool for estimation of membrane absorption. *J. Pharm. Sci.*, 94, 25–37.

138. Cheng, Y.Y., Song, J.C., Hanlan, L., Pidgeon, C. (1997). Immobilized Artificial Membranes—screens for drug membrane interactions. *Adv. Drug Delivery Rev.*, 23, 229–256.

139. Liu, H., Ong, S., Glunz, L., Pidgeon, C. (1995). Predicting drug-membrane interactions by HPLC: structural requirements of chromatographic surfaces. *Anal. Chem.*, 67, 3550–3557.

140. Ong, S., Liu, H., Pidgeon, C. (1996). Immobilized-artificial-membrane chromatography: measurements of membrane partition coefficient and predicting drug membrane permeability. *J. Chromatogr., A*, 728, 113–128.

141. Ong, S., Liu, H., Qiu, X., Bhat, G., Pidgeon, C. (1995). Membrane partition coefficients chromatographically measured using immobilized artificial membrane surfaces. *Anal. Chem.*, 67, 755–762.

142. Ong, S., Pidgeon, C. (1995). Thermodynamics of solute partitioning into immobilized artificial membranes. *Anal. Chem.*, 67, 2119–2128.

143. Pidgeon, C., Ong, S., Liu, H., Qiu, X., Pidgeon, M., Dantzig, A.H., Munroe, J., Hornback, W.J., Kasher, J.S., Glunz, L., et al. (1995). IAM chromatography: an screen for predicting drug membrane permeability. *J. Med. Chem.*, 38, 590–594.

144. Shaowei, O., Hanlan, L., Pidgeon, C. (1996). Immobilized-artificial-membrane chromatography: measurements of membrane partition coefficient and predicting drug membrane permeability. *J. Chromatogr., A*, 728, 113–128.

145. Beigi, F., Gottschalk, I., Lagerquist Hagglund, C., Haneskog, L., Brekkan, E., Zhang, Y., Osterberg, T., Lundahl, P. (1998). Immobilized liposome and biomembrane partitioning chromatography of drugs for prediction of drug transport. *Int. J. Pharm.*, 164, 129–137.

146. Beigi, F., Lundahl, P. (1999). Immobilized biomembrane chromatography of highly lipophilic drugs. *J. Chromatogr., A*, 852, 313–317.

147. Beigi, F., Yang, Q., Lundahl, P. (1995). Immobilized-liposome chromatographic analysis of drug partitioning into lipid bilayers. *J. Chromatogr., A*, 704, 315–321.

148. Lundahl, P., Beigi, F. (1997). Immobilized liposome chromatography of drugs for model analysis of drug-membrane interactions. *Adv. Drug Delivery Rev.*, 23, 221–227.

149. Loidl-Stahlhofen, A., Eckert, A., Hartmann, T., Schottner, M. (2001). Solid-supported lipid membranes as a tool for determination of membrane affinity: high-throughput screening of a physicochemical parameter. *J. Pharm. Sci.*, 90, 599–606.

150. Loidl-Stahlhofen, A., Hartmann, T., Schottner, M., Rohring, C., Brodowsky, H., Schmitt, J., Keldenich, J. (2001). Multilamellar liposomes and solid-supported lipid membranes (TRANSIL): screening of lipid-water partitioning toward a high-throughput scale. *Pharm. Res.*, 18, 1782–1788.

151. Avdeef, A. (2010). Leakiness and size exclusion of paracellular channels in cultured epithelial cell monolayers-interlaboratory comparison. *Pharm. Res.*, 27, 480–489.

152. Neuhoff, S., Ungell, A.-L., Zamora, I., Artursson, P. (2003). pH-dependent bidirectional transport of weakly basic drugs across Caco-2 monolayers: implications for drug-drug interactions. *Pharm. Res.*, 20, 1141–1148.

153. Avdeef, A., Nielsen, P.E., Tsinman, O. (2004). PAMPA–a drug absorption model*1: 11. Matching the unstirred water layer thickness by individual-well stirring in microtitre plates. *Eur. J. Pharm. Sci.*, 22, 365.

154. Wils, P., Warnery, A., Phung-Ba, V., Legrain, S., Scherman, D. (1994). High lipophilicity decreases drug transport across intestinal epithelial cells. *J. Pharmacol. Exp. Ther.*, 269, 654–658.

155. Krishna, G., Chen, K.-J., Lin, C.-C., Nomeir, A.A. (2001). Permeability of lipophilic compounds in drug discovery using in-vitro human absorption model, Caco-2. *Int. J. Pharm.*, 222, 77–89.

156. Neuhoff, S., Artursson, P., Ungell, A.L. (2007). Advantages and disadvantages of using bovine serum albumin and/or Cremophor EL as extracellular additives during transport studies of lipophilic compounds across Caco-2 monolayers. *J. Drug Delivery Sci. Technol.*, 17, 259–266.

157. Neuhoff, S., Artursson, P., Zamora, I., Ungell, A.-L. (2006). Impact of extracellular protein binding on passive and active drug transport across Caco-2 cells. *Pharm. Res.*, 23, 350–359.

158. Sawada, G.A., Ho, N.F., Williams, L.R., Barsuhn, C.L., Raub, T.J. (1994). Transcellular permeability of chlorpromazine demonstrating the roles of protein binding and membrane partitioning. *Pharm. Res.*, 11, 665–673.

159. Yamashita, S., Furubayashi, T., Kataoka, M., Sakane, T., Sezaki, H., Tokuda, H. (2000). Optimized conditions for prediction of intestinal drug permeability using Caco-2 cells. *Eur. J. Pharm. Sci.*, 10, 195–204.

160. Aungst, B.J., Nguyen, N.H., Bulgarelli, J.P., Oates-Lenz, K. (2000). The influence of donor and reservoir additives on Caco-2 permeability and secretory transport of HIV protease inhibitors and other lipophilic compounds. *Pharm. Res.*, 17, 1175–1180.

161. Liu, T., Chang, L.J., Uss, A., Chu, I., Morrison, R.A., Wang, L., Prelusky, D., Cheng, K.C., Li, C. (2010). The impact of protein on Caco-2 permeability of low mass balance compounds for absorption projection and efflux substrate identification. *J. Pharm. Biomed. Anal.*, 51, 1069–1077.

162. Yamashita, S., Tanaka, Y., Endoh, Y., Taki, Y., Sakane, T., Nadai, T., Sezaki, H. (1997). Analysis of drug permeation across Caco-2 monolayer: implication for predicting drug absorption. *Pharm. Res.*, 14, 486–491.

163. Saha, P., Kou, J.H. (2000). Effect of solubilizing excipients on permeation of poorly water-soluble compounds across Caco-2 cell monolayers. *Eur. J. Pharm. Biopharm.*, 50, 403–411.

164. Takahashi, Y., Kondo, H., Yasuda, T., Watanabe, T., Kobayashi, S., Yokohama, S. (2002). Common solubilizers to estimate the Caco-2 transport of poorly water-soluble drugs. *Int. J. Pharm.*, 246, 85–94.

165. Volpe, D.A. (2008). Variability in Caco-2 and MDCK cell-based intestinal permeability assays. *J. Pharm. Sci.*, 97, 712–725.

166. Naruhashi, K., Tamai, I., Li, Q., Sai, Y., Tsuji, A. (2003). Experimental demonstration of the unstirred water layer effect on drug transport in caco-2 cells. *J. Pharm. Sci.*, 92, 1502–1508.

167. Putnam, W.S., Ramanathan, S., Pan, L., Takahashi, L.H., Benet, L.Z. (2002). Functional characterization of monocarboxylic acid, large neutral amino acid, bile acid and peptide transporters, and P-glycoprotein in MDCK and Caco-2 cells. *J. Pharm. Sci.*, 91, 2622–2635.

168. Takano, R., Furumoto, K., Shiraki, K., Takata, N., Hayashi, Y., Aso, Y., Yamashita, S. (2008). Rate-limiting steps of oral absorption for poorly water-soluble drugs in dogs; prediction from a miniscale dissolution test and a physiologically-based computer simulation. *Pharm. Res.*, 25, 2334–2344.

169. Lee, Y.C., Zocharski, P.D., Samas, B. (2003). An intravenous formulation decision tree for discovery compound formulation development. *Int. J. Pharm.*, 253, 111–119.

170. Bittner, B., Mountfield, R.J. (2002). Intravenous administration of poorly soluble new drug entities in early drug discovery: the potential impact of formulation on pharmacokinetic parameters. *Curr. Opin. Drug Discov. Devel.*, 5, 59–71.

171. Akimoto, M., Nagahata, N., Furuya, A., Fukushima, K., Higuchi, S., Suwa, T. (2000). Gastric pH profiles of beagle dogs and their use as an alternative to human testing. *Eur. J. Pharm. Biopharm.*, 49, 99–102.

172. Sagawa, K., Li, F., Liese, R., Sutton, S.C. (2009). Fed and fasted gastric pH and gastric residence time in conscious beagle dogs. *J. Pharm. Sci.*, 98, 2494–2500.

173. Polentarutti, B., Albery, T., Dressman, J., Abrahamsson, B. (2010). Modification of gastric pH in the fasted dog. *J. Pharm. Pharmacol.*, 62, 462–469.

174. Lentz, K.A. (2008). Current methods for predicting human food effect. *AAPS J.*, 10, 282–288.

175. Lentz, K.A., Quitko, M., Morgan, D.G., Grace, J.E. Jr., Gleason, C., Marathe, P.H. (2007). Development and validation of a preclinical food effect model. *J. Pharm. Sci.*, 96, 459–472.

176. Sagara, K., Kawata, M., Mizuta, H., Shibata, M. (1994). Utility of gastrointestinal physiology regulated-dogs: bioavailability study of a commercial sustained-release dosage form of theophylline. *Biol. Pharm. Bull.*, 17, 931–934.

177. Sagara, K., Nagamatsu, Y., Yamada, I., Kawata, M., Mizuta, H., Ogawa, K. (1992). Bioavailability study of commercial sustained-release preparations of diclofenac sodium in gastrointestinal physiology regulated-dogs. *Chem. Pharm. Bull. (Tokyo)*, 40, 3303–3306.

178. Sagara, K., Yamada, I., Matsuura, Y., Kawata, M., Shibata, M. (1996). Gastrointestinal physiology-regulated dogs for bioavailability evaluation of an oral controlled-release dosage form composed of pulsatile release granules. *Biol. Pharm. Bull.*, 19, 1184–1188.

179. Cao, X., Gibbs, S.T., Fang, L., Miller, H.A., Landowski, C.P., Shin, H.C., Lennernas, H., Zhong, Y., Amidon, G.L., Yu, L.X., Sun, D. (2006). Why is it challenging to predict intestinal drug absorption and oral bioavailability in human using rat model. *Pharm. Res.*, 23, 1675–1686.

CHAPTER 8

VALIDATION OF MECHANISTIC MODELS

"The aim of science is not to open the door to infinite wisdom, but to set a limit to infinite error."

—Bertolt Brecht

Biopharmaceutical modeling is not perfect. Therefore, it is important to understand its limitations. For example, some of the physiological data has large uncertainty. The solubilities of a drug in artificial GI fluids can be different from those in *in vivo* GI fluids. There are many other factors that should be improved in the future (Chapter 16). Therefore, it is important to know the limitations of current biopharmaceutical modeling before applying it to practical uses in drug discovery and development.

In this section, the GUT framework is used as an example.[1] All the equations in the GUT framework have been published and available for everyone. The drug and physiological data used in this section are all published ones. In addition, to increase the transparency of validation processes, the simplest equation is used as long as it is sufficient. This policy is also in accordance with Occam's razor principle.

In this section, we focus on the validation of *in vivo* results. The reliability of each primary equation has already been discussed in Section 2.5, therefore

---

[1]For commercial programs employing the other model equations, please ask the vendors for the thorough validation results.

Biopharmaceutics Modeling and Simulations: Theory, Practice, Methods, and Applications, First Edition. Kiyohiko Sugano.
© 2012 John Wiley & Sons, Inc. Published 2012 by John Wiley & Sons, Inc.

it is not repeated in this section. Usually, the mechanistic equation of each primary process has been validated by comparison with well-controlled *in vitro* experiments. For example, the Henderson–Hasselbalch (HH) equation was validated with experimental pH–solubility profiles [1]. Generally speaking, physical equations such as the HH equation were well validated for a wide range of physical conditions, covering the physiological conditions in the GI tract (e.g., from pH 1 to 9).

8.1 CONCERNS RELATED TO MODEL VALIDATION USING *IN VIVO* DATA

The current status of biopharmaceutical modeling is that a perfect a priori prediction of Fa% (e.g., <30% error from *in vitro* data) is in principle unattainable because of (i) differences between *in vivo* and *in vitro* drug data (e.g., real intestinal fluid vs FaSSIF, *in vivo* intestinal membrane vs Caco-2), (ii) uncertainty of GI physiological data (e.g., fluid volume, fluid dynamics, transporter expression level), and (iii) imperfect theoretical equations (e.g., nucleation theory, first-pass metabolisms). In contrast, there were many publications seemingly suggesting perfect predictions. However, it is misleading to take these publications as validation of biopharmaceutical modeling. We discuss this point in depth in Chapter 16.

In many of the publications suggesting perfect predictions, the plasma concentration (C_p)–time profiles of one or a few drugs were selected as the target of simulation. However, the use of C_p–time profiles for the validation of biopharmaceutical modeling has some issues. As an *in vivo* PK model is additionally required, the simulation processes for a C_p–time profile have become more complicated than those for Fa%, making it difficult to validate the simulation processes. It could distract us from the essential points of oral absorption and focus too much on nonessential points (such as the subtle nuance in the shape of a C_p–time profile). When this type of "all in all" validation is employed, it is often difficult to be aware of the pitfalls in the simulation processes. In addition, the estimation of Fg and Fh has large uncertainty even when starting with *in vivo* CL data. In many cases of drugs with low solubility, i.v. PK data is not available.

8.2 STRATEGY FOR TRANSPARENT AND ROBUST VALIDATION OF BIOPHARMACEUTICAL MODELING

To avoid the above-mentioned concerns, for the validation of the GUT framework, we use the following principles:

- The simplest model equation required for each category of drugs (Occam's razor principle)

- To keep transparency, the simplest model should be used for validation. The use of unnecessary complex model decreases the transparency of validation process. Considering the variation of *in vivo* data used for validation, it would be impossible to prove the subtle advantage of a complex model. Parameter fitting is not performed unless the physiological parameter is not available in the literature. When parameter fitting is inevitable, the parameter is optimized with more than four Fa% data.

- Fa% data (but neither BA% nor C_p–time data)

  Fa% data were used for validation to avoid interference from the first-pass metabolisms and other uncertainties. For drugs with low solubility, the method explained in Section 5.5 was used to calculate Fa% from *in vivo* data.

- A large number of *in vivo* Fa% data for structurally and physicochemically diverse drugs (Table 8.1)

  Hundreds of Fa% data were used to increase the robustness of validation. This type of validation became possible, as Fa% data has been accumulated in the literature. Especially, the Fa% data of drugs with low solubility became available by introducing several calculation criteria as discussed in Section 5.5.

- Cross-validation with different data set

  The GUT framework is validated by several different experimental observations, such as *in vivo/in situ/in vitro* studies in humans/dogs/rats. This increases the robustness of the validation.

- Step-by-step validation

  A step-wise validation is pursued. The models are validated from the simplest one to the more complicated one, that is, (i) permeability-limited cases (Section 8.4), (ii) dissolution-rate and solubility-permeability-limited cases without the stomach effect (Section 8.5), and (iii) cases with the stomach effect (Section 8.6).

Validation of other specific processes such as colonic absorption and carrier-mediated absorption are discussed in the later sections.

8.3   PREDICTION STEPS

Before moving on to the validation processes, the prediction process step (PPS) is introduced to roughly categorize the available input data [2].

PPS I: Chemical structure only (*in silico* in a narrow sense)

PPS II: PPS I + *in vitro* data

A: Simple *in vitro* data (e.g., solubility, Caco-2)

B: Complex *in vitro* data (e.g., dissolution test, intestinal perfusion)

TABLE 8.1 Fa% Values and Physicochemical Properties of Drugs

Name	MW	$\log P_{oct}{}^{a}$	$pK_a{}^{b}$	log D, pH 6.5^{c}	Fa%	References
AAFC	243	$-1.3(\pm 1)^{d}$	—	-1.3	32	3
Acarbose	645	-6.8	—	-6.8	1	4
Acebutolol	336	2.0	9.5 (B)	-1.0	89.5	4
Acefylline	238	$-0.8(\pm 0.52)^{d}$	3.7 (A)^{e}	-3.6	<10	5
Acetaminophen	151	0.3	—	0.3	100	4
Acetylsalicylic acid	180	0.9	3.5 (A)	-2.1	84	3
Acrivastatine	348	—	2.2 (A), 9.6 (B)	-0.1(pH 6.5)	88	3
Acyclovir	225	-1.7	—	-1.7	29	6
Adefovir	273	0.8	2.6 (A)^{g}	-3.1	16	4
Adinazolam	351	4.4	5.7 (B)	4.3	100	4
Alfentanil	417	2.4	6.5 (B)	2.1	100	4
Alizapride	315	1.8	9.0 (B)	-0.7	100	4
Allopurinol	136	-1.0	—	-1.0	90	4
Alprazolam	308	2.6	—	2.6	92	4
Alprenolol	249	3.0	9.5 (B)	0.0	93	4
Amantadine	151	2.4	10.5 (B)	-1.6	95	4
Amiloride	229	-0.3	8.7 (B)	-2.5	50	6
Aminopyrine	231	0.9	5.1 (B)	0.8	100	3
Amiodarone	645	7.8	9.1 (B)	5.2	100	4
Amisulpride	369	1.1	9.0 (B)	-1.4	48	4
Amitriptyline	277	4.8	9.5 (B)	1.8	95	4
Amlodipine	408	3.7	9.3 (B)	1.0	95	4
Amoxicillin	365	—	2.6 (A), 7.3 (B)	-1.9(pH 7.4)	93	4
Amphetamine	135	1.8	10.1 (B)	-1.8	90	3
Amphotericin B	923	—	5.7 (A), 10.0 (B)	—	5	4
Ampicillin	349	—	2.6 (A), 7.1 (B)	-1.4(pH 7.0)	57.6	7
Amrinone	187	$-0.2(\pm 0.67)^{d}$	—	-0.2	93	3
Antipyrine	188	0.7	—	0.7	97	4
Ascorbic acid	176	-1.9	4.1 (A)	-4.3	35	3
Atenolol	266	0.2	9.5 (B)	-2.8	50	4
Atomoxetine	255	3.7	9.2 (B)	1.0	100	4
Atovaquone	366	5.1	—	5.1	6	4
Atropine	289	1.9	9.8 (B)	-1.5	98	4
Azithromycin	749	3.9	8.8 (B), 8.1 (B)	0.0	60	4
Azosemide	370	1.3 $(\pm 0.8)^{d}$	3.8 (A)^{f}	-1.4	> 10	3
Aztreonam	435	$-1.5(\pm 1.6)^{d}$	-2.6(A)^{h}	-10.6	1	4
Balsalazide	357	2.8 $(\pm 0.58)^{d}$	2.7 (A), 4.4 (A)^{e}	-3.2	< 10	5
Benazepril	424	—	3.1 (A)	-0.2(pH 7.4)	37	5
Benserazide	257	-1.7	7.1 (B)	-2.4	70	5
Benzylpenicillin	334	1.5	2.5 (A)	-2.5	15–30	3
Betaxolol	307	2.4	9.4 (B)	-0.5	100	4
Biperiden	311	4.1	9.7 (B)^{f}	0.9	100	4
Bisoprolol	325	2.2	9.6 (B)	-0.9	95	4
Bornaprine	329	4.5 $(\pm 0.63)^{d}$	9.9 (B)^{f}	1.1	100	3
Bretylium tosylate	242	—	(Q)	—	23	3
Bromazepam	315	1.7	—	1.6	84	4
Bromfenac	333	3.4	4.3 (A)	1.2	100	4
Bromocriptine	653	4.2	5.4 (B)	4.2	28	6

(continued)

TABLE 8.1 (*Continued*)

Name	MW	$\log P_{oct}{}^a$	$pK_a{}^b$	log D, pH 6.5[c]	Fa%	References
Budesonide	430	1.9	—	1.9	100	4
Buflomedil	307	2.4 (± 0.37)[d]	10.0 (B)[f]	−1.1	100	4
Bufuralol	261	3.5	8.9 (B)	1.1	100	4
Bumetanide	364	4.1	4.0 (A)	1.6	90	4
Bupivacaine	288	3.6	8.1 (B)	2.0	90	4
Bupropion	240	3.0	7.9 (B)	1.6	87	6
Busulphan	246	−0.3	—	−0.3	94	4
Caffeine	194	0.1	—	0.1	100	4
Camazepam	371	2.7	—	2.7	100	3
Captopril	217	0.3	3.7 (A)	−2.5	84	4
Carfecillin	454	3.0	2.9 (A)	−0.6	99	3
Carvedilol	406	4.1	8.0 (B)	2.7	65	4
Cefaclor	367	—	1.6 (A), 7.2 (B)	—	90	7
Cefadroxil	363	−0.1	2.6 (A), 7.2 (B)	−4.0	100	4
Cefatrizine	463	—	2.6 (A), 7.0 (B)	—	76	4
Cefazolin	454	−1.5	2.3 (A)	−5.7	6	8
Cefcanel daloxate	478	1.2 (± 0.91)[d]	7.0 (B)[e]	0.5	42	4
Cefetamet pivoxil	397	1.8	—	1.8	52	4
Cefixime	453	−0.3(± 0.45)[d]	2.1 (A), 3.7 (A)	−4.7	30	4
Cefotiam	525	—	4.6 (A), 7.0 (B)	—	3.1	7
Cefpodoxime pivoxil	427	0.2	—	0.2	50	5
Ceftibuten	446	−1.0	2.2 (A), 3.7 (A)	−5.3	70.5	7
Ceftizoxime	383	0.0 (± 0.45)[d]	3.0 (A)	−3.6	72	3
Ceftriaxone	554	−1.7	3.2 (A), 4.3 (A)	−7.2	1	4
Cefuroxime	424	−0.8	2.1 (A)	−5.2	5	6
Cephalexin	347	—	2.6 (A), 7.1 (B)	−1.0(pH 6.5)	90	7
Cephaloridine	415	—	(A), (Q)	−1.52	< 5	44
Cephalothin	398	0	2.4 (A)	−4.1	< 5	9
Cephradine	349	—	2.6 (A), 7.3 (B)	−1.6(pH 7.4)	94	7
Cerivastatin	459	3.4	4.9 (A)	1.8	100	4
Ceronapril	440	—	1.9 (A), 4.2 (A), 1018.0 (B)	—	76	10
Cetirizine	389	—	2.9 (A), 8.0 (B)	1.5 (pH 6.5)	> 80	11
Chlorambucil	304	3.4	5.8 (A)	2.6	100	4
Chloramphenicol	322	1.1	—	1.1	90	4
Chlordiazepoxide	299	1.7	—	1.7	100	4
Chloroquine	319	4.7	10.4 (B), 8.4 (B)	−1.2	100	4
Chlorothiazide	295	−0.2	—	−0.2	56	12
Chlorpheniramine	202	3.4	9.3 (B)	0.6	94	4
Chlorpromazine	319	5.3	9.2 (B)	2.6	100	4
Chlorpropamide	319	5.3	9.2 (B)	2.6	100	4
Chlortetracycline	479	—	—	−0.9(pH 7.5)	60	5
Chlorthalidone	338	1.3	—	1.3	82	4
Cibenzoline	262	3.4 (± 0.6)[d]	9.4 (B)[f]	0.6	100	4
Cicaprost	374	2.9 (± 0.63)[d]	3.4 (A)[f]	−0.2	100	3
Cidofovir	279	−3.9	2.6 (A)[g]	−7.8	3	6
Cilazapril	435	—	3.3 (A), 6.5 (B)	−0.2(pH 7.4)	90	13, 14
Cilazaprilate	389	—	(A), (A), (B)	−2.2(pH 7.4)	19	13, 14
Cilomilast	343	3.5 (± 0.62)d	4.6 (A)	1.6	100	4

TABLE 8.1 (*Continued*)

Name	MW	log P_{oct} [a]	pK_a [b]	log D, pH 6.5 [c]	Fa%	References
Cimetidine	252	0.4	7.1 (B)	−0.2	68	4
Ciprofloxacin	331	—	8.6 (B), 6.2 (A)	−1.1(pH 7.4)	63	4
Cisapride	465	3.3	7.8 (B)	2.0	100	3
Citalopram	324	3.9	9.6 (B)	0.8	100	4
Clarithromycin	747	3.2	8.5 (B)	1.2	89	4
Clavulanic acid	199	−1.4(±0.67) [d]	2.7 (A)	−5.2	75	4
Clinafloxacin	366	—	5.3 (A), 9.0 (B)	−0.4(pH 7.0)	100	4
Clindamycin	424	1.6	7.5 (B)	0.6	100	4
Clofibrate	242	3.7	—	3.7	97	3
Clonazepam	315	3.0	—	3.0	98	4
Clonidine	229	1.6	8.1 (B)	0.0	95	3
Cloxacillin	435	3.0	2.8 (A)	−0.7	49	6
Clozapine	327	3.2	7.9 (B)	1.8	55	4
Codeine	299	1.1	8.2 (B)	−0.6	95	3
Conivaptan	498	6.3	—	6.3	100	4
Corticosterone	346	2.3	—	2.3	100	3
Cotinine	176	0.1	—	0.1	90	4
Creatinine	113	−2.2	—	−2.2	80	6
Cromolyn sodium	468	2.0	2.2 (A), 2.2 (A)	−6.7	0.5	15
Cyclacillin	341	—	2.7 (A), 7.5 (B)	−2.5(pH 7.4)	95	7
Cyclophosphamide	260	0.8	—	0.8	90	4
Cycloserine	102	−0.9	7.4 (B)	−1.9	73	3
Cyclosporine	1,203	3.5	—	3.5	86	4
Cymarin	548	0.6	—	0.6	47	6
Cyproterone acetate	374	3.8 (±0.47) [d]	—	3.8	100	3
Cytarabine	243	−2.8	—	−2.8	20	6
Dapsone	248	0.9	—	0.9	100	4
Demeclocycline	464	—	—	−0.7(pH 6.6)	66	5
Desferrioxamine	561	−2.2	8.0 (B), 9.1 (B), 9.9 (B)	−6.3	2	4
Desipramine	266	3.8	10.2 (B)	0.1	100	4
Dexamethasone	392	1.1	—	1.1	90	4
Dexloxiglumide	461	4.5	4.5 (A)	2.5	95	4
Diazepam	285	2.9	—	2.9	100	4
Diazoxide	230	1.3	—	1.3	91	4
Diclofenac	295	4.5	4.0 (A)	2.0	100	4
Dicloxacillin	469	3.7	2.8 (A)	0.0	55	6
Didanosine	236	−0.2	—	−0.2	50	4
Digoxin	781	1.3	—	1.3	81	4
Dihydrocodeine	301	1.8 (±0.33) [d]	8.8 (B)	−0.5	89	3
Diltiazem	415	3.2	8.0 (B)	1.7	90	4
Diltiazem	415	3.2	8.0 (B)	1.7	80	6
Diprophylline	254	−1.5	—	−1.5	95	4
Disopyramide	339	2.4	8.4 (B)	0.5	83	4
Distigmine bromide	578	—	—	—	8	3
Disulfiram	296	1.9	—	1.9	97	3
Dofetilide	441	2.1	7.0 (B)	1.5	96	4
Domperidone	426	2.4	7.8 (B)	1.1	93	4
Doxapram	378	3.6	6.7 (B)	3.2	100	4

(*continued*)

TABLE 8.1 (*Continued*)

Name	MW	$\log P_{\text{oct}}$[a]	pK_a[b]	$\log D$, pH 6.5[c]	Fa%	References
Doxifluridine	246	−1.4	—	−1.4	90	4
Doxorubicin	544	1.4	8.3 (B)	−0.4	12	4
Doxycycline	444	—	8.9 (B)	−0.2(pH 7.5)	100	4
Drotaverine	398	4.7 (±0.76)	—	4.7	100	4
Eflornithine	182	—	0.1 (A), 10.4 (B), 6.4 (B)	−3.3(pH 7.4)	55	3
Enalapril	376	—	5.4 (B), 2.9 (A)	−1.8(pH 7.0)	66	6
Enalaprilat	376	—	7.8 (B), 3.2 (A), 1.3 (A)	—	10	15
Encainide	352	4.0	10.2 (B)	0.3	95	4
Entacapone	305	2.0	4.5 (A)	0.0	96	4
Epristeride	400	4.7 (±0.48)[d]	4.8 (A)	3.0	93	4
Eprosartan	424	—	4.1 (A), 5.7 (A), 8.7 (B)	−1.3(pH 7.2)	15	4
Erythritol	122	−2.3	—	−2.3	90	6
Erythromycin	733	2.5	8.8 (B)	0.2	50	4
Ethambutol	204	−0.3	9.2 (B), 6.1 (B)	−3.1	80	6
Ethinylestradiol	296	3.4	—	3.4	100	3
Ethionamide	166	0.5	—	0.5	80	6
Etilefrine	181	0.3	9.0 (B)	−2.2	100	4
Etoposide	589	0.5	—	0.5	52	4
Famciclovir	321	0.6	—	0.6	77	3
Famotidine	337	−0.6	7.1 (B)	−1.3	38	6
Faropenem	312	−1.5	3.5 (A)	−4.5	20	16
Felbamate	238	0.3	—	0.3	90	3
Felodipine	383	4.3	—	4.3	88	4
Fenclofenac	297	4.8	4.4 (A)	2.6	100	3
Fenoterol	303	1.2 (±0.39)[d]	8.5 (B)	−0.8	60	6
Fenspiride	260	2.0 (±0.21)[d]	9.4 (B)[f]	−0.9	100	4
Fexofenadine	502	—	4.3 (A), 9.5 (B)	0.3 (pH 7.0)	34	17
Finasteride	372	4.7	—	4.7	80	4
Flecainide	414	4.6	9.3 (B)	1.8	81	4
Fleroxacin	369	—	5.5 (A), 8.0 (B)	−0.6(pH 7.4)	100	4
Fluconazole	306	0.5	—	0.5	95	4
Flucytosine	129	−1.1	—	−1.1	88	4
Fludarabine	365	−2.8	1.2 (A), 6.1 (A)	−8.6	75	5
Flumazenil	303	1.6	—	1.6	95	4
Flupirtine	304	2.5 (±0.2)[d]	5.3 (B)	2.5	100	4
Fluvastatin	411	4.0	4.3 (A)	1.8	100	4
Folinic acid	473	−1.6	3.1 (A), 4.6 (A)	−6.9	36	4
Foscarnet	126	−2.1	2.6 (A)[g]	−6.0	17	4
Fosfomycin	138	−1.6	2.6 (A)[g]	−5.5	31	4
Fosinopril	563	5.6	3.8 (A)	2.8	36	3
Fosmidomycin	183	−2.2(±1.1)[d]	2.6 (A)[g]	−6.1	30	3
Frovatriptan	243	0.9	9.9 (B)	−2.5	40	4
Furosemide	330	2.6	3.5 (A)	−0.4	61	4
Gabapentin	171	—	3.7 (A), 10.7 (B)	−1.3(pH 7.4)	60	4
Gallopamil	485	4.4 (±0.88)[d]	10.5 (B)	0.4	100	3
Ganciclovir	255	−1.7	—	−1.7	5.6	12
Gatifloxacin	375	—	6.0 (A), 9.2 (B)	−0.9(pH 6.9)	96	4
Genaconazole	331	0.7 (±0.94)[d]	—	0.7	100	4

TABLE 8.1 (*Continued*)

Name	MW	$\log P_{oct}{}^a$	$pK_a{}^b$	log D, pH 6.5[c]	Fa%	References
Gentamicin	477	−3.1	8.6 (B)	−5.2	0	4
Ginkgolide A	408	−0.1(±1.33)[d]	—	−0.1	90	4
Ginkgolide B	424	−0.8(±1.23[d]	—	−0.8	90	4
Glibenclamide	494	4.4	6.8 (A)	4.2	100	4
Gliclazide	323	2.6	5.8 (A)	1.8	97	3
Glimepiride	490	3.5	6.2 (A)	3.0	100	4
Glipizide	445	2.6	5.1 (A)	1.2	100	4
Glycine	75	—	2.3 (A), 9.6 (B)	—	100	3
Glycopyrrolate	318	—	(Q)	—	10–25	5
Granisetron	312	2.6	9.4 (B)	−0.3	100	4
Guanabenz	230	3.0	8.1 (B)	1.4	75	6
Guanfacine	245	1.7	7.1 (B)	1.0	100	4
Guanoxan	207	0.4 (±0.2)[d]	13.6 (B)	−6.7	50	3
Haloperidol	376	3.6	8.4 (B)	1.7	100	4
HBED	388	—	0.9 (A), 1.6 (A), 8.3 (B)	—	5	6
Hydrochlorothiazide	297	0.0	—	0.0	67	6
Hydrocortisone	362	1.8	—	1.8	91	6
Hydroflumethazide	331	0.5	—	0.5	62	4
Hydroxyurea	76	−1.6	—	−1.6	100	4
Ibuprofen	206	3.5	4.5 (A)	1.4	95	4
Idarubicin	497	1.8	8.0 (B)	0.3	30	5
Idazoxan	204	1.1 (±0.33)[d]	8.8 (B)	−1.2	95	4
Ifosfamide	260	0.8	—	0.8	100	4
Imipenem	299	—	3.2 (A), 10.8 (B)	—	2.5	4
Imipramine	280	4.4	9.5 (B)	1.4	100	6
Indomethacin	358	4.3	4.4 (A)	2.2	100	4
Iothalamate sodium	613	2.2 (±0.95)[d]	1.1 (A)	−3.2	1.9	3
Iotroxic acid	1216	4.5	1.1 (A), 1.7 (A)	−5.6	< 10	5
Isoniazid	137	−0.8	—	−0.8	80	6
Isosorbide-5-mononitrate	236	−0.9	—	−0.9	100	4
Isoxicam	335	2.8	3.9 (A)	0.3	100	4
Isradipine	371	2.9	—	2.9	92	3
Itraconazole	704	5.7	—	5.7	85	4
Kanamycin	484	−6.3	7.2 (B)	−7.1	1	3
Ketanserin	395	3.3	7.5 (B)	2.3	100	4
Ketoprofen	254	3.2	4.0 (A)	0.6	92	4
Ketorolac	255	5.0	3.5 (A)	2.0	100	4
k-Strophanthoside	872	−2.4(±1.11)[d]	—	−2.4	16	3
Labetalol	328	—	9.4 (B)	0.3 (pH 6.5)	95	3
Lactulose	342	−4.3	—	−4.3	0.6	6
Lamivudine	229	−1.4	—	−1.4	100	4
Lamotrigine	256	2.1	5.7 (B)	2.0	100	4
Lansoprazole	369	1.9	—	1.9	100	4
Letrozole	285	2.5	—	2.5	100	4
Levodopa	197	−1.8	2.3 (A)	−6.0	86	3
Levofloxacin	361	—	6.1 (A), 8.1 (B)	−0.3(pH 7.0)	100	4
Levomepromazine	328	4.7	9.2 (B)	2.0	100	18
Levonorgestrel	312	3.8	—	3.8	100	3

(*continued*)

TABLE 8.1 (*Continued*)

Name	MW	$\log P_{oct}{}^a$	$pK_a{}^b$	log D, pH 6.5[c]	Fa%	References
Levoprotiline	293	3.4 ($\pm$0.37)[d]	9.6 (B)[f]	0.3	100	4
Lincomycin	406	0.6	7.6 (B)	−0.6	28	6
Linezolid	337	0.9	—	0.9	100	4
Lisinopril	405	—	4.0 (A), 4.0 (A), 6.7 (B), 10.1 (B)	—	28	4
Loracarbef	349	—	2.0 (A), 7.3 (B)	—	>86	3
Lorazepam	320	2.5	—	2.5	100	4
Lorcainide	371	4.2	9.4 (B)	1.2	100	4
Lormetazepam	335	2.7	—	2.7	100	4
Lornoxicam	372	2.6	4.7 (A)	0.8	100	3
Losartan	422	2.9	4.3 (A)	0.7	80	4
Lovastatin	423	3.9	—	3.9	31	4
Loxiglumide	460	3.7 ($\pm$0.39)[d]	4.5 (A)[f]	1.6	100	4
Mannitol	182	−3.9	—	−3.9	16–80	19
Mebendazole	295	3.1	—	3.1	100	4
Melagatran	429	—	11.5 (B), 2.0 (A)	−1.3(pH 9.7)	15	4
Meloxicam	351	3.4	4.2 (A)	1.1	90	4
Mesna	142	−1.1($\pm$0.74)[d]	−2.6(A)[h]	−10.2	77	3
Metaproterenol	211	0.6 ($\pm$0.49)[d]	8.6 (B)	−1.5	44	6
Metformin	129	−0.5	12.4 (B)	−6.4	52	4
Methadone	309	4.2	8.9 (B)	1.8	100	4
Methotrexate	454	−0.1	4.0 (A), 3.3 (A), 5.4 (B)	−2.6	70	4
Methyldopa	211	—	2.2 (A), 9.2 (B)	—	40	4
Methylprednisolone	374	2.1	—	2.1	82	6
Metoclopramide	300	2.4	9.2 (B)	−0.3	100	4
Metolazone	365	4.1	—	4.1	64	4
Metoprolol	267	2.0	9.6 (B)	−1.1	98	4
Metronidazole	171	0.0	—	0.0	100	4
Mibefradil	495	5.4 ($\pm$0.56)[d]	5.5 (B)	5.4	69	3
Midazolam	325	3.2	6.2 (B)	3.1	90	4
Mifobate	358	1.2 ($\pm$0.6)[d]	—	1.2	82	3
Miglitol	207	−2.7	—	−2.7	59	4
Milrinone	211	0.4	—	0.4	100	4
Minocycline	457	—	9.5 (B)	0.0 (pH 7.5)	100	4
Minoxidil	209	0.6	—	0.6	98	3
Mirtazapine	265	3.0	7.1 (B)	2.3	80	4
Moclobemide	268	1.5	6.2 (B)	1.3	98	4
Montelukast	585	2.9	6.5 (A)	2.6	80	4
Morphine	285	0.9	8.2 (B)	−0.8	85	3
Moxifloxacin	401	—	6.4 (A), 9.5 (B)	−0.6(pH 7.0)	90	4
Moxonidine	242	0.9	7.4 (B)	0.0	99	4
Nadolol	309	0.9	9.7 (B)	−2.3	35	6
Naloxone	327	2.2	7.9 (B)	0.8	91	3
Naltrexone	341	0.7	8.1 (B)	−0.9	96	6
Naproxen	230	3.3	4.2 (A)	1.0	99	6
Naratriptan	335	2.0	9.7 (B)	−1.3	80	4

TABLE 8.1 (*Continued*)

Name	MW	$\log P_{\text{oct}}{}^a$	$pK_a{}^b$	log D, pH 6.5^c	Fa%	References
Nateglinide	317	3.9	3.1 (A)	0.5	90	4
Nedocromil	371	2.2	2.8 (A), 3.5 (A)	−4.5	< 10	5
Nefazodone	469	4.7	6.8 (B)	4.2	100	4
Neomycin	614	−7.8	9.3 (B), 8.8 (B), 8.2 (B), 7.6 (B)	−12.9	1	3
Neostigmine	223	—	(Q)	—	5	4
Netivudine	282	−1.1(±0.28)^d	—	−1.1	28	3
Nevirapine	266	2.5	—	2.5	100	4
Nicardipine	479	3.8	7.1 (B)	3.1	95	4
Nicotine	162	1.3	8.1 (B)	−0.3	100	4
Nicotinic acid	123	0.2	2.2 (A)	−4.1	88	3
Nifedipine	346	3.2	—	3.2	100	4
Nimodipine	418	2.7	—	2.7	90	4
Nisoldipine	388	3.1	—	3.1	90	4
Nitrazepam	281	2.4	—	2.4	78	4
Nitrendipine	360	3.6	—	3.6	88	3
Nizatidine	331	1.1	6.8 (B)	0.7	100	4
Nomifensine	238	3.4 (±0.4)^d	8.5 (B)^f	1.4	100	4
Nordiazepam	270	3.2	—	3.2	99	3
Norfloxacin	319	—	8.5 (B), 6.2 (A)	−1.0(pH 7.4)	34	6
Nortriptyline	263	4.4	10.1 (B)	0.8	100	4
Ofloxacin	361	—	5.7 (A), 7.9 (B)	−0.44(pH 7.4)	100	4
Olsalazine	302	2.3	2.5 (A), 2.5 (A)	−5.7	2	6
Omeprazole	345	1.8	—	1.8	95	4
Ondansetron	293	2.4	7.4 (B)	1.4	100	4
Oseltamivir	312	1.2	7.8 (B)	−0.1	80	4
Ouabain	584	−1.2	—	−1.2	1.4	3
Oxacillin	401	2.4	2.8 (A)	−1.3	33	6
Oxatomide	427	3.2	7.2 (B)	2.4	100	3
Oxazepam	286	2.8	—	2.8	92.8	4
Oxiracetam	158	−2.2(±0.42)^d	—	−2.2	75	4
Oxprenolol	265	2.5	9.6 (B)	−0.6	95	3
Oxyfedrine	313	2.5 (±0.23)^d	8.2 (B)^f	0.8	85	3
Oxytetracycline	460	—	9.1 (B)	—	60	6
Pafenolol	337	1.8	9.4 (B)	−1.1	> 29	3
Pantoprazole	383	1.3	—	1.3	100	4
Papaverine	339	3.0	6.4 (B)	2.7	100	4
Paricalcitol	416	4.6	—	4.6	86.1	4
Paromomycin	615	−7.4	8.9 (A), 8.2 (B), 7.6 (B), 7.1 (B)	−9.9	3	20
Pefloxacin	333	—	6.2 (A), 7.9 (B)	0.18 (pH 7.4)	95	4
Penciclovir	253	−1.1	—	−1.1	10	4
Phencyclidine	243	4.7	8.3 (B)	2.9	95	4

(*continued*)

TABLE 8.1 *(Continued)*

Name	MW	$\log P_{\text{oct}}{}^{a}$	$pK_a{}^{b}$	log D, pH 6.5[c]	Fa%	References
Phenethicillin	402	2.2	2.8 (A)	−1.5	78	21
Phenglutarimide	288	2.1 (±0.32)[d]	10.0 (B)[f]	−1.4	100	3
Phenobarbital	232	1.5	—	1.5	100	4
Phenoxymethylpenicillin	350	2.1	2.8 (A)	−1.6	38	4
Phenytoin	252	2.5	—	2.5	90	4
Pindolol	248	1.8	9.5 (B)	−1.2	100	4
Pirbuterol	240	0.2 (±0.36)[d]	10.3 (B)	−3.7	60	3
Pirmenol	338	3.3	10.2 (B)	−0.4	95	4
Piroxicam	331	2.0	5.1 (A)	0.5	100	3
Piroximone	217	0.5 (±0.25)[d]	—	0.5	81	3
Practolol	266	0.8	9.5 (B)	−2.2	100	4
Pralidoxime	137	—	(Q)	—	< 30	5
Pravastatin	424	2.2	4.6 (A)	0.3	34	4
Praziquantel	312	2.4	—	2.4	100	3
Prazosin	383	1.4	7.1 (B)	0.7	86	4
Prednisolone	358	1.7	—	1.7	99	4
Prednisone	358	1.7	—	1.7	95	4
Probenecid	285	2.9	3.4 (A)	−0.2	100	4
Procainamide	235	1.2	9.2 (B)	−1.5	85	4
Procyclidine	287	4.2	10.2 (B)[f]	0.5	100	4
Progesterone	314	3.6	—	3.6	100	3
Propiverine	367	5.0	8.6 (B)	3.0	84	3
Propranolol	259	2.9	9.5 (B)	−0.1	99	4
Propylthiouracil	170	0.4	—	0.4	90	4
Proxyphylline	238	−0.1	6.4 (B)	−0.4	100	22
Pyridostigmine	181	—	(Q)	—	10	4
Quinapril	438	—	2.8 (A), 5.4 (B)	−0.5(pH 7.4)	61	4
Quinidine	324	2.9	8.6 (B)	0.8	100	4
Quinine	324	2.9	8.6 (B)	0.8	80	4
Rabeprazole	359	2.3	—	2.3	90	4
Raffinose	504	−5.5(±1.02)[d]	—	−5.5	0.3	6
Ramipril	416	—	3.1 (A), 5.6 (B)	0.1 (pH 7.0)	60	10
Ranitidine	314	−0.1	8.4 (B)	−2.0	50	6
Reboxetine	313	3.1	8.3 (B)	1.3	100	4
Recainam	263	2.4 (±0.37)[d]	10.0 (B)[e]	−1.1	80	4
Remoxipride	370	2.9	8.9 (B)	0.5	100	4
Repaglinide	452	—	4.0 (A), 6.2 (B)	3.7 (pH 6.5)	95	4
Reproterol	389	0.4	8.2 (B)[e]	−1.3	60	3
Ribavirin	244	−2.2	—	−2.2	33−> 52	3
Rifabutin	846	4.6	6.9 (B)	4.0	53	4
Rifampin	822	2.7	7.9 (B)	1.3	100	4
Rimiterol	223	0.9 (±0.47)[d]	8.7 (B)	−1.4	48	3
Risedronate	283	−3.6	2.6 (A)[g]	−7.5	0.63	4
Risperidone	410	2.8	8.2 (B)	1.1	100	4
Ritonavir	693	4.3	—	4.3	70	4
Roquinimex	308	2.3 (±0.67)[d]	4.3 (A)[e]	0.1	100	4
Rosiglitazone	357	—	6.1 (B), 6.8 (A)	2.6 (pH 7.4)	100	4
Rosuvastatin	481	2.5	4.6 (A)	0.6	50	4

TABLE 8.1 (*Continued*)

Name	MW	$\log P_{oct}{}^a$	$pK_a{}^b$	log D, pH 6.5^c	Fa%	References
Saccharin	183	0.9	4.0 (A)	−1.6	88	3
salbutamol	239	1.4	9.3 (B)	−1.4	100	4
Salicylicacid	138	2.4	2.9 (A)	−1.2	100	3
Saquinavir	671	4.1	7.0 (B)	3.5	80	4
Scopolamine	303	0.8	7.7 (B)	−0.4	95	4
Selegiline	187	2.7	6.9 (B)	2.2	100	4
Sematilide	313	—	9.5 (B)	−1.0(pH 7.4)	65	4
Sildenafil	474	1.9	6.8 (B)	1.4	92	4
Sitafloxacin	410	—	5.7 (A), 9.2 (B)	−0.6(pH 7.0)	95	4
Sitagliptin	407	1.5	—	1.5	95	4
Solifenacin	480	3.2	8.5 (B)	1.2	100	4
Sorivudine	349	−1.0(±0.39)^d	—	−1.0	82	3
Sotalol	272	−0.5	8.3 (B)	−2.3	95	4
Sparfloxacin	392	—	6.3 (A), 8.8 (B)	−0.1(pH 6.8)	100	4
Spironolactone	416	3.3	—	3.3	73	3
Stavudine	224	−0.8	—	−0.8	100	3
Streptomycin	581	−6.4	10.0 (B)	−9.9	1	3
Sudoxicam	337	1.6	5.3 (A)	0.4	100	3
Sufentanil	386	2.8	8.0 (B)	1.3	90	4
Sulfadiazine	250	−0.1	6.4 (A)	−0.5	85	4
Sulfamethoxazole	270	0.9	—	0.9	100	4
Sulfasalazine	398	3.6	2.4 (A)	−0.6	13	6
Sulfinpyrazone	404	3.6	3.3 (A)	0.3	93	4
Sulfisoxazole	267	1.0	5.0 (A)	−0.5	100	4
Sulindac	356	3.6	4.1 (A)	1.2	90	6
Sulpiride	341	0.6	9.0 (B)	−1.9	44	4
Sultopride	354	1.1	9.1 (B)	−1.5	89	3
Sumatriptan	295	1.3	9.6 (B)	−1.8	57	4
Suprofen	260	2.4	3.9 (A)	−0.2	92	4
Suramin	1,296	−0.9(±2.74)^d	−2.6(A)^h	< −10.0	0	4
Tacrolimus	803	3.3	—	3.3	15	4
Talinolol	363	3.1	9.4 (B)	0.2	65	4
Tamsulosin	408	2.3	8.4 (B)	0.4	100	4
Tegaserod	301	2.6	11.5 (B)^e	−2.4	50	4
Telmisartan	514	3.2	4.1 (A)	0.8	90	4
Tenidap	321	4.0	3.1 (A)	0.5	89	3
Tenoxicam	337	1.9	5.5 (A)	0.9	100	4
Terazosin	387	2.3	7.0 (B)	1.6	90	4
Terbutaline	225	−0.1	8.7 (B)	−2.3	62	4
Terodiline	281	5.1 (±0.26)^d	9.3 (B)	2.3	100	4
Tesaglitazar	408	3.1 (±0.46)^d	3.6 (A)^f	0.2	100	4
Testosterone	288	3.0	—	3.0	100	3
Tetracycline	444	—	9.6 (B)	−1.4(pH 7.5)	78	6
Theophylline	180	0.0	—	0.0	100	4
Thiacetazone	236	1.5	5.8 (B)	1.4	> 20	3
Tiacrilast	262	1.3 (±0.36)^d	4.4 (A)^f	−0.8	99	23
Tiagabine	375	—	3.3 (A), 9.4 (B)	1.6 (pH 7.0)	95	4
Tilidine	273	3.2 (±0.38)^d	8.3 (B)	1.4	100	4

(*continued*)

TABLE 8.1   *(Continued)*

Name	MW	$\log P_{oct}{}^a$	$pK_a{}^b$	log D, pH 6.5^c	Fa%	References
Timolol	316	2.1	—	2.1	95	4
Tinidazole	247	0.7	—	0.7	100	4
Tizanidine	253	1.4	7.4 (B)	0.4	100	4
Tocainide	192	1.1	7.8 (B)	−0.2	100	4
Tolbutamide	270	2.2	5.2 (A)	0.8	85	4
Tolmesoxide	214	1.2 $(\pm 0.48)^d$	—	1.2	100	3
Tolterodine	325	5.6	9.9 (B)	2.2	> 77	4
Topiramate	339	0.6	—	0.6	86	3
Toremifene	405	6.8	8.0 (B)	5.3	100	3
Torsemide	348	2.3	—	2.2	96	4
Tramadol	263	2.7	9.5 (B)	−0.3	90	4
Tranexamic acid	157	—	4.5 (A), 10.7 (B)	—	55	6
Trapidil	205	1.4	—	1.4	97	3
Trazodone	372	3.5	6.8 (B)	3.0	100	4
Triazolam	342	5.5	—	5.5	85	4
Trimethoprim	290	0.8	7.1 (B)	0.2	97	4
Trovafloxacin	416	—	5.9 (A), 8.1 (B)	0.3 (pH 6.5)	95	4
Urapidil	387	1.6	7.1 (B)	0.9	100	4
Valproic Acid	144	2.6	4.8 (A)	0.9	100	4
Valsartan	435	3.9	3.6 (A), 4.7 (A)	−0.8	55	4
Vancomycin	1447	−3.1	8.6 (B), 7.5 (B), 2.7 (A)	−6.3	5	4
Vardenafil	488	3.4	6.7 (B)	3.0	90	4
Venlafaxine	277	3.6	9.4 (B)	0.7	97	4
Verapamil	455	4.2	9.1 (B)	1.6	100	4
Vigabatrin	129	—	4.7 (A), 8.6 (B)	—	58	3
Viloxazine	237	1.8	8.1 (B)	0.2	98	3
Warfarin	308	3.1	4.8 (A)	1.4	98	4
Xamoterol	339	0.0	7.9 (B)^e	−1.4	5	4
Ximoprofen	261	2.7 $(\pm 0.41)^d$	4.4 (A)^f	0.6	98	3
Xipamide	355	2.8	4.6 (A)	0.9	97	24
Zalcitabine	211	−1.3	—	−1.3	100	4
Zaleplon	305	0.9	—	0.9	100	4
Zanamivir	332	—	13.0 (B), 2.4 (A)	—	11	4
Zidovudine	267	−0.1	—	−0.1	100	6
Ziprasidone	412	3.8 $(\pm 0.65)^d$	6.5 (B)	3.5	90	4
Zofenopril	430	4.4	3.5 (A)	1.4	96	10
Zolmitriptan	287	1.6	9.5 (B)	−1.4	92	4
Zolpidem	307	1.2	6.2 (B)	1.0	100	4
Zopiclone	388	1.5	6.8 (B)	1.0	100	4

^{a}Experimental value unless otherwise noted.
^{b}Experimental value unless otherwise noted. (A) acid, (B) base, and (Q) quaternary ammonium.
^{c}Calculated from $\log P_{oct}$ and pK_a. For zwitter ions, experimental values at a pH.
^{d}Calculated by $A \log P$s (http://www.vcclab.org/lab/alogps/start.html). $A \log P$s is the consensus-based estimation.
^{e}Calculated by SPARC (http://archemcalc.com/sparc/).
^{f}Calculated by ACD.
^{g}Assumed to be same as n-butylphosphonate.
^{h}Assumed to be same as mesylate.

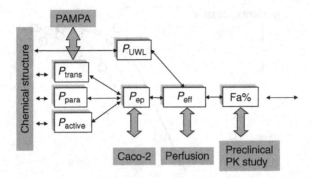

Figure 8.1 Prediction process steps for intestinal membrane permeability.

PPS III: PPS II + *in vivo* animal data
PPS IV: PPS III + human data

Overall prediction error becomes larger as the prediction step becomes longer. Predictability largely depends on the quality of the available data and the compound characteristics. PPS I has the maximum prediction error, whereas PPS IV has the minimum error. PPS I and IIA predictions are mainly used in the drug discovery stages, whereas PPS IIB and III are mainly used at the early developmental stages. PPS IV is used in the late developmental stages (after the phase I study) and the product enhancement stages. When considering the validation of a prediction scheme, it is important to be explicitly conscious regarding what type of prediction process is involved (Fig. 8.1).

8.4 VALIDATION FOR PERMEABILITY-LIMITED CASES

8.4.1 Correlation Between Fa% and P_{eff} Data for Humans (Epithelial Membrane Permeability-Limited Cases PL-E)

The first validation step is to check the predictability of human Fa% from human P_{eff}. This corresponds to the PPS IV. The experimental human P_{eff} and Fa% data were used to validate the model equation. As shown in Figure 8.2, the analytical solutions for Fa% calculation are almost identical between the one-compartment model and the S1I7C3 model.

$$\text{Fa} = 1 - \left(1 + \frac{2}{7R_{GI}}\text{DF} \cdot P_{eff} \cdot T_{si}\right)^{-7} \approx 1 - \exp\left(-\frac{2}{R_{GI}}\text{DF} \cdot P_{eff} \cdot T_{si}\right) \quad (8.1)$$

The intestinal transit time (T_{si}) is set to 3.5 h. The intestinal radius (R_{GI}) is set to 1.5 cm. These physiological data were consistent among many reports and thought to be highly reliable (Chapter 6). The contribution of colonic absorption on Fa% was neglected, as Fa% < 80% data determine the validity of the

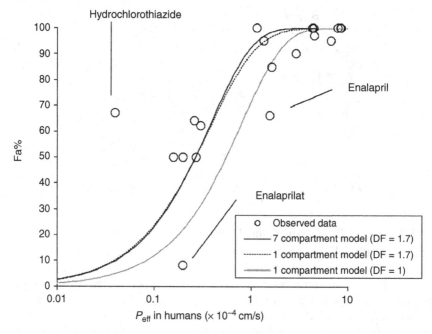

Figure 8.2 P_{eff}—Fa% correlation in humans.

model and in this Fa% region, the drugs have low colonic permeability (c.f. the contribution of colonic absorption on Fa% is <20%). From the standpoint of mechanistic modeling, the degree of flatness (DF) should be independently obtained from the shape of the intestinal tube. However, no reliable data on the intestinal tube shape is available. Therefore, DF had to be obtained by fitting Equation 8.1 to the experimental P_{eff}–Fa% profile. To avoid overlearning, P_{eff} and Fa% data were collected from the literature as much as possible. Theoretically, DF is 1 for a cylindrical tube (hence, $2DF/R_{GI}(= SA_{GI}/V_{GI})$ becomes 1.3 for humans). However, because the small intestine is like a deflated tube, DF should be larger than 1.

The P_{eff} and Fa% data are summarized in Table 8.2. The optimum DF was found to be 1.7 (hence, $2DF/R_{GI}(= SA_{GI}/V_{GI})$ becomes 2.3 for humans). This value is in good agreement with the deflated tube shape. The $2DF/R_{GI}$ model explains well the species differences (similarity) of Fa% between humans and rats (Section 13.5), that is, even though the rat P_{eff} is ca. sixfold smaller than the human P_{eff}, Fa% of a drug in rats and humans becomes similar, because of the smaller R_{GI} values in rats (Fig. 13.4).

Because of the variation in the human P_{eff} values, further refinement of the GI model (e.g., the difference of DF and R_{GI} in each GI region) was impossible by this data set. For comparison, the DF = 1 case ($2DF/R_{GI} = 1.3$) is also shown in Figure 8.2.

TABLE 8.2 Observed P_{eff} and Fa%

Compound[a]	MW	pKa[b,c]	log P_{oct}[b]	P_{eff} Humans[d]	P_{eff} Monkey[l]	P_{eff} Dog[e]	P_{eff} Rat[f]	Fa% Human[a]	Fa% Monkey[m]	Fa% Dog[g]	Fa% Rat[h]
Acetaminophen	151	—	0.2	—	-3.8	—	-4.1[k]	100	—	—	—
Amiloride	230	8.65 (B)	-1.03[a]	-3.8	—	—	—	50	—	—	—
Antipyrine	188	—	0.56	-3.3	-3.7	—	-4.2	97	—	—	100
Atenolol	266	9.54 (B)	0.22	-4.7	-4.4	—	-4.8	50	45	100	49
Carbamazepine	236	—	2.45	-3.4	—	—	-4.2	—	100	—	—
Cimetidine	241	6.93 (B)	0.48	-4.6	—	—	-4.3	64	—	98	100
Creatinine	113	—	-1.82[a]	-4.5	—	—	—	80	—	—	—
Desipramine	266	10.16 (B)	3.79	-3.3	—	—	—	100	—	—	—
Fluvastatine	411	4.31 (A)[a]	4.17	-3.6	—	—	—	100	—	100	100[g]
Furosemide	331	3.52 (A)	2.56	-4.8[i]	—	—	-4.5	61	63	54	60
Hydrochlorothiazide	298	—	-0.03	-5.4	—	—	-4.7	67	—	—	65
Ketoprofen	254	3.98 (A)	3.16	-3.1	—	—	-4.0	100	—	—	100
Metoprolol	267	9.56 (B)	1.95	-3.9	—	—	-4.5	95	92	—	—
Midazolam	—	—	—	—	-3.8	—	—	—	—	—	—

(*continued*)

TABLE 8.2 (Continued)

Compound[a]	MW	pKa[b,c]	log P_oct[b]	P_eff				Fa%			
				Humans[d]	Monkey[l]	Dog[e]	Rat[f]	Human[a]	Monkey[m]	Dog[g]	Rat[h]
Naproxen	230	4.18 (A)	3.24	−3.1	—	—	−3.7[j]	99	—	—	92
Piroxicam	331	5.07 (A)	1.98	−3.2	−3.6	—	−4.1	100	—	—	—
Propranolol	259	9.53 (B)	3.48	−3.5	−4.0	−4.2	−4.3	90	100	100	99
Ranitidine	314	8.31 (B)	1.28	−4.6	—	—	−4.7	50	—	100	63
Terbutaline	225	8.67 (B)	−0.08	−4.5	—	—	−5.3[j]	62	—	78	60
Verapamil	454	9.1 (B)	4.2	−3.2	−4.0	—	—	100	—	—	—

[a]Compound set from Obata et al. [25].
[b]Data from Avdeef, A., 2003 [26] unless otherwise noted.
[c](A), acid (pK_a < 6.5); (B), base (pK_a > 6.5).
[d]Data from Lennernas [27].
[e]Data from Lipka et al. [28].
[f]Data from Zakeri-Milani et al. [29].
[g]Data from Chiou et al. [30].
[h]Data from Chiou and Barve [31] unless otherwise noted.
[i]Data from Knutson et al. [32].
[j]Data from Fagerholm et al. [33].
[k]Data from Kalantzi et al. [34]
[l]Data from Takahashi et al. [35].
[m]Data from Chiou et al. [36].

8.4.2   Correlation Between *In Vitro* Permeability and P_{eff} and/or Fa% (PL-E Cases)

Prediction of human P_{eff} and Fa% from *in vitro* permeability data (e.g., Caco-2, MDCK, and rat SPIP) has been extensively investigated (Fig. 8.3).

A simple empirical linear relationship has been widely used to correlate P_{app} to P_{eff} (Fig. 7.27).

$$P_{eff} = aP_{app}^b \qquad (8.2)$$

where a and b are fitting coefficients. In many reports, P_{app} and Fa were correlated by Equation 8.3, in which the prepermeability coefficient (A) and intestinal transit time (T_{si}) is lumped in the fitting coefficient (A').

$$Fa = 1 - \exp(-A'P_{app}) \qquad (8.3)$$

However, these types of empirical equations cannot handle many characteristics of *in vivo* membrane permeation, such as species difference, bile-micelle effect (food effect), microclimate pH effect, unstirred water layer effect, difference in the paracellular pathways, and particle drifting effect. Mechanistic equations used in the GUT framework can handle these cases (Chapter 4). In addition, the contribution of each process can also be estimated, leading to better understanding of the permeation mechanism of a drug.

8.4.2.1   *Caco-2.*

Figure 8.4 shows the Fa% predictability from Caco-2 data. The paracellular component was corrected using the Renkin's electric field model in the same manner as the GUT framework (Section 4.8.3). Transporter substrates are excluded from the analysis.

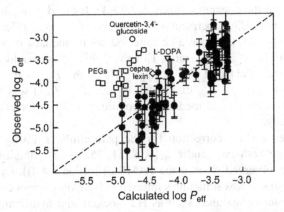

Figure 8.3 P_{eff} prediction from Caco-2 after correction for the paracellular pathway and UWL contribution. Source: Adapted from Reference 37 with permission.

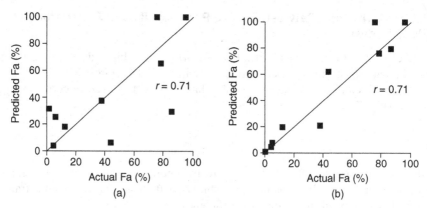

Figure 8.4 Fa% prediction from Caco-2 after correction for the paracellular pathway contribution. (a) Paracellular pathway not corrected, (b) Corrected. *Source:* Adapted from Reference 8 with permission.

The contribution of the paracellular pathway and the UWL were quantified for the drugs whose P_{eff} were reported [37]. Figure 8.5 shows the percentage of drugs categorized by the main permeability determinant. The contribution of the paracellular pathway and the UWL was estimated to be larger than usually thought. For example, for metoprolol ($P_{eff} = 1.3 \times 10^{-4}$ cm/s) [27], which is a marker compound for high/low boundary permeability, the UWL resistance was estimated to be about 50% of the total permeation resistance, suggesting that the UWL would be the main permeation barrier for BCS (biopharmaceutical classification system) drugs with high permeability. The UWL determines the upper limit of P_{eff} and should be taken into account in the case of lipophilic compounds ($\log D_{oct} > 0.5$–2). An *in vitro* membrane permeation study, such as Caco-2, can have various UWL thickness values depending on the agitation strength and the size and shape of the apparatus (Section 7.9.8.1). It could coincidentally give an appropriate *in vivo* UWL permeability value, as the excess thickness of UWL *in vitro* ($\approx$1500–3000 μm) could be canceled out by the lack of villi expansion, resulting in similar P'_{ep}/P_{UWL} ratio. However, this point should not be misapprehended as the effect of UWL is negligible in the $P_{app} - P_{eff}$ extrapolation. The empirical $\log P_{app} - P_{eff}$ extrapolation line (Fig. 7.27) was validated only for compounds with low to medium lipophilicity and not for compounds with high lipophilicity.

As discussed earlier, correction for the paracellular pathway improved the predictability for both Fa% and P_{eff} [6, 8, 11, 25, 37–41] (this improvement is more explicitly observed when using PAMPA (Section 8.4.4)). Even though the paracellular pathway was sometimes referred to have only minor contribution, for many blockbuster compounds such as H2 blockers and hydrophilic β-blockers, the contribution of paracellular pathway is estimated to be significant (>50% of total permeability).

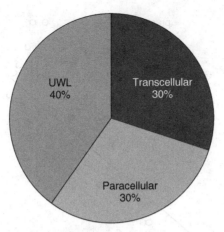

Figure 8.5 Theoretically estimated main P_{eff} determinant of the drugs for which human P_{eff} has been measured. The paracellular markers such as PEGs are excluded from the analysis [37].

From $P_{app} - P_{eff}$ correlation, plica–villi expansion coefficient (PE × VE) was back-estimated to be ca. 33 [37]. This is in good agreement with the anatomical value for humans (3 × 10 = 30).

8.4.2.2 PAMPA. As discussed in Section 7.9.4, many versions of PAMPA have been reported in the literature. In this section, the biomimetic PAMPA is used as an example [6, 38, 42, 43]. As clearly shown in Figures 8.6 and 8.7, because a PAMPA membrane does not possess the paracellular pathway, the correction for the paracellular pathway is one of the key factors to improve the predictability of PAMPA (Fig. 8.6).

8.4.2.3 Experimental log P_{oct} and pK_a. Octanol–water partition coefficient (P_{oct}) can be used as a surrogate for $P_{trans,0}$. Considering the fact that log P_{oct} prediction from the chemical structure has an average error of 1 log unit, the use of experimental value is recommended for biopharmaceutical modeling. Figure 8.8 shows the relationship between log D_{oct} (pH 6.5) and Fa% in humans. When log D_{oct} of a drug is larger than 0, Fa% becomes >50%. In the case of small MW molecules, Fa% tends to be higher than expected from that obtained using log D_{oct}, especially in the case of cationic drugs. This is due to the contribution of the paracellular pathway (Fig. 4.15).

Figure 8.9 shows the predictions of Fa% and P_{eff} from the experimental log P_{oct} data [44]. In addition to human P_{eff}, species differences in P_{eff} are also well predicted by the GUT framework (Sections 6.1 and 13.5.1).

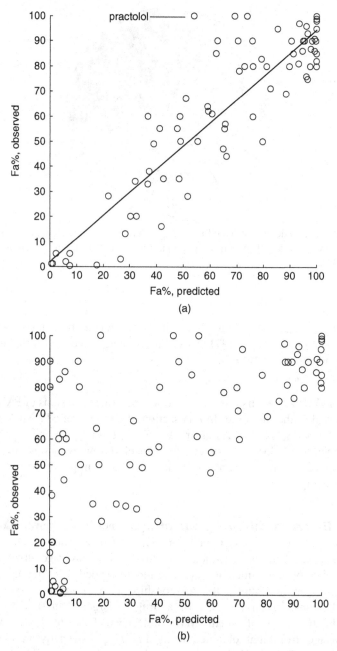

Figure 8.6 Fa% prediction from PAMPA data (a) with and (b) without correction for the paracellular pathway contribution. *Source:* Adapted from Reference 6 with permission.

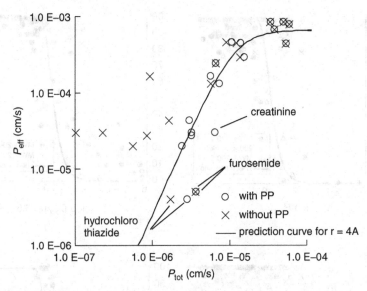

Figure 8.7 Human P_{eff} prediction from PAMPA data with and without the correction for the paracellular pathway contribution (PP: paracellular pathway correction). *Source:* Adapted from Reference 38 with permission.

8.4.3 P_{eff} for UWL Limited Cases[2]

Only a limited number of experimental P_{eff} values for highly lipophilic drugs are available in the literature. In addition, these P_{eff} values were measured in the absence of bile micelles. Therefore, the following equation was used to back-calculate P_{eff} from Fa% for highly lipophilic drugs. In the case of solubility-permeability-limited absorption, P_{eff} can be back-calculated from Fa, $S_{dissolv}$, and dose strength (Dose) as

$$P_{eff} = \frac{Fa \times Dose}{DF \cdot \frac{2}{R_{GI}} \cdot V_{GI} \cdot S_{dissolv} \cdot T_{si}} \qquad (8.4)$$

The Fa values at high dose strength (>5 mg/kg) were excluded from the analysis since particle drifting in the UWL would possibly reduce the effective thickness of the UWL (Section 4.7.2). $DF = 1.7, R_{GI} = 1.5$ cm, $T_{si} = 3.5$ h, and $V_{GI} = 250$ ml were used for the calculation of P_{eff} from the clinical Fa values.

Both P_{UWL} and P_{eff} estimated by Equations 4.24 and 4.2, respectively, showed good correlation with *in vivo* P_{eff} estimated by Equation 8.4 (Fig. 8.10). However, no relationship was observed with the apparent Caco-2 permeability (data not shown). This result further supports the fact that P_{eff} of these compounds with

---

[2]Estimation of P_{UWL} is not important for permeability-limited cases with Fa% < 90%, as epithelial membrane permeability is the rate-limiting step for these cases. However, P_{UWL} affect Fa% for solubility-permeability-limited cases. Therefore, before moving onto the validation for solubility-permeability-limited cases, the validation of P_{UWL} is discussed here.

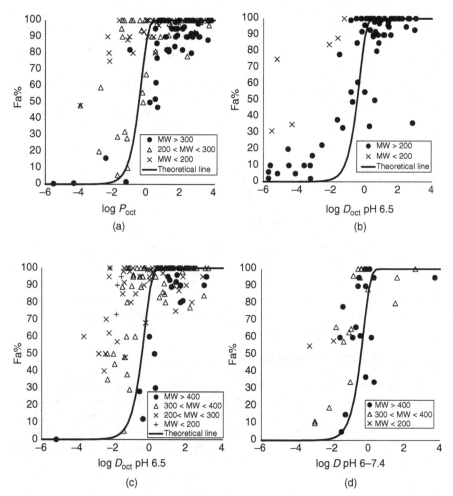

Figure 8.8 Relationship between experimental log D_{oct} and Fa% in humans. (a) Undissociable, (b) monoacid, (c) monobase, and (d) zwitter ion. Low solubility drugs and transporter substrates are excluded from the analysis.

low solubility was mainly determined by the UWL but not by the epithelial membrane. In addition, this result also suggests that bile-micelle binding reduces P_{UWL} permeability in humans (cf. Eq. 4.24) (cf. the reduction of P_{UWL} by bile-micelle binding has been demonstrated using rat and *in vitro* models [45, 46]).

8.4.4 Chemical Structure to P_{eff}, Fa%, and Caco-2 Permeability

Prediction of Fa% and P_{eff} from the chemical structures of drugs has been investigated using the mechanistic models by Obata et al. [25, 48], followed by Reynolds et al. [41]. Calculated log P_{oct}, pK_a, and MW were put into the mechanistic models for the prediction of Fa% and P_{eff} (Chapter 4) (corresponding to PPS I).

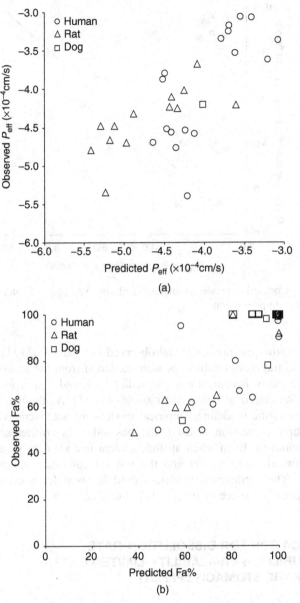

Figure 8.9 Fa and P_{eff} prediction from experimental $\log P_{oct}$ and pK_a. $P_{trans,0}$ was predicted from $\log P_{oct}$ by Equation 4.34, which was independently derived from the Caco-2 data. Other model equations and physiological parameters were the same as those used in previous independent validation (e.g., DF = 1.7). *Source:* Adapted from Reference 44 with permission.

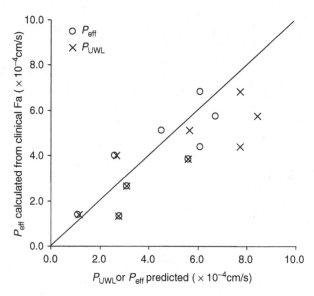

Figure 8.10   Correlation between simulated and observed P_{UWL}. *Source:* Adapted from Reference 47 with permission.

Figure 8.11 shows the predicted and observed Fa% and P_{eff}%. Drugs with low solubility and transporter substrates were excluded from the analysis.

There are many investigations to predict Fa% and P_{eff} from the chemical structure using empirical regression models [49–51]. As the main focus of this book is mechanistic modeling, empirical models are not discussed in this book. When multiple regression is used, the possibility of overlearning should be carefully examined. Even when an independent test set data is separately used for validation, the training set and the test set can share structurally similar compounds. These empirical models should be used for a compound that is within the chemical space of the validation data set.

8.5   VALIDATION FOR DISSOLUTION-RATE AND SOLUBILITY-PERMEABILITY-LIMITED CASES (WITHOUT THE STOMACH EFFECT)

8.5.1   Fa% Prediction Using *In Vitro* Dissolution Data

As discussed in Section 3.2, accurate estimation of k_{diss} from the solubility and other parameters of a drug is not easy task. The estimation errors of each component of k_{diss} accumulatively propagate to the error in the k_{diss} value. Therefore, a practical approach would be to obtain k_{diss} directly from the *in vitro* dissolution experiment and use it for biopharmaceutical modeling (corresponding to PPS IIB). For this purpose, an *in vitro* dissolution test should be performed

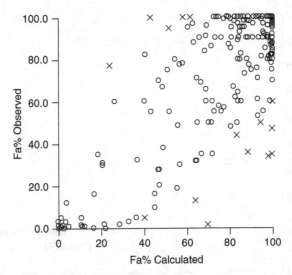

Figure 8.11 Prediction of Fa% from calculated $\log P_{oct}$. *Source:* Adapted from Reference 25 with permission.

under a sink condition. To obtain k_{diss}, the initial linear slope of the dissolved amount–time data is divided by the dose, or Equation 8.5 can be fitted to the dissolved amount–time curve. When a nonsink condition is used, the estimation error for k_{diss} can become significant, as a saturated concentration is quickly achieved [52].

$$\frac{dX_t}{dt} = -k_{diss} \cdot X_{t=0}^{2/3} \cdot X_t^{1/3} \left(1 - \frac{X_{dissolv}}{V_{fluid} S_{dissolv}} \right) \tag{8.5}$$

$$k_{diss} = \frac{3 D_{eff} S_{surface}}{r_p h} = k'_{diss} S_{surface}$$

$$= k''_{diss} D_{eff} S_{surface} \left(k'_{diss} = \frac{3 D_{eff}}{r_p h}, k''_{diss} = \frac{3}{r_p h} \right) \tag{8.6}$$

Fa% predictability of this approach was investigated by Takano et al. [53] for structurally diverse BCS II drugs. Fa% of undissociable compounds, free acids, and free bases (with the high pH stomach) were used for validation. By combined use of the simple *in silico* P_{UWL} prediction and one-compartment GI model, the Fa% values of BCS II drugs were appropriately predicted (Fig. 8.12).

In this pivotal investigation by Takano et al. [53, 54], the following points were concluded:

1. It is critical to consider the effect of the UWL on P_{eff}. Without this, in more than half of the cases, Fa% is significantly overestimated, suggesting that

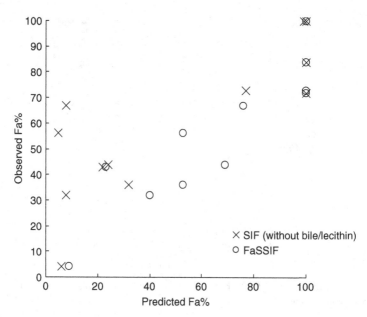

Figure 8.12   Prediction of Fa% using k'_{diss} value obtained from the mini-paddle dissolution test with FaSSIF [53].

the majority of BCS class II drugs are categorized as solubility—UWL-permeability limited, rather than dissolution-rate limited. Caco-2 permeability was found to be inappropriate to be used for drugs with low solubility.

2. The use of a simulated intestinal fluid with bile micelles (FaSSIF) is critical for appropriate Fa% prediction. The use of a simple buffer without bile micelles resulted in significant underestimation of Fa%.

3. A speed of 50 rpm in the minipaddle method (corresponds to 10–25 rpm in a compendium dissolution test) gave an appropriate agitation strength, whereas 25 and 100 rpm under- and overestimated Fa%, respectively.

It should be noted that in this investigation, each drug formulation was added to the vessel after gently crushing the drug products. Therefore, the disintegration process was not reflected in the results.

8.5.2 Fa% Prediction Using *In Vitro* Solubility and Permeability Data

The most frequent use of biopharmaceutical modeling in drug discovery is to estimate *in vivo* Fa% from solubility, particle size, and *in vitro* permeability data for drug candidates with low solubility (corresponds to PPSII A). Therefore, this process is discussed in detail in this section [12]. It should be noted that this discussion became possible after the permeability model had been validated, as discussed in the earlier sections.

TABLE 8.3 Drugs Used to Validate PPSII Type Simulation for DRL and SL Cases

Drug	MW	z^a	pK_a	$\log P_{oct}$	Solubility, mg/ml pH 6.5	FaSSIF	FeSSIF	Caco-2, $\times 10^{-6}$ cm/s	References
Acyclovir	225	0	–	-1.7	2.5	2.5^d	–	0.38	42, 55, 56
Albendazole	265	0	4.2	3.1	0.00055	0.0021	–	–	57, 58
Aprepitant	534	0	4.2^b	4.8	0.0008	0.021^e	–	–	59, 60
Atovaquone	367	0	–	5.1	0.00043	0.0024	–	–	61, 62
AZ0865	366	0	6.1	4.2	0.00185	0.0057	–	–	63
Carbamazepine (anhydrate)	236	0	–	1.8	0.120	0.185, 0.220	–	–	64, 65
Carbamazepine (Dihydrate)	236	0	–	1.8	0.08^f	0.013	–	–	—
Celecoxib	381	0	–	(>) 3	0.0032	0.0462	0.103	–	66
Chlorothiazide	265	0	–	-0.24	0.73	0.87	0.83	0.92	8, 26, 67
Cilostazole	369	0	–	2.7	0.0063	$0.0064, 0.008^e$	0.014^e	-	68
Cinnarizine	369	+	7.45	5.7	0.0014	$0.013, 0.021^e, 0.013^f, 0.021^{e,f}$	–	–	58
Danazol	337	0	–	4.5	0.0002	$0.018, 0.020^e$	0.047	–	47, 69, 70
Digoxin	780	0	–	1.3	0.016	0.017	–	1.3	55, 71, 72
Dipyridamole	505	0	6.2	3.9	0.006	$0.017, 0.024^e$	–	–	53, 69
Efavirentz	316	0	–	4.1	0.01	0.194	–	–	53
EMD57033	425	0	–	2.7	0.0047	0.0075	–	–	73
Felodipine	384	0	–	4.3	0.00086	0.077^e	–	–	69, 74
Fenofibrate	362	0	–	5.2	0.0002	0.014	0.037	–	75, 76
FTI-2600	448	0	–	3.2	0.0037	0.033^e	–	–	77
Ganciclovir	255	0	–	-1.7	4.3	4.3^d	–	0.23	55, 78
Gefitinib	447	+	7.2	4.1	0.0041	$0.085, 0.083^f$	–	–	79, 80
Glibenclamide	494	–	5.9	3.1	0.0045	$0.0046, 0.0027^f$	–	–	58
Griseofulvin	353	0	–	2.5	0.01	$0.015, 0.018^e$	–	–	47, 69, 70

(continued)

TABLE 8.3 (Continued)

Drug	MW	z^a	pK_a	$\log P_{oct}$	Solubility, mg/ml			Caco-2, $\times 10^{-6}$ cm/s	References
					pH 6.5	FaSSIF	FeSSIF		
Irbesartan	429	–	4.4	4.0^c	0.11	$0.21, 0.11^f$	0.29	127	67, 81–83
Indomethacin	358	–	4.2	4.3	0.22	$0.59, 0.74^e$	–	–	58
Ivermectine	875	0	–	3.2	0.0007	0.12	–	–	53
Ketoconazole	531	+	6.5	4.3	0.012	$0.021, 0.027^e$	–	–	26, 53, 62
Lobucavir	265	0	–	–1.2	0.8	0.8^d	–	0.88	55, 78
LY-2157299	369	0	4.34	1.73	0.082	1.8	–	–	84
N74	353	–	–	3.1	0.041	0.12	–	–	85
Nifedipine	346	0	–	3.2	0.013	0.031^e	–	–	86
Nitrendipine	360	0	–	3.3	0.004	0.016	–	–	53
Panadiplon	335	0	–	1.2^b	0.077	$0.085 d,e$	0.13^e	–	87
Phenitoin	252	0	–	2.5	0.039	0.043	0.059	–	69
Pranlukast	491	–	3.4	4.2^b	0.0033	$0.088, 0.086^f$	$0.8, 0.8^f$	25	67, 88
Spironolactone	417	0	–	3.3	0.03	0.042	–	–	53
Tolfenamic acid	262	–	4.8	5.7	0.027	$0.063, 0.040^f$	–	–	58

[a] Dominant charge at pH 6.5 (>50% dissociated cases were assigned as + or –).

[b] Calculated value (ACD/Labs Software V8.14).

[c] Calculated from pK_a and log $D_{pH7.4}$.

[d] Estimated from blank buffer solubility and log P_{oct}.

[e] For dogs.

[f] Estimated from the solubility ratio of anhydrate and dehydrate at pH 1.2.

TABLE 8.4 Simulated and Observed Fa% by PPSII Type Simulation for DRL and SL Cases

Drug	Species	State	Dose, mg	d50ᵃ, μm	Dn	Do	Pn	Predicted Fa%	Type	Observed Fa%	Method[b]	References
Acyclovir	Human	Fasted	200	50[a]	353.3	0.6	0.3	27	PL	29	(VI)	89–91
Acyclovir	Human	Fasted	400	50	353.3	1.2	0.3	23	SL-E	21	(VI)	
Acyclovir	Human	Fasted	800	50	353.3	2.5	0.3	13	SL-E	12	(VI)	
Albendazole	Human	Fasted	1400	10	1.9	5142.8	46	1.9	SL-U	2.7	(II)	92, 93
Aprepitant	Dog	Fasted	20	0.2	9434.5	51.4	48.1	82	SL-U	57	(III)	59, 94
Aprepitant	Dog	Fasted	20	2	94.3	51.4	6.6	21	SL-U	33	(II)	
Aprepitant	Dog	Fasted	20	5	15.1	51.4	3.7	12	SL-U	28	(II)	
Aprepitant	Dog	Fasted	20	26	0.6	51.4	2.7	7	SL-U	18	(II)	
Atovaquone	Human	Fasted	500	0.3	1468.2	1607.1	242.1	33	SL-U	39	(VI)	95–98
Atovaquone	Human	Fasted	1000	0.3	1468.2	3214.2	311.3	23	SL-U	30	(VI)	
Atovaquone	Human	Fasted	1500	0.3	1468.2	4821.3	344.2	18	SL-U	17	(VI)	
AZ0865	Human	Fasted	100	2.5	87.2	134.4	20.1	27	SL-U	49	(II), (IV), (V)	63
Carbamazepine (form I)	Dog	Fasted	40	14	126.6	10.7	11.0	78	SL-U	87	(II), (IV)	65, 99
Carbamazepine (Dihydrate)	Dog	Fasted	40	13	99.4	15.8	11.4	68	SL-U	90	(II), (IV)	
Carbamazepine (form I)	Dog	Fasted	200	14	126.6	53.3	26.3	60	SL-U	62	(II), (IV)	
Carbamazepine (dihydrate)	Dog	Fasted	200	13	99.4	78.8	27.0	49	SL-U	30	(II), (IV)	
Carbamazepine (Tagretol)	Dog	Fasted	200	2.5	2688.0	78.8	40.1	63	SL-E	90	(II), (IV)	
Carbamazepine (Tagretol)	Dog	Fasted	200	150	1.2	49.0	9.0	21	SL-U	48	(II), (IV)	
Carbamazepine (Tagretol)	Human	Fasted	200	2.5	7267.7	8.3	48.9	100	SL-U	100	(III)	
Carbamazepine (Tagretol)	Human	Fasted	400	150	2.0	16.7	15.9	55	SL-U	70	(III)	
Celecoxib	Human	Fasted	5	2	279.4	0.8	4.1	98	PL	94	(III), (VI)	100, 101
Celecoxib	Human	Fasted	25	2	279.4	4.2	4.7	75	SL-U	87	(III), (VI)	
Celecoxib	Human	Fasted	50	2	279.4	8.3	5.8	63	SL-U	69	(III), (VI)	
Celecoxib	Human	Fasted	100	2	279.4	16.7	9.1	58	SL-U	67	(III), (VI)	
Celecoxib	Human	Fasted	200	2	279.4	33.4	14.3	53	SL-U	86	(III), (VI)	

(continued)

TABLE 8.4 (*Continued*)

Drug	Species	State	Dose, mg	d50^a,μm	Dn	Do	Pn	Predicted Fa%	Type	Observed Fa%	Method^b	References
Celecoxib	Human	Fasted	400	2	279.4	66.8	21.3	46	SL-U	51	(III, VI)	102, 103
Celecoxib	Human	Fasted	600	2	279.4	100.2	25.9	40	SL-U	72	(III, VI)	
Celecoxib	Human	Fasted	900	2	279.4	150.3	30.4	34	SL-U	55	(III, VI)	
Celecoxib	Human	Fasted	1200	2	279.4	200.4	33.3	30	SL-U	44	(III, VI)	
Celecoxib	Human	Fed	200	2	1378.5	12.5	17.1	88	SL-U	107	(III, VI)	
Celecoxib	Human	Fed	400	2	1378.5	25.0	25.2	82	SL-U	81	(III, VI)	
Chlorothiazide	Human	Fasted	50	50	96.1	0.4	0.6	47	PL	56	(I)	102, 103
Chlorothiazide	Human	Fasted	500	50	96.1	4.4	0.6	17	SL-E	15	(I)	
Chlorothiazide	Human	Fed	500	50	97.6	3.9	0.7	19	SL-E	29	(I)	
Cilostazole	Dog	Fasted	100	0.22	21,476.3	675	401.1	76	SL-U	100	(III, VI)	68, 104, 105
Cilostazole	Dog	Fasted	100	13	6.2	675	29.8	9	SL-U	20	(III, VI)	
Cilostazole	Dog	Fasted	100	2.4	180.5	675	88.1	27	SL-U	21	(III, VI)	
Cilostazole	Dog	Fed	100	0.22	25,318.8	321.4	240.8	82	SL-U	95	(III, VI)	
Cilostazole	Dog	Fed	100	13	7.3	321.4	17.8	11	SL-U	32	(III, VI)	
Cilostazole	Dog	Fed	100	2.4	212.7	321.4	53.9	31	SL-U	75	(III, VI)	
Cilostazole	Human	Fasted	50	10	17.8	60.3	20.8	47	SL-U	40	(II)	
Cilostazole	Human	Fasted	100	10	17.8	120.5	22.9	31	SL-U	31	(II)	
Cilostazole	Human	Fasted	200	10	17.8	241.1	29.0	22	SL-U	25	(II)	
Cinnarizine	Dog	Fasted	25	25	0.8	64.3	3.1	7	SL-U	5	(IV), (VI)	106, 107
Cinnarizine	Human	Fasted	25	25	0.7	14.8	4.8	24	SL-U	27	(IV)	
Cinnarizine	Human	Fasted	25	60	0.1	14.8	4.8	9	DRL	13	(IV)	
Danazol	Dog	Fasted	2	5	11.9	5.4	2.4	43	SL-U	30	(II)	59, 108–111
Danazol	Dog	Fasted	20	5	11.9	54	3.3	11	SL-U	12	(II)	
Danazol	Dog	Fasted	20	229	0	54	2.3	0.35	DRL	2	(II)	
Danazol	Dog	Fasted	200	0.16	11,582.9	540	127.2	43	SL-U	77	(II)	

Danazol	Dog	Fasted	200	10	3	540	8.3	3	SL-U	4.8	(II)	
Danazol	Human	Fasted	100	4.46	7.7	42.9	4	15	SL-U	18	(II), (III)	
Danazol	Human	Fasted	200	4.46	7.7	85.7	5.6	12	SL-U	14	(II), (III)	
Danazol	Human	Fed	100	4.46	111.9	13.7	6.4	52	SL-U	58	(II), (III)	112
Digoxin	Human	Fasted	0.5	7	65.8	0.2	1	62	PL	78	(II)	
Digoxin	Human	Fasted	0.5	13	19.1	0.2	1	60	PL	96	(II)	
Digoxin	Human	Fasted	0.5	102	0.3	0.2	1	10	DRL	37	(II)	
Dipyridamole	Human	Fasted	50	75	0.3	22.7	8	16	DRL	36	(IV), (VI)	113–115
Dipyridamole	Dog	Fasted	75	75	0.2	166	4.6	3	SL-U	11	(IV)	
Efavirentz	Human	Fasted	600	3	444.4	23.9	20	75	SL-U	82	(III)	116, 117
Efavirentz	Human	Fasted	1200	3	444.4	47.7	27.4	65	SL-U	59	(III)	
EMD57033	Dog	Fasted	30	15	3.3	216.0	9.7	8	SL-U	10	(II)	73
Felodipine	Dog	Fasted	3	8	17.9	2.1	2.4	66	SL-U	72	(II)	74
Felodipine	Dog	Fasted	3	125	0.1	2.1	2.3	4	DRL	5	(II)	
Fenofibrate	Human	Fasted	145	0.4	811	79.9	28.6	50	SL-U	70	Other[c]	118–120
Fenofibrate	Human	Fasted	200	2.2	26.8	110.2	8.9	15	SL-U	51	Other	
Fenofibrate	Human	Fed	67	2.2	364	11.6	7.6	63	SL-U	84	Other	
Fenofibrate	Human	Fed	145	0.4	11,010.5	25.2	57.8	100	SL-U	79	Other	
Fenofibrate	Human	Fed	200	2.2	364	34.7	16.5	57	SL-U	72	Other	
FTI-2600	Dog	Fasted	30	1	931	49.7	21.4	55	PL	28	(II)	77
Ganciclovir	Human	Fasted	500	50	574.1	0.9	0.2	18	PL	5.6	(VI)	121
Ganciclovir	Human	Fasted	750	50	574.1	1.3	0.2	14	SL-E	4.5	(VI)	
Ganciclovir	Human	Fasted	1000	50	574.1	1.8	0.2	10	SL-E	4.5	(VI)	

(continued)

TABLE 8.4 (Continued)

Drug	Species	State	Dose, mg	d50^a,μm	Dn	Do	Pn	Predicted Fa%	Type	Observed Fa%	Method^b	References
Ganciclovir	Human	Fasted	1250	50	574.1	2.2	0.2	9	SL-E	2.6	(VI)	—
Gefitinib	Human	Fasted	250	30	1.6	22.7	4	21	SL-U	39	(III), (IV), (VI)	80, 122, 123
Glibenclamide	Human	Fasted	5	50	0.3	8.4	16.8	22	DRL	45	(I)	—
Griseofulvin	Dog	Fasted	2	7	35.8	6	7.5	81	SL-U	85	(II)	59, 124, 125
Griseofulvin	Dog	Fasted	20	118	0.1	60	7.4	7	SL-U	2.9	(II)	—
Griseofulvin	Dog	Fasted	20	7	35.8	60	10.7	28	SL-U	46.9	(II)	—
Griseofulvin	Human	Fasted	125	4	181.8	64.3	28.8	57	SL-U	45	(III)	—
Griseofulvin	Human	Fasted	500	4	181.8	257.1	78.5	49	SL-U	43	(I)	—
Indomethacin	Dog	Fasted	25	150	1.5	2.3	4.4	59	DRL	46	(IV),(VI)129	126, 127
Irbesartan	Human	Fasted	25	20	39.8	0.9	9.4	100	PL	99	(II), (VI)	128–130
Irbesartan	Human	Fasted	50	20	39.8	1.8	9.5	100	SL-U	83	(II), (VI)	—
Irbesartan	Human	Fasted	100	20	39.8	3.7	9.9	100	SL-U	75	(II), (VI)	—
Irbesartan	Human	Fasted	150	20	39.8	5.5	10.2	91	SL-U	71	(II), (VI)	—
Irbesartan	Human	Fasted	200	20	39.8	7.3	10.6	86	SL-U	64	(II), (VI)	—
Irbesartan	Human	Fasted	300	20	39.8	11	11.6	78	SL-U	78	(II), (VI)	—
Irbesartan	Human	Fasted	600	20	39.8	22	15.8	69	SL-U	59	(II), (VI)	—
Irbesartan	Human	Fasted	900	20	39.8	33.1	19.8	65	SL-U	54	(II), (VI)	—
Irbesartan	Human	Fed	25	20	62.2	0.6	8.1	100	PL	83	(II), (VI)	—
Irbesartan	Human	Fed	300	20	62.2	6.7	9.5	85	SL-U	90	(II), (VI)	—
Ivermectine	Human	Fasted	6	25	1.2	0.4	2.8	52	DRL	54	(II), (III)	53, 131–133
Ivermectine	Human	Fasted	12	25	1.2	0.8	2.8	52	DRL	52	(II), (III)	—
Ivermectine	Human	Fasted	15	25	1.2	1	2.8	52	DRL	51	(II), (III)	—
Ivermectine	Human	Fasted	30	25	1.2	1.9	2.8	53	DRL	53	(II), (III)	—
Ivermectine	Human	Fasted	60	25	1.2	3.9	2.8	43	SL-U	46	(II), (III)	—

Ivermectine	Human	Fasted	90	25	1.2	5.8	2.9	36	SL-U	30	(II), (III)	—
Ivermectine	Human	Fasted	120	25	1.2	7.7	2.9	31	SL-U	35	(II), (III)	—
Ketoconazole	Human	Fasted	200	200	0.1	73.5	11.1	5	DRL	6	(II)	115, 134
Ketoconazole	Dog	Fasted	200	200	0	400	6.3	2	SL-U	3.3	(IV)	—
Lobucavir	Human	Fasted	20	50	105	0.2	0.7	51	PL	48	(VI)	78
Lobucavir	Human	Fasted	70	50	105	0.7	0.7	51	PL	53	(VI)	—
Lobucavir	Human	Fasted	200	50	105	1.9	0.7	31	SL-E	42	(VI)	—
Lobucavir	Human	Fasted	400	50	105	3.9	0.7	21	SL-E	28	(VI)	—
Lobucavir	Human	Fasted	700	50	105	6.7	0.7	14	SL-E	14	(VI)	—
LY-2157299	Dog	Fasted	500	10	363.1	14.8	3.3	30	SL-E	20	(II)	84
N74	Dog	Fasted	10	120	0.5	4.5	5.4	35	DRL	29	(II)	85
Nitrendipine	Human	Fasted	20	10	12.1	9.6	7.3	65	SL-U	76	(II)	53, 135
Nifedipine	Dog	Fasted	10	50	1.0	17.4	6.3	29	SL-U	39	(II)	136
Nifedipine	Dog	Fasted	30	30	2.7	52.3	6.9	19	SL-U	31	(II)	137
Nifedipine	Dog	Fasted	40	10	24.0	69.7	11.3	27	SL-U	34	Other[e]	138
Panadiplon	Dog	Fasted	10	9	161.5	6.4	7.7	81	SL-U	84	(VI)	87
Panadiplon	Dog	Fasted	10	25	20.9	6.4	7.3	77	SL-U	77	(VI)	
Panadiplon	Dog	Fasted	10	100	1.3	6.4	7.1	51	SL-U	25	(VI)	
Panadiplon	Dog	Fed	10	9	176.3	3.6	5.6	84	SL-U	100	(VI)	
Panadiplon	Dog	Fed	10	25	22.9	3.6	5.4	81	SL-U	91	(VI)	
Panadiplon	Dog	Fed	10	100	1.4	3.6	5.3	56	DRL	35	(VI)	
Phenitoin	Human	Fasted	280	4	819.7	50.2	81.3	95	SL-U	81	(II), (VI)	139–142
Phenitoin	Human	Fasted	200	50	5.2	35.9	22	56	SL-U	60	(II), (VI)	
Phenitoin	Human	Fasted	350	190	0.4	62.8	21.2	18	SL-U	14	(II), (VI)	—
Phenitoin	Human	Fed	350	190	0.4	38.5	16.9	21	DRL	31	(II), (VI)	—
Pranlukast	Human	Fasted	50	2	309.6	4.4	0.7	18	SL-E	20	Other[d]	143–146
Pranlukast	Human	Fasted	100	2	309.6	8.8	0.7	11	SL-E	13	Other	

(continued)

TABLE 8.4 (Continued)

Drug	Species	State	Dose, mg	d50[a], μm	Dn	Do	Pn	Predicted Fa%	Type	Observed Fa%	Method[b]	References
Pranlukast	Human	Fasted	300	2	309.6	26.3	0.8	5	SL-E	7.2	Other	
Pranlukast	Human	Fasted	600	2	309.6	52.6	0.8	3	SL-E	5	Other	
Pranlukast	Human	Fed	112.5	2	9408.9	0.9	0.1	8	PL	12	Other	
Pranlukast	Human	Fed	225	2	9408.9	1.8	0.1	5	SL-E	11	Other	
Pranlukast	Human	Fed	300	2	9408.9	2.4	0.1	4	SL-E	11	Other	
Pranlukast	Human	Fed	337.5	2	9408.9	2.7	0.1	4	SL-E	7.1	Other	
Pranlukast	Human	Fed	450	2	9408.9	3.6	0.1	3	SL-E	12	Other	
Pranlukast	Human	Fed	562.5	2	9408.9	4.5	0.1	2	SL-E	9.8	Other	
Pranlukast	Human	Fed	675	2	9408.9	5.4	0.1	2	SL-E	7.6	Other	
Spironolactone	Human	Fasted	200	10	80.8	36.7	21.2	64	SL-U	58	(III)	147, 148
Tolfenamic acid	Human	Fasted	200	6	159.5	24.5	24.5	81	SL-U	60	(VI)	149–151
Tolfenamic acid	Human	Fasted	100	18	17.7	12.2	12.4	77	SL-U	82	(VI)	
Tolfenamic acid	Human	Fasted	200	18	17.7	24.5	13.7	60	SL-U	59	(VI)	
Tolfenamic acid	Human	Fasted	400	18	17.7	49	17.8	48	SL-U	61	(VI)	
Tolfenamic acid	Human	Fasted	800	18	17.7	98	31	44	SL-U	68	(VI)	

[a]For acyclovir, chlorothiazide, ganciclovir, and lobucavir, the particle size was assumed to be $50^r\,\mu m$. Predicted Fa% did not depend on the particle size. For cinnarizine, EMD57033, dipyridamole, gefitinib, indomethacin, ivermectine, ketoconazole, N74, nifedipine, and nitrendipine, the particle size was estimated from the dissolution data.

[b]The method used to estimate Fa% (see text for detail): (I), Fa% reported in the literature; (II), relative bioavailability of solution versus solid form formulation; (III) relative bioavailability in the fasted versus the fed state (especially when Do < 1 at the fed state); (IV) relative bioavailability with the low/high pH in the stomach when Do < 1 in the stomach (for basic drugs) (IV); (V), dose-normalized relative bioavailability at Do < 1 versus Do > 1 when the terminal elimination half-life is consistent; (VI), from absolute bioavailability (F) and hepatic clearance using Fa $= F/(1 - CL_h/Q)$ (VI).

[c]Estimated using the PK of acid parent drug.

[d]Estimated from the total metabolite amount in urine and the unchanged drug in the feces.

[e]Powder versus solid dispersion.

Drugs with low solubility for which the effect of the stomach on Fa% is negligible are the simplest ones to simulate Fa%. Undissociable and free acid drugs are such cases. In addition, Fa% of free base drugs in high pH stomach cases (such as when coadministered with antacids) was also included, to increase the number of model drugs. As the effect of the stomach is negligible, a simple Fa% equation ($Fa_{SS.corr}$) was used for validation (Section 5.3.5).[3] In total, 29 structurally diverse drugs were used as model drugs (Table 8.3). Fa% data at several doses and particle sizes in humans and dogs were collated from the literature (Table 8.4). In the original investigation, a total of 110 Fa% data were used. In addition, several test set drugs were newly added in this book [LY-2157299, nabumetone, AZ0865, nitrendipine, celecoxib, acyclovir (800 mg, human fed), N74, nifedipine, indomethacin].

As typical input data solubility in biorelevant media (FaSSIF, FeSSIF), molecular weight, experimental log P_{oct}, experimental pK_a, Caco-2 permeability, dose, and particle size were used. For clarification, the mechanistic model equations used for this investigation are summarized as follows (see Chapter 2 for details):

- Fa%[4]

$$Fa = 1 - \exp\left(-\cfrac{1}{\cfrac{1}{k_{diss}} + \cfrac{k_{perm}}{Do}}T_{si}\right) = 1$$

$$- \exp\left(-\cfrac{1}{\cfrac{1}{Dn} + \cfrac{Do}{Pn}}\right) \quad \text{if } Do < 1, Do = 1$$

$$Pn = k_{perm}T_{si}, Dn = k_{diss}T_{si}, Do = \frac{Dose}{S_{dissolv}V_{GI}}$$

- Dissolution

$$k_{diss} = \frac{3D_{eff}S_{surface}}{\rho}\sum^{i}\frac{f_i}{r_{p,i}^2}$$

$$f_{mono} = \frac{S_{blank}}{S_{dissolv}}$$

$$D_{mono}(cm^2/s) = 9.9 \times 10^{-5}MW^{-0.453}$$

$$D_{eff} = D_{mono} \cdot f_{mono} + D_{bm}(1 - f_{mono})$$

---

[3] Occams razor. See Section 8.2.
[4] Plus correction factors (Section 5.3.5).

- Permeation

$$k_{perm} = \frac{2DF}{R_{GI}} P_{eff}$$

$$P_{eff} = \frac{PE}{\dfrac{1}{P'_{ep}} + \dfrac{1}{P_{UWL}}}$$

$$= \frac{PE}{\dfrac{1}{f_{mono}\,(f_0 P_{trans,0} + P_{para}) \cdot VE} + \dfrac{1}{\dfrac{D_{eff}}{h_{UWL}} + P_{WC}}}$$

$$P_{trans,0}\,(cm/s) = 2.36 \times 10^{-6} P_{oct}^{1.1}$$

$$P_{para}\,(cm/s) = 3.9 \times 10^{-4} \cdot \frac{1}{MW^{1/3}}$$

$$\cdot\, RK\left(\frac{MW^{1/3}}{8.46}\right)\left(f_0 + \sum_{z\,(z \neq 0)} f_z \frac{2.39z}{1 - e^{-2.39z}}\right)$$

$$h_{UWL} = h_{fam} \cdot \left(1 - RK\left(\frac{r_{p,mean}}{R_{mucus}}\right)\right) + h_{pd} - \frac{1}{2} h_{pd} R_{SA} \qquad R_{SA} \leq 1$$

$$h_{UWL} = h_{fam} \cdot \left(1 - RK\left(\frac{r_{p,mean}}{R_{mucus}}\right)\right) + \frac{1}{2}\frac{h_{pd}}{R_{SA}} \qquad R_{SA} > 1$$

$$R_{SA} = \frac{3 \cdot C_{pd} \cdot h_{pd} Dose}{\cdot} V_{GI} \cdot \rho \sum_i \frac{f_i}{r_{p,i}}$$

$$RK(x) = (1 - x)^2 (1 - 2.104\,x + 2.09\,x^3 - 0.95\,x^5)\,x < 1$$

The following drug parameters were used (see Chapters 2 and 7 for details):

- $S_{dissolv}$: The solubility values in FaSSIF and FeSSIF [152]. The pH of FeSSIF was set to 6.5 according to the recent update [88, 153]. TCs of 3, 5, 15, and 18 mM were used for fasted humans, fasted dogs, fed humans, and fed dogs, respectively. TC/PC ratio was 4:1. When the solubility value for dogs was not available, it was estimated from human FaSSIF or FeSSIF data correcting for the bile-micelle concentration.
- $S_{surface}$: Calculated by the Mooney–Stella equation and HH equation (Section 3.2.6).

- D_{bm}: 0.13, 0.56, 1.12, and 1.14 $\times$ 10^{-6} cm^2/s for 3, 5, 15, and 18 mM TC, respectively (Section 3.1.2). D_{bm} at 3 mM TC was multiplied threefold for P_{UWL} calculation [154].
- ρ: 1.2 g/cm^3.
- P_{ep}: In the case of lipophilic drugs (log $D_{oct,pH\ 6.5} > 2$), P_{ep} was estimated from log P_{oct}, pK_a, and MW because their permeability is expected to be UWL limited, and the Caco-2 study with a standard condition often underestimates the permeability of highly lipophilic drugs (Section 7.9.8). In the case of log $D_{oct,pH\ 6.5} < 2$, Caco-2 permeability was used if available in the literature.
- r_p: Assumed log-normal distribution with ln 2 standard deviation ($\Sigma f_i/r_{p,i}$ and $\sum f_i/r_{p,i}^2$ becomes ca. $1.4/r_{p,mean}$ and $3.3/r_{p,mean}^2$, respectively). When the particle size data is not available, it is back-estimated from the *in vitro* dissolution data.

The following physiological parameters were used (see Chapter 6 for details): DF = 1.7 (independently obtained from human P_{eff}–Fa% relationship), VE = 10 and h_{fam} = 15 μm for both humans and dogs; PE = 3 and 1, R_{GI} = 1.5 and 0.5 cm, and T_{si} = 3.5 and 2 h, P_{WC} = 0.23 and 0.29 $\times$ 10^{-4} cm/s, V_{GI} = 130 and 18.6 ml for humans and dogs, respectively. V_{GI} in the fed state was set 1.2-fold larger than that in the fasted state [67]. R_{mucus}, C_{pd}, and h_{UWL} were assumed to be the same in humans and dogs and were set to 2.9, 2.2, and 300 μm, respectively. Because R_{mucus} and C_{pd} are not available in the literature, they are optimized in the original investigation [12].[5]

The results were shown in Figure 8.13. In approximately 80% of the cases, the difference in simulated and observed error was within twofold, suggesting that the GUT framework has practical predictability for drug discovery but not for drug development.

The majority of drugs with low solubility (Do > 1) used in this study was categorized as SL-U (Fig. 8.14) but not DRL. This point is discussed later in Section 10.2.2.

Permeation resistance from the UWL has often been ignored in oral absorption simulation, and infinite fast permeation has sometimes been assumed. However, when permeation resistance from the UWL was ignored, Fa% of the SL-U cases were overestimated. This is in good agreement with the previous findings [53, 54, 59].

Interestingly, in many articles regarding the BCS, it was speculated that BCS II cases would be dissolution-rate limited and that *in vitro–in vivo* correlation

---

[5]Therefore, strictly speaking, this simulation is not a "prediction" for the cases in the original paper when the particle drifting effect is significant (i.e., SL-U, dose > 5 mg/kg, d_p < 5 μm). However, the number of Fa% data (> 11) is much larger than that of fitted parameter (two). Other cases can be taken as "prediction," as all the physiological data were independently determined and no fitting is employed. The data for the drugs newly added in this book can be interpreted as the independent test set.

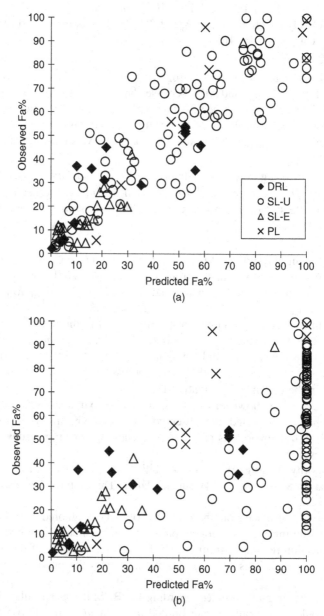

Figure 8.13 Simulated and observed Fa% for drugs with low solubility. (a) UWL considered and (b) UWL neglected.

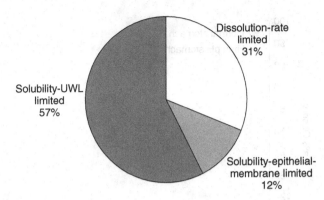

Figure 8.14 Percentage of DRL, SL-E, and SL-U (Do > 1 cases).

should be anticipated for this class. However, the result of this study suggested that the majority of BCS II drugs are likely to be solubility–permeability limited rather than dissolution-rate limited, especially, when the dose is larger than 20 mg.

8.6 VALIDATION FOR DISSOLUTION-RATE AND SOLUBILITY-PERMEABILITY-LIMITED CASES (WITH THE STOMACH EFFECT)

8.6.1 Difference Between Free Base and Salts

Since pH in the stomach is lower than that in the small intestine, a base drug shows higher solubility in the stomach than in the small intestine. Therefore, in the case of a basic drug, the drug molecule once dissolved in the stomach can precipitate out in the small intestine. However, the precipitation mechanism is different depending on the solid form of the active pharmaceutical ingredient (API), that is, free base or salt [2].

8.6.2 Simulation Model for Free Base

As a simpler case, the oral absorption of a free base drug is first discussed in this section [155]. The gastric pH provides a favorable environment to dissolve a free base. However, because the gastric emptying rate follows first-order kinetics, a portion of drug particles exits from the stomach into the small intestine before completely dissolving in the stomach.[6] As the gastric fluid (which contains both dissolved drug molecules and undissolved drug particles) pours into the small intestine, the pH is neutralized, and the dissolved drug concentration (C_{dissolv}) in the small intestine becomes transiently higher than the equilibrium solubility of a

---

[6]If the solid surface pH of a free base were not taken into account, the dissolution rate in the stomach would be overestimated.

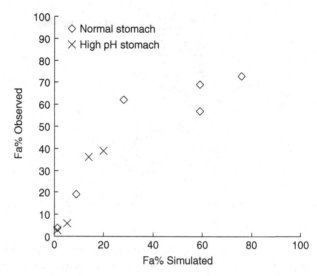

Figure 8.15 Simulated versus observed Fa% for free bases. *Source:* Adapted from Reference 159 with permission.

drug in the small intestine. Owing to the negative concentration gradient around the particles, the particles grow in the small intestine (Fig. 3.17a). This particle growth reduces $C_{dissolv}$ in the small intestine [156]. Therefore, in biopharmaceutical modeling, both the dissolution rate in the stomach and the particle growth rate in the intestine have to be simulated appropriately.

The Nernst–Brunner (NB) equation can be used for both the dissolution and particle growth of API [156].[7] The API particles dissolve or grow depending on the concentration gradient (ΔC) around a particle, that is, ΔC is positive for dissolution and negative for particle growth. Appropriate estimation of the solid surface solubility of a free base is one of the key factors for appropriate simulation. For free base drugs, the solid surface solubility of a drug can become significantly smaller than the bulk solubility in the stomach (>100-fold) (Fig. 3.16). The Mooney–Stella equation can be used to calculate the solid surface pH (Section 3.2.6). The solid surface pH can also be experimentally obtained (Section 7.6.3.3) [157, 158]. In addition, the NB equation has to be modified as Equation 3.53 to differentiate the solid surface solubility from bulk solubility.

To model the pH change between the stomach and the small intestine, a compartment model is required. In addition, the position of undissolved particles will affect the concentration reduction rate in the small intestine. Therefore, biopharmaceutical modeling was performed using the S1I7C1 model.

---

[7]Particle growth is the reverse process of dissolution.

8.6.3 Simulation Results

Albendazole, aprepitant, dipyridamol, gefitinib, and ketoconazole were used as model drugs to validate this mechanism (all free base APIs (not salts)). Fa% of these drugs was appropriately simulated (Fig. 8.15). On the basis of the simulation results, it was suggested that the dissolution patterns in the gastrointestinal tract were significantly different depending on the dose–solubility ratio in the stomach. The oral absorption patterns of free bases can be roughly categorized into the following two types:

- When the dose number in the stomach is greater than 1 ($Do_{stomach} > 1$), saturated solubility is rapidly achieved in the stomach and further dissolution does not occur (Figs. 8.16 and 8.17). Therefore, most of the drug particles reach the small intestine before being completely dissolved (Fig. 8.18), and the regrowth of these particles rapidly reduces $C_{dissolv}$ in the small intestine.
- When the dose number in the stomach is less than 1 ($Do_{stomach} < 1$), saturated solubility is not achieved in the stomach (Fig. 8.16). However, some portions of drugs reach the small intestine before being completely dissolved in the stomach. The effect of stomach pH on Fa% is larger than that for $Do_{stomach} > 1$ cases (Section 13.1). Since both the dissolution rate in the stomach and the concentration reduction rate in the small intestine become faster as the particle size of a drug is reduced, it was theoretically suggested that there is an optimal particle size to effectively utilize the stomach fluid to dissolve a weak base drug. The relatively large particle sizes of dipyridamol, ketoconazole, and gefitinib might be explained by this mechanism.

8.7 SALTS

After dosing a salt form, a free form (not the salt) precipitates out in the small intestine (Figs. 3.17 and 3.18). The precipitation of the free base is initiated by a nucleation process, and then the nuclei particles grow and $C_{dissolv}$ is reduced in the small intestine. The model equations to simulate nucleation are discussed in Section 3.3. The categorization of precipitation patterns is discussed later in Section 11.1.

Owing to the lack of appropriate *in vitro* precipitation models [63], the validation of the GUT framework for salts has not been achieved yet. As a first step to handle nucleation, the classical nucleation theory has been introduced to the GUT framework [2, 160]. However, this approach should be validated carefully in the future. Currently (as of 2011), none of the commercial software can handle the nucleation process.

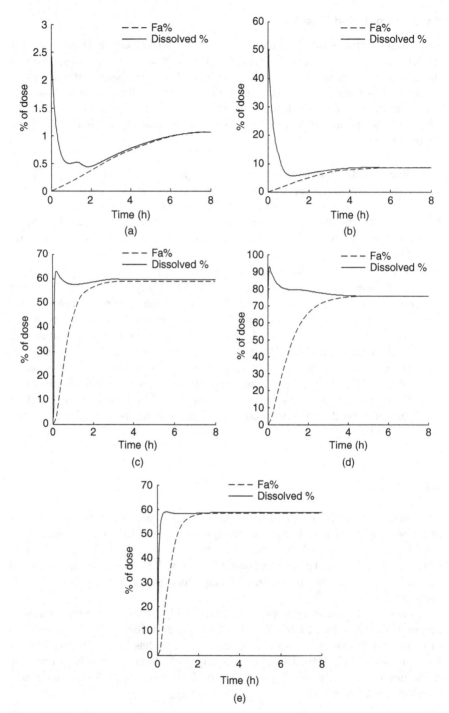

Figure 8.16 Simulated dissolved %. (a) Albendazole, (b) arepitant, (c) dipyridamole, (d) gefitinib, and (e) ketoconazole. *Source:* Adapted from Reference 159 with permission.

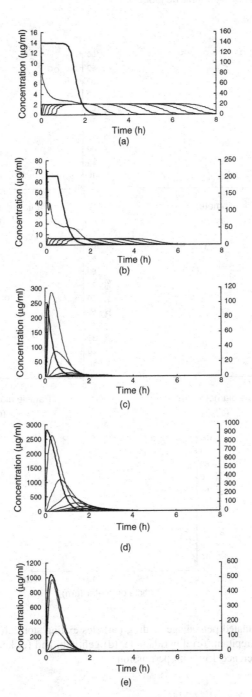

Figure 8.17 Simulated GI concentration. The lines from the left to the right: stomach (bold line), intestine compartments (1 to 7, proximal to distal). Axis: RHS stomach, LHS intestine. (a) Albendazole, (b) arepitant, (c) dipyridamole, (d) gefitinib, and (e) ketoconazole. *Source:* Adapted from Reference 159 with permission.

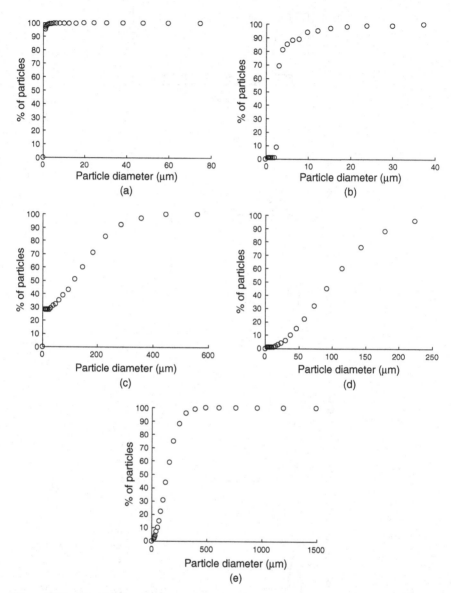

Figure 8.18 Simulated percentage of drug particles exiting stomach as undissolved. (a) Albendazole, (b) arepitant, (c) dipyridamole, (d) gefitinib, and (e) ketoconazole. *Source:* Adapted from Reference 159 with permission.

TABLE 8.5 BCS-Based Assessment of the Feasibility of Biopharmaceutical Modeling

BCS Class	API form/APermeation Pathway	I	II A	II B	III	IV
BCS I		Δ^b– ○	○^{b}	○^{b}	◎^{b}	◎^{b}
BCS II (dissolution limited)	Neutral	×^{b}	Δ	○	○	◎
	Free acid	×	Δ	○	○	◎
	Free base	×	× – Δ	Δ	Δ	◎
	Salts	×	×	× – Δ	Δ	○
BCS II (solubility limited)	Neutral	×	○	○	○	◎
	Free acid	×	○	○	○	◎
	Free base	×	× – Δ	× – Δ	Δ	○
	Salts	×	×	×	Δ	Δ
BCS III (permeability limited)	Passive	×	○	○	○	◎
	Active	×	Δ	Δ	Δ	○
BCS IV	—	×	×	×	Δ	○
Special formulations^c	—	×	×	×	Δ	○

Prediction Process Step^a spans columns I, II A, II B, III, IV.

^{a} See text.
^{b} ×, Poor predictability; Δ, marginal predictability; ○, reasonable predictability (e.g., with in twofold error with 70% probability); ◎, Excellent predictability.
^{c} SEDDS, solid dispersion, nano API particle, controlled release, etc.

8.8 RELIABILITY OF BIOPHARMACEUTICAL MODELING

As per the above discussions, the predictability of biopharmaceutical modeling is guesstimated based on the BCS (Table 8.5). BCS categorizes drugs into four classes based on the permeability and dose number. The theoretical basis of BCS is discussed in the next chapter. BCS is quite useful to navigate the strategy in drug discovery and development. BCS has been used as a common language among disciplines. Therefore, the BCS system is used as guidance for the reliability of biopharmaceutical modeling [2].

REFERENCES

1. Volgyi, G., Baka, E., Box, K.J., Comer, J.E., Takacs-Novak, K. (2010). Study of pH-dependent solubility of organic bases. Revisit of Henderson-Hasselbalch relationship. *Anal. Chim. Acta*, 673, 40–46.

2. Sugano, K. (2009). Introduction to computational oral absorption simulation. *Expert Opin. Drug Metab. Toxicol*, 5, 259–293.

3. Zhao, Y., Le, J., Abraham, M.H., Hersey, A., Eddershaw, P.J., Luscombe, C.N., Boutina, D., Beck, G., Sherborne, B., Cooper, I., Platts, J.A. (2001). Evaluation

of human intestinal absorption data and subsequent derivation of a quantitative structure-activity relationship (QSAR) with the Abraham descriptors. *J. Pharm. Sci.*, 90, 749–784.

4. Varma, M.V., Obach, R.S., Rotter, C., Miller, H.R., Chang, G., Steyn, S.J., El-Kattan, A., Troutman, M.D. (2010). Physicochemical space for optimum oral bioavailability: contribution of human intestinal absorption and first-pass elimination. *J. Med. Chem.*, 53, 1098–1108.

5. Zmuidinavicius, D., Didziapetris, R., Japertas, P., Avdeef, A., Petrauskas, A. (2003). Classification structure-activity relations (C-SAR) in prediction of human intestinal absorption. *J. Pharm. Sci.*, 92, 621.

6. Sugano, K., Takata, N., Machida, M., Saitoh, K., Terada, K. (2002). Prediction of passive intestinal absorption using bio-mimetic artificial membrane permeation assay and the paracellular pathway model. *Int. J. Pharm.*, 241, 241–251.

7. Shimizu, R., Sukegawa, T., Tsuda, Y., Itoh, T. (2008). Quantitative prediction of oral absorption of PEPT1 substrates based on *in vitro* uptake into Caco-2 cells. *Int. J. Pharm.*, 354, 104–110.

8. Saitoh, R., Sugano, K., Takata, N., Tachibana, T., Higashida, A., Nabuchi, Y., Aso, Y. (2004). Correction of permeability with pore radius of tight junctions in Caco-2 monolayers improves the prediction of the dose fraction of hydrophilic drugs absorbed by humans. *Pharm. Res.*, 21, 749.

9. Bretschneider, B., Brandsch, M., Neubert, R. (1999). Intestinal transport of beta-lactam antibiotics: analysis of the affinity at the H+/peptide symporter (PEPT1), the uptake into Caco-2 cell monolayers and the transepithelial flux. *Pharm. Res.*, 16, 55–61.

10. Ranadive, S.A., Chen, A.X., Serajuddin, A.T. (1992). Relative lipophilicities and structural-pharmacological considerations of various angiotensin-converting enzyme (ACE) inhibitors. *Pharm. Res.*, 9, 1480–1486.

11. Tam, K.Y., Avdeef, A., Tsinman, O., Sun, N. (2010). The permeation of amphoteric drugs through artificial membranes–an in combo absorption model based on paracellular and transmembrane permeability. *J. Med. Chem.*, 53, 392–401.

12. Sugano, K. (2011). Fraction of a dose absorbed estimation for structurally diverse low solubility compounds. *Int. J. Pharm.*, 405, 79–89.

13. Williams, P.E., Brown, A.N., Rajaguru, S., Francis, R.J., Walters, G.E., McEwen, J., Durnin, C. (1989). The pharmacokinetics and bioavailability of cilazapril in normal man. *Br. J. Clin. Pharmacol.*, 27 Suppl 2, 181S–188S.

14. Cilazapril. Interview form. http://www.info.pmda.go.jp.

15. Wessel, M.D., Jurs, P.C., Tolan, J.W., Muskal, S.M. (1998). Prediction of human intestinal absorption of drug compounds from molecular structure. *J. Chem. Inf. Comput. Sci.*, 38, 726–735.

16. Faropenem. Interview form. http://www.info.pmda.go.jp.

17. Lappin, G., Shishikura, Y., Jochemsen, R., Weaver, R.J., Gesson, C., Houston, B., Oosterhuis, B., Bjerrum, O.J., Rowland, M., Garner, C. (2010). Pharmacokinetics of fexofenadine: evaluation of a microdose and assessment of absolute oral bioavailability. *Eur. J. Pharm. Sci.*, 40, 125–131.

18. Bagli, M., Hoflich, G., Rao, M.L., Langer, M., Baumann, P., Kolbinger, M., Barlage, U., Kasper, S., Moller, H.J. (1995). Bioequivalence and absolute bioavailability of oblong and coated levomepromazine tablets in CYP2D6 phenotyped subjects. *Int. J. Clin. Pharmacol. Ther.*, 33, 646–652.

19. Wei, Y., Neves, L.A., Franklin, T., Klyuchnikova, N., Placzek, B., Hughes, H.M., Curtis, C.G. (2009). Vascular perfused segments of human intestine as a tool for drug absorption. *Drug Metab. Dispos.*, 37, 731–736.

20. Balon, K., Riebesehl, B.U., Muller, B.W. (1999). Drug liposome partitioning as a tool for the prediction of human passive intestinal absorption. *Pharm. Res.*, 16, 882–888.

21. Sugano, K., Artificial membrane technologies to assess transfer and permeation of drugs in drug discovery, in: B. Testa, H. van de Waterbeemd (Eds.) Comprehensive medicinal chemistry II Volume 5 ADME-Tox approach, Elsevier, Oxford, 2007, pp. 453–487.

22. Selvig, K. (1981). Pharmacokinetics of proxyphylline in adults after intravenous and oral administration. *Eur. J. Clin. Pharmacol.*, 19, 149–155.

23. Kansy, M., Senner, F., Gubernator, K. (1998). Physicochemical high throughput screening: parallel artificial membrane permeation assay in the description of passive absorption processes. *J. Med. Chem.*, 41, 1007–1010.

24. Knauf, H., Mutschler, E. (1984). Pharmacodynamics and pharmacokinetics of xipamide in patients with normal and impaired kidney function. *Eur. J. Clin. Pharmacol.*, 26, 513–520.

25. Obata, K., Sugano, K., Saitoh, R., Higashida, A., Nabuchi, Y., Machida, M., Aso, Y. (2005). Prediction of oral drug absorption in humans by theoretical passive absorption model. *Int. J. Pharm.*, 293, 183–192.

26. Avdeef, A., Absorption and Drug Development, Wiley-Interscience, NJ, Hoboken, 2003.

27. Lennernaes, H. (2007). Intestinal permeability and its relevance for absorption and elimination. *Xenobiotica*, 37, 1015–1051.

28. Lipka, E., Spahn-Langguth, H., Mutschler, E., Amidon, G.L. (1998). *In vivo* nonlinear intestinal permeability of celiprolol and propranolol in conscious dogs: evidence for intestinal secretion. *Eur. J. Pharm. Sci.*, 6, 75–81.

29. Zakeri-Milani, P., Valizadeh, H., Tajerzadeh, H., Azarmi, Y., Islambolchilar, Z., Barzegar, S., Barzegar-Jalali, M. (2007). Predicting human intestinal permeability using single-pass intestinal perfusion in rat. *J. Pharm. Pharm. Sci.*, 10, 368–379.

30. Chiou, W.L., Jeong, H.Y., Chung, S.M., Wu, T.C. (2000). Evaluation of using dog as an animal model to study the fraction of oral dose absorbed of 43 drugs in humans. *Pharm. Res.*, 17, 135–140.

31. Chiou, W.L., Barve, A. (1998). Linear correlation of the fraction of oral dose absorbed of 64 drugs between humans and rats. *Pharm. Res.*, 15, 1792–1795.

32. Knutson, T., Fridblom, P., Ahlstrom, H., Magnusson, A., Tannergren, C., Lennernas, H. (2008). Increased understanding of intestinal drug permeability determined by the LOC-I-GUT approach using multislice computed tomography. *Mol. Pharm.*, 6, 2–10.

33. Fagerholm, U., Johansson, M., Lennernaes, H. (1996). Comparison between permeability coefficients in rat and human jejunum. *Pharm. Res.*, 13, 1336–1342.

34. Kalantzi, L., Reppas, C., Dressman, J.B., Amidon, G.L., Junginger, H.E., Midha, K.K., Shah, V.P., Stavchansky, S.A., Barends, D.M. (2006). Biowaiver monographs for immediate release solid oral dosage forms: acetaminophen (paracetamol). *J. Pharm. Sci.*, 95, 4–14.

35. Takahashi, M., Washio, T., Suzuki, N., Igeta, K., Yamashita, S. (2010). Investigation of the intestinal permeability and first-pass metabolism of drugs in cynomolgus monkeys using single-pass intestinal perfusion. *Biol. Pharm. Bull.*, 33, 111–116.

36. Chiou, W.L., Buehler, P.W. (2002). Comparison of oral absorption and bioavailability of drugs between monkey and human. *Pharm. Res.*, 19, 868–874.

37. Avdeef, A., Tam, K.Y. (2010). How well can the Caco-2/Madin-Darby canine kidney models predict effective human jejunal permeability? *J. Med. Chem*, 53, 3566–3584.

38. Sugano, K., Nabuchi, Y., Machida, M., Aso, Y. (2003). Prediction of human intestinal permeability using artificial membrane permeability. *Int. J. Pharm.*, 257, 245–251.

39. Avdeef, A. (2010). Leakiness and size exclusion of paracellular channels in cultured epithelial cell monolayers-interlaboratory comparison. *Pharm. Res.*, 27, 480–489.

40. Avdeef, A., Bendels, S., Di, L., Faller, B., Kansy, M., Sugano, K., Yamauchi, Y. (2007). Parallel artificial membrane permeability assay (PAMPA)-critical factors for better predictions of absorption. *J. Pharm. Sci.*, 96, 2893–2909.

41. Reynolds, D.P., Lanevskij, K., Japertas, P., Didziapetris, R., Petrauskas, A. (2009). Ionization-specific analysis of human intestinal absorption. *J. Pharm. Sci.*, 98, 4039–4054.

42. Sugano, K., Hamada, H., Machida, M., Ushio, H. (2001). High throuput prediction of oral absorption: Improvement of the composition of the lipid solution used in parallel artificial membrane permeation assay. *J. Biomol. Screen*, 6, 189–196.

43. Sugano, K., Hamada, H., Machida, M., Ushio, H., Saitoh, K., Terada, K. (2001). Optimized conditions of bio-mimetic artificial membrane permeation assay. *Int. J. Pharm.*, 228, 181–188.

44. Sugano, K. (2009). Theoretical investigation of passive intestinal membrane permeability using Monte Carlo method to generate drug-like molecule population. *Int. J. Pharm.*, 373, 55–61.

45. Poelma, F.G.J., Breas, R., Tukker, J.J., Crommelin, D.J.A. (1991). Intestinal absorption of drugs. The influence of mixed micelles on the disappearance kinetics of drugs from the small intestine of the rat. *J. Pharm. Pharmacol.*, 43, 317–324.

46. Amidon, G.E., Higuchi, W.I., Ho, N.F.H. (1982). Theoretical and experimental studies of transport of micelle-solubilized solutes. *J. Pharm. Sci.*, 71, 77–84.

47. Sugano, K. (2009). Oral absorption simulation for low solubility compounds. *Chem. Biodivers.*, 6, 2014–2029.

48. Sugano, K., Obata, K., Saitoh, R., Higashida, A., Hamada, H. (2006). Processing of biopharmaceutical profiling data in drug discovery. Pharmacokinetic Profiling in Drug Research: Biological, Physicochemical, and Computational Strategies, [LogP2004, Lipophilicity Symposium], 3rd; 2004 Feb 29 Mar 4; Zurich, Switzerland. pp. 441–458.

49. Winiwarter, S., Bonham, N.M., Ax, F., Hallberg, A., Lennernas, H., Karlen, A. (1998). Correlation of human jejunal permeability (*in vivo*) of drugs with experimentally and theoretically derived parameters. A multivariate data analysis approach. *J. Med. Chem.*, 41, 4939–4949.

50. Hou, T., Wang, J., Li, Y. (2007). ADME evaluation in drug discovery. 8. The prediction of human intestinal absorption by a support vector machine. *J. Chem. Inf. Model*, 47, 2408–2415.

51. Shen, J., Cheng, F., Xu, Y., Li, W., Tang, Y. (2010). Estimation of ADME properties with substructure pattern recognition. *J. Chem. Inf. Model.*, 50, 1034–1041.

52. Fujioka, Y., Kadono, K., Fujie, Y., Metsugi, Y., Ogawara, K.-i., Higaki, K., Kimura, T. (2007). Prediction of oral absorption of griseofulvin, a BCS class II drug, based on GITA model: utilization of a more suitable medium for in-vitro dissolution study. *J. Controlled Release*, 119, 222–228.

53. Takano, R., Sugano, K., Higashida, A., Hayashi, Y., Machida, M., Aso, Y., Yamashita, S. (2006). Oral absorption of poorly water-soluble drugs: computer simulation of fraction absorbed in humans from a miniscale dissolution test. *Pharm. Res.*, 23, 1144–1156.

54. Takano, R., Doctoral Thesis, Setsunan University, 2009.

55. Matsson, P., Bergstroem, C.A.S., Nagahara, N., Tavelin, S., Norinder, U., Artursson, P. (2005). Exploring the role of different drug transport routes in permeability screening. *J. Med. Chem.*, 48, 604–613.

56. Sawyer, M.H., Webb, D.E., Balow, J.E., Straus, S.E. (1988). Acyclovir-induced renal failure. Clinical course and histology. *Am. J. Med.*, 84, 1067–1071.

57. Escher, B., Berger, C., Bramaz, N., Kwon, J.H., Richter, M., Tsinman, O., Avdeef, A. (2008). Membrane-water partitioning, membrane permeability and baseline toxicity. *Environ. Toxicol. Chem.*, 27, 909–918.

58. Fagerberg, J.H., Tsinman, O., Sun, N., Tsinman, K., Avdeef, A., Bergstrom, C.A.S. (2010). Dissolution rate and apparent solubility of poorly soluble drugs in biorelevant dissolution media. *Mol. Pharm.*, ACS ASAP.

59. Takano, R., Furumoto, K., Shiraki, K., Takata, N., Hayashi, Y., Aso, Y., Yamashita, S. (2008). Rate-limiting steps of oral absorption for poorly water-soluble drugs in dogs; prediction from a miniscale dissolution test and a physiologically-based computer simulation. *Pharm. Res.*, 25, 2334–2344.

60. Aprepitant (2009). Aprepitant Interview form. http://www.info.pmda.go.jp.

61. Singh, B.N. (2005). A quantitative approach to probe the dependence and correlation of food-effect with aqueous solubility, dose/solubility ratio, and partition coefficient (Log P) for orally active drugs administered as immediate-release formulations. *Drug Dev. Res.*, 65, 55–75.

62. Vertzoni, M., Fotaki, N., Kostewicz, E., Stippler, E., Leuner, C., Nicolaides, E., Dressman, J., Reppas, C. (2004). Dissolution media simulating the intraluminal composition of the small intestine: physiological issues and practical aspects. *J. Pharm. Pharmacol.*, 56, 453–462.

63. Carlert, S., Palsson, A., Hanisch, G., von Corswant, C., Nilsson, C., Lindfors, L., Lennernas, H., Abrahamsson, B. (2010). Predicting intestinal precipitation–a case example for a basic BCS class II drug. *Pharm. Res.*, 27, 2119–2130.

64. Schwebel, H.J., van Hoogevest, P., Leigh, M.L., Kuentz, M. (2011). The apparent solubilizing capacity of simulated intestinal fluids for poorly water-soluble drugs. *Pharm. Dev. Technol.*, 16, 278–286.

65. Kobayashi, Y., Ito, S., Itai, S., Yamamoto, K. (2000). Physicochemical properties and bioavailability of carbamazepine polymorphs and dihydrate. *Int. J. Pharm.*, 193, 137–146.

66. Shono, Y., Jantratid, E., Janssen, N., Kesisoglou, F., Mao, Y., Vertzoni, M., Reppas, C., Dressman, J.B. (2009). Prediction of food effects on the absorption of celecoxib based on biorelevant dissolution testing coupled with physiologically based pharmacokinetic modeling. *Eur. J. Pharm. Biopharm.*, 73, 107–114.

67. Sugano, K., Kataoka, M., da Costa Mathews, C., Yamashita, S. (2010). Prediction of food effect by bile micelles on oral drug absorption considering free fraction in intestinal fluid. *Eur. J. Pharm. Sci.*, 40, 118–124.

68. Jinno, J.-I., Kamada, N., Miyake, M., Yamada, K., Mukai, T., Odomi, M., Toguchi, H., Liversidge, G.G., Higaki, K., Kimura, T. (2006). Effect of particle size reduction on dissolution and oral absorption of a poorly water-soluble drug, cilostazol, in beagle dogs. *J. Controlled Release*, 111, 56–64.

69. Glomme, A., März, J., Dressman, J., Predicting the intestinal solubility of poorly soluble drugs in: B. Testa, S. Krämer, H. Wunderli-Allenspach, G. Folkers (Eds.) Pharmacokinetic Profiling in Drug Research, Wiley-VCH, Zurich, 2006, pp. 259–280.

70. Okazaki, A., Mano, T., Sugano, K. (2008). Theoretical dissolution model of polydisperse drug particles in biorelevant media. *J. Pharm. Sci.*, 97, 1843–1852.

71. Alsenz, J., Kansy, M. (2007). High throughput solubility measurement in drug discovery and development. *Adv. Drug Delivery Rev.*, 59, 546–567.

72. Dzimiri, N., Fricke, U., Klaus, W. (1987). Influence of derivatization on the lipophilicity and inhibitory actions of cardiac glycosides on myocardial sodium-potassium ATPase. *Br. J. Pharmacol.*, 91, 31–38.

73. Schamp, K., Schreder, S.-A., Dressman, J. (2006). Development of an *in vitro/in vivo* correlation for lipid formulations of EMD 50733, a poorly soluble, lipophilic drug substance. *Eur. J. Pharm. Biopharm.*, 62, 227–234.

74. Scholz, A., Abrahamsson, B., Diebold, S.M., Kostewicz, E., Polentarutti, B.I., Ungell, A.-L., Dressman, J.B. (2002). Influence of hydrodynamics and particle size on the absorption of felodipine in labradors. *Pharm. Res.*, 19, 42–46.

75. Hanafy, A., Spahn-Langguth, H., Vergnault, G., Grenier, P., Tubic Grozdanis, M., Lenhardt, T., Langguth, P. (2007). Pharmacokinetic evaluation of oral fenofibrate nanosuspensions and SLN in comparison to conventional suspensions of micronized drug. *Adv. Drug Delivery Rev.*, 59, 419–426.

76. Buch, P., Langguth, P., Kataoka, M., Yamashita, S. (2009). IVIVC in oral absorption for fenofibrate immediate release tablets using a dissolution/permeation system. *J. Pharm. Sci.*, 98, 2001–2009.

77. Takano, R., Takata, N., Saitoh, R., Furumoto, K., Higo, S., Hayashi, Y., Machida, M., Aso, Y., Yamashita, S. (2010). Quantitative analysis of the effect of supersaturation on *in vivo* drug absorption. *Mol. Pharm.*, 7, 1431–1440.

78. Yang, Z., Manitpisitkul, P., Sawchuk, R.J. (2006). *In situ* studies of regional absorption of lobucavir and ganciclovir from rabbit intestine and predictions of dose-limited absorption and associated variability in humans. *J. Pharm. Sci.*, 95, 2276–2292.

79. Wilson, C.G., O'Mahony, B., Connolly, S.M., Cantarini, M.V., Farmer, M.R., Dickinson, P.A., Smith, R.P., Swaisland, H.C. (2009). Do gastrointestinal transit parameters influence the pharmacokinetics of gefitinib? *Int. J. Pharm.*, 376, 7–12.

80. Gefitinib (2009). Gefitinib Interview form. http://www.info.pmda.go.jp.

81. Tosco, P., Rolando, B., Fruttero, R., Henchoz, Y., Martel, S., Carrupt, P.-A., Gasco, A. (2008). Physicochemical profiling of sartans: a detailed study of ionization constants and distribution coefficients. *Helv. Chim. Acta*, 91, 468–482.

82. Young, A.M., Audus, K.L., Proudfoot, J., Yazdanian, M. (2006). Tetrazole compounds: the effect of structure and pH on Caco-2 cell permeability. *J. Pharm. Sci.*, 95, 717–725.

83. Irbesartan (2009). Irbesartan Interview form. http://www.info.pmda.go.jp.

84. Bhattachar, S.N., Perkins, E.J., Tan, J.S., Burns, L.J. (2011). Effect of gastric pH on the pharmacokinetics of a bcs class II compound in dogs: utilization of an artificial stomach and duodenum dissolution model and gastroplus, simulations to predict absorption. *J. Pharm. Sci.*, 100(11), 4756–4765.

85. Lehto, P., Kortejarvi, H., Liimatainen, A., Ojala, K., Kangas, H., Hirvonen, J., Tanninen, V.P., Peltonen, L. (2011). Use of conventional surfactant media as surrogates for FaSSIF in simulating *in vivo* dissolution of BCS class II drugs. *Eur. J. Pharm. Biopharm.*, 78, 531–538.

86. Clarysse, S., Psachoulias, D., Brouwers, J., Tack, J., Annaert, P., Duchateau, G., Reppas, C., Augustijns, P. (2009). Postprandial changes in solubilizing capacity of human intestinal fluids for BCS Class II drugs. *Pharm. Res.*, 26, 1456–1466.

87. Nishihata, T., Ishizaka, M., Yokohama, S., Martino, A.C., Gordon, R.E. (1993). Effects of particle size of bulk drug and food on the bioavailability of U-78875 in dogs. *Drug Dev. Ind. Pharm.*, 19, 2679–2698.

88. Kataoka, M., Masaoka, Y., Yamazaki, Y., Sakane, T., Sezaki, H., Yamashita, S. (2003). *In vitro* system to evaluate oral absorption of poorly water-soluble drugs: simultaneous analysis on dissolution and permeation of drugs. *Pharm. Res.*, 20, 1674–1680.

89. Steingrimsdottir, H., Gruber, A., Palm, C., Grimfors, G., Kalin, M., Eksborg, S. (2000). Bioavailability of aciclovir after oral administration of aciclovir and its prodrug valaciclovir to patients with leukopenia after chemotherapy. *Antimicrob. Agents Chemother.*, 44, 207–209.

90. Vergin, H., Kikuta, C., Mascher, H., Metz, R. (1995). Pharmacokinetics and bioavailability of different formulations of aciclovir. *Arzneim.-Forsch.*, 45, 508–515.

91. Acyclovir. Interview form. http://www.info.pmda.go.jp.

92. Rigter, I.M., Schipper, H.G., Koopmans, R.P., Van Kan, H.J.M., Frijlink, H.W., Kager, P.A., Guchelaar, H.J. (2004). Relative bioavailability of three newly developed albendazole formulations: a randomized crossover study with healthy volunteers. *Antimicrob. Agents Chemother.*, 48, 1051–1054.

93. Schipper, H.G., Koopmans, R.P., Nagy, J., Butter, J.J., Kager, P.A., Van Boxtel, C.J. (2000). Effect of dose increase or cimetidine co-administration on albendazole bioavailability. *Am. J. Trop. Med. Hyg.*, 63, 270–273.

94. Wu, Y., Loper, A., Landis, E., Hettrick, L., Novak, L., Lynn, K., Chen, C., Thompson, K., Higgins, R., Batra, U., Shelukar, S., Kwei, G., Storey, D. (2004). The role of biopharmaceutics in the development of a clinical nanoparticle formulation of MK-0869: a Beagle dog model predicts improved bioavailability and diminished food effect on absorption in human. *Int. J. Pharm.*, 285, 135–146.

95. Webpage, The electronic Medicines Compendium Wellvone 750mg, http://www.medicines.org.uk/EMC/medicine/777/SPC/Wellvone+750mg+5ml+oral+suspension/.

96. Rolan, P.E., Mercer, A.J., Weatherley, B.C., Holdich, T., Meire, H., Peck, R.W., Ridout, G., Posner, J. (1994). Examination of some factors responsible for a food-induced increase in absorption of atovaquone. *Br. J. Clin. Pharmacol.*, 37, 13–20.

97. Freeman, C.D., Klutman, N.E., Lamp, K.C., Dall, L.H., Strayer, A.H. (1998). Relative bioavailability of atovaquone suspension when administered with an enteral nutrition supplement. *Ann. Pharmacother.*, 32, 1004–1007.

98. Dixon, R., Pozniak, A.L., Watt, H.M., Rolan, P., Posner, J. (1996). Single-dose and steady-state pharmacokinetics of a novel microfluidized suspension of atovaquone in human immunodeficiency virus-seropositive patients. *Antimicrob. Agents Chemother.*, 40, 556–560.

99. Zhang, X., Lionberger, R.A., Davit, B.M., Yu, L.X. (2011). Utility of physiologically based absorption modeling in implementing Quality by Design in drug development. *AAPS J.*, 13, 59–71.

100. Dolenc, A., Kristl, J., Baumgartner, S., Planinsek, O. (2009). Advantages of celecoxib nanosuspension formulation and transformation into tablets. *Int. J. Pharm.*, 376, 204–212.

101. Davies, N.M., McLachlan, A.J., Day, R.O., Williams, K.M. (2000). Clinical pharmacokinetics and pharmacodynamics of celecoxib: a selective cyclo-oxygenase-2 inhibitor. *Clin. Pharmacokinet.*, 38, 225–242.

102. Welling, P.G., Barbhaiya, R.H. (1982). Influence of food and fluid volume on chlorothiazide bioavailability: comparison of plasma and urinary excretion methods. *J. Pharm. Sci.*, 71, 32–35.

103. Dressman, J.B., Fleisher, D., Amidon, G.L. (1984). Physicochemical model for dose-dependent drug absorption. *J. Pharm. Sci.*, 73, 1274–1279.

104. Bramer, S.L., Forbes, W.P. (1999). Relative bioavailability and effects of a high fat meal on single dose cilostazol pharmacokinetics. *Clin. Pharmacokinet.*, 37, 13–23.

105. Bramer, S.L., Forbes, W.P., Mallikaarjun, S. (1999). Cilostazol pharmacokinetics after single and multiple oral doses in healthy males and patients with intermittent claudication resulting from peripheral arterial disease. *Clin. Pharmacokinet.*, 37 Suppl 2, 1–11.

106. Yamada, I., Goda, T., Kawata, M., Ogawa, K. (1990). Use of gastric acidity-controlled beagle dogs in bioavailability studies of cinnarizine. *Yakugaku Zasshi*, 110, 280–285.

107. Ogata, H., Aoyagi, N., Kaniwa, N., Ejima, A., Sekine, N., Kitamura, M., Inoue, Y. (1986). Gastric acidity dependent bioavailability of cinnarizine from two commercial capsules in healthy volunteers. *Int. J. Pharm.*, 29, 113–120.

108. Liversidge, G.G., Cundy, K.C. (1995). Particle size reduction for improvement of oral bioavailability of hydrophobic drugs: I. Absolute oral bioavailability of nanocrystalline danazol in beagle dogs. *Int. J. Pharm.*, 125, 91–97.

109. Sunesen, V.H., Vedelsdal, R., Kristensen, H.G., Christrup, L., Muellertz, A. (2005). Effect of liquid volume and food intake on the absolute bioavailability of danazol, a poorly soluble drug. *Eur. J. Pharm. Sci.*, 24, 297–303.

110. Charman, W.N., Rogge, M.C., Boddy, A.W., Berger, B.M. (1993). Effect of food and a monoglyceride emulsion formulation on danazol bioavailability. *J. Clin. Pharmacol.*, 33, 381–386.

111. Lloyd-Jones, J.G. (1977). Danazol plasma concentration in man. *J. Int. Med. Res.*, 5 Suppl 3, 18–24.

112. Jounela, A.J., Pentikainen, P.J., Sothmann, A. (1975). Effect of particle size on the bioavailability of digoxin. *Eur. J. Clin. Pharmacol.*, 8, 365–370.

113. Bjornsson, T.D., Mahony, C. (1983). Clinical pharmacokinetics of dipyridamole. *Thromb. Res.*, 93–104.

114. Russell, T.L., Berardi, R.R., Barnett, J.L., O'Sullivan, T.L., Wagner, J.G., Dressman, J.B. (1994). pH-Related changes in the absorption of dipyridamole in the elderly. *Pharm. Res.*, 11, 136–143.

115. Zhou, R., Moench, P., Heran, C., Lu, X., Mathias, N., Faria, T.N., Wall, D.A., Hussain, M.A., Smith, R.L., Sun, D. (2005). pH-dependent dissolution *in vitro* and absorption *in vivo* of weakly basic drugs: development of a canine model. *Pharm. Res.*, 22, 188–192.

116. Merck, FDA approval document for sustiva, http://www.accessdata.fda.gov/scripts/cder/drugsatfda/index.cfm.

117. Gao, J.Z., Hussain, M.A., Motheram, R., Gray, D. A. B., Benedek, I.H., Fiske, W.D., Doll, W.J., Sandefer, E., Page, R.C., Digenis, G.A. (2007). Investigation of human pharmacoscintigraphic behavior of two tablets and a capsule formulation of a high dose, poorly water soluble/highly permeable drug (Efavirenz). *J. Pharm. Sci.*, 96, 2970–2977.

118. Sauron, R., Wilkins, M., Jessent, V., Dubois, A., Maillot, C., Weil, A. (2006). Absence of a food effect with a 145mg nanoparticle fenofibrate tablet formulation. *Int. J. Clin. Pharmacol. Ther.*, 44, 64–70.

119. Zhu, T., Ansquer, J.-C., Kelly Maureen, T., Sleep Darryl, J., Pradhan Rajendra, S. (2010). Comparison of the gastrointestinal absorption and bioavailability of fenofibrate and fenofibric Acid in humans. *J. Clin. Pharmacol.*, 50, 914–921.

120. Guivarc'h, P.-H., Vachon, M.G., Fordyce, D. (2004). A new fenofibrate formulation: results of six single-dose, clinical studies of bioavailability under fed and fasting conditions. *Clin. Ther.*, 26, 1456–1469.

121. Spector, S.A., Busch, D.F., Follansbee, S., Squires, K., Lalezari, J.P., Jacobson, M.A., Connor, J.D., Jung, D., Shadman, A., Mastre, B., Buhles W., Drew W. L., AIDS Clinical Trials Group, and Cytomegalovirus Cooperative Study Group. (1995). Pharmacokinetic, safety, and antiviral profiles of oral ganciclovir in persons infected with human immunodeficiency virus: a phase I/II study. *J. Infect. Dis.*, 171, 1431–1437.

122. Bergman, E., Forsell, P., Persson, E.M., Knutson, L., Dickinson, P., Smith, R., Swaisland, H., Farmer, M.R., Cantarini, M.V., Lennernaes, H. (2007). Pharmacokinetics of gefitinib in humans: the influence of gastrointestinal factors. *Int. J. Pharm.*, 341, 134–142.

123. Tashtoush, B.M., Al-Qashi, Z.S., Najib, N.M. (2004). *In vitro* and *in vivo* evaluation of glibenclamide in solid dispersion systems. *Drug Dev. Ind. Pharm.*, 30, 601–607.

124. Ahmed, I.S., Aboul-Einien, M.H., Mohamed, O.H., Farid, S.F. (2008). Relative bioavailability of griseofulvin lyophilized dry emulsion tablet vs. immediate release tablet: a single-dose, randomized, open-label, six-period, crossover study in healthy adult volunteers in the fasted and fed states. *Eur. J. Pharm. Sci.*, 35, 219–225.

125. Chiou, W.L., Riegelman, S. (1971). Absorption characteristics of solid dispersed and micronized griseofulvin in man. *J. Pharm. Sci.*, 60, 1376–1380.

126. Hosny, E.A., El-Sayed, Y.M., Al-Meshal, M.A., Al-Angary, A.A. (1994). Effect of food on bioavailability of bioadhesive-containing indomethacin tablets in dogs. *Int. J. Pharm.*, 112, 87–91.

127. Jung, M.S., Kim, J.S., Kim, M.S., Alhalaweh, A., Cho, W., Hwang, S.J., Velaga, S.P. (2010). Bioavailability of indomethacin-saccharin cocrystals. *J. Pharm. Pharmacol.*, 62, 1560–1568.

128. Vachharajani, N.N., Shyu, W.C., Mantha, S., Park, J.S., Greene, D.S., Barbhaiya, R.H. (1998). Lack of effect of food on the oral bioavailability of irbesartan in healthy male volunteers. *J. Clin. Pharmacol.*, 38, 433–436.

129. Hirlekar, R.S., Sonawane, S.N., Kadam, V.J. (2009). Studies on the effect of water-soluble polymers on drug-cyclodextrin complex solubility. *AAPS PharmSciTech.*, 10, 858–863.

130. Irbesartan, Interview form, http://www.info.pmda.go.jp.

131. Guzzo, C.A., Furtek, C.I., Porras, A.G., Chen, C., Tipping, R., Clineschmidt, C.M., Sciberras, D.G., Hsieh, J. Y. K., Lasseter, K.C. (2002). Safety, tolerability, and pharmacokinetics of escalating high doses of ivermectin in healthy adult subjects. *J. Clin. Pharmacol.*, 42, 1122–1133.

132. Ivermectine, Interview form, http://www.info.pmda.go.jp.

133. Merck, F. D. A., approval document for ivermectin, in.

134. Lelawongs, P., Barone, J.A., Colaizzi, J.L., Hsuan, A. T. M., Mechlinski, W., Legendre, R., Guarnieri, J. (1988). Effect of food and gastric acidity on absorption of orally administered ketoconazole. *Clin. Pharm.*, 7, 228–235.

135. Mikus, G., Fischer, C., Heuer, B., Langen, C., Eichelbaum, M. (1987). Application of stable isotope methodology to study the pharmacokinetics, bioavailability and metabolism of nitrendipine after i.v. and p.o. administration. *Br. J. Clin. Pharmacol.*, 24, 561–569.

136. Sugimoto, M., Okagaki, T., Narisawa, S., Koida, Y., Nakajima, K. (1998). Improvement of dissolution characteristics and bioavailability of poorly water-soluble drugs by novel cogrinding method using water-soluble polymer. *Int. J. Pharm.*, 160, 11–19.

137. Hoshi, N., Kida, A., Hayashi, T., Murakami, Y. (2007). Development of PVA copolymer capsules II. *Pharm. Tech Jpn.*, 23, 75–80.

138. Sugimoto, I., Kuchiki, A., Nakagawa, H., Tohgo, K., Kondo, S., Iwane, I., Takahashi, K. (1980). Dissolution and absorption of nifedipine from nifedipine-polyvinylpyrrolidone coprecipitate. *Drug Dev. Ind. Pharm.*, 6, 137–160.

139. Lund, L., Alvan, G., Berlin, A., Alexanderson, B. (1974). Pharmacokinetics of single and multiple doses of phenytoin in man. *Eur. J. Clin. Pharmacol.*, 7, 81–86.

140. Mizuno, N., Shinkuma, D., Hamaguchi, T. (2003). Variance of bioavailability of pharmaceutical preparations and analysis of factors affecting it. *Yakugaku Zasshi*, 123, 477–493.

141. Yakou, S., Umehara, K., Sonobe, T., Nagai, T., Sugihara, M., Fukuyama, Y. (1984). Particle size dependency of dissolution rate and human bioavailability of phenytoin in powders and phenytoin-polyethylene glycol solid dispersions. *Chem. Pharm. Bull.*, 32, 4130–4136.

142. Hamaguchi, T., Shinkuma, D., Irie, T., Yamanaka, Y., Morita, Y., Iwamoto, B., Miyoshi, K., Mizuno, N. (1993). Effect of a high-fat meal on the bioavailability of phenytoin in a commercial powder with a large particle size. *Int. J. Clin. Pharmacol., Ther. Toxicol.*, 31, 326–330.

143. Nakajima, M., Kanamaru, M., Umematsu, T., Tsubokura, S. (1993).. A phase I clinical study of a Leukotriene C4, D4 and E4 receptor antagonist; ONO-1078 in healthy volunteers. *Rynsho Iyaku*, 9 Suppl 1, 3–29.

144. Brocks, D.R., Upward, J.W., Georgiou, P., Stelman, G., Doyle, E., Allen, E., Wyld, P., Dennis, M.J. (1996). The single and multiple dose pharmacokinetics of pranlukast in healthy volunteers. *Eur. J. Clin. Pharmacol.*, 51, 303–308.

145. Brocks, D.R., Upward, J., Davy, M., Howland, K., Compton, C., McHugh, C., Dennis, M.J. (1997). Evening dosing is associated with higher plasma concentrations of pranlukast, a leukotriene receptor antagonist, in healthy male volunteers. *Br. J. Clin. Pharmacol.*, 44, 289–291.

146. Pranlukast, Interview form, http://www.info.pmda.go.jp.

147. Overdiek, H. W. P. M., Merkus, F. W. H. M. (1986). Influence of food on the bioavailability of spironolactone. *Clin. Pharmacol. Ther.*, 40, 531–536.

148. Barber, D., Keuter, J., Kravig, K. (1998). A logical stepwise approach to laser diffraction particle size distribution analysis methods development and validation. *Pharm. Dev. Technol.*, 3, 153–161.

149. Pentikaeinen, P.J., Neuvonen, P.J., Backman, C. (1981). Human pharmacokinetics of tolfenamic acid, a new antiinflammatory agent. *Eur. J. Clin. Pharmacol.*, 19, 359–365.

150. Neuvonen, P.J., Kivisto, K.T. (1988). Effect of magnesium hydroxide on the absorption of tolfenamic and mefenamic acids. *Eur. J. Clin. Pharmacol.*, 35, 495–501.

151. Pedersen, S.B. (1994). Biopharmaceutical aspects of tolfenamic acid. *Pharmacol. Toxicol. (Oxford, UK)*, 75, 22–32.

152. Galia, E., Nicolaides, E., Horter, D., Lobenberg, R., Reppas, C., Dressman, J.B. (1998). Evaluation of various dissolution media for predicting *in vivo* performance of class I and II drugs. *Pharm. Res.*, 15, 698–705.

153. Jantratid, E., Janssen, N., Reppas, C., Dressman, J.B. (2008). Dissolution media simulating conditions in the proximal human gastrointestinal tract: an update. *Pharm. Res.*, 25, 1663–1676.

154. Li, C.-Y., Zimmerman, C.L., Wiedmann, T.S. (1996). Diffusivity of bile salt/phospholipid aggregates in mucin. *Pharm. Res.*, 13, 535–541.

155. Sugano, K. (2010). Computational oral absorption simulation of free base drugs. *Int. J. Pharm.*, 398, 73–82.

156. Johnson, K.C. (2003). Dissolution and absorption modeling: model expansion to simulate the effects of precipitation, water absorption, longitudinally changing intestinal permeability, and controlled release on drug absorption. *Drug Dev. Ind. Pharm.*, 29, 833–842.

157. Vertzoni, M., Pastelli, E., Psachoulias, D., Kalantzi, L., Reppas, C. (2007). Estimation of intragastric solubility of drugs. *Pharm. Res.*, 24, 909–917.

158. Pudipeddi, M., Zannou, E.A., Vasanthavada, M., Dontabhaktuni, A., Royce, A.E., Joshi, Y.M., Serajuddin, A.T.M. (2008). Measurement of surface pH of pharmaceutical solids: a critical evaluation of indicator dye-sorption method and its comparison with slurry pH method. *J. Pharm. Sci.*, 97, 1831–1842.

159. Sugano, K. (2010). Computational oral absorption simulation of free base drugs. *Int. J. Pharm.*, 398(1–2), 73–82.

160. Sugano, K. (2009). A simulation of oral absorption using classical nucleation theory. *Int. J. Pharm.*, 378, 142–145.

CHAPTER 9

BIOEQUIVALENCE AND BIOPHARMACEUTICAL CLASSIFICATION SYSTEM

"By far the best proof is experience."

—Francis Bacon

9.1 BIOEQUIVALENCE

The equivalence of bioavailabilities from two different formulations of the same drug is referred to as *bioequivalence* (BE). Even when two formulations contain the same drug, the C_p–time profiles after dosing these formulations could be different. Therefore, it is critically important to confirm the BE of C_p–time profiles when the formulation is changed during drug development (including generic drug development).

A standard BE study employs a crossover design in 12–24 healthy volunteers. A crossover design is employed to avoid the interindividual variations in drug disposition processes. The bioavailability of a drug product (both rate and extent of oral absorption) should be identical between the two formulations (Fig. 9.1). Definition of *in vivo* BE is

$$80\% < C_{max} < 125\% \text{ (with 90\% confidence interval)}$$

$$80\% < AUC < 125\% \text{ (with 90\% confidence interval)}.$$

Biopharmaceutics Modeling and Simulations: Theory, Practice, Methods, and Applications,
First Edition. Kiyohiko Sugano.
© 2012 John Wiley & Sons, Inc. Published 2012 by John Wiley & Sons, Inc.

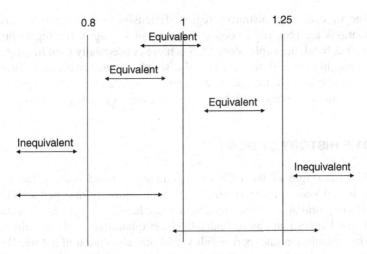

Figure 9.1 90% confidence interval and bioequivalence.

However, it is practically impossible to confirm BE by a clinical study every time the formulation is changed. The clinical BE study is expensive (ca. $100,000–250,000) and time consuming, which could in return be reflected in the drug price. In addition, it is ethically preferable to reduce the number of clinical studies with healthy volunteers. Therefore, the appropriate use of an *in vitro* dissolution test to waive (be exempted from) a clinical BE study would be of great benefit for both patients and industries [1]. However, it is well known that an *in vitro* dissolution test is not versatile for all drug products. Therefore, a guidance on when and for what case an *in vitro* study can be used to ensure BE is important.

The Biopharmaceutical classification system (BCS) was used as such guidance, first by the US FDA, and later by EMEA (EMA) and WHO. BCS has been widely known as a concept to classify a drug molecule on the basis of equilibrium solubility and effective permeability. Since the original publication in 1995 by Amidon and coworkers, this concept has been applied to various situations all through drug discovery and development [2, 3]. At present, BCS is used as a common language in the pharmaceutical industries, regulatory agencies and academia. At the same time, the discussion about BCS is often confused, as it is interpreted from different points of view.

BCS was derived from the same theories used in biopharmaceutical modeling. Therefore, in this section, as an important application of biopharmaceutical modeling, the BCS concept and its position in drug discovery and development are discussed. The concept of BCS is currently used for both regulatory and exploratory drug discovery perspectives, named regulatory BCS and exploratory BCS, respectively. The regulatory BCS is used in regulatory submission for biowaiver.[1] The formal BCS criteria are strictly defined in the regulatory

---

[1] After the candidate selection, especially after FIH, people tend to use the word "BCS" in this context.

guideline of each administrative region. Extensive and rigorous experimental investigations are required to define the class of a drug in the regulatory BCS. On the other hand, the exploratory BCS is more conceptually used in drug discovery and roughly defined on the basis of a simple *in vitro* experiment or even an *in silico* prediction.[2] In the following sections, we start with the original articles from the Amidon's group and then move forward to recent progresses.

9.2 THE HISTORY OF BCS

Probably, the origin of the BCS concept may be traced back to the 1960s or earlier. It had been well recognized that both solubility and permeability of a drug affect its oral absorption. Since then, there have been various theoretical and experimental investigations to understand the quantitative relationship between solubility, dissolution rate, permeability, and oral absorption of a drug. However, it remained unclear as to what parameters are essential to characterize the oral absorption of a drug. Especially, the dual role of solubility, that is, to determine both the maximum dissolved drug concentration and the dissolution rate, might have made it difficult to comprehend the relationships between each parameter.

In 1993, a pivotal paper was published by Amidon and coworkers [4]. They theoretically proved that three dimensionless parameters, that is, the dose number (Do), the dissolution number (Dn), and the absorption number (An), are sufficient to determine the oral absorption of a drug (for the cases without precipitation). They applied the plug flow model and rearranged the dissolution and permeability equations by introducing the above three dimensionless parameters. The following pair of differential equations was derived (Eqs. 9.1 and 9.2).[3]

$$\frac{dr^*}{dz^*} = -\frac{Dn}{3}(1 - C^*)\frac{C^*}{r^*} \tag{9.1}$$

$$\frac{dC^*}{dz^*} = Do \cdot Dn \cdot r^*(1 - C^*) - 2AnC^* \tag{9.2}$$

where

$$z^* = \frac{z}{L_{GI}}, C* = \frac{C_{dissolv}}{S_{dissolv}}, r* = \frac{r_p(t)}{r_{p,ini}} \tag{9.3}$$

$$Do = \frac{Dose}{S_{dissolv} \cdot V_{GI}} \tag{9.4}$$

$$Dn = k_{diss}T_{si} = \frac{3D_{eff}S_{dissolv}}{r_{p,ini}^2 \rho}T_{si} \tag{9.5}$$

[2]Before the candidate selection in drug discovery, people tend to use the word "BCS" in this context.
[3]As a courtesy for the original paper, An is used here. In the other parts in this book, permeation number (Pn) is used to simplify the equation.

$$\text{An} = \frac{1}{2}k_{\text{perm}}T_{\text{si}} \left(= \frac{1}{2}\text{Pn} \right) \tag{9.6}$$

where z^*, C^*, and r^* are the dimensionless variants representing the position of the API particle in the GI tract, C_{dissolv}, and r_p at the position, respectively. By the plug flow model, the time after oral administration was converted to the position of API particles in the GI tract at the time (z^*) (cf. Eq. 5.2).

Even though Equations 9.1 and 9.2 are still sequential differential equations, all the coefficients are grouped into the three dimensionless parameters.[4] This means that the oral absorption of a drug is sufficiently described by these three dimensionless parameters.

$$\text{Fa} = f(\text{Do}, \text{Dn}, \text{Pn}) \tag{9.7}$$

This is the most important conclusion of the 1993 paper. This finding means that if the identity of Dn, Do, and Pn between the two formulations were shown, the BE of the two formulations could then be proved.[5] This congruent condition for BE is discussed in Section 9.3).

In the 1993 paper, the pair of the equations was then numerically solved[6] to investigate the shape of Equation 9.7 (Fig. 9.2). At present, we have an approximate analytical solution as [5, 6]

$$\text{Fa}_{\text{SS}} = 1 - \exp\left(-\frac{1}{\dfrac{1}{k_{\text{diss}}} + \dfrac{\text{Do}}{k_{\text{perm}}}} \cdot T_{\text{si}} \right)$$

$$= 1 - \exp\left(-\frac{1}{\dfrac{1}{\text{Dn}} + \dfrac{\text{Do}}{\text{Pn}}} \right) \quad \text{If Do} < 1, \text{Do} = 1 \tag{9.8}$$

In 1995, on the basis of the above-mentioned theoretical analysis,[7] the BCS classification was proposed by Amidon and coworkers [7]. In the original BCS paper, solubility, rather than the dose number, was first used for classification. Furthermore, the low solubility/high permeability class (today, this corresponds to BCS II) was described as "the cases where An is high and dissolution number

[4]This is in a similar situation of the Reynolds number (Re) in the Navier–Stokes equation. The parameters of the flow system, for example, main flow velocity (U), fluid viscosity (μ), fluid density (ρ), and representative length (L), are lumped into Re as $\text{Re} = UL\rho/\mu$.

[5]This is something as proving the congruence of triangle by Angel-Side-Angle theorem.

[6]This is one of the earliest applications of computational biopharmaceutical modeling.

[7]The title of the first paper that underwrites the BCS is "Theoretical bases for BCS," however, not "BCS as theoretical bases of oral absorption." Sometimes BCS is referred to as a theory. However, this is misleading because BCS is the consequence of a theory but not the theory itself. The theoretical bases of BCS is Equations 9.1–9.6.

(Dn) is low." Currently, the dose number (Do) is used for low/high solubility definition. The quadrants of the BCS panel (Do-Pn[8] panel) were assigned a BCS class I–IV as (Fig. 9.3)

$$\text{BCS I} : \text{Do} < 1, \ \text{Pn} > 3$$

$$\text{BCS II} : \text{Do} > 1, \ \text{Pn} > 3$$

$$\text{BCS III} : \text{Do} < 1, \ \text{Pn} < 3$$

$$\text{BCS IV} : \text{Do} > 1, \ \text{Pn} < 3.$$

In 1999, another classification scheme was introduced by Yu et al. [8]. In the BCS classification, the dissolution number (Dn) is not taken into account. In Yu's classification, the dissolution-rate-limited (DRL) and solubility-permeability limited cases are separated. Currently, we define them as

$$\text{Dissolution-rate limited} : \text{Dn} < \ \text{Pn}/\text{Do}$$

$$\text{Permeability limited} : \ \text{Pn} < \text{Dn}, \text{Do} < 1$$

$$\text{Solubility–permeability limited} : \ \text{Pn}/\text{Do} < \text{Dn}, \text{Do} > 1.$$

A drug being classified as BCS II does not mean that its oral absorption is categorized as "DRL." Actually, the majority of BCS class II drugs are "solubility–permeability limited" (Section 9.5.2). Furthermore, even in the case of BCS class I and III drugs (i.e., Do < 1, high solubility), the oral absorption could be "DRL." For example, for a drug with a dose strength of 1 mg, solubility of 0.05 mg/ml, particle diameter of 200 μm, and $P_{eff} = 3 \times 10^{-4}$ cm/s, the oral absorption would be DRL even though Do is less than 1 (Do = 0.2, Dn = 0.4, Pn = 8.6).

9.3 REGULATORY BIOWAIVER SCHEME AND BCS

The regulatory BCS is used in the biowaiver scheme (BWS) for a BE study. Currently, the following two-step strategy is employed as the BWS in several regulatory bodies.

BWS step 1: BCS classification

BWS step 2: *In Vitro* dissolution test.

---

[8]The original criteria of permeability is defined by Fa% (high permeability is Fa% > 90%). If there is no solubility/dissolution-rate limitation and absorption occurs homogeneously in the small intestine, there is one to one relationship between Fa% and Pn as Fa = 1 − exp(−Pn). Therefore, in this book, Pn is used instead of Fa%. Fa% is often not available, especially for the solubility-limited and DRL cases. Therefore, Pn is more realistic as a permeability parameter. Caco-2 permeability has been used as the surrogate of Fa% in regulatory submission. As you see in this section, the use of Pn makes the discussion much more straightforward and comprehensive. Fa% is a time-dependent parameter (T_{si} dependent) but not a thermodynamic (equilibrium) parameter.

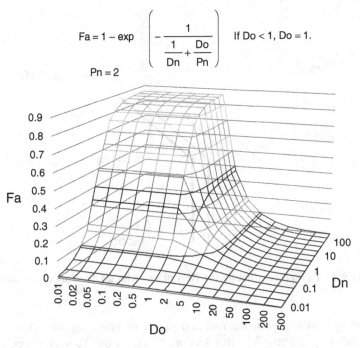

$$Fa = 1 - \exp\left(-\cfrac{1}{\cfrac{1}{Dn}+\cfrac{Do}{Pn}}\right) \quad \text{If } Do < 1, Do = 1.$$

$$Pn = 2$$

Figure 9.2 Shape of Fa function calculated by Fa_{SS} equation.

The first step is the classification of an active pharmaceutical ingredient (API) by dose/solubility ratio and permeability. BCS I drugs are granted permission to proceed to the second step (FDA guideline).[9] The second step is a dissolution test. An official dissolution test apparatus is used to confirm the identity of the dissolution process (e.g., USP paddle, 50 rpm, 900 ml, 85% dissolution in 30 min).

However, the scientific rationale behind applying this two-step process is not self-evident. Why is it acceptable to use an *in vitro* dissolution test for BCS I drugs but not for BCS II–IV drugs? In the following sections, this point is discussed in detail.

9.3.1 Elucidation of BCS Criteria in Regulatory Biowaiver Scheme

In the original BCS paper published in 1995, it was written that "(this analysis) clarifies the regime of the drug absorption process and offers a basis for determining when and under which condition *in vitro*–in vivo correlation are to be expected." [7]. Later in 2002, Yu of FDA wrote [9]: "When combined with the *in vitro* dissolution characteristics of the drug product, the BCS takes into account three major factors: solubility, intestinal permeability, and dissolution

---

[9] A clinical BE study is required for BCS II–IV drugs.

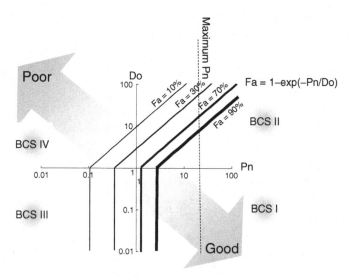

Figure 9.3 Fa% contour line in the BCS plane (with no dissolution-rate limitation).

rate, all of which govern the rate and extent of oral drug absorption from IR solid oral-dosage forms." In this section, based on the Yu's assertion, a further elucidation of the BCS criteria is attempted.[10]

9.3.1.1 Congruent Condition of Bioequivalence.

Let us assume that a compendium *in vitro* dissolution test can be used to prove the equivalence of the *in vivo* dissolution number (Dn) as in the BWS step 2.[11] If Do and Pn were proved to be equivalent between the test and reference products, the two drug products can be proved to be bioequivalent by the congruent condition of BE (Fig. 9.4). The next question is to define the conditions by which a formulation change would not affect Do and Pn.

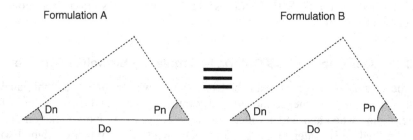

Figure 9.4 The congruent condition of bioequivalence.

[10] The following discussions are personal opinions.
[11] But this assumption is questionable.

9.3.1.2 Equivalence of Dose Number (Do).

When the solubility of an API is sufficient to completely dissolve the drug in the stomach and the small intestine, the dose number becomes less than 1. In the approximate Fa% equation (Eq. 9.8), if Do is less than 1, regardless of the Do value, it is reset to 1. This means that when Do < 1, it does not affect the Fa%. Therefore, the equivalence of Do in Fa% equation can be proved if Do < 1 for both the drug products. Usually, excipients do not reduce the solubility of a drug. Therefore, it is sufficient to show the Do value of an API to be less than 1. The Do value for regulatory BCS is calculated based on the equilibrium solubility of a drug at physiological gastrointestinal pHs (pH 1.2–6.8 or 7.4) at 37° C, the highest dose strength, and a fluid volume of 250 ml.[12]

9.3.1.3 Equivalence of Permeation Number (Pn).

Similarly, we can discuss the conditions in which Pn is not affected by the formulation. As discussed in Chapter 4, the rate-limiting process of membrane permeation can be categorized into the unstirred water layer (UWL) and epithelial membrane permeations. The UWL diffusion is a simple diffusion process through the aqueous layer, and it is highly unlikely that any excipient will change the diffusion rate through this layer. On the other hand, it is possible that some excipients affect the epithelial membrane permeability by changing the lipid membrane fluidity or by affecting the carrier-mediated transport of a drug. The effective permeability (P_{eff}) becomes UWL limited when $P_{eff} > 2 \times 10^{-4}$ cm/s. Therefore, Pn > 5.5 would be sufficient to show the equivalence of Pn between the two drug products.[13] Currently, metoprolol ($P_{eff} = 1.3 \times 10^{-4}$ cm/s, Pn = 3.7) is used as a marker for high/low permeability. For methanol, it was suggested that about 50% of the permeation resistance was from the UWL [10]. Originally, the permeability criteria was defined based on Fa% in humans. In FDA regulatory guidance, Fa% > 90% is used as the permeability criteria, which corresponds to Pn = 2.3.

In the biopharmaceutical drug disposition classification system (BDDCS) [11, 12], when the total amount of oxidative and conjugate metabolites is > 90%, the drug is categorized as high permeability (cf. drug metabolism usually occurs after absorption into the body).

In addition, Pn also affects the criteria setting of Dn equivalence in two different meanings: (i) the setoff effect of dissolution rate difference between two formulations and (ii) the maintenance of sink condition *in vivo*. These points are discussed in the next section.

9.3.1.4 Equivalence of Dissolution Number (Dn).

Once the equivalences of Do and Pn are proved in BWS step 1, we can proceed to BWS step 2, the dissolution test. If the dissolution numbers (Dn) of the two drug products are

---

[12]The equilibrium solubility at a pH is basically identical, regardless of the starting material being a salt or free from. On the other hand, the intrinsic dissolution rate depends on the API being free or salt. Therefore, the intrinsic dissolution rate cannot be used for BCS.

[13]Extension of permeability criteria to low–moderate permeability (BCS class III) is possible, if we can prove that the excipients used in the formulation do not alter the permeability of a drug.

proved equivalent in BWS step 2,[14] as the equivalences of Do and Pn have already been proved in BWS step 1, we can then prove the *in vivo* BE of the two formulations in accordance with the congruent condition for BE. However, unlike Do and Pn, a mechanistic consideration cannot be used to show the equivalence of Dn. Therefore, the equivalence of Dn has to be proved by an *in vitro* dissolution test. For this purpose, the *in vitro* dissolution test should reflect the *in vivo* conditions. The dissolution process of a drug product *in vivo* is affected by various factors such as pH, buffer species, surfactant, shear force, and destructive force. However, a simple compendium dissolution test cannot capture all the factors of the *in vivo* dissolution. Therefore, we should carefully design a dissolution test. Usually, the discrimination power of a dissolution test is as follows:

- Weak agitation > strong agitation
- Less solubilizer > more solubilizer
- Sink condition > nonsink condition.

If the Dns of the two formulations are diagnosed as equivalent under the conditions that are more discriminative than the *in vivo* situation, we can expect that the two formulations will show the same dissolution profiles *in vivo*. However, because of uncertainty in the similarity of *in vitro* and *in vivo* conditions, a safer criterion is used in regulatory guidelines.

Rapid dissolution (>85% dissolution in 30 min) is employed in the FDA, EMEA, and WHO guidelines for BCS I. In addition, very rapid dissolution (>85% dissolution in 15 min) is also used in the WHO guideline for BCS III. The rationale of the rapid and very rapid dissolution criteria is that if the mean dissolution time (MDT) of the two formulations is much smaller than the intestinal transit time (ca. 210 min), the effect of the difference of the dissolution rates on Fa% would be minimum (hence Dn can be considered to be equivalent).

The relationship between the dissolution rate, permeability, and BE has been investigated using biopharmaceutical modeling [13–15]. Figure 9.5 shows the effect of mean dissolution time (MDT $= 1/k_{\text{diss}}$) and mean permeation time (MPT $= 1/k_{\text{perm}}$) on the maximum difference of Fa% (i.e., instant dissolution vs 85% dissolution at 15 or 30 min) (Do < 1). When permeability is higher (MPT is smaller), the difference in Fa% becomes smaller. When the very rapid dissolution criterion is used (85% dissolution at 15 min), the difference in Fa% becomes less than 20%, regardless of the permeability of the drug. When the rapid dissolution criterion is used (85% dissolution at 30 min), the permeability number of the drug needs to be larger than 2.3 ($P_{\text{eff,human}} > 0.8 \times 10^{-4}$ cm/s) for the difference of Fa% to be less than 20%.

Currently (as of September, 2011), in the FDA, EMEA, and WHO guidelines, a sink condition is required for the dissolution test. A sink condition is defined as the dissolved drug concentration being less than 30% of the equilibrium solubility in the fluid. The Do < 1 condition in BWS step 1 automatically guarantees a sink

---

[14]Here, we include the disintegration process in Dn.

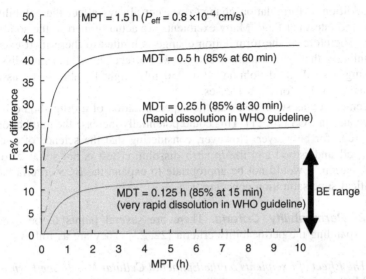

Figure 9.5 The relationship between Fa% difference, MPT, and MDT.

condition in the 900-ml dissolution test (cf. Do is calculated based on 250 ml volume). However, Do < 1 does not guarantee a sink condition *in vivo*, especially when the permeability of a drug is low (therefore, the criterion should be Do < 0.3 for BCS III). The high permeability (Pn > 3) works to maintain a sink condition *in vivo*.

9.3.2 Possible Extension of the Biowaiver Scheme

Historically, the BCS criteria was set conservative and the biowaiver was granted only for BCS class I drugs. At the same time, the expansion of applicable BCS category has been investigated.

9.3.2.1 Dose Number Criteria. Currently, Do is calculated on the basis of the minimum equilibrium solubility between pH 1.2 and 7.4 (or 6.8). However, as the main absorption site is the small intestine, Do < 1 at neutral pH in the small intestine is expected to be sufficient to prove the BE. Many NSAIDs that have Do > 1 in the stomach and Do < 1 in the intestine show a complete oral absorption after oral administration [16–18].

The use of a biorelevant media such as FaSSIF would be more suitable to judge the dose number for drugs with low solubility [19].

Ideally, both *in vitro* and *in vivo* dissolutions should be under a sink condition. Therefore, Do < 0.3 would be safer than Do < 1. Considering that absorption of the dissolved drug into the body can enhance the *in vivo* sink condition, Sn < 0.3 would be a more suitable criteria to judge the *in vivo* sink condition (cf. Sn = 1/(1 + Pn/(Dn × Do)), Eq. 5.32).

In addition, a formulation change does not always affect the solubility of a drug in the intestinal fluid. Many excipients are actually inert to the solubility of a drug. Therefore, if the formulation change is limited to these inert excipients, it is unlikely that a formulation change will affect Do. A nonsink dissolution test using a small fluid volume (100–250 ml) might be able to be assess the equivalence of Do for Do >1 cases.

Recently, it was suggested that the supersaturation of a drug should be taken into account in BCS [20, 21]. This could potentially increase the number of applicable drugs for biowaiver. However, considering that the science of nucleation is not well understood and the *in vitro* dissolution test is not suitable to assess the nucleation, it would not be appropriate to expand the BCS criteria based on the critical supersaturation concentration.

9.3.2.2 Permeability Criteria. There are several points to be considered when expanding the permeability criteria [22, 23]. They are as follows:

1. *The Effect of Excipients on the Epithelial Cellular Membrane Permeability.* Most excipients are actually inert to the permeability for passive transport case. However, the effect of excipients on carrier-mediated transports is not well known. In addition, the effect of excipients on the GI physiology (such as GI mobility) is also not well known and needs further investigations [24].
2. *The Relationship with the Dissolution-Rate Criterion.* As discussed above, theoretically, the permeability criterion affects the dissolution test criterion.
3. *Maintenance of Sink Condition by Permeability.* For drugs with low permeability, its absorption is not effective to maintain a sink condition in the *in vivo* small intestine. Therefore, Do < 0.3 would be a safer criterion to guarantee a sink condition *in vivo* for drugs with low permeability.

9.3.3 Another Interpretation of the Theory

In the previous section, the mainstream opinions about the BWS, the BCS BWS, are discussed. In this section, this topic is discussed with a different logical plot.

9.3.3.1 Another Assumption about Dissolution Test. The discussion about the BCS BWS is based on an assumption that the equivalence of the dissolution number (Dn) can be assessed by a compendium dissolution test. However, most of the practical formulation scientists think that it may not be a valid assumption. Considering the simple paddle apparatus and artificial dissolution test media being in contrast to the complex *in vivo* GI physiology, it is obvious that the *in vitro* paddle method cannot represent all factors of the *in vivo* dissolution. The 50-rpm paddle method is most often used in the dissolution test. However, it was reported that the agitation strength in humans corresponds to 10–30 rpm (Section 6.2.3). At present, extensive investigations are underway to develop more biorelevant dissolution tests [25]. On the other hand, as long as standard excipients, which are usually inert for equilibrium solubility and permeability of a drug, are used, the dose number (Do) and permeation number (Pn) should not be affected by the difference of the two formulations. Therefore, the proof of the equivalence for the dissolution number (Dn) would be the most uncertain among the three parameters. Once this assumption is agreed upon, the next question is what kinds of drugs are less sensitive to the uncertainty of the Dn equivalence.

9.3.3.2 *Assessment of Suitability of Dissolution Test Based on Rate-Limiting Process.* As discussed in the previous sections, the oral absorption of drug products can be categorized as DRL, permeability limited (PL), and solubility–permeability limited (SL). Solubility–permeability limited can be further categorized by the rate-limiting process in permeability, that is, solubility UWL limited (SL-U) and solubility epithelial membrane permeability limited (SL-E).

Even though it is counterintuitive, theoretically, the oral absorption of an SL drug should be less sensitive to the uncertainty of the Dn equivalence, as Pn/Do dominates the oral absorption of the drug. This class of compound corresponds to BCS II or IV. When we compare UWL and epithelial-membrane-limited cases in this class (i.e., SL-U and SL-E, respectively), the former case is possibly sensitive to the particle size of the API because of the particle drifting effect. Therefore, SL-E should be most insensitive to a change in formulation. In addition, the solubility of drugs in this class is less sensitive to the surfactant, as the main reason for low solubility would be high crystallinity but not lipophilicity (Section 2.3.7). SL-E corresponds to BCS class IV. Therefore, BCS class IV would be the most probable case where *in vitro* equivalences of the three parameters can be translated to *in vivo* equivalence. This is the opposite of what is suggested by the BCS BWS.

The DRL case is most sensitive to the differences between *in vitro* and *in vivo* dissolution conditions. Therefore, if an *in vitro* dissolution test is not a good representation of an *in vivo* situation, an appropriate IVIVC should not be observed. In a permeability-limited case (Pn < Dn), the dissolution rate can affect the C_{max}, as the flux $= C_{dissolv} \times P_{eff}$ and $C_{dissolv}$ in the early stages of oral absorption largely depends on the dissolution rate. If the *in vitro* dissolution rate of a drug is threefold faster than the *in vivo* dissolution rate, 85% dissolution in 30 min *in vitro* could be 30% dissolution *in vivo*. Figure 9.6 shows such a case.

9.3.4   Validation of Biowaiver Scheme by Clinical BE Data

The most conservative criterion for Do and Pn, that is, "Do < 1 and Pn > 2.3," was originally adopted by the FDA. As discussed above, this BCS BWS is based on the theoretical consideration, and therefore, needs to be validated experimentally. What percentage of biowaivered drug products actually shows clinical BE in healthy volunteers (and even in patients)? This type of investigation is critical for the future improvements of the BCS BWS.

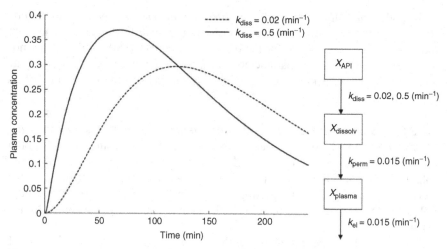

Figure 9.6 Effect of dissolution rate on C_{max} for a BCS III drug. Simulation results based on three sequential first-order kinetics (k_{diss}, k_{perm}, and k_{el}).

Recently, the result of a validation study of the BCS scheme was reported [26]. The results of 124 clinical BE studies were statistically analyzed based on the BCS classes. As expected from both the BCS and rate-limiting process discussions, BCS II showed the largest percentage of clinical inequivalence. However, BCS I showed ca. 15% false-positive results. All of them failed BE in C_{max} but not in AUC. This ratio is similar for BCS class III. Surprisingly, even though the number of samples is small, six out of seven BCS IV cases showed clinical BE.

9.3.5 Summary for Regulatory BCS Biowaiver Scheme

In summary, even though the final clause of the BCS BWS looks different for each regulatory body, the basic concept for biowaiver is the same, that is, "Fa% is determined by Dn, Do and Pn. If a formulation change has no effect on all Dn, Do and Pn, the two products will be bioequivalent" [9]. In the BCS-based BWS, the BCS classification is used to diagnose unlikeliness that a formulation change would affect Do and Pn. The compendium dissolution test is used to diagnose equivalence in Dn. Even though FDA, EMA, and WHO have the same structure of the BWS, that is, BCS + dissolution test, each regulatory agency has different criteria. Furthermore, another logical scenario can be derived from the same theory of oral absorption.

The BCS BWS should be further experimentally validated in the future. Meanwhile, for the safety of patients, it might be another good judgment to request a clinical BE study for the first launch of a generic drug product or after a significant change in formulation and manufacture process.

Even though the scientific basis is the same, the regulatory scheme in each administrable region can be different depending on the tolerance of the nation for the risk and cost, which depends on the culture, history, ethnic difference, medical care and insurance schemes, etc. The regulatory scheme should be determined by the sovereignty of the nation. In addition, the patients have the right to know whether the drug product is approved based on the BWS or a clinical BE study [27],[15] and the freedom of choice.

9.4 EXPLORATORY BCS

The BCS concept has been widely used in drug discovery. In the lead optimization process, the BCS plane can be used to navigate the SAR. Combination of PAMPA and high throughput solubility screening was found to be able to give appropriate BCS classification [28].

The BCS concept is also applied to judge the developability of a drug [29]. The BCS plane can be used to diagnose whether the standard particle size reduction would result in a good Fa% or a special formulation will be required for the development. Particle size reduction down to 10 μm is usually achieved using a standard milling technology and will not be a development issue. In Equation 9.8, if the Do/Pn term is greater than 1, even when particle size is reduced (Dn ≫ 1), the Fa% would not exceed 60% (as 1/Dn + Do/Pn cannot exceed 1). This criterion is determined by the ratio of Do and Pn. In other words, high permeability can compensate low solubility to give adequate Fa%. This concept is basically the same as that proposed by Lipinski based on the MAD calculation, which suggests that low/high solubility criteria for drug development change with the permeability and the dose strength of a drug [30].

9.5 *IN VITRO–IN VIVO* CORRELATION

IVIVC can be used as a biowaiver approach for extended-release formulations, as the release process becomes the rate-limiting step, but not the solubility and permeation.

9.5.1 Levels of IVIVC

The levels of IVIVC have been defined in the FDA guidelines as follows:

- Level A correlation is based on the relationship between *in vitro* and *in vivo* dissolved %. *In Vivo* dissolved % can be obtained by a deconvolution method such as the Wagner–Nelson, Loo–Riegelman, and model-independent numerical deconvolution methods (Section 5.5.4).
- Level B correlation is the relationship between the mean *in vitro* dissolution time ($MDT_{in\ vitro}$) of a product and the mean *in vivo* residence time (MRT) or the mean *in vivo* dissolution time ($MDT_{in\ vivo}$).

---

[15]In Japan, this information is available in the label or the interview form of generic products.

- Level C correlation is the relationship between one dissolution time point (e.g., $t_{50\%}$) and one mean pharmacokinetic parameter such as AUC, T_{max}, or C_{max}.

9.5.2 Judgment of Similarity Between Two Formulations (f2 Function)

The $f2$ function is most often used to quantify the similarity between the dissolution profiles of two formulations. The similarity factor ($f2$) can be calculated as

$$f2 = 50 \times \log_{10} \left(\left(1 + \frac{1}{n} \sum_{t=1}^{n} (R_t - T_t)^2 \right)^{-0.5} \times 100 \right) \qquad (9.9)$$

where n is the number of the sampling time points and R_t and T_t are the dissolved % values at time t for reference and test formations, respectively. The $f2$ becomes 100 when the dissolution profiles of two formulations are identical. When the dissolved fraction differs by 10% at each sample point, $f2 = 50$. When $50 < f2 < 100$, the two formulations are thought to have equivalent dissolution profiles.

9.5.3 Modeling the Relationship Between f2 and Bioequivalence

The relationship between the *in vitro* similarity ($f2$) and *in vivo* BE has been recently investigated using computational simulation [31]. In this section, a simpler approach is taken to correlate *in vitro* similarity and *in vivo* equivalence.

An IVIVC is expected most likely in the cases of DRL absorption. Therefore, by replacing k_a with k_{disso} in Equation 5.41, we obtain

$$C_p(t) = \frac{\text{Dose} \times \text{FgFh}}{V_d} \cdot \frac{k_{diss}}{k_{diss} - k_{el}} (\exp(-k_{el} \cdot t) - \exp(-k_{diss} \cdot t)) \cdots t \leq T_{si}$$

$$(9.10)$$

$$C_p(t) = C_p(T_{si}) \exp(-k_{el} \cdot (t - T_{si})) \cdots t > T_{si} \qquad (9.11)$$

$$T_{max} = \frac{\ln(k_{disso}/k_{el})}{k_{disso} - k_{el}} \qquad (9.12)$$

The $f2$ was calculated after calculating the Dissolved % at the time points of 1/4, 1/2, 3/4, and 1 of the time of 85% dissolution.

$$\text{Dissolved\%} = 1 - \exp(-k_{diss} \cdot t) \qquad (9.13)$$

These equations are used to calculate C_{max} of test and reference formulations with $k_{disso,test}$ and $k_{disso,reference}$, respectively. As shown in Figure 9.7, the range of $80\% < C_{max,test}/C_{max,reference} < 125\%$ overlaps the range of $f2 > 50$. Therefore, $f2 > 50$ is a good criterion to predict BE in clinical studies.

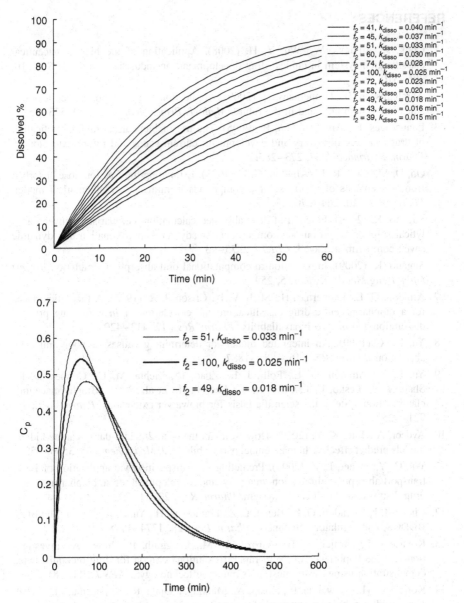

Figure 9.7 f_2 function and bioequivalence.

9.5.4 Point-to-Point IVIVC

The total amount dissolved until time t *in vitro* ($A_{in\,vitro}$) and the total amount absorbed until time t ($A_{in\,vivo}$) is often related using the following function.

$$A_{in\,vivo} = a1 + a2 \times A_{in\,vitro}(b1 + b2 \times t) \qquad (9.14)$$

REFERENCES

1. Cook, J., Addicks, W., Wu, Y. H. (2008). Application of the biopharmaceutical classification system in clinical drug development–an industrial view. *AAPS J.*, 10, 306–310.
2. Abrahamsson, B., Lennernaes, H. (2009). Application of the biopharmaceutics classification system now and in the future. *Methods Princ. Med. Chem*, 40, 523–558.
3. Lennernaes, H., Abrahamsson, B. (2005). The use of biopharmaceutic classification of drugs in drug discovery and development: current status and future extension. *J. Pharm. Pharmacol.*, 57, 273–285.
4. Oh, D. M., Curl, R. L., Amidon, G. L. (1993). Estimating the fraction dose absorbed from suspensions of poorly soluble compounds in humans: a mathematical model. *Pharm. Res.*, 10, 264–270.
5. Sugano, K. (2009). Fraction of dose absorbed calculation: comparison between analytical solution based on one compartment steady state approximation and dynamic seven compartment model. *CBI J.*, 9, 75–93.
6. Sugano, K. (2009). Introduction to computational oral absorption simulation. *Expert Opin. Drug Metab. Toxicol*, 5, 259–293.
7. Amidon, G. L., Lennernas, H., Shah, V. P., Crison, J. R. (1995). A theoretical basis for a biopharmaceutic drug classification: the correlation of *in vitro* drug product dissolution and *in vivo* bioavailability. *Pharm. Res.*, 12, 413–420.
8. Yu, L. X. (1999). An integrated model for determining causes of poor oral drug absorption. *Pharm. Res.*, 16, 1883–1887.
9. Yu, L. X., Amidon, G. L., Polli, J. E., Zhao, H., Mehta, M. U., Conner, D. P., Shah, V. P., Lesko, L. J., Chen, M.-L., Lee, V. H. et al. (2002). Biopharmaceutics classification system: the scientific basis for biowaiver extensions. *Pharm. Res.*, 19, 921–925.
10. Avdeef, A., Tam, K. Y. (2010). How well can the caco-2/madin-darby canine kidney models predict effective human jejunal permeability?. *J. Med. Chem.*, 53, 3566–3584.
11. Wu, C. Y., Benet, L. Z. (2005). Predicting drug disposition via application of BCS: transport/absorption/elimination interplay and development of a biopharmaceutics drug disposition classification system. *Pharm. Res.*, 22, 11–23.
12. Chen, M. L., Amidon, G. L., Benet, L. Z., Lennernas, H., Yu, L. X. (2011). The BCS, BDDCS, and regulatory guidances. *Pharm. Res.*, 28, 1774–1778.
13. Kovacevi, I., Parojci, J., Tubi-Grozdanis, M., Langguth, P. (2009). An investigation into the importance of "very rapid dissolution" criteria for drug bioequivalence demonstration using gastrointestinal simulation technology. *AAPS J.*, 11, 381–384.
14. Kortejarvi, H., Shawahna, R., Koski, A., Malkki, J., Ojala, K., Yliperttula, M. (2010). Very rapid dissolution is not needed to guarantee bioequivalence for biopharmaceutics classification system (BCS) I drugs. *J. Pharm. Sci.*, 99, 621–625.
15. Tsume, Y., Amidon, G. L. (2010). The biowaiver extension for BCS class III drugs: the effect of dissolution rate on the bioequivalence of BCS class III immediate-release drugs predicted by computer simulation. *Mol. Pharm.*, 7, 1235–1243.
16. Chuasuwan, B., Binjesoh, V., Polli, J. E., Zhang, H., Amidon, G. L., Junginger, H. E., Midha, K. K., Shah, V. P., Stavchansky, S., Dressman, J. B., Barends, D. M. (2009). Biowaiver monographs for immediate release solid oral dosage forms: diclofenac sodium and diclofenac potassium. *J. Pharm. Sci.*, 98, 1206–1219.

17. Potthast, H., Dressman, J. B., Junginger, H. E., Midha, K. K., Oeser, H., Shah, V. P., Vogelpoel, H., Barends, D. M. (2005). Biowaiver monographs for immediate release solid oral dosage forms: ibuprofen. *J. Pharm. Sci.*, 94, 2121–2131.

18. Yazdanian, M., Briggs, K., Jankovsky, C., Hawi, A. (2004). The "high solubility" definition of the current FDA Guidance on Biopharmaceutical Classification System may be too strict for acidic drugs. *Pharm. Res.*, 21, 293–299.

19. Zaki, N. M., Artursson, P., Bergstrom, C. A. (2010). A modified physiological BCS for prediction of intestinal absorption in drug discovery. *Mol. Pharm.*, 7, 1478–1487.

20. Box, K., Comer, J. E., Gravestock, T., Stuart, M. (2009). New ideas about the solubility of drugs. *Chem. Biodivers.*, 6, 1767–1788.

21. Box, K. J., Comer, J. E. (2008). Using measured pKa, LogP and solubility to investigate supersaturation and predict BCS class. *Curr. Drug Metab.*, 9, 869–878.

22. Rege, B. D., Yu, L. X., Hussain, A. S., Polli, J. E. (2001). Effect of common excipients on Caco-2 transport of low-permeability drugs. *J. Pharm. Sci.*, 90, 1776–1786.

23. Stavchansky, S. (2008). Scientific perspectives on extending the provision for waivers of *in vivo* bioavailability and bioequivalence studies for drug products containing high solubility-low permeability drugs (BCS-Class 3). *AAPS J.*, 10, 300–305.

24. Schulze, J. D., Ashiru, D. A., Khela, M. K., Evans, D. F., Patel, R., Parsons, G. E., Coffin, M. D., Basit, A. W. (2006). Impact of formulation excipients on human intestinal transit. *J. Pharm. Pharmacol.*, 58, 821–825.

25. McAllister, M. (2010). Dynamic dissolution: a step closer to predictive dissolution testing? *Mol. Pharm.*, 7, 1374–1387.

26. Ramirez, E., Laosa, O., Guerra, P., Duque, B., Mosquera, B., Borobia, A. M., Lei, S. H., Carcas, A. J., Frias, J. (2010). Acceptability and characteristics of 124 human bioequivalence studies with active substances classified according to the Biopharmaceutic Classification System. *Br. J. Clin. Pharmacol.*, 70, 694–702.

27. Benet, L. Z., Larregieu, C. A. (2010). The FDA should eliminate the ambiguities in the current BCS biowaiver guidance and make public the drugs for which BCS biowaivers have been granted. *Clin. Pharmacol. Ther.*, 88, 405–407.

28. Obata, K., Sugano, K., Machida, M., Aso, Y. (2004). Biopharmaceutics classification by high throughput solubility assay and PAMPA. *Drug Dev. Ind. Pharm.*, 30, 181.

29. Butler, J. M., Dressman, J. B. (2010). The developability classification system: application of biopharmaceutics concepts to formulation development. *J. Pharm. Sci.*, 99, 4940–4954.

30. Lipinski, C., Aqueous solubility in discovery, chemistry and assay changes, in: H. Vande Waterbeemd, H. Lennernaes, P. Artursson (Eds.) *Drug bioavailability*, Wiley-VCH Verlag GmbH & Co. KgaA, Weinheim, 2003, pp. 215–231.

31. Duan, J. Z., Riviere, K., Marroum, P. (2011). *In Vivo* bioequivalence and *in vitro* similarity factor (f2) for dissolution profile comparisons of extended release formulations: how and when do they match? *Pharm. Res.*, 28, 1144–1156.

CHAPTER 10

DOSE AND PARTICLE SIZE DEPENDENCY

"The whole of science is nothing more than a refinement of everyday thinking."
—Albert Einstein

Predictions of dose and particle size dependency are everyday requests in drug discovery and development. In preclinical toxicology and first-in-human (FIH) studies, a dose escalation study is usually performed. Compared to pharmacological studies, the maximum dose strength for these studies are significantly higher. For a preclinical toxicology study, 1000–2000 mg/kg dose is often required. For an FIH study, 1000 mg/dose or higher (>30 mg/kg) is often required. A preliminary toxicokinetic (TK) study is usually performed before the toxicological studies in each animal species. If the exposure is not sufficient, enabling formulation options are pursued (Chapter 11). In addition, simulation of particle size dependency is often requested in drug development, as the particle size of an API often becomes one of the key quality attributes.

10.1 DEFINITIONS AND CAUSES OF DOSE NONPROPORTIONALITY

In this book, the terms *dose linear* and *dose proportional* are used in the same meaning. When an increase in dose strength (e.g., two-, four-, and eightfold) results in a proportional increase in C_{max} and AUC (i.e., two-, four-, and

Biopharmaceutics Modeling and Simulations: Theory, Practice, Methods, and Applications,
First Edition. Kiyohiko Sugano.
© 2012 John Wiley & Sons, Inc. Published 2012 by John Wiley & Sons, Inc.

eightfold), the pharmacokinetics (PK) is said to be "dose linear" and/or "dose proportional". A nonlinear PK can be caused by several reasons listed in the following.

Subproportional Exposure

- solubility-permeability-limited absorption;
- saturation of influx transporter in the intestine.

Supraproportional Exposure

- saturation of efflux transporters in the intestine;
- saturation of intestinal and liver first-pass metabolism;
- saturation of disposition CL (hepatic and renal clearances).

10.2 ESTIMATION OF THE DOSE AND PARTICLE SIZE EFFECTS

The dose and particle size dependency of Fa% can be estimated from the rate-limiting step of the oral drug absorption (Fig. 1.3) [1, 2].

10.2.1 Permeability-Limited Cases (PL)

In the permeability-limited absorption range (Do < 1, Pn < Dn), Fa% is usually independent of both dose and particle size, except for the cases in which a transporter is involved in the permeation process. The AUC and C_{max} linearly increase as the dose increases. However, as the dose exceeds a certain point, the dose number becomes larger than 1 and the absorption pattern could change from PL to solubility-limited (SL) absorption.

10.2.2 Dissolution-Rate-Limited (DRL) Cases

In dissolution-rate-limited (DRL) absorption (Dn < Pn/Do), Fa% should be dose independent, but particle size dependent.[1] Particle size reduction would be effective in increasing the oral absorption of a drug. However, as the dose increases or particle size decreases, the regime of oral absorption could change from DRL to solubility-permeability-limited absorption.

The critical particle size discriminating DRL and SL can be calculated as follows. The criterion to discriminate DRL and SL, that is, 1/Dn >Do/Pn (for Do >1), can be rearranged to

$$\frac{1}{\text{Dn}} = \frac{r_p^2 \rho}{3 \cdot D_{eff} \cdot S_{dissolv} \cdot T_{si}} > \frac{\text{Do}}{\text{Pn}} = \frac{\text{Dose}}{S_{dissolv} \cdot V_{GI}} \frac{R_{GI}}{2\text{DF} \cdot P_{eff} \cdot T_{si}} \quad (10.1)$$

---

[1]However, particle size dependency of AUC and C_{max} is not a sufficient condition to prove that the oral absorption is dissolution rate limited. The particle size could also affect the UWL permeability of a drug (particle drifting effect (PDE) (Section 4.7.2)).

By rearranging this equation, the critical radius to become DRL can be calculated as,

$$r_p > \sqrt{\frac{3D_{eff} \cdot Dose \cdot R_{GI}}{2 \cdot V_{GI} \cdot DF \cdot P_{eff} \cdot \rho}} \tag{10.2}$$

$S_{dissolv}$ is canceled out from the both sides of Equation 10.1, suggesting that the critical particle size does not depend on the solubility of a drug for Do >1 cases. This point can be interpreted as follows. When the solubility is low, the dissolution rate becomes slow, and at the same time, the ceiling of the dissolved drug concentration (=saturated solubility) becomes low. On the other hand, when the solubility is high, the dissolution rate becomes fast and the ceiling of the dissolved drug concentration becomes high. Therefore, the tendency of $C_{dissolv}$ reaching the saturated solubility (=becoming SL absorption) does not depend on the solubility of a drug (in other words, the tendency to deviate from the sink condition does not depend on $S_{dissolv}$).

Using a conventional milling process, the mean particle size can be reduced to 10 μm or less. The particle diameter of drugs with low solubility in the marketed formulation is often less than 10 μm. Therefore, according to Equation 10.2, even for relatively high P_{eff} cases such as 5×10^{-4} cm/s (before applying PDE), when the dose is greater than 20 mg (>0.3 mg/kg), the oral absorption becomes SL. As discussed in Section 8.5.2, the majority of BCS II drugs shows SL, but not DRL absorption. This is in good agreement with our real-life experiences in drug industries that a level A IVIVC (*in vitro* (dissolution)–*in vivo* correlation) is difficult to obtain for medium- to high-dose cases of drugs with low solubility (cf. DRL absorption is a prerequisite for a good IVIVC). During drug development, particle size reduction is usually used to remove dissolution rate limitation if incomplete oral absorption is anticipated.

It is often speculated that the particle size reduction would not be effective when the particle size is smaller than a critical value (i.e., oral absorption becomes solubility-permeability limited). However, this speculation is in contradiction with the experimental observations for the solubility-UWL-limited (SL-U) cases (Table 8.3). This point is discussed in Section 10.2.4.

10.2.3 Solubility–Epithelial Membrane Permeability Limited (SL-E) Cases

In this compound class, a steep dose dependency of Fa% is observed usually at a dose higher than that gives the dose number (Do) greater than 1. Figure 10.1 shows the dose dependency of Fa% for several solubility–epithelial membrane permeability limited (SL-E) drugs. When a Fa% information at a dose of Do < 1 is available, this data can be used to back-calculate the permeation number (Pn) (Section 7.9.1). This Pn is then used to calculate the Fa% at Do > 1 as Fa $= 1 - \exp(-Pn/Do)$.

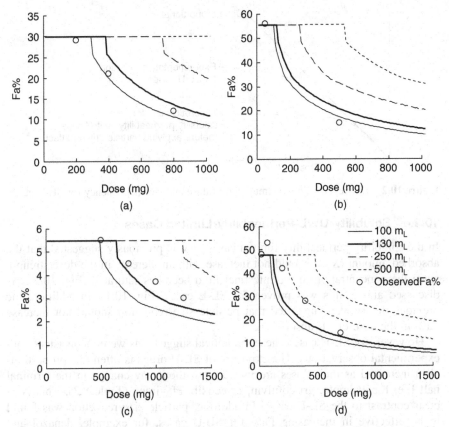

Figure 10.1 Dose dependency of Fa% for SL-E cases: (a) acyclovir, (b) chlorothiazide, (c) ganciclovir, and (d) lobucavir.

As shown in Figure 10.1, for the quantitative estimation of dose dependency for SL-E cases, it is critically important to use a correct V_{GI} value (100–250 ml) (Section 6.3.1.2). This V_{GI} corresponds to 5–15% of the full capacity of the small intestine (Fig. 4.3).

Example The inflection dose strength at which Fa% starts to decrease for acyclovir ($S_{dissolv} = 2.5$ mg/ml) can be calculated as

$$\text{Dose} > S_{dissolv} \times V_{GI} = 2.5 \times 130 = 325 \text{ mg}$$

In humans, Fa at 200-mg dose (Do < 1) is 0.29. As Fa $= 1 - \exp(-Pn) \approx$ Pn for Do < 1, Pn = 0.29. Fa for 800-mg dose (Do > 1) is then estimated as

$$\text{Fa} = 1 - \exp(-Pn/\text{Do}) \approx \frac{Pn}{\text{Do}} = \frac{0.29}{800/325} = 0.12$$

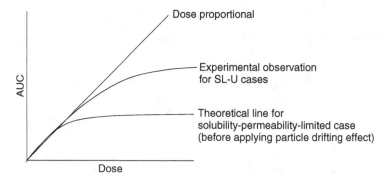

Figure 10.2   Discrepancy in the simulation of dose and size dependency for SL-U cases.

10.2.4   Solubility-UWL-Permeability-Limited Cases

In the solubility-permeability-limited cases, it was previously suggested that the absorbed amount (X_{abs}) should not increase with an increase in the dose strength since the concentration in the intestinal fluid becomes saturated (Fig. 10.2). As discussed above, this was proven for SL-E cases (Fig. 10.1). In addition, the previous theory also suggested that particle size reduction should not increase Fa% in the case of SL absorption.

However, for SL-U cases, these theoretical suggestions were inconsistent with experimental observations. The exposure of SL-U drugs is often (subproportionally) increased as their doses are increased without any change in the terminal half-life, for example, griseofulvin, celecoxib, efavirenz (Table 8.3). This is in clear contrast to the SL-E cases. In addition, particle size reduction was found to be effective in increasing Fa% for SL-U cases, for example, danazol and cilostazol (Table 8.3; Section 11.2, nano-API).[2]

These discrepancies may be due to overlooking the point that the drug particles can drift into the UWL (Section 4.7.2; Fig. 4.6). The PDE suggests that Pn could depend on the particle size and dose of a drug. Once this effect is taken into account, the dose and particle size dependency were reasonably simulated (Figs. 10.3–10.5; the other examples are found in Table 8.3). Using the same theoretical scheme, the effectiveness of particle nanomization to improve Fa% can be also elucidated (Section 11.2). A superficial rank order correlation (but not level A IVIVC) between the dissolution rate and *in vivo* oral absorption for SL-U cases can be a superficial correlation intermediated by the PDE.

10.3   EFFECT OF TRANSPORTERS

Dose-dependent absorption can be observed for a transporter substrate.[3] This point is discussed in detail in Chapter 14.

---

[2]This should not be confused with DRL.

[3]This does not mean that a transporter substrate always shows dose-dependent absorption. Apparent K_m could be higher or lower than the concentration range in the GI tract.

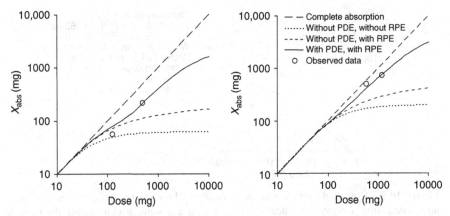

Figure 10.3 Dose dependency of Fa% for SL-U cases. RPE, remaining particle effect. (a) griseofulvin and (b) efavirenz. *Source*: Adapted from Reference [3] with permission.

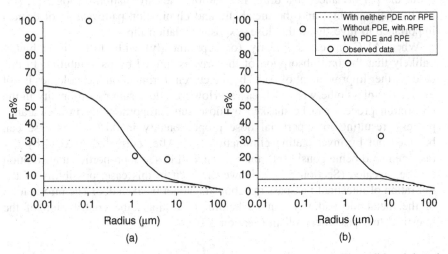

Figure 10.4 Particle size dependency of Fa% of cilostazol in dogs. The solid and dotted lines are the theoretical prediction with and without considering the particle drifting effect, respectively. (a) Fasted state and (b) fed state. *Source:* Adapted from Reference 3 with permission.

10.4   ANALYSIS OF *IN VIVO* DATA

In many cases, *in vivo* PK data at multiple dose strengths are available in drug discovery. If these data are carefully analyzed,[4] they give us a lot of information

---

[4]The formulation for PK and TK studies should be carefully prepared and well characterized (Section 7.10.1).

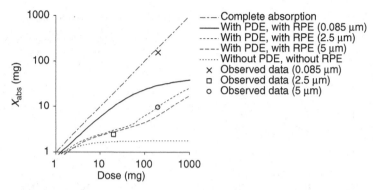

Figure 10.5 Dose and particle size dependency of Fa% of danazol in dogs. The solid and dotted lines are the theoretical prediction with and without considering the particle drifting effect, respectively. *Source:* Adapted from Reference [3] with permission.

about the performance of a drug. In addition, the information on log P_{oct}, solubility, permeability, and the metabolic and elimination pathways is of critical importance to investigate the dose–exposure relationship.

When AUC increases linearly (or supralinearly) with doses, it is highly unlikely that the oral absorption of the drug is limited by its solubility. In this case, further improvement of AUC by the current formulation technologies is not expected (unless otherwise DRL cases). However, dose subproportionality in the absorption process can be masked by dose supraproportionality in a clearance process, resulting in superficial dose proportionality in AUC. This case can be ruled out by investigating elimination $t_{1/2}$. After normalizing AUC by $t_{1/2}$ (assuming Vd being consistent), the existence of dose subproportional absorption can be revealed (Section 5.5.3). However, even in this case, possibility of the saturation of intestinal fast-pass metabolism cannot be excluded. The information of the metabolic pathway can be helpful to evaluate the contribution of the intestinal first-pass metabolism (Section 4.10).

REFERENCES

1. Yu, L. X. (1999). An integrated model for determining causes of poor oral drug absorption. *Pharm. Res.*, 16, 1883–1887.
2. Sugano, K., Okazaki, A., Sugimoto, S., Tavornvipas, S., Omura, A., Mano, T. (2007). Solubility and dissolution profile assessment in drug discovery. *Drug Metab. Pharmacokinet.*, 22, 225–254.
3. Sugano, K. (2010). Computational oral absorption simulation of free base drugs. *Int. J. Pharm.*, 398(1–2), 73–82.

CHAPTER 11

ENABLING FORMULATIONS

"If an elderly but distinguished scientist says that something is possible he is almost certainly right, but if he says that it is impossible he is very probably wrong."
—Arthur C. Clarke

Biopharmaceutical modeling is expected to be a useful tool for design and selection of an enabling formulation. The suitability of an enabling formulation is different for each drug. A trial and error approach has been undertaken to find a suitable enabling formulation. However, there is a high demand to improve the efficiency of drug discovery and development. By understanding the rate-limiting process, rational design and selection of an enabling formulation would become possible. In this chapter, each enabling technique is reviewed from the viewpoint of biopharmaceutical modeling.

11.1 SALTS AND COCRYSTALS: SUPERSATURATING API

Salt formation is most widely used as a measure to overcome the dissolution rate and/or solubility-permeability-limited absorptions for dissociable drugs. After dissolution of the salt, a supersaturated drug concentration can be induced in the intestine (Fig. 11.1). This transient supersaturated drug concentration can be

Biopharmaceutics Modeling and Simulations: Theory, Practice, Methods, and Applications,
First Edition. Kiyohiko Sugano.
© 2012 John Wiley & Sons, Inc. Published 2012 by John Wiley & Sons, Inc.

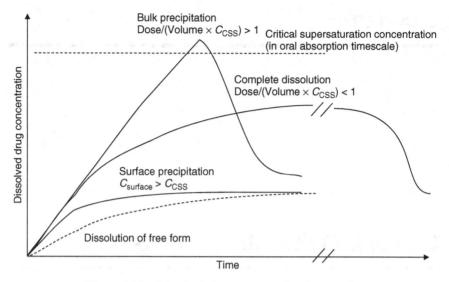

Figure 11.1 Dissolved drug concentration from a salt.

maintained during the intestinal transit time[1] and can enhance the oral absorption of a drug. Figure 11.2 shows the schematic presentation of the dose–AUC profile. In most cases, a salt form significantly outperforms a free form.

For biopharmaceutical modeling of a salt, an appropriate nucleation model is required to predict the precipitation *in vivo*. The use of classical nucleation theory would be just a starting point to incorporate the nucleation process into

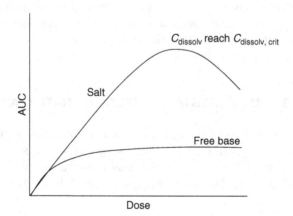

Figure 11.2 Dose–AUC pattern theoretically predicted for a salt.

[1]The equilibrium solubility of a drug at a pH in the pH-controlled region becomes the same value, regardless of the starting material being a salt or a free form (Section 2.3).

biopharmaceutical modeling (Section 3.3). In addition, none of the *in vitro* dissolution models have been successful in predicting the supersaturation *in vivo* [1].[2] The nucleation of a free form can occur not only in the bulk fluid but also at the solid surface of the drug [2–5].

In this section, we first discuss the three possible scenarios for the oral absorption of a salt. Some case examples are then discussed. A case by case strategy of biopharmaceutical modeling is then discussed. The discussion about a salt can be also applicable for cocrystals, anhydrates, and amorphous APIs (supersaturating APIs) (see also spring and parachute approach; Fig. 11.14).

11.1.1 Scenarios of Oral Absorption of Salt

There are several possible scenarios for the oral absorption of a salt (Fig. 11.1) [6].

(A) The dissolved drug concentration ($C_{dissolv}$) does not reach the critical supersaturation concentration ($C_{dissolv, crit}$) because the dose is not high enough and/or a high permeation clearance reduces $C_{dissolv}$. The nucleation induction time is longer than the intestinal transit time. The dose number based on $C_{dissolv, crit}$ ($Do_{supersaturation} = Dose/(V_{GI} \times C_{dissolv, crit})$) is less than 1. Precipitation of the free form does not occur both in the bulk fluid and solid surface.

(B) The nucleation induction time is shorter than the intestinal transit time, but the supersaturated concentration is maintained for several minutes to hours.

(C) As the salt form of a drug dissolves, the concentration of the drug reaches $C_{dissolv, crit}$ in the GI tract ($Do_{supersaturation} > 1$), and a free form immediately precipitates out (mostly as fine particles). The precipitated free form redissolves rapidly (faster than absorption flux), and therefore, $C_{dissolv}$ is maintained at the saturated solubility of the precipitant (free form) during the absorption process. The solid form of the precipitant can be a stable form (crystalline) or semistable form (amorphous).

(D) A free form precipitates out at the surface of dissolving salt as an insoluble layer.

  (D-1) The precipitated free form forms a loose and porous layer on the surface of the salt. The dissolution of the drug continues, however, at a somewhat slower rate than the original salt because of the extra barrier for dissolution.

  (D-2) The precipitated free form completely covers the surface of a salt. Further dissolution is controlled by the solubility of the free form on the solid surface. Although the supersaturable form exists below the surface layer, it is not available for dissolution.

---

[2]Using a nonsink dissolution test, a rank-order comparison of various salts might be possible.

11.1.2 Examples

11.1.2.1 Example 1: Salt of Basic Drugs. AZ0865 mesylate (45–159 mg/dose) [1] and indinavir sulfate (250–500 mg/m^2) [7] might be the case for scenario (A). In this dose range, the oral absorption of these drugs is dose-linear (Figs. 7.23 and 11.3).

FTI-2600 might be the case for scenario (C). In the *in vitro* dissolution test, after the HCl salt was dissolved, the free base immediately precipitated out in an amorphous form. However, it was not further converted to a crystalline form (Fig. 11.4). In this case, $C_{dissolv}$ in the small intestine is determined by the solubility of the amorphous form.[3]

Ziprasidone HCl and mesylate are also likely to be the cases for scenario (C). The solubility values of these salts in the unbuffered water are 0.08 and 0.73 mg/ml, respectively [9], suggesting that if there is no precipitation, Fa% should be 100% at 40-mg dose in humans. The equilibrium solubility of ziprasidone in a pH 7.4 buffer is 0.0008 μg/ml. The relative bioavailability in humans in the fasted state is ca. 30–50% compared to that in the fed state and other solubility-enhanced formulations (Table 11.1) [10]. At 20–80 mg, the oral absorption is dose-subproportional in the fasted state, but it is dose-proportional in the fed state [11]. These observations suggest that precipitation occurred *in vivo* in the fasted state. As the particle size of the HCl salt had only a little effect on the oral absorption (20 vs 105 μm), it is unlikely that precipitation of the free base occurred at the solid surface (but this is not conclusive) [12]. Interestingly,

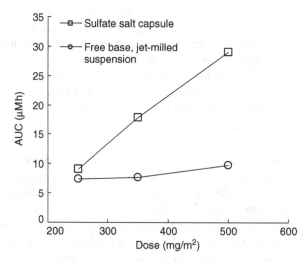

Figure 11.3 Dose dependency of AUC after administration of indinavir sulfate in humans [7].

---

[3]This concentration could be much higher compared to the solubility of a crystalline form. Therefore, the concentration of the drug is supersaturated against a crystalline.

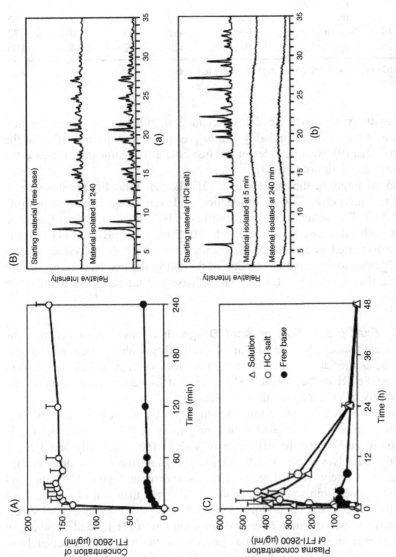

Figure 11.4 FTI-2600. (a) Dissolution profile of FTI-2600 crystalline free base and HCl salt in FaSSIF. (b) PXRD pattern of the initial and precipitated solids. Initial material: (a) crystalline free base and (b) HCl salt. (C) *In vivo* PK profile. Mean ± SD plasma concentrations of FTI-2600 following oral administration in achlorhydric beagle dogs ($n = 5$) under fasted conditions at a dose of 3 mg/kg. Δ, FTI-2600 crystalline free base dissolved in 10% HCO60 solution; ○, a mixture of FTI-2600 HCl salt and lactose encapsulated in hard gelatin capsules; ●, FTI-2600 crystalline free base suspended in 5% gum arabic. *Source:* Adapted from Reference 8 with permission.

TABLE 11.1   Bioavailabilities of Ziprasidone Salts and Formulations

API	Dose, mg	Formulation	Fasted/Fed	AUC, ng h/ml	BA%	Fa% (Fh Model)	Fa%[a]
HCl	40	Capsule	Fasted	481	23	55	38
HCl	40	HPMC-coated tablet	Fasted	822	39	93	66
Free	40	Nanosuspension	Fasted	962	45	109	77
HCl	20	Capsule	Fed	627	59	142	100

[a]On the basis of the AUC of 20-mg capsule in the fed state.

HPMC (hydroxypropylmethylcellulose) coating significantly increased the oral absorption of the HCl salt probably due to precipitation inhibiting effect of the HPMC polymer [9]. Nanoparticles of the free base also significantly increase the oral absorption of ziprasidone [9].

REV 5901 might be the case for D-2) [2]. The pH–solubility profiles of both the base and the salt at 37°C were identical and were in agreement with a pK_a value of 3.67. The solubility of the drug (ca. 0.002 mg/ml at pH 6) increased gradually with a decrease in pH and reached 0.95 mg/ml at pH 1. At pH < 1, the solubility decreased as a result of the common-ion effect. At pH values greater than pH_{max}, due to the rapid conversion of the salt to the free base at the surface of the salt, the dissolution rates of both the base and the salt were found to be identical.

11.1.2.2 *Example 2: Salt of Acid Drugs.* It is often speculated that the salt of an acid should have a similar bioavailability with the free acid, as the salt will be immediately converted to a free acid when it comes into contact with the acidic pH in the stomach. However, salt formation often increases the bioavailability of acid drugs with low solubility.

The oral absorption of phenytoin sodium might be the case for scenario (C). Phenytoin is an acidic compound with a pK_a value of 8.4, and its solubility is 35–40 µg/ml at 37°C in the pH range of 1–7.4. Therefore, only about 5 mg of the drug dissolves in the GI fluid (~130 ml) and the excess drug precipitates out in a finely divided state [13]. As shown in Figure 11.5, the oral absorption of phenytoin sodium is significantly higher than that of free acid (of 50–100 µm particle size) at 400-mg dose (5.7 mg/kg) in humans. As no supersaturation was observed in an *in vitro* dissolution test at pH 1.2 and 5 (50 mg in 500 ml), phenytoin sodium would be converted to the free acid immediately in the stomach and/or in the small intestine [14]. Interestingly, the oral absorption from the fine particles of phenytoin free acid (4 µm) and the sodium salt was found to be similar in humans at 280- (4 mg/kg) and 210-mg (3 mg/kg) doses, respectively [14].

In dogs, the oral absorption from phenytoin sodium was ca. twofold higher than that of fine particles (4 µm) at 50 mg/kg [14].

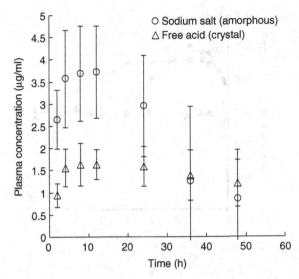

Figure 11.5 Plasma concentration–time profile of phenytoin in humans after administration of 400-mg dose. Sodium salt: amorphous form with 1–3 μm particle size. Free acid: crystalline with 50–100 μm particle size.

11.1.2.3 *Example 3: Other Supersaturable API Forms.* As an anhydrate has higher solubility than a hydrate, it can induce supersaturation. Figure 11.6 shows the dissolution and the C_p–time profiles of carbamazepine in dogs. The conversion rate from anhydrate to hydrate in the water is slow and is inhibited by the bile-micelles [4]. Four anhydrate forms have been identified [15], and one of them is used in a marketed drug product [16].

Recently, cocrystals attracted a lot of attention in pharmaceutical industries. Implementation of high throughput solid form screening increased the success rate of finding cocrystals [18]. Cocrystals can behave like salts, so that after fast dissolution in the GI tract, a supersaturated concentration can be maintained. However, a limited number of oral absorption data is available in the literature [19–21]. Figure 11.7 shows the case examples for which an increase in oral absorption is observed by forming a cocrystal [16].

An amorphous form is often discussed as the API form to increase Fa%. However, a naked amorphous API is often not stable and is not suitable for drug development. Therefore, the amorphous state is often stabilized as solid dispersion formulations.

11.1.3 Suitable Drug for Salts

11.1.3.1 *pK_a Range.* For the development of a salt, the balance of bioavailability and storage stability should be considered. Long-term physical and chemical stability over a 2-year period at room temperature is usually required for marketing. For a base drug, no compound with $pK_a < 4.6$ has been marketed as

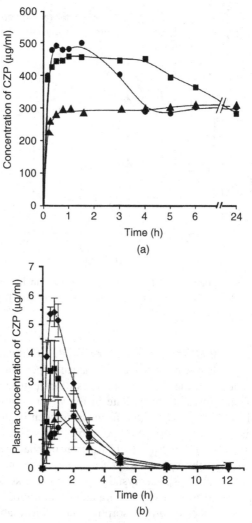

Figure 11.6 (a) Dissolution and (b) C_p-time profiles of carbamazepine polymorphs and dihydrate. (a) pH 1.2 at 37°C under nonsink conditions. (b) Plasma concentration-time curves after oral administration of 400 mg to dogs ($n = 4$; mean $\pm$ S.E.). ■, anhydrate form I; ●, anhydrate form III; ▲, dehydrate; and ◆, solution. CZP, carbamazepine. *Source:* Adapted from Reference 17 with permission.

a salt in the past (Tables 11.2 and 11.3) [22]. This does not necessarily mean that a compound with a $pK_a < 4.6$ cannot be marketed as a salt. But the development of a compound with low pK_a values might be more challenging, as it has an inherent risk of disproportionation. Figure 11.8 shows the pK_a values of drugs and its counterions for the marketed drugs. It is commonly believed that when the difference between the pK_a of an acid and a base is greater than 2, a

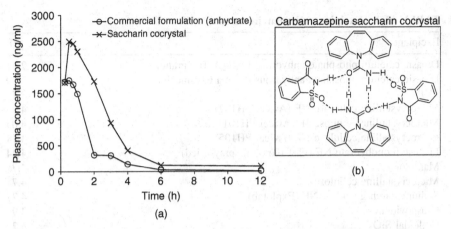

(b)

(a)

Figure 11.7 C_p–time profiles of carbamazepine (200 mg) in fasted beagle dogs ($n = 4$). (a) Commercial formulation (anhydrate) versus saccharin cocrystal. (b) Structure of carbamazepine–saccharin cocrystal. *Source:* Replotted from Reference 16.

TABLE 11.2   Classification of Acids and Bases According to their Strength[a]

| | pK_a | |
Attribute	Acids	Bases
Very strong	<0	14
Strong	0–4.5	9.5–14
Weak	4.5–9.5	4.5–9.5
Very weak	9.5–14	0–4.5
Extremely weak	14	<0

[a]Reference 22.

stable salt can be formed ("rule of two") [23]. If the pH_{max} of a salt is lower than the microenvironmental pH of the excipients, the risk of disproportionation (conversion to a free base) becomes higher. Even a small portion of a free base (<0.1%) can induce catastrophic precipitation (Fig. 11.9) [3]. However, quantitative detection of a trace amount of a free base is practically impossible. A nonsink dissolution test may be used to investigate the stability of a salt [24].

11.1.3.2 *Supersaturability of Drugs.* By the kinetic pH titration method (Section 7.8.1), Box et al. [25] identified some chemical structural characteristics of supersaturable and nonsupersaturable drugs. Typical chemical features are listed in Table 11.4. In the case of nonsupersaturable drugs, an amorphous solid (or oil) precipitated out and this amorphous form did not get converted to a crystalline form during the experimental time.[4] Recently, it was demonstrated that

---

[4]Salt formation is often used to obtain a crystalline material when the free form does not crystallize. In addition, in the case of a base, salt formation can avoid absorption of CO_2 from the air.

TABLE 11.3   Excipient Microenvironmental pH[a]

Excipient	pH
Dibasic calcium phosphate anhydrous USP (A-Tab granules)	2.21
Dibasic calcium phosphate anhydrous (Sigma Chemicals)	3.59
PVP	3.7
Microcrystalline cellulose NF (Avicel PH102)	4.07
Microcrystalline cellulose JP (Avicel PH101)	4.03
Microcrystalline cellulose NF (Avicel PH105)	4.14
Lactose monohydrate NF (Fast Flo 316, spray-dried)	4.24
Mannitol	4.7
Microcrystalline cellulose	4.7
Sodium starch glycolate NF (Explotab)	4.77
Crospovidone	4.9
Colloidal SiO$_2$	5.2
Sodium croscarmellose	5–7
Lactose	6.1
Maize starch	6.3
Calcium carbonate USP (Vicron 75-17-FG)	6.58
Magnesium stearate	7.1
Carbonate carbonate USP (Calcipure GCC300)	7.20
Magnesium stearate NF	7.45
Hydrogenated castor oil	7.5
Calcium carbonate USP (Precarb 150)	7.69
Calcium carbonate USP (Vicality Medium PCC)	8.07

[a]Reference 22.

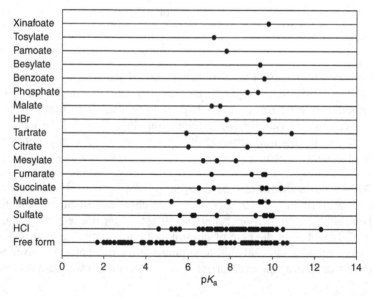

Figure 11.8 Graph depicting the most basic pK_a of an active ingredient versus the counter ion chosen as in its product. *Source:* Adapted from Reference 22 with permission.

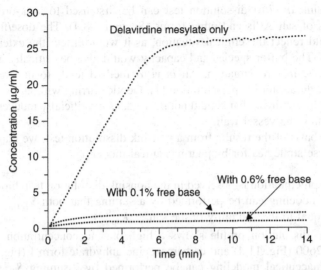

Figure 11.9 Rotating disk dissolution data for delavirdine mesylate at pH 2 spiked with 0%, 0.1%, and 0.6% w/w of delavirdine free base. *Source:* Adapted from Reference 3 with permission.

TABLE 11.4 Typical Features of Chasers and Nonchasers[a]

Supersaturable Drugs	Nonsupersaturable Drugs
• Can be acids, bases, and ampholytes • Sum of H-bond donor + acceptor is 3 or above • Solid form of precipitant tends to be crystalline • High melting point of free form • Solubility usually increases with temperature	• Only observed for bases • Little capacity for H-bonding; most have no H-bond • Low melting point of free form; mainly liquid at 25° C • Solubility unchanged or decreases with temperature

[a]Reference 25.

the nucleation induction time is related to the effectiveness of a supersaturable formulation to increase the oral absorption of a drug [26].

11.1.4 Biopharmaceutical Modeling of Supersaturable API Forms

Given the lack of any appropriate *in vitro* dissolution test and computational model, the current best practice to predict the clinical performance of a salt form is to carefully perform *in vivo* experiments and interpret the data. Dogs would be practically the most appropriate species to investigate the oral absorption of a salt (Section 7.10).

A nonsink *in vitro* dissolution test can be first used to rank-order the performances of salt APIs and other forms (Section 7.8.4). The dose/fluid volume ratio should reflect the clinical situation, as it would affect the extent of supersaturation. The buffer species and capacity would also be critically important to represent the *in vivo* situation. An *in vitro* method tends to underestimate the extent and duration of supersaturation [1]. Gentle stirring without using a paddle is preferable. A stirring bar should not be used, as it artificially induces nucleation by scratching the vessel wall.

On the basis of the results from a nonsink dissolution test, we may be able to follow these strategies for biopharmaceutical modeling.

- If no precipitation is observed in the nonsink dissolution test, biopharmaceutical modeling can be performed by assuming that both $S_{dissolv}$ and $S_{surface}$ are equal to the solubility of the salt ($=K_{sp}^{0.5}$).
- If the dissolution profile shows a high plateau concentration, such as in FTI-2600 (Fig. 11.4) and carbamazepine anhydrate form I (Fig. 11.6), biopharmaceutical modeling can be performed by assuming $S_{dissolv}$ is equal to the plateau concentration and $S_{surface}$ is the theoretical solubility of the administered solid (e.g., $K_{sp}^{0.5}$ for a salt).
- If the dissolution profile of a salt is identical to that of the free form, biopharmaceutical modeling can be performed in the same manner as the free form.
- When the supersaturation duration is within 3.5 h (such as in carbamazepine anhydrate form III; Fig. 11.6), the preexponential and surface energy parameters of the nucleation equation (Section 3.3) can be obtained by curve fitting the *in vitro* data. Then, these parameters are used to estimate the *in vivo* oral absorption.

It should be remembered that *in vitro* tests tend to underestimate supersaturation. Therefore, the above modeling strategy will give a pessimistic estimation. One of the typical mistakes in biopharmaceutical modeling for a salt is that the equilibrium solubility of a salt in a buffer at a pH is used as the solubility input. This would result in a dramatic underestimation of the oral absorption of a salt.

Manufacturability is critically important as well. For robust manufacturing processes and long-term storage stability, it is preferable to select the most stable form among the polymorphs. Salt formation can improve the manufacturability by increasing the stability of the API form [27].

11.2 NANOMILLED API PARTICLES

Nanomilling technology has been proven to be effective in increasing the oral absorption of the solubility-UWL-limited cases, although it is often speculated that nanomilling is only effective in dissolution-rate-limited cases (Fig. 11.10). As discussed in Section 10.2.2, the oral absorption of a drug with low solubility

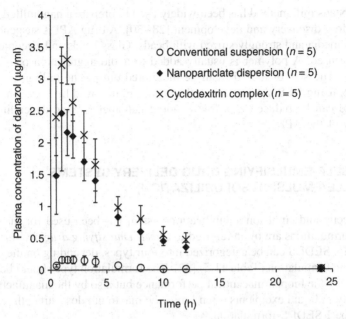

Figure 11.10 Effect of formulations on the oral absorption of danazol in fasted dogs (20 mg/kg). The particle sizes of conventional and nanosuspension were 10 and 0.16 μm, respectively. *Source:* Adapted from Reference 31 with permission.

becomes solubility-permeability limited when the dose is larger than 20 mg and particle size is smaller than 10 μm. Considering the dose of many drugs with low solubility (Table 8.3), the oral absorption of these drugs should be solubility-permeability limited. In addition, an increase in solubility by nanosizing (cf. the Ostwald–Freundlich equation) was also speculated as the reason for enhancing oral absorption. However, this mechanism is unlikely both theoretically and experimentally. The Ostwald–Freundlich equation predicts that this effect becomes significant only when the particle size is less than 100 nm even assuming highest surface tension for a drug (such as that of alkanes) (Section 2.3.9). This point was recently experimentally confirmed for drugs with low solubility (Section 7.6.3.4).

As an alternative explanation, the particle drifting effect (PDE) was introduced (Section 4.7.2). API particles can be drifted into the UWL, and the drug molecules diffuse into the epithelial membrane from the surface of the API particles in the UWL. Even though the PDE was first introduced to explain the oral absorption of SL-U drugs from conventional formulations, this effect would be larger for nanoparticles.

Figures 10.4 and 10.5 show simulated Fa% of danazol and cilostazol in dogs. Introduction of the PDE significantly decreased the discrepancy between simulated and observed Fa%. The Fa% of atovaquone, fenofibrate, and aprepitant nanoparticle formulations was also appropriately simulated (Table 8.3).

The beads mill method has been widely used to prepare a nanomilled formulation in drug discovery and development [28–30]. A drug API is suspended in an aqueous media and strongly stirred with beads. Glass beads and zirconium beads are often used. A polymer is usually added to avoid aggregation of nanomilled particles. The size of the API can be monitored during the milling process, for example, using DLS. After milling, the beads are removed by filtration. The particle size can be reduced to a few hundred nanometer range depending on the property of the API.

11.3 SELF-EMULSIFYING DRUG DELIVERY SYSTEMS (MICELLE/EMULSION SOLUBILIZATION)

The micelle and emulsion solubilization system has been used for many drugs. These formulations are often referred to as *self-emulsifying drug delivery systems* (*SEDDS*). SEDDS can be categorized into four types, depending on the composition of the formulation (Table 11.5) [32]. The formulation type should be selected not only by the biopharmaceutical performance but also by the manufacturability. Solubility in liquid excipients often limits the maximum dose strength, especially for a type I SEDDS formulation.

Once in contact with the GI fluid, the SEDDS forms dispersed micelles. For type I and II formulations, bile-micelle solubilization and the digestion of lipid components by lipase largely affect the performance of these formulations (Fig. 11.11) [33]. The drug concentration in the mixed micelle phase after digestion of the formulation was found to correlate with the exposure of a drug [32, 34]. After entering the intestinal enterocytes, a lipophilic compound of log $P_{oct} > 5$ can be carried by the lymphatic system (Fig. 11.12) [35, 36]. The lymphatic flow is significantly slower than the blood flow. Therefore, the appearance of the drug in the systemic circulation is usually slow. It is well known that the lipid components affect the lymphatic absorption. For example in rats, the lymphatic absorption of halofantrine is 2%, 6%, and 16% from the short-, medium-, and long-chain fatty acid triglyceride formulations, respectively (Table 11.6) [37]. The liver first-pass effect can be avoided via lymphatic transport.

Owing to its complex absorption mechanism, no mechanistic computational modeling has been reported (as of 2011). Construction of an *in vitro* model is also challenging. Therefore, preclinical animal models would be required to assess the performance of SEDDS formulations. The droplet size of emulsions (especially after lipid digestion) seems to have a significant effect on their performance. The drug molecules dissolved in micelles with less than 400 nm size were suggested to be effective for permeation, probably because it can readily defuse the UWL.

Micelle-solubilized drugs can diffuse the UWL, and the unbound fraction of a drug can then permeate the epithelial membrane [35]. Therefore, the UWL and unbound fraction should be at least taken into account for biopharmaceutical modeling of SEDDS. The micelle size (hence diffusion coefficient) could change depending on the excipient component, lipid digestion, and interaction

TABLE 11.5 Type I, II, IIIA, and IIIB Lipid Formulations

Type	I	II	IIIA	IIIB	IV
Typical composition, %					
Triglycerides or mixed glycerides	100	40–80	40–80	<20	—
Water-insoluble surfactants (HLB <12)	—	20–60	—	—	0–20
Water-soluble surfactants (HLB >12)	—	—	20–40	20–50	30–80
Hydrophilic cosolvents (e.g., PEG)	—	—	0–40	20–50	0–50
Oral absorption characteristics					
Particle size of aqueous dispersion, nm	Coarse	100–250	100–250	50–100	50–100
Loss of solubilization capacity	Solvent capacity unaffected	Solvent capacity unaffected	Some loss of solvent capacity	Potential loss of solvent capacity	Potential loss of solvent capacity
Requirement of lipase digestibility	Crucial	Not crucial but likely to occur	Not crucial but may be inhibited	Not required and unlikely to occur	Not required and unlikely to occur

Abbreviation: HLB, hydrophilic–lipophilic balance.

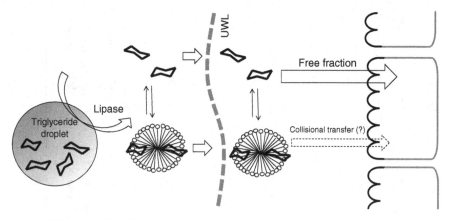

Figure 11.11   Oral absorption process of the lipid-based formulations.

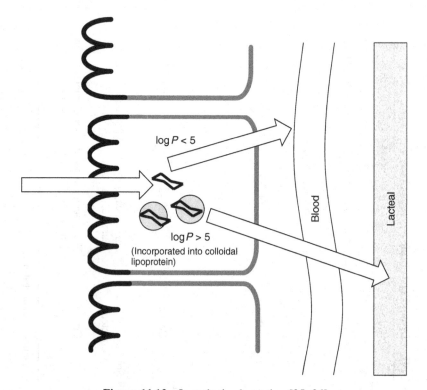

Figure 11.12   Lymphatic absorption [35, 36].

with endogenous bile-micelles. The unbound fraction of a drug in the mixed micelle phase after digestion by lipase should also be considered (Fig. 11.13). If the drug is absorbed via the lymphatic route, the lymphatic flow rate should be taken into account. Even though an API drug is fully solubilized in the

TABLE 11.6 Bioavailability of Halofantrine Free Base (Mean% Dose ± SD, $n = 4$) in Lymph-Cannulated Rats after Oral Administration[a]

Formulation	Lymphatic Transport	Total
LCT (C_{18})	15.8 ± 2.2	22.7 ± 4.0
MCT (C_{8-10})	5.5 ± 1.5	19.2 ± 4.5
SCT (C_4)	2.2 ± 1.8	15.2 ± 3.1
Aqueous suspension	0.34 ± 0.5	6.4 ± 0.8

Cumulative mass of halofantrine recovered over 12 h in mesenteric lymph calculated as a percentage of dose.

The lymph flow (g/12 h) in each experimental group was $13.8 \pm 2.2, 10.0 \pm 2.8, 7.82 \pm 0.7$, and 4.20 ± 2.2 g/12 h, respectively, for groups dosed with LCT, MCT, SCT, or the aqueous suspension formulation.

[a]Reference 37.

1. Carry out *in vitro* digestion of formulation using a pH-stat
2. Ultracentrifuge the resultant dispersion (after 0, 15, and 60 min of digestion). Long-chain TG oil gives four phases
3. Separate (as best as possible) the component phases and measure volumes
4. Assay each phase for drug. Carry out mass balance if possible

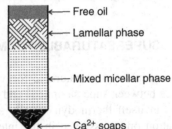

Figure 11.13 Lipase digestion study and components of digestion. TG, triglyceride. *Source:* Adapted from Reference 32 with permission.

formulation, after dispersed in the GI fluid, it can precipitate out in the GI tract. Simulation of this precipitation phenomenon is also a challenging area.

11.4 SOLID DISPERSION

It is well known that solid dispersions and amorphous formulations can significantly improve the oral absorption of drugs with low solubility [38, 39]. As this type of formulations can increase the unbound drug concentration, it would be effective for both SL-E and SL-U cases [40]. Drugs can also exist in the polymer micelles after the erosion of solid dispersion. For biopharmaceutical modeling, considering the proposed mechanism of oral absorption from solid dispersion [40], both unbound molecules and polymer-micelle-bound molecules should be explicitly taken into account. Owing to its complex absorption mechanism, no mechanistic computational modeling has been reported in the literature (as of 2011).

Solid dispersions can be prepared by spray drying, freeze-drying, rapid evaporation, etc. The drug API is dissolved in an organic solvent with polymers, and then the organic solvent is removed. Freeze-drying and rapid evaporation would be a convenient method to prepare a small-scale sample. A miniscale spray dryer is commercially available and can be used in drug discovery. Hot melt extrusion can also be used to prepare a solid dispersion. As a polymer, HPMC, HPMC-AS, PVP, etc. are often used.

One drawback of the solid dispersion formulation is its storage stability. Crystallization is often observed during storage, resulting in a change in the dissolution profile. It could be kinetically stable to survive more than 2 or 3 years, but a large amount of polymer would be required to stabilize the formulation. Prediction of long-term stability of solid dispersion is a challenging area.

When administering the solid dispersions as a suspension in an aqueous media, the stability of the solid dispersion in the vehicle should be carefully checked. A rapid crystallization is often observed. In addition, dissolution performance should be checked by a dissolution test. A nonsink dissolution test should be used to investigate the supersaturation duration.

11.5 SUPERSATURABLE FORMULATIONS

The concept of supersaturable formulation emerged recently [41–44]. The difference between supersaturated[5] and supersaturable formulations is that the latter one is in itself thermodynamically stable but induces supersaturated drug concentration once dissolved in the intestinal fluid. Figure 11.14 shows the spring and parachute concept for the supersaturable formulations.

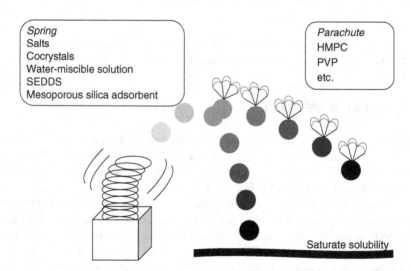

Figure 11.14 Spring and parachute concept.

[5]For example, solid dispersion.

Salts, cocrystals, liquid formulation (including type IV SEDDS), and meso-porous silica adsorbents [45–49] have been used as the "spring" to induce the supersaturated drug concentration [44]. Various polymers have been used to pro-long the duration of supersaturation ("parachute"). As this type of formulation can increase the unbound drug concentration, it would be effective for both SL-E and SL-U cases. For biopharmaceutical modeling, the nucleation theory should be taken into account. However, little is known about the mechanism of the inhibition of supersaturation by a polymer. Inhibition of nucleation process was previously suggested as an inhibition mechanism. However, recently, inhibition of crystal growth was suggested as an inhibition mechanism as well [50]. Biopharmaceutical modeling for supersaturable formulations is the subject of future investigation.

11.6 PRODRUGS TO INCREASE SOLUBILITY

To increase the aqueous solubility of drugs with low solubility, a hydrophilic group can be attached to a drug molecule. A phosphate prodrug has been used to increase the solubility of amprenavir (fosamprenavir) (Fig. 11.15). The phosphate moiety is cleaved to the parent drug at the surface of the epithelial membrane, which then permeates the epithelial membrane.

The oral absorption of phenytoin was found to be significantly increased by water-soluble prodrugs (Table 11.7) [51, 52]. Solubility of these phenytoin pro-drugs are ca. 150 mg/ml (cf. the solubility of free acid is 0.04 mg/ml).

Biopharmaceutical modeling of the oral absorption of this type of prodrug has not been reported. The rat mucous layer scrap and Caco-2 cells were found to cleave the phosphate prodrug, whereas MDCK cells do not [53].

11.7 PRODRUGS TO INCREASE PERMEABILITY

Practically, a formulation approach to improve membrane permeability has not been successful in the past[6] because an effective enhancer often shows toxicity

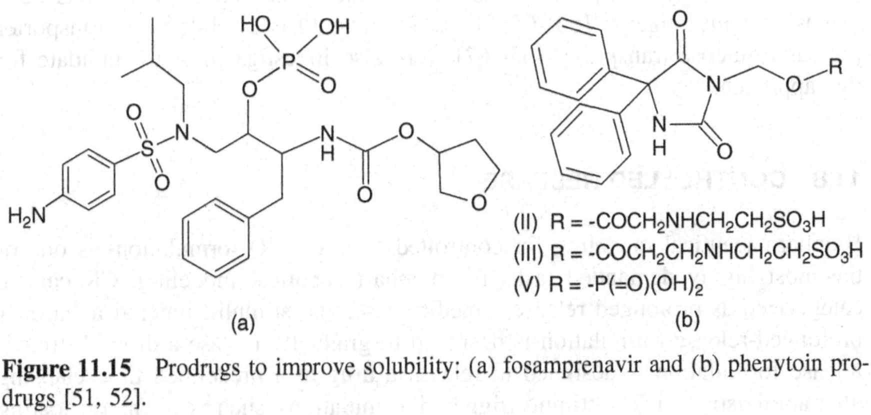

(II) R = -COCH$_2$NHCH$_2$CH$_2$SO$_3$H
(III) R = -COCH$_2$CH$_2$NHCH$_2$CH$_2$SO$_3$H
(V) R = -P(=O)(OH)$_2$

(a)   (b)

Figure 11.15 Prodrugs to improve solubility: (a) fosamprenavir and (b) phenytoin pro-drugs [51, 52].

[6]Capric acid formulation for rectal administration is an exception.

TABLE 11.7 Bioavailability of Phenytoin Prodrugs

	BA%
Prodrug II	65 ± 23
Prodrug III	76 ± 45
Prodrug IV	51 ± 6
Sodium salt	14 ± 3
Free acid	10^a

[a]Predicted value for 190 μm.

to the intestine. Therefore, prodrug approaches are usually pursued to improve the membrane permeability of a drug.

11.7.1 Increasing Passive Permeation

Most of the prodrugs in the market were designed to increase the passive transcellular permeation of a parent drug by masking hydrophilic functional groups, such as carboxyl, hydroxyl, and guanidine groups [54, 55]. In many cases, prodrugs are converted to the parent drugs by esterase [54]. Animal models may not be suitable to evaluate the performance of a prodrug due to the species difference in carboxyl esterase [54]. In addition, Caco-2 cells express different types of carboxyl esterase from the *in vivo* human intestine [54, 56, 57].

Although not yet investigated, biopharmaceutical modeling will be soon applicable for prodrugs. Estimation of the conversion rate in the intestinal lumen and enterocyte is of particular importance. Mizuma [58] summarized the relationship between the conversion clearance and absorption clearance.

11.7.2 Hitchhiking the Carrier

Valacyclovir is a prodrug of acyclovir (Fig. 11.16) [59]. Valacyclovir is designed to hitchhike PEP-T1 expressed in the small intestine. This approach has been extensively investigated [60–64]. In addition to PEP-T1, bile acid transporter [62] and glucose transporter [65–67] were also investigated as a candidate for this approach.

11.8 CONTROLLED RELEASE

Biopharmaceutical modeling for controlled-release (CR) formulations is one of the most highly demanded tasks for biopharmaceutical modeling. CR can be categorized as prolonged release, timed release, and stimuli-triggered release. A prolonged-release formulation is designed to gradually release a drug. A timed-release formulation is designed to release a drug at a predefined time elapsing after administration. The stimuli-triggered formulations, such as an enteric coating formulation, are designed to release a drug by a specific stimulus at the desired GI

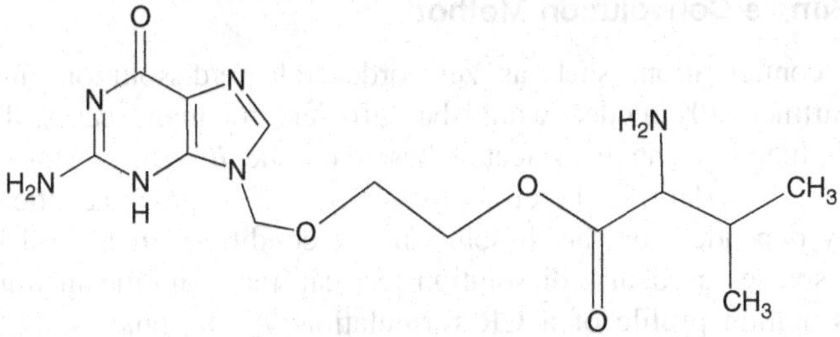

Figure 11.16 Valacyclovir.

position, for example, pH. In the following sections, each category is discussed in detail, as well as the key aspects of biopharmaceutical modeling.

The objectives of biopharmaceutical modeling for a CR development can be divided into (A) mechanistic simulation of release profile from the formulation and (B) convolution of the release pattern with the PK profile. For (A), various factors had to be taken into account, for example, the mechanism of water penetration into the formulation, erosion of the excipient, dissolution of a drug, and the effect of shear force. This type of investigation is important for designing the formulation and manufacture process. On the other hand, (B) is often used to figure out the release pattern required to achieve a desirable PK profile. Even though (A) and (B) can be merged in the future, currently these two are separately investigated. In the following sections, we first discuss (B) and then briefly discuss (A).

11.8.1 Fundamentals of CR Modeling

For a CR formulation to work, the following two points are fundamental:

- CR formulation is designed to show a robust release profile against the variations in the physiological environment, such as pH, bile concentration, and agitation strength.
- The rate-limiting process of drug absorption should be the drug release process from the formulation, rather than intestinal membrane permeability.

These trivial points mean that the use of complicated physiological biopharmaceutical modeling is not required in most cases. Even though the CR function is provided in commercial modeling software, these programs only calculate the convolution of user-defined release profile and PK profile. Currently, little or no mechanistic biopharmaceutical modeling has been reported, in which the effect of physiological environment on the release profile of CR formulation has been taken into account. Therefore, a convolution of drug release and drug disposition functions might be sufficient for biopharmaceutical modeling (the use of a complicated physiological GI model may not be required or should even be avoided considering the transparency of the model).

11.8.2   Simple Convolution Method

A simple configuration, such as zero-order release/dissolution function plus one compartment PK model, would be sufficient for many cases. The release/dissolution function can be selected based on the *in vitro* release/dissolution profile of the formulation. Therefore, the success of biopharmaceutical modeling is critically dependent on the dissolution test conditions. It is well known that the buffer species used in a dissolution test can have significant impact on the release/dissolution profile of a CR formulation. A phosphate buffer, which is most widely used as a dissolution media (including FaSSIF and FeSSIF), may not be suitable, whereas a bicarbonate buffer would be more suitable [68, 69].

11.8.3   Advanced Controlled-Release Modeling

It is very difficult to incorporate the effect of biological factors into the modeling of CR formulation. To do this task, a mechanistic model that can handle the effect of physiological factors on the release profile is required. Currently, mechanistic simulation of drug release from a matrix-type CR formulation is under extensive investigation [70–72]. Jia and Williams used the computational fluid dynamic (CFD) simulation to investigate the dissolution behavior of a tablet. X-ray microtomography (XMT) was used to provide the structural input [73] for CFD.

11.8.4   Controlled-Release Function

In biopharmaceutical modeling, the release profile can be represented by a CR function, which is linked to the virtual particle bins (Section 5.4.3). For prolonged- and timed-release formulations, the binary CR function can be programmed to activate the dissolution of the particles as a function of time after oral administration. For triggered-release formulations, the binary CR function can be programmed to activate the dissolution of the particle by a specific physiological condition or elapsed time, such as pH (Section 5.4.3).

11.8.5   Sustained Release

11.8.5.1   Objectives to Develop a Sustained-Release Formulation.   The key objectives for prolonged release could be to

- reduce the dosing frequency to increase compliance;
- decrease the systemic side effects by lowering the C_{max}/C_{min} ratio;
- avoid degradation by the acidic pH of the stomach;
- deliver the drug to fit to the circadian rhythm of a disease.

If CR is needed to reduce C_{max}-related side effects, the dosage form might have a 4–6 h delivery duration. If the objective is to avoid degradation of acid-labile drugs, enteric coating formulations can also be used. The timed- or prolonged-release formulation can be used to adjust the C_p–time profile with the circadian rhythm of a disease.

11.8.5.2 Suitable Drug Character for Sustained Release. Feasibilities
of a drug for a CR formulation are summarized in Table 11.8 (except enteric
coating formulation) [74]. Among these properties, mathematical biopharmaceutical models can support the assessment of P_{eff}, absorption mechanism, first-pass
metabolism, etc. The drug should have reasonable solubility and permeability
along the GI tract. The assessment of regional differences is discussed in detail
in Section 13.6.

11.8.5.3 Gastroretentive Formulation. The gastroretentive formulation
gained a lot of interest, as it can continuously supply drug to the upper small
intestine. Therefore, this technology can be applied to a drug that shows
site-specific and/or saturable membrane permeation in the upper small intestine,
especially the ones with little colonic absorption, such as gabapentin (Fig. 11.17).
Ofloxacin, metformine, ciprofloxacin, gabapentin, morphine, prazosin, cefaclor,
tramadol, baclofen, carvedilol, levodopa, diazepam, and misoprostol have been
marketed as gastroretentive formulation [75].

Swelling [77] and floating [75] systems are most often used. The swelling
system formulation increases its size larger than the pylorus diameter when it
is exposed to the gastric fluid. As erosion of the swelled formulation occurs,
the size of the formulation reduces and the formulation eventually exits into the
small intestine. The initial formulation size is typically ca. 10 mm, and the size
expands a few fold in the stomach.

The floating system has sufficient buoyancy to float over the gastric contents
and remain in the stomach for a prolonged period. While the system floats over
the gastric contents, the drug is slowly released [75]. Floating systems can be
further classified as effervescent and noneffervescent systems.

Biopharmaceutical modeling would be beneficial to support the design of
release profile. The gastric emptying time of a formulation can be modified to
represent the *in vivo* situation.

11.8.6 Triggered Release

11.8.6.1 Time-Triggered Release. Time-triggered release (pulsate release)
is of particular interest for chronotherapy [78, 79]. Single unit and multiple
unit systems have been investigated. Biopharmaceutical modeling for multiple
unit systems are straightforward, as the release from a granule can be easily
represented by the conditional binary CR function (Section 5.4.3). For single unit
system, the migrating motor complex affects the gastric emptying time (Section
6.2.2).

11.8.6.2 pH-Triggered Release. Enteric coating is often used to avoid
degradation of a drug in the stomach and/or to protect the stomach from
irritation by a drug. The coating polymer is usually an acid polymer that does
not dissolve at an acidic pH but dissolves in a neutral pH of around 5–6.
Polymethacrylic resins are widely used as pH-sensitive polymers for the purpose

TABLE 11.8 Suitability for Controlled-Release Formulation

Dose, mg	<1	Greater development complexity (potential drug content uniformity issue)
	10–250	Average degree of difficulty
	≫250–300	Could need more than one tablet to accommodate the drug load
Dose Number	<0.004	Several technology options exist for CR development
	0.004<, <0.4	Average degree of difficulty
	0.4<, <4	CR development will be challenging but feasible
	4<, <40	Need solubilization; CR development will be difficult
	>40	CR development is practically impossible
Absorption Mechanism	Transcellular passive diffusion	Average degree of difficulty
	Other mechanisms including efflux	Performance could be difficult to predict
Permeability (P_{eff}), cm/s	$< 0.3 \times 10^{-4}$	CR formulations with prolonged delivery duration may not be feasible; likely will not be bioequivalent to IR
	$0.3<, <3 \times 10^{-4}$	CR development challenging but feasible; might not be bioequivalent to IR
	$>3 \times 10^{-4}$	CR development should be feasible; likely to be bioequivalent to IR
Metabolism and Efflux	High presystemic or first-pass metabolism	Relative BA of CR formulation might be low
	Compound is P-gp or CYP3A4 substrate	CR performance difficult to predict
PK or PD Half-Life	<1–2 h	Half-life too short for CR development
	2–10 h	Acceptable half-life
	>10 h	Compound might not need CR for reducing dosing frequency

IR, immediate release.

of enteric coating and colon targeting, for example, commercially available ones such as Eudragit®. Different types of Eudragit, whether water insoluble or water soluble, are used for colon targeting. Eudragit L dissolves at pH $\geq$ 6, whereas Eudragit S dissolves at pH $\geq$ 7 because of the presence of a higher amount of esterified groups than carboxylic groups.

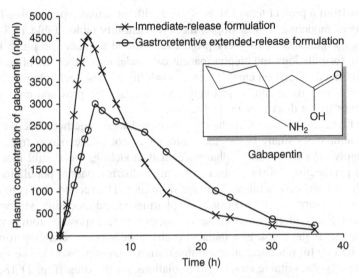

Figure 11.17 Gabapentin plasma concentration (mean ± SE)-time profiles following single-dose oral administration of the drug (600 mg) as immediate-release and gastroretentive extended-release formulations under fed state (1000 kcal, ~50% from fat). *Source:* Replotted from Reference 76.

The pH-triggered formulation for colonic targeting has been investigated. Compared to enteric coating, colon targeting by a pH-sensitive polymer is difficult because of the intra- and interindividual variation in the intestinal and colonic pH.

Biopharmaceutical modeling for pH-sensitive formulations is relatively straightforward. The CR function can be programmed to activate as the virtual particle bins sense the pH environment (Section 5.4.3). The postprandial pH change in the stomach should be taken into account when investigating the food effect on the pH-triggered CR formulation.

11.8.6.3 *Position-Triggered Release.* The diazo functional group is liable for bacterial degradation in the colon. This property can be used to deliver an active drug to the colon. The prodrug approach has been most successful in the past, for example, sulfasalazine. Bacteria-degradable polymers have also been investigated [80, 81]. Biopharmaceutical modeling can be performed in the same manner with the pH-triggered formulation.

11.9 COMMUNICATION WITH THERAPEUTIC PROJECT TEAM

Biopharmaceutical modeling is often requested from a project team to investigate the feasibility of enabling formulations. This request should be responded starting with consultation. In more than 50% cases, probably more than 80% cases, the requests from a project team can be solved without actually performing biopharmaceutical modeling. For example, the CR feasibility table (Table 11.8) can be used as the guidance. Discovery project teams tend to place too much hope on enabling formulations and biopharmaceutical modeling, as they are often exposed to exaggerated advertisements about the capability of these technologies. The subject matter experts should objectively communicate the pros and cons of these techniques to the discovery project teams.

The first step is to listen to the customers and work together to derive a problem statement. In many cases, the customer is not aware of the true problem and simply asks us to run biopharmaceutical modeling. We should first discuss various perspectives of the project (e.g., target disease, patient population, available PK and physicochemical data, and deadline). The second step is to identify the cause of inappropriate exposure. Biopharmaceutical modeling will be helpful to quantitatively identify the cause of inappropriate exposure from a standard formulation. If the cause is a metabolic clearance process, enabling formations cannot be helpful (an alternative administration route may work). The third step is to identify the suitable enabling formulations for the drug (Fig. 11.18).

The last step is the assessment of the effect of an enabling formulation on oral absorption of a drug. However, because the absorption enhancement mechanisms of the enabling formulations are complicated, biopharmaceutical modeling might not be applicable. In addition, there might not exist any appropriate *in vitro* method. Therefore, an *in vivo* test should also be considered. In the preclinical stage, *in vivo* dog models would be practically the most appropriate method to test the performance of formulations. These points should be well communicated to the other disciplines that are overexpecting the ability of current commercial biopharmaceutical modeling programs.

For CR simulation, the tabled data of release profile obtained from an *in vitro* dissolution test is often used for simulation. When a commercial program is used in this way, it should be remembered that the effect of physiological factors are

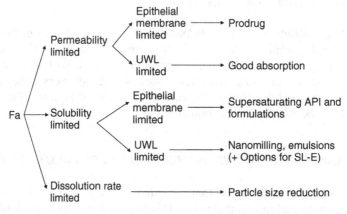

Figure 11.18 Decision tree for enabling formulation.

not taken into account for the release profile from the formulation. A simple combination of release kinetics and disposition kinetics would be sufficient for many cases, as the dissolution (of API) and membrane permeability is usually not the rate-limiting step for a CR drug product.

REFERENCES

1. Carlert, S., Palsson, A., Hanisch, G., von Corswant, C., Nilsson, C., Lindfors, L., Lennernas, H., Abrahamsson, B. (2010). Predicting intestinal precipitation–a case example for a basic BCS class II drug. *Pharm. Res.*, 27, 2119–2130.

2. Serajuddin, A. T., Sheen, P. C., Mufson, D., Bernstein, D. F., Augustine, M. A. (1986). Preformulation study of a poorly water-soluble drug, alpha-pentyl-3-(2-quinolinylmethoxy)benzenemethanol: selection of the base for dosage form design. *J. Pharm. Sci.*, 75, 492–496.

3. Hawley, M., Morozowich, W. (2010). Modifying the diffusion layer of soluble salts of poorly soluble basic drugs to improve dissolution performance. *Mol. Pharm.*, 7, 1441–1449.

4. Lehto, P., Aaltonen, J., Tenho, M., Rantanen, J., Hirvonen, J., Tanninen, V. P., Peltonen, L. (2009). Solvent-mediated solid phase transformations of carbamazepine: effects of simulated intestinal fluid and fasted state simulated intestinal fluid. *J. Pharm. Sci.*, 98, 985–996.

5. Boetker, J. P., Savolainen, M., Koradia, V., Tian, F., Rades, T., Mullertz, A., Cornett, C., Rantanen, J., Ostergaard, J. (2011). Insights into the early dissolution events of amlodipine using UV imaging and Raman spectroscopy. *Mol. Pharm.*, 8, 1372–1380.

6. Serajuddin, A. T. M. (2007). Salt formation to improve drug solubility. *Adv. Drug Delivery Rev.*, 59, 603–616.

7. Mueller, B. U., Sleasman, J., Nelson, R. P. Jr., Smith, S., Deutsch, P. J., Ju, W., Steinberg, S. M., Balis, F. M., Jarosinski, P. F., Brouwers, P., Mistry, G., Winchell, G., Zwerski, S., Sei, S., Wood, L. V., Zeichner, S., Pizzo, P. A. (1998). A phase I/II study of the protease inhibitor indinavir in children with HIV infection. *Pediatrics*, 102, 101–109.

8. Takano, R., Takata, N., Saitoh, R., Furumoto, K., Higo, S., Hayashi, Y., Machida, M., Aso, Y., Yamashita, S. (2010). Quantitative analysis of the effect of supersaturation on in vivo drug absorption. *Mol. Pharm.*, 7, 1431–1440.

9. Busch, F. R., Rose, C. A., Shine, R. J. (1999). Mesylate dihydrate salts of 5-(2-(4-(1,2-benzisothiazol-3-yl)-1-piperazinyl)-ethyl)-6-chloro-1,3-dihyd   ro-2(1H)-indol-2-one (= ziprasidone), its preparation and its use as dopamine D2 antagonist.

10. Curatolo, W. J., Herbig, S. M., Hombre, A. G., Shah, J. C., Shamblin, S. L., Lukas, T., Caldwell, W. B., Friesen, D. T., Lyon, D. K., Craig, C. D. (2009). Methods, dosage forms and kits for administering ziprasidone without food.

11. Miceli, J. J., Glue, P., Alderman, J., Wilner, K. (2007). The effect of food on the absorption of oral ziprasidone. *Psychopharmacol. Bull.*, 40, 58–68.

12. Arenson, D. R., Busch, F. R., Hausberger, A. G., Rasadi, B. (1999). Ziprasidone formulations.

13. Dill, W. A., Glazko, A. J., Kazenko, A., Wolf, L. M. (1956). Studies on 5, 5′-diphenylhydantoin (dilantin) in animals and man. *J. Pharmacol. Exp. Ther.*, 118, 270–279.

14. Shinkuma, D., Hashimoto, H., Yamanaka, Y., Murata, Y., Mizuno, N. (1979). Bioavailability of phenytoin. *Yakugaku Zasshi*, 39, 121–128.

15. Grzesiak, A. L., Lang, M., Kim, K., Matzger, A. J. (2003). Comparison of the four anhydrous polymorphs of carbamazepine and the crystal structure of form I. *J. Pharm. Sci.*, 92, 2260–2271.

16. Hickey, M. B., Peterson, M. L., Scoppettuolo, L. A., Morrisette, S. L., Vetter, A., Guzman, H., Remenar, J. F., Zhang, Z., Tawa, M. D., Haley, S., Zaworotko, M. J., Almarsson, O. (2007). Performance comparison of a co-crystal of carbamazepine with marketed product. *Eur. J. Pharm. Biopharm.*, 67, 112–119.

17. Kobayashi, Y., Ito, S., Itai, S., Yamamoto, K. (2000). Physicochemical properties and bioavailability of carbamazepine polymorphs and dihydrate. *Int. J. Pharm.*, 193, 137–146.

18. Takata, N., Shiraki, K., Takano, R., Hayashi, Y., Terada, K. (2008). Cocrystal screening of stanolone and mestanolone using slurry crystallization. *Cryst. Growth Des.*, 8, 3032–3037.

19. McNamara, D. P., Childs, S. L., Giordano, J., Iarriccio, A., Cassidy, J., Shet, M. S., Mannion, R., O'Donnell, E., Park, A. (2006). Use of a glutaric acid cocrystal to improve oral bioavailability of a low solubility API. *Pharm. Res.*, 23, 1888–1897.

20. Bak, A., Gore, A., Yanez, E., Stanton, M., Tufekcic, S., Syed, R., Akrami, A., Rose, M., Surapaneni, S., Bostick, T., King, A., Neervannan, S., Ostovic, D., Koparkar, A. (2008). The co-crystal approach to improve the exposure of a water-insoluble compound: AMG 517 sorbic acid co-crystal characterization and pharmacokinetics. *J. Pharm. Sci.*, 97, 3942–3956.

21. Jung, M. S., Kim, J. S., Kim, M. S., Alhalaweh, A., Cho, W., Hwang, S. J., Velaga, S. P. (2010). Bioavailability of indomethacin-saccharin cocrystals. *J. Pharm. Pharmacol.*, 62, 1560–1568.

22. Stephenson, G. A., Aburub, A., Woods, T. A. (2011). Physical stability of salts of weak bases in the solid-state. *J. Pharm. Sci.*, 100, 1607–1617.

23. Childs, S. L., Stahly, G. P., Park, A. (2007). The salt-cocrystal continuum: the influence of crystal structure on ionization state. *Mol. Pharm.*, 4, 323–338.

24. Gu, C. H., Gandhi, R. B., Tay, L. K., Zhou, S., Raghavan, K. (2004). Importance of using physiologically relevant volume of dissolution medium to correlate the oral exposure of formulations of BMS-480188 mesylate. *Int. J. Pharm.*, 269, 195–202.

25. Box, K., Comer, J. E., Gravestock, T., Stuart, M. (2009). New ideas about the solubility of drugs. *Chem. Biodivers.*, 6, 1767–1788.

26. Ozaki, S., Minamisono, T., Yamashita, T., Kato, T., Kushida, I. (2011). Supersaturation-nucleation behavior of poorly soluble drugs and its impact on the oral absorption of drugs in thermodynamically high-energy forms. *J. Pharm. Sci.*, 101(1), 214–22.

27. Kojima, T., Sugano, K., Onoue, S., Murase, N., Sato, M., Kawabata, Y., Mano, T. (2008). Solid form selection of zwitterionic 5-HT4 receptor agonist. *Int. J. Pharm.*, 350, 35–42.

28. Tanaka, Y., Inkyo, M., Yumoto, R., Nagai, J., Takano, M., Nagata, S. (2009). Nanoparticulation of poorly water soluble drugs using a wet-mill process and physicochemical properties of the nanopowders. *Chem. Pharm. Bull. (Tokyo)*, 57, 1050–1057.

29. Takatsuka, T., Endo, T., Jianguo, Y., Yuminoki, K., Hashimoto, N. (2009). Nanosizing of poorly water soluble compounds using rotation/revolution mixer. *Chem. Pharm. Bull. (Tokyo)*, 57, 1061–1067.

30. Niwa, T., Miura, S., Danjo, K. (2011). Universal wet-milling technique to prepare oral nanosuspension focused on discovery and preclinical animal studies - development of particle design method. *Int. J. Pharm.*, 405, 218–227.

31. Liversidge, G. G., Cundy, K. C. (1995). Particle size reduction for improvement of oral bioavailability of hydrophobic drugs: I. Absolute oral bioavailability of nanocrystalline danazol in beagle dogs. *Int. J. Pharm.*, 125, 91–97.

32. Pouton, C. W. (2006). Formulation of poorly water-soluble drugs for oral administration: physicochemical and physiological issues and the lipid formulation classification system. *Eur. J. Pharm. Sci.*, 29, 278–287.

33. MacGregor, K. J., Embleton, J. K., Lacy, J. E., Perry, E. A., Solomon, L. J., Seager, H., Pouton, C. W. (1997). Influence of lipolysis on drug absorption from the gastrointestinal tract. *Adv. Drug Delivery Rev.*, 25, 33–46.

34. Dahan, A., Hoffman, A. (2007). The effect of different lipid based formulations on the oral absorption of lipophilic drugs: the ability of in vitro lipolysis and consecutive ex vivo intestinal permeability data to predict in vivo bioavailability in rats. *Eur. J. Pharm. Biopharm.*, 67, 96–105.

35. Porter, C. J. H., Trevaskis, N. L., Charman, W. N. (2007). Lipids and lipid-based formulations: optimizing the oral delivery of lipophilic drugs. *Nat. Rev. Drug Discov.*, 6, 231–248.

36. Trevaskis, N. L., Charman, W. N., Porter, C. J. (2008). Lipid-based delivery systems and intestinal lymphatic drug transport: a mechanistic update. *Adv. Drug Delivery Rev.*, 60, 702–716.

37. Caliph, S. M., Charman, W. N., Porter, C. J. (2000). Effect of short-, medium-, and long-chain fatty acid-based vehicles on the absolute oral bioavailability and intestinal lymphatic transport of halofantrine and assessment of mass balance in lymph-cannulated and non-cannulated rats. *J. Pharm. Sci.*, 89, 1073–1084.

38. Chiou, W. L., Riegelman, S. (1971). Pharmaceutical applications of solid dispersion systems. *J. Pharm. Sci.*, 60, 1281–1302.

39. Serajuddin, A. T. (1999). Solid dispersion of poorly water-soluble drugs: early promises, subsequent problems, and recent breakthroughs. *J. Pharm. Sci.*, 88, 1058–1066.

40. Friesen, D. T., Shanker, R., Crew, M., Smithey, D. T., Curatolo, W. J., Nightingale, J. A. (2008). Hydroxypropyl methylcellulose acetate succinate-based spray-dried dispersions: an overview. *Mol. Pharm.*, 5, 1003–1019.

41. Gao, P., Rush, B. D., Pfund, W. P., Huang, T., Bauer, J. M., Morozowich, W., Kuo, M. S., Hageman, M. J. (2003). Development of a supersaturable SEDDS (S-SEDDS) formulation of paclitaxel with improved oral bioavailability. *J. Pharm. Sci.*, 92, 2386–2398.

42. Gao, P., Guyton, M. E., Huang, T., Bauer, J. M., Stefanski, K. J., Lu, Q. (2004). Enhanced oral bioavailability of a poorly water soluble drug PNU-91325 by supersaturatable formulations. *Drug Dev. Ind. Pharm.*, 30, 221–229.

43. Gao, P., Morozowich, W. (2006). Development of supersaturatable self-emulsifying drug delivery system formulations for improving the oral absorption of poorly soluble drugs. *Expert Opin. Drug Deliv.*, 3, 97–110.

44. Brouwers, J., Brewster, M. E., Augustijns, P. (2009). Supersaturating drug delivery systems: the answer to solubility-limited oral bioavailability? *J. Pharm. Sci.*, 98, 2549–2572.

45. Qian, K. K., Bogner, R. H. (2011). Application of mesoporous silicon dioxide and silicate in oral amorphous drug delivery systems. *J. Pharm. Sci.*, 75(3), 354–365.

46. Van Speybroeck, M., Mols, R., Mellaerts, R., Thi, T. D., Martens, J. A., Van Humbeeck, J., Annaert, P., Van den Mooter, G., Augustijns, P. (2010). Combined use of ordered mesoporous silica and precipitation inhibitors for improved oral absorption of the poorly soluble weak base itraconazole. *Eur. J. Pharm. Biopharm.*, 75, 354–365.

47. Van Speybroeck, M., Mellaerts, R., Mols, R., Thi, T. D., Martens, J. A., Van Humbeeck, J., Annaert, P., Van den Mooter, G., Augustijns, P. (2010). Enhanced absorption of the poorly soluble drug fenofibrate by tuning its release rate from ordered mesoporous silica. *Eur. J. Pharm. Sci.*, 41, 623–630.

48. Mellaerts, R., Aerts, A., Caremans, T. P., Vermant, J., Van den Mooter, G., Martens, J. A., Augustijns, P. (2010). Growth of itraconazole nanofibers in supersaturated simulated intestinal fluid. *Mol. Pharm.*, 7, 905–913.

49. Mellaerts, R., Mols, R., Kayaert, P., Annaert, P., Van Humbeeck, J., Van den Mooter, G., Martens, J. A., Augustijns, P. (2008). Ordered mesoporous silica induces pH-independent supersaturation of the basic low solubility compound itraconazole resulting in enhanced transepithelial transport. *Int. J. Pharm.*, 357, 169–179.

50. Lindfors, L., Forssen, S., Westergren, J., Olsson, U. (2008). Nucleation and crystal growth in supersaturated solutions of a model drug. *J. Colloid Interface Sci.*, 325, 404–413.

51. Varia, S. A., Schuller, S., Sloan, K. B., Stella, V. J. (1984). Phenytoin prodrugs III: water-soluble prodrugs for oral and/or parenteral use. *J. Pharm. Sci.*, 73, 1068–1073.

52. Varia, S. A., Stella, V. J. (1984). Phenytoin prodrugs V: in vivo evaluation of some water-soluble phenytoin prodrugs in dogs. *J. Pharm. Sci.*, 73, 1080–1087.

53. Yuan, H., Li, N., Lai, Y. (2009). Evaluation of in vitro models for screening alkaline phosphatase-mediated bioconversion of phosphate ester prodrugs. *Drug Metab. Dispos.*, 37, 1443–1447.

54. Imai, T., Ohura, K. (2010). The role of intestinal carboxylesterase in the oral absorption of prodrugs. *Curr. Drug Metab.*, 11, 793–805.

55. Sun, J., Dahan, A., Amidon, G. L. (2010). Enhancing the intestinal absorption of molecules containing the polar guanidino functionality: a double-targeted prodrug approach. *J. Med. Chem.*, 53, 624–632.

56. Ohura, K., Sakamoto, H., Ninomiya, S., Imai, T. (2010). Development of a novel system for estimating human intestinal absorption using Caco-2 cells in the absence of esterase activity. *Drug Metab. Dispos.*, 38, 323–331.

57. Ohura, K., Nozawa, T., Murakami, K., Imai, T. (2011). Evaluation of transport mechanism of prodrugs and parent drugs formed by intracellular metabolism in Caco-2 cells with modified carboxylesterase activity: temocapril as a model case. *J. Pharm. Sci.*, 100, 3985–3994.

58. Mizuma, T. (2008). Pharmacokinetic strategy for designing orally effective prodrugs overcoming biological membrane barriers: proposal of kinetic classification and criteria for membrane-permeable prodrug-likeness. *Chem. Bioinform. J.*, 8, 25–32.

59. Balimane, P. V., Tamai, I., Guo, A., Nakanishi, T., Kitada, H., Leibach, F. H., Tsuji, A., Sinko, P. J. (1998). Direct evidence for peptide transporter (PepT1)-mediated uptake of a nonpeptide prodrug, valacyclovir. *Biochem. Biophys. Res. Commun.*, 250, 246–251.

60. Ma, K., Hu, Y., Smith, D. E. (2011). Peptide transporter 1 is responsible for intestinal uptake of the dipeptide glycylsarcosine: studies in everted jejunal rings from wild-type and Pept1 null mice. *J. Pharm. Sci.*, 100, 767–774.

61. Omkvist, D. H., Trangbaek, D. J., Mildon, J., Paine, J. S., Brodin, B., Begtrup, M., Nielsen, C. U. (2011). Affinity and translocation relationships via hPEPT1 of H-X aa-Ser-OH dipeptides: evaluation of H-Phe-Ser-OH as a pro-moiety for ibuprofen and benzoic acid prodrugs. *Eur. J. Pharm. Biopharm.*, 77, 327–331.

62. Rais, R., Fletcher, S., Polli, J. E. (2011). Synthesis and in vitro evaluation of gabapentin prodrugs that target the human apical sodium-dependent bile acid transporter (hASBT). *J. Pharm. Sci.*, 100, 1184–1195.

63. Gupta, S. V., Gupta, D., Sun, J., Dahan, A., Tsume, Y., Hilfinger, J., Lee, K. D., Amidon, G. L. (2011). Enhancing the intestinal membrane permeability of zanamivir: a carrier mediated prodrug approach. *Mol. Pharm.*, 8(6), 2358–2367.

64. Yan, Z., Sun, J., Chang, Y., Liu, Y., Fu, Q., Xu, Y., Sun, Y., Pu, X., Zhang, Y., Jing, Y., Yin, S., Zhu, M., Wang, Y., He, Z. (2011). Bifunctional peptidomimetic prodrugs of didanosine for improved intestinal permeability and enhanced acidic stability: synthesis, transepithelial transport, chemical stability and pharmacokinetics. *Mol. Pharm.*, 8, 319–329.

65. Mizuma, T., Ohta, K., Hayashi, M., Awazu, S. (1992). Intestinal active absorption of sugar-conjugated compounds by glucose transport system: implication of improvement of poorly absorbable drugs. *Biochem. Pharmacol.*, 43, 2037–2039.

66. Mizuma, T., Awazu, S. (1998). Intestinal Na+/glucose cotransporter-mediated transport of glucose conjugate formed from disaccharide conjugate. *Biochim. Biophys. Acta*, 1379, 1–6.

67. Mizuma, T., Nagamine, Y., Dobashi, A., Awazu, S. (1998). Factors that cause the beta-anomeric preference of Na+/glucose cotransporter for intestinal transport of monosaccharide conjugates. *Biochim. Biophys. Acta*, 1381, 340–346.

68. Liu, F., Merchant, H. A., Kulkarni, R. P., Alkademi, M., Basit, A. W. (2011). Evolution of a physiological pH 6.8 bicarbonate buffer system: application to the dissolution testing of enteric coated products. *Eur. J. Pharm. Biopharm.*, 78, 151–157.

69. Fadda, H. M., Merchant, H. A., Arafat, B. T., Basit, A. W. (2009). Physiological bicarbonate buffers: stabilisation and use as dissolution media for modified release systems. *Int. J. Pharm.*, 382, 56–60.

70. Siepmann, J., Gopferich, A. (2001). Mathematical modeling of bioerodible, polymeric drug delivery systems. *Adv. Drug Delivery Rev.*, 48, 229–247.

71. Borgquist, P., Korner, A., Piculell, L., Larsson, A., Axelsson, A. (2006). A model for the drug release from a polymer matrix tablet–effects of swelling and dissolution. *J. Controlled Release*, 113, 216–225.

72. Kaunisto, E., Abrahmsen-Alami, S., Borgquist, P., Larsson, A., Nilsson, B., Axelsson, A. (2010). A mechanistic modelling approach to polymer dissolution using magnetic resonance microimaging. *J. Controlled Release*, 147, 232–241.

73. Jia, X., Williams, R. A. (2007). A hybrid mesoscale modelling approach to dissolution of granules and tablets. *Chem. Eng. Res. Des.*, 85, 1027–1038.

74. Thombre, A. G. (2005). Assessment of the feasibility of oral controlled release in an exploratory development setting. *Drug Discov. Today*, 10, 1159–1166.

75. Pawar, V. K., Kansal, S., Garg, G., Awasthi, R., Singodia, D., Kulkarni, G. T. (2011). Gastroretentive dosage forms: a review with special emphasis on floating drug delivery systems. *Drug Deliv.*, 18, 97–110.

76. Chen, C., Cowles, V. E., Hou, E. (2011). Pharmacokinetics of gabapentin in a novel gastric-retentive extended-release formulation: comparison with an immediate-release formulation and effect of dose escalation and food. *J. Clin. Pharmacol.*, 51, 346–358.

77. Berner, B., Cowles, V. E. (2006). Case studies in swelling polymeric gastric retentive tablets. *Expert Opin. Drug deliv.*, 3, 541–548.

78. Youan, B. B. (2004). Chronopharmaceutics: gimmick or clinically relevant approach to drug delivery? *J. Controlled Release*, 98, 337–353.

79. Gandhi, B. R., Mundada, A. S., Gandhi, P. P. (2011). Chronopharmaceutics: as a clinically relevant drug delivery system. *Drug Deliv.*, 18, 1–18.

80. Van den Mooter, G. (2006). Colon drug delivery. *Expert Opin. Drug Deliv.*, 3, 111–125.

81. Shah, N., Shah, T., Amin, A. (2011). Polysaccharides: a targeting strategy for colonic drug delivery. *Expert Opin. Drug Deliv.*, 8, 779–796.

CHAPTER 12

FOOD EFFECT

"It is not just food. It is M&S food."

—Marks & Spencer TV ad.

The modeling and simulation (M&S) of the food effect on oral drug absorption is one of the key areas where biopharmaceutical modeling can be applied. It is preferable to design a compound and formulation that is less susceptible to the food effect. In addition to meals, fruit juice and alcohol also affect the oral absorption of a drug.

12.1 PHYSIOLOGICAL CHANGES CAUSED BY FOOD

The changes in physiological conditions by food intake have already been discussed in Chapter 6 and are only briefly described here. The bile acid concentration in the GI fluid increases from ca. 3 mM in the fasted state to ca. 15 mM in the fed state. The stomach pH is increased from 1.5 to 6 immediately after food intake and gradually decreases to the fasted pH in 1 h [1]. In the small intestine, pH in the fed state is about 6, which is slightly lower than that in the fasted state (pH 6.5). The stomach emptying time ($T_{1/2}$) increases from ca. 10 min in the fasted state to ca. 60 min in the fed state. Food intake increases the intestinal motility and intestinal and hepatic blood flows. Among these physiological changes, the increase of bile micelles is the most significant postprandial

Biopharmaceutics Modeling and Simulations: Theory, Practice, Methods, and Applications,
First Edition. Kiyohiko Sugano.
© 2012 John Wiley & Sons, Inc. Published 2012 by John Wiley & Sons, Inc.

change that affects the oral absorption of a drug. The development of a simulated intestinal fluid to mimic the postprandial state has been extensively investigated.

12.1.1 Food Component

Food components have a significant impact on the food effect. FDA recommends that food effect studies should be conducted using meal conditions that are expected to provide the greatest food effect. A high fat (~50% of total caloric content of the meal) and high calorie (~800–1000 kcal) meals is recommended as a test meal for food effect studies. This test meal should derive approximately 150, 250, and 500–600 kcal from protein, carbohydrate, and fat, respectively. An example test meal would be two eggs fried in butter, two strips of bacon, two slices of toast with butter, 4 oz of hash brown potatoes, and 8 oz of whole milk (Table 12.1) [2].

The contraction of the gallbladder is stimulated by a small amount of lipid ingested. Carbohydrates increase the motility of the intestinal tract but not the gallbladder contraction [3]. Typical viscosities of meals lie in the range of 10 to 100,000 cP. Marciani and coworkers utilized echo planar magnetic resonance imaging (MRI) in humans to monitor the changes in viscosity of meals and demonstrated significant and rapid reductions in viscosity with time due to dilution by the gastric fluids [4]. Figure 12.1 shows the effect of food component on the stomach pH [5]. Protein increased the gastric pH, whereas carbohydrate (Moducal) and lipid did not.

12.1.2 Fruit Juice Components

Recently, fruit juice–drug interaction has been extensively investigated. Grapefruit is known to affect the oral absorption of CYP3A4 and OATP substrates. Figure 12.2 shows the major flavonoids in the grapefruit juice. Table 12.2 shows

TABLE 12.1 Examples of Meals Used in Food Effect Studies

Standard Breakfast Meal[a]	Ensure Plus[b]
One English muffin with butter	Energy, kJ, 1263
One fried egg	Energy, kcal, 300
One slice of cheese	Carbohydrate, g, 40.4
One slice of Canadian bacon	Protein, g, 12.5
One serving of hash browned (fried shredded)	Total fat, g, 8.4
potatoes	Saturated fatty acids, g, 0.98
6 oz orange juice	Essential fatty acids, g, 2.9
8 oz whole milk	Dietary fiber, g, 0
Carbohydrate 73 g, 292 kcal, 1222 kJ, 45% of calories	Water, g, 155
Protein 29 g, 116 kcal, 485 kJ, 18% of calories	Minerals, vitamins
Fat 27 g, 240 kcal, 1004 kJ, 37% of calories	

[a]FDA office of generic drugs.
[b]Nutritive value per 200 ml.

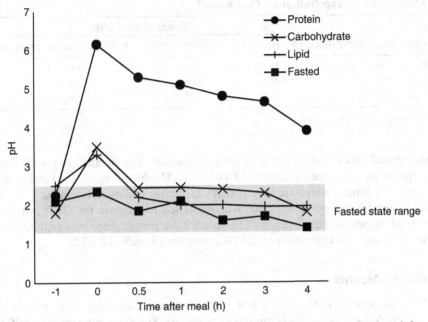

Figure 12.1 Stomach pH changes after meal administration. *Source:* Replotted from Reference 5.

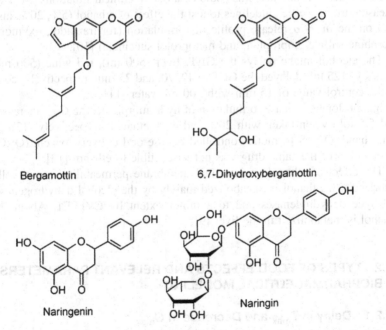

Figure 12.2 Structures of flavonoids and furanocoumarins present in grapefruit juice. *Source:* Adapted from Reference 8 with permission.

TABLE 12.2 Grapefruit Juice Component[a]

Type of Grapefruit Juice	Concentration, μM		
	Naringin	Bergamottin	6′,7′-Dihydroxybergamottin
Pink (3 brands)	782 ± 113	10.0 ± 2.9	0.6 ± 0.3
White (5 brands)	1010 ± 287	24.5 ± 7.6	14.5 ± 22.1
Red (6 brands)	473 ± 277	9.5 ± 6.3	5.6 ± 6.5

[a]References 6 and 8.

the typical concentration range of these flavonoids. The interaction via CYP3A is due to its high concentrations of DHB (6′,7′-dihydroxybergamottin) and/or the spiroester dimers, which are very potent irreversible inhibitors of enteric CYP3A [6]. Concentrated grapefruit juice was suggested to increase the GET, whereas normal grapefruit juice does not [7]. In addition, orange juice was suggested to decrease the oral absorption of OATP substrates (Section 12.2.3.2).

12.1.3 Alcohol

The concomitant intake of alcohol can cause an uncontrolled rapid release of a controlled-release formulation (dose dumping). Since a controlled-release formulation usually contains a larger drug amount than an IR formulation, if this amount is released at once, this could be a risk in clinical situations [9]. The FDA released drug-specific guidelines to test the effect of ethanol (5%, 20%, and 40% v/v) on the *in vitro* release profile of formulation (for tramadol, oxymorphone, morphine sulfate, bupropion, and metoprolol succinate) [10].

The alcohol intake delays the GET. Beer (500 ml), red wine (500 ml), and whiskey (125 ml) delayed the GET to 40, 70, and 25 min, respectively, compared to the control value of 15 min with 500 ml water [11].

In a prolonged-release formulation of hydromorphone, the C_{max} increased 1.9- and 5.5-fold when taken with 20% and 40% ethanol, respectively [12]. On the other hand, OROS [osmotic-controlled release oral delivery system (OROS[TM])] formulation of the same drug was not susceptible to ethanol [13].

The effect of ethanol on intestinal membrane permeability is not well characterized [9]. Ethanol is metabolized mainly by the alcohol dehydrogenases and aldehyde dehydrogenases and to a minor extent by CYP2E1. About 99% of ethanol is metabolized in the liver [9].

12.2 TYPES OF FOOD EFFECTS AND RELEVANT PARAMETERS IN BIOPHARMACEUTICAL MODELING

12.2.1 Delay in T_{max} and Decrease in C_{max}

The delay in stomach emptying occurs, regardless of the drug property. However, the delay in T_{max} and reduction in C_{max} are often not observed for BCS II drugs, as an increase in drug solubility in the intestine in the fed state masks these effects.

To investigate the appropriateness of the kinetic model for gastric emptying, biopharmaceutical modeling of acetaminophen was investigated, as shown in Figure 12.3 [14–16]. Acetaminophen is often used as a marker to investigate the GET. By setting the GET $T_{1/2}$ to 60 min, oral PK profile of acetaminophen in the fed state is appropriately reproduced (Fig. 12.3).

12.2.2 Positive Food Effect

A drug that shows a positive food effect usually has a dose number greater than 1 [18, 19] and high permeability (BCS II) [20, 21].

12.2.2.1 Bile Micelle Solubilization.
Bile micelle solubilization has been suggested to be the major reason for a positive food effect for compounds with low solubility with Do > 1 (solubility-permeability-limited (SL) cases). However, this looks contradicting to the free fraction theory, as bile micelle solubilization would not increase the concentration of unbound drug (Section 2.3.3). This contradiction can be dispelled by considering the difference between the UWL- and epithelial-membrane-limited cases (SL-U and SL-E, respectively).

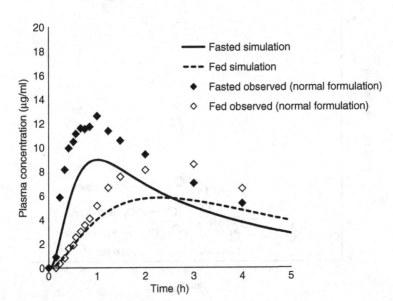

Figure 12.3   Food effect on acetaminophen PK. Dose = 1000 mg, $S_{dissolv}$ = 23.7 mg/ml, k_{perm} = 0.038 min^{-1} (estimated from rat SPIP data [14], FgFh = 0.8 [14], d_p = 1 μm (immediate dissolution), k_{12} = 0.95 h^{-1}, k_{21} = 1.41 h^{-1}, k_{13} = 0.51 h^{-1}, and V_1 = 0.6 l/kg [17]. Gastric $T_{1/2}$ = 10 min (fasted) and 60 min (fed). *Source:* Observed data from Reference 15.

The drug molecules bound to bile micelles can pass through the UWL. Once carried close to the epithelial membrane, the drug molecules, which are in rapid dynamic equilibrium between the bound and unbound states, then permeate the epithelial membrane. In the case of solubility-UWL-limited drugs (SL-U), the former process is slower than the latter process and becomes the rate-limiting step. Bile micelles increase the solubility of a drug (S_{dissolv}) (i.e., increase the dissolved drug concentration (C_{dissolv})). At the same time, as the diffusion of bile-micelle-bound drug molecules is slower than that of unbound drug molecules, bile micelle binding reduces the effective diffusion coefficient (D_{eff}) of a drug in the UWL (Section 8.4.6). However, the D_{eff} does not become zero (cf. $D_{\text{eff}} = f_u \times D_{\text{mono}} + (1 - f_u) \times D_{\text{bm}}$). Consequently, the flux across the UWL is increased by bile micelle solubilization of a drug (cf. flux $= C_{\text{dissolv}} \times P_{\text{UWL}}$). For example, P_{UWL} of griseofulvin would be slightly decreased (0.6-fold), while its solubility is increased 2.3-fold, resulting in a net positive food effect (1.6-fold). Reduction in the effective permeability of griseofulvin by bile binding was experimentally observed [22].

Figure 12.4 shows the relationship between the lipophilicity of a drug and the clinical food effect for SL-U cases (undissociable drugs). A positive food effect

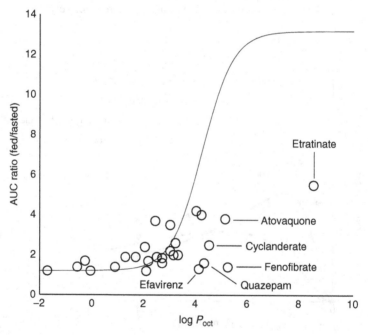

Figure 12.4   Relationship between lipophilicity of a drug and clinical food effect for SL-U cases (undissociable drugs). The solid line indicates an a priori theoretical line derived from $\log K_{\text{bm}} - \log P_{\text{oct}}$ and $\log P_{\text{trans,0}} - \log P_{\text{oct}}$ relationships. D_{mono} and D_{bm} for the fasted and fed states were set to 7, 0.5, and 1.1×10^{-6} cm^2/s, respectively. V_{GI} ratio was set to 1.2.

by bile micelle solubilization would be observed for a compound with its $\log P_{oct}$ greater than 2. The theoretical line in Figure 12.4 shows an *a priori* prediction derived from the $\log K_{bm}$–$\log P_{oct}$ equation (Eq. 2.17), the $\log P_{trans,0}$–$\log P_{oct}$ equation (Eq. 4.34), and the diffusion coefficient of bile micelles. This theoretical line corresponds to the maximum food effect, so that when Fa% in the fed state is 100%, the fed/fasted AUC ratio can become less than the predicted values (Fig. 12.5). For example, if a drug has Fa% = 50% in the fasted state, the fed/fasted AUC ratio cannot exceed 2. Atovaquone (Fa% in the fasted state = 30%, the hereinafter the same), fenofibrate (51%), efavirenz (82%), cyclandelate (>40%), quazepam (>56%), and etretinate (30–70%) [23] would be such cases (Table 12.3). The positive food effect can be more than 10-fold, for example, halofantrine HCl (13-fold, 250 mg in dogs, $\log P_{oct}$ = 8.9) [24] and indomethacin farnesil (>50-fold, 150 mg in humans, calculated $\log P_{oct}$ = 9.6) [25]. The relationship between solubility ratio (FeSSIF/FaSSIF) and clinical food effect for SL-U cases is shown in Figure 12.5.

On the other hand, in the case of solubility–epithelial membrane limited drugs (SL-E), the oral absorption would not be increased by bile micelle solubilization. The bile-micelle-bound fraction cannot permeate across the epithelial cell membranes. Therefore, the flux through the epithelial membrane (the rate-limiting step) would not be increased (flux = $S_{dissolv} \times f_u P_{ep} = S_{blank}/f_u \times f_u P_{ep} = S_{blank} \times P_{ep}$). Pranlukast was suggested to be a typical example for this case (Tables 8.2 and 8.3). The solubility of pranlukast is increased ca. ninefold

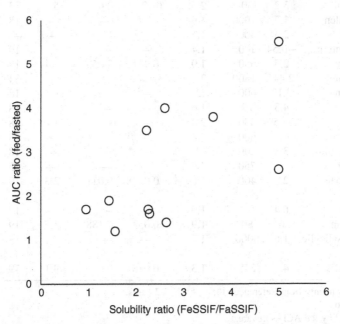

Figure 12.5 Relationship between solubility ratio (FeSSIF/FaSSIF) and clinical food effect for SL-U cases. (a) I.V. and (b) P.O.

TABLE 12.3 Food Effect for undissociable and Free Acid Drugs with Low Solubility[a]

				Solubility, mg/ml			References	
	$\log P_{oct}$	Dose, mg	Food Effect (Fed/Fasted)[b]	FaSSIF	FeSSIF	Solubility Ratio	Food Effect	Solubility
Indissociable								
Atovaquone	5.1	1000	3.8	0.0024	0.0087	3.6	19	26
Bropirimine	1.3[c]	500	1.9	—	—	—	19	—
Carbamazepine	2.1	400	1.2	0.185	0.29	1.6	18	27
Celecoxib	3	400	3.5	0.0462	0.103	2.2	28	29
Chlorothiazide	−0.24	500	1.7	0.87	0.83	0.95	18	26
Cyclandelate	4.49[c]	100	2.5	—	—	—	30	—
Danazol	4.2	100	4	0.018	0.047	2.6	19	26
Dicoumarol	2.7	250	1.85	—	—	—	18	—
Efavirenz	4.1	600	1.3	—	—	—	19	—
Etretinate	8.48	100	5.5	0.0034	0.017	5	18	31
Fenofibrate	5.2	200	1.4	0.014	0.037	2.6	—	32
FK-143	3	500	2.2	—	—	—	18	—
Ganciclovir	−1.7	1000	1.2	—	—	—	19	—
Griseofulvin	2.18	125	1.7	0.015	0.034	2.3	19	26
Hydrochloro-thiazide	−0.03	50	1.2	—	—	—	19	—
Ivermectin	3.2	30	2.6	0.12	0.6	5	33	26
Methoxsalen	1.7	1000	1.9	—	—	—	18	—
Lopinavir	2.3	400	1.7	—	—	—	—	—
Nitrofurantoin	−0.54	100	1.4	—	—	—	19	—
Phenytoin	2.5	350	1.9	0.041	0.059	1.4	18	26
Praziquantel	2.44[c]	1800	3.7	—	—	—	34	—
Proquazone	3.13	600	2	—	—	—	18	—
Quazepam	4.3	20	1.6	—	—	—	18	—
Repirinast	2.05[c]	300	2.4	—	—	—	18	—
Rufinamide	0.9	600	1.4	—	—	—	18	—
Spironolactone	3.3	200	2	—	—	—	18	—
Telaprevir	4	750	4.2	—	—	—	35	—
Troglitazone	2.7	400	1.6	0.0048	0.011	2.3	19	31
Free acid								
Acitretin	6.4	25	1.9	—	—	—	19	—
Isotretinoin	6	80	1.9	0.053	0.188	3.5	19	31
p-Aminosalicylic acid	1.6	6000	1.7	—	—	—	19	—
Pranlukast	4.2	225	1.3	0.088	0.8	9.1	19	26

[a] Compiled mainly from References 18, 19 for ≥ 1.2 cases.
[b] AUC ratio.
[c] Calculated by the ACD software.

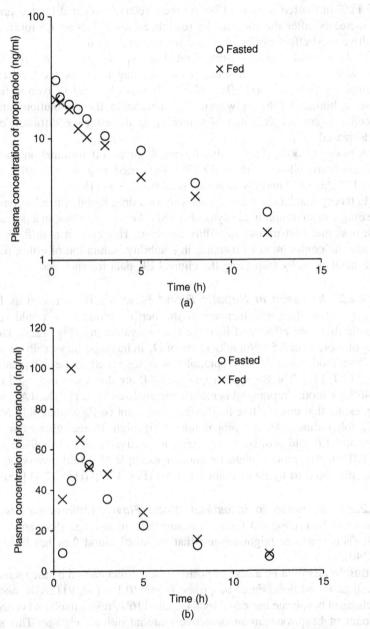

Figure 12.6 Plasma concentration-time curves for racemic propranolol after simultaneous dosing with 80-mg oral (p.o.) (b) and 0.1 mg/kg intravenous (i.v.) doses (a) (dotted line, fasted state; solid line, fed state). Mean ± SE; $n = 6$. *Source:* Adapted from Reference 41 with permission.

in the fed state. However, the food effect is only a 1.5-fold increase at 300 mg (cf. Fa% in the fed state is 11%). As the effective intestinal fluid volume would be increased after the food intake (estimated to be 1.2- to 1.5-fold), a slightly positive food effect can be observed for this class of drugs.

In the case of dissolution-rate-limited absorption, the bile micelle solubilization would increase the dissolution rate, leading to a positive food effect. For example, a positive food effect (2.6-fold) was observed in ivermectin (30-mg dose in humans) [36]. However, the increase in the dissolution rate by bile micelles is smaller than that of solubility as the effective diffusion coefficient is decreased [37].

A positive food effect is also observed for an oil formulation such as fenretinide (corn oil-polysorbate 80 [38], fed/fasted ratio = 3.2 [18]), pleconaril (MCT, 2.23) [39], and cyclosporine (emulsion, 3.8) [18].

In theory, the increase in the solubility of a drug by bile micelles may increase the drug concentration in the cytosol for SL-U cases, resulting in a decrease in the first-pass metabolism and the efflux transport. However, it is difficult to differentiate the contribution of increase in solubility, saturation of efflux transporter, and metabolism by inspecting the clinical PK data for such cases.

12.2.2.2 *Increase in Hepatic Blood Flow.*

Fg is expressed as $Fg = 1 - CL_h/Q_h$. Therefore, the increase of the hepatic blood flow would reduce the hepatic first-pass effect and increase the bioavailability (Fig. 12.8). Drugs with CL_h of more than 6.5 ml/min/kg (32% of Q_h in humans) may exhibit a significant positive food effect [40]. Propranolol was suggested to be a typical example (Fig. 12.7) [41]. The BA% of propranolol (80-mg dose) was increased from 27% to 46% by food. Propranolol is mainly metabolized by CYP2D6, 1A2, and 2C19, suggesting that this positive food effect would not be Fg related [42]. Metoprolol [43], tolterodine [44], and propafenone [40] might be the other examples (1.4-, 1.5-, and 1.6-fold positive food effect, respectively; all metabolized mainly by CYP2D6). Rizatriptan might be another example (1.2-fold positive food effect [18], metabolized by monoamine oxidase) (Fig. 12.7; Table 12.4) [45].

12.2.2.3 *Increase in Intestinal Blood Flow.*

Little or no positive food effect has been observed for atrovastatin [87], nisoldipine [88], and midazolam [89]. This evidence might suggest that intestinal blood flow has little effect on Fg [40].

Buspirone might be a case of positive food effect caused by the increase in the intestinal blood flow. Fg of buspirone is low (0.16) [90, 91]. AUC and C_{max} of unchanged buspirone increased by 84% and 116%, respectively, whereas the total amount of buspirone immunoreactive material did not change. This suggested that the presystemic metabolic clearance of buspirone was decreased by the food effect. As the dose number of buspirone is less than 0.5 (dose 20 mg, solubility >0.2 mg/ml), the solubility increase would not be the reason for the positive food effect. Deramciclane might be another example. AUC and C_{max} of unchanged deramciclane increased by 30% and 20%, respectively, whereas the total amount

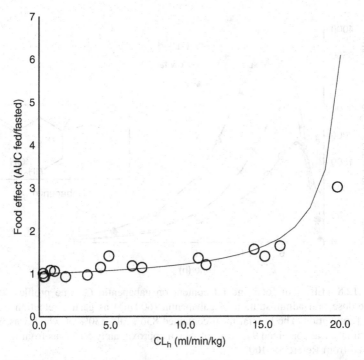

Figure 12.7   Hepatic clearance and food effect. The line indicates the theoretical prediction by $Fh = 1 - CL_h/Q_h$.

of metabolite did not change [92]. Chloroquine and clarithromycin show positive food effects (1.4- and 1.2-fold, respectively) [18, 40], and CYP3A4 is involved in their metabolism. Fg of clarithromycin was estimated to be 0.87 from the grapefruit juice effect [93]. However, it is difficult to exclude the possibility of increase in Fh of these drugs. For drugs with low solubility and low Fg such as saquinavir, it is difficult to identify the main reason for the positive food effect.

12.2.2.4   *Inhibition of Efflux Transporter and Gut Wall Metabolism.* The components of grapefruit juice inhibit the CYP3A4 metabolism in the gut wall and significantly increase the exposure of a drug, which undergoes the gut wall metabolism. The inhibition of CYP3A4 by grapefruit juice occurs in the intestinal wall, but not in the liver [94]. Therefore, the grapefruit effect on bioavailability of a drug was suggested to be a good surrogate to estimate Fg [94]. The mean recovery half-life of intestinal CYP3A4 is 23 ± 10 h, which is shorter than that in hepatic CYP3A4 (1–6 d) [94].

To the best of the author's knowledge, little or no clinical evidence showing inhibition of P-gp by fruit juice has been reported [95]. With 220 ml single-strength grapefruit juice, digoxin AUC 0–24 was minimally increased to 1.1-fold, compared with water (not statistically significant) [96, 97]. *In vitro*, fruit juices moderately inhibited the P-gp effect [98].

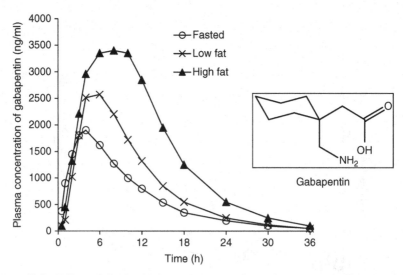

Figure 12.8 Effect of food and fat content on gabapentin C_p-time profiles following a single-dose oral administration of gabapentin (600 mg) as gastric retention extended-release formulation. The low fat meal contained 836 kcal, <30% of which was from fat. The high fat meal contained 945 kcal, of which approximately 50% was from fat. *Source:* Replotted from Reference 100.

TABLE 12.4 Positive Food Effect via Increase in Hepatic Blood Flow

	CL_h, ml/min/kg	Food Effect (Fed/Fasted)	References
Chloroquine	4.6	1.4	40
Diazepam	0.4	0.9	40
Diprafenone	10.6	1.4	40
Fluconazole	0.3	0.9	40
Labetalol	27.0	1.4	116
Metoprolol	15.0	1.4	40
Oxycodone	11.1	1.2	18
Pindolol	4.1	1.2	40
Prednisolone	1.0	1.1	40
Primaquine	6.8	1.1	40
Propafenone	14.3	1.6	40
Propranolol	16.0	1.6	40
Pyrazinamide	0.3	1.0	40
Quinidine	3.2	1.0	40
Selegiline	19.8	3	117
Stavudine	1.7	0.9	40
Theophylline	0.7	1.1	40
Timolol	6.2	1.2	40

Even though it has been theoretically suggested that the bile acids and food components can inhibit apical efflux transporters, little or no clinical evidence was reported.

In biopharmaceutical modeling, Fg estimation would be the key factor to estimate the effect of grapefruit juice on exposure of a drug (Section 4.10).

12.2.2.5 Desaturation of Influx Transporter. From the theoretical point of view, a slow gastric emptying can reduce the concentration of a drug in the upper intestine and increase the permeability of a drug via an uptake transporter. Together with the prolonged exposure of a drug to an upper-intestine-specific transporter, this could result in an increase in Fa%.

Gabapentin is absorbed via an L-amino acid transporter. This drug showed a dose-subproportional oral absorption. When dosed after a meal containing fat, the exposure of gabapentin was increased by 12% [99]. Interestingly, the food effect is more significant when dosed as a gastric retention formulation (Fig. 12.9) [100]. As this drug is very hydrophilic and zwitterionic, it is unlikely that pH and bile had affected its solubility in the intestine. Capsule and solution administration gave an identical oral absorption [99]. Therefore, the increase in exposure in the fed state would be due to the desaturation of uptake transport of gabapentin.

Ribavirin [101] and riboflavin [102] also show a positive food effect (both 1.4-fold). These compounds were also absorbed via influx transporters [103, 104].

12.2.3 Negative Food Effect

A drug that shows a negative food effect usually has a dose number less than 1 [18, 19] and low permeability (BCS III) [20, 21]. When compared to the positive food effects, the reasons for the negative food effects would be more complex. Two or more reasons may be acting simultaneously.

12.2.3.1 Bile Micelle Binding/Food Component Binding. Bile micelle binding has been suggested to be the reason for a negative food effect in drugs with low permeability and Do < 1 [22, 26, 31, 105–111]. Bile micelle binding reduces the unbound drug concentration at the epithelial surface and reduces the effective permeability of a drug (Fig. 12.9). In many low to moderately lipophilic base drugs, the food intake reduces the C_{max} and AUC. In spite of their hydrophilicity, nadolol and atenolol were found to bind to bile micelles and the effective intestinal permeability was reduced due to the reduction in the unbound fraction [112]. The extent of the negative food effect was found to quantitatively correlate with the free fraction ratio in FeSSIF/FaSSIF [31].

It is interesting that many compounds that show a negative food effect (Table 12.5) also show a bimodal PK profile [113], for example, pafenolol [108], talinolol [114] (Fig. 12.10), and maraviroc [115] (Fig. 12.11).[1] The second peak

---

[1]These drugs are also P-gp substrates and show dose-supralinear exposure (Section 14.2). A slower gastric emptying in the fed state may desaturate the efflux and decrease oral absorption of these drugs.

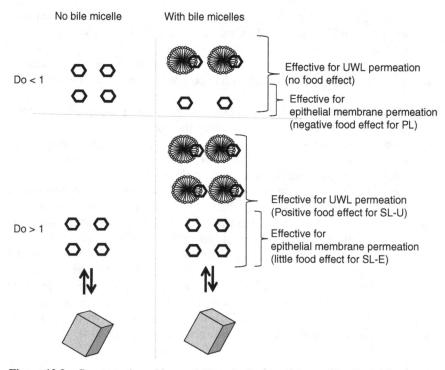

Figure 12.9 Concentration of free and bile-micelle-bound drug molecules in the presence and absence of undissolved solid drug. The bile-micelle-bound fraction is 50% for both Do > 1 and Do < 1 cases.

was found to be larger than the first peak, suggesting that the enterohepatic recirculation is not the reason for the bimodal PK profile. It was suggested that the drug molecules once bound to bile micelles in the upper small intestine would be released at the end of ileum as the bile acids are almost completely reabsorbed by a site-specific bile acid transporter (Fig. 12.12; Section 13.6.3.2) [108].

The oral absorption of bisphosphonates is significantly reduced when taken with food. Complex formation with Ca^{2+} would be the reason for this negative food effect.

12.2.3.2 Inhibition of Uptake Transporter.
Fruit juice components can inhibit the uptake of a transporter substrate at the intestinal epithelial membrane. The oral absorptions of intestinal OATP substrates such as fexofenadine (Fig. 12.13) [118], celiprolol [119], talinolol [114], and aliskiren [120] are reduced when they are coadministered with grapefruit juice by 63%, 84%, 44%, and 61%, respectively. Inhibition of OATP uptake of these drugs by grapefruit components was suggested as the mechanism for clinical observation. It should be noted that orange juice is often taken in a food effect study (Table 12.1).

TABLE 12.5   Negative Food Effect

Drug	Food Effect[a]	Comments	References
5-Aminosalicylic acid	0.52	—	19
6-Thioguanine	0.41	—	18
Alendronate	<0.15	Bisphosphonate	129
Aliskiren	0.32	—	130
Ambenonium chloride	0.3	Quaternary amine	18
Amoxicillin	0.55	—	18
Aspirin	0.768	—	18
Atenolol	0.8	—	18
Bisamide	0.73	—	18
Bromazepam	0.67	—	18
Capecitabine	0.69	—	18
Captopril	0.44	—	18
Clodronate	0.7	Bisphosphonate	19
Didanosine	0.45	—	19
Delavirdine	0.74	—	65
Endralazine	0.33	—	131
Entecavir	0.79	—	19
Eptastigmine	0.63	—	19
Estramustine	0.674, 0.411	Alkylating agent	18
Etidronate	0	Bisphosphonate	132
Fenoldopam	0.35	Desaturation of metabolism	121
Fexofenadine	0.73[b]	—	133
Furosemide	0.55	—	19
Hydralazine	0.45	—	18
Indinavir sulfate	0.57	—	31
Isoniazid	0.57	—	19
Ketoprofen	0.78	—	18
Maraviroc	0.76	—	115
Melagatran	0.14	—	134
Melphalan	0.45	Alkylating agent	18
Metformin	0.76	—	18
Methotrexate	0.77	—	18
Nadolol	0.74	—	135
Nimodipine	0.62	—	18
Pafenolol	0.6	—	108
Penicillamine	0.49	—	18
Pidotimod	0.51	—	19
Pravastatin	0.69	—	19
Riluzole	0.8	—	31
Risedronate	0.44	Bisphosphonate	136
Sotalol	0.8	—	19
Sulpiride	0.71	—	18
Tacrine	0.79	—	18
Talinolol	0.5	—	137
Tamsulosin	0.7	—	19

(continued)

TABLE 12.5   (*Continued*)

Drug	Food Effect[a]	Comments	References
Tegaserod	0.45	—	138
Telmisartan	0.7	Solid dispersion formulation	139
Tetracycline	0.6	—	18
Tyramine	0.41	—	18
Voriconazole	0.56	—	125
Zafirlukast	0.78	Solubilized formulation	140
Zidovudine	0.67	—	18

[a]Compiled mainly from References 18, 19 for ≤ 0.8 cases.
[b]No orange juice included in the food study.

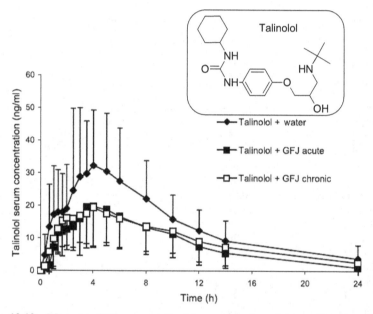

Figure 12.10   Mean ($\pm$ SD) serum talinolol concentration–time profiles ($n = 24$) for orally administered talinolol (50 mg) with 300 ml of water, with 300 ml of grapefruit juice (GFJ acute), or after ingestion of 300 ml of grapefruit juice thrice daily for 6 d (GFJ chronic). *Source:* Adapted from Reference 114 with permission.

12.2.3.3 *Desaturation of First-Pass Metabolism and Efflux Transport.*
Because of the slow stomach emptying, the dissolved drug concentration in the intestine in the fed state becomes lower than that in the fasted state, leading to desaturation of the first-pass metabolism (both at liver and gut wall) and the efflux transport in the intestine. Fenoldopam might be an example for this case [121]. The mean relative bioavailabilities (fed/fasted) were 35% and 81%, respectively, for fenoldopam and its sulfate metabolite (SK&F 87782) (Fig. 12.14).

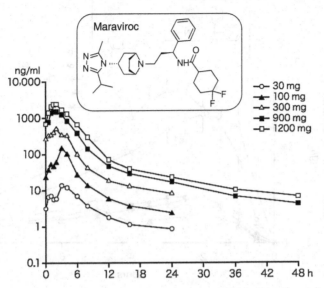

Figure 12.11 Mean plasma maraviroc concentration–time profiles after oral administration of maraviroc. *Source:* Adapted from Reference 115.

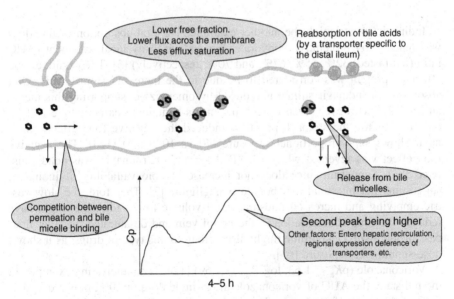

Figure 12.12 Bimodal PK and bile-micelle binding.

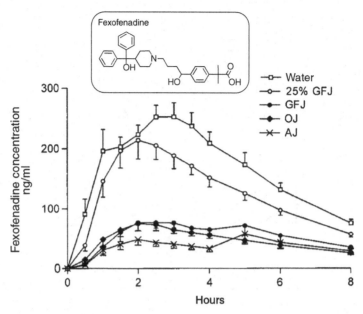

Figure 12.13 Mean plasma fexofenadine concentration-time profiles (n = 10) for orally administered fexofenadine (120 mg) with 300 ml water, grapefruit juice (GFJ) at 25% of regular strength (25% GFJ), GFJ, orange juice (OJ), or apple juice (AJ) followed by 150 ml of the same fluid every 0.5-3 h (total volume, 1.2 l). *Source:* Adapted from Reference 118 with permission.

Indinavir sulfate might be another example. The oral absorption of this drug was reduced by protein, carbohydrate, fat, and viscosity meal treatment (AUC ratio (fed/fasted) 32%, 55%, 67%, and 70%, respectively) [5]. The negative food effect by protein was considered to be due to the increased stomach pH. Oral absorption of indinavir sulfate is reduced by omeprazole, supporting this mechanism [122]. However, even though the meals containing carbohydrate and fat did not increase the stomach pH, they induced the negative food effects. Indinavir shows supraproportional exposure (40 vs 1000 mg) [123]. The negative food effect was reversed when a CYP3A4 inhibitor, ritonavir, was coadministered [86]. Grapefruit juice does not increase the bioavailability of indinavir, suggesting that intestinal metabolism is negligible [7]. Therefore, the slow gastric emptying and increased intestinal fluid volume in the fed state might have reduced the drug concentration in the portal vein and desaturated the liver first-pass metabolism. Delavirdine might also belong to this type of drugs, as it shows dose-supralinear exposure [63].

Voriconazole ($pK_a = 1.63$, log $P_{oct} = 1.69$) [124] is an interesting example. In the fed state, the AUC of voriconazole after single dose of 200 mg is reduced to 57% of that in the fasted state. This negative food effect is less significant after multiple doses (78% at day 7) [125]. The bioavailability of voriconazole is 100% in the fasted state, and hence, there is no first-pass metabolism in the fasted state

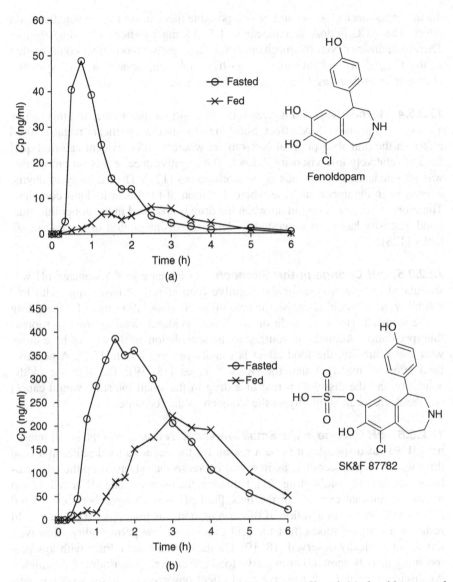

Figure 12.14 Mean plasma concentration (C_p)-time profile of (a) fenoldopam and (b) SK&F 87782 in humans in the fasted and fed states. *Source:* Replotted from Reference 121.

[124]. The solubility is similar in FaSSIF (0.66 mg/ml) and FeSSIF (0.73 mg/ml) (i.e., unbound fraction is similar), and the dose number is 1.2 (based on FaSSIF solubility and 200-mg dose) [31]. The gastric pH had no effect on oral absorption [126]. Therefore, the reduction of solubility in the stomach and permeability in the small intestine can be excluded from the possible mechanisms. Desaturation of

the first-pass metabolism would be one possible mechanism for the negative food effect. The AUC is dose-supralinear in 1.5–6.0 mg/kg after i.v. administration. Therefore, another possible mechanism for the negative food effect could be that as the C_{max} decreases due to slow gastric emptying, desaturation of systemic clearance (non-first-pass) occurred, leading to a decrease in AUC.

12.2.3.4   Viscosity. Food increases the viscosity of the chyme, and this can be a cause for a negative food effect. Solid meals caused a significant negative food effect on the oral absorption of bidisomide, whereas an equivalent caloric liquid food of relatively low viscosity did not. The negative meal effect on bidisomide was also generated by viscous zero-calorie meals [127]. The viscosity of chyme is greatest in the upper intestine where digestion of food is at its least complete. Therefore, viscosity is important when the drug is absorbed in the upper intestine. Food viscosity has been suggested to delay the disintegration of a paracetamol tablet [128].

12.2.3.5   pH Change in the Stomach. An increase in the stomach pH was speculated to be a reason for the negative food effect for base drugs with low solubility, as it would decrease the solubility and dissolution rate of a base drug in the stomach. However, little or no clinical evidence was reported to support this speculation. Actually, in contrast to the speculation, in the case of base drugs with low solubility, the food effect is usually positive (Table 12.6). A negative food effect is merely found for Do > 1 cases [18, 19]. The increase in the solubility and the dissolution rate of a drug in the small intestine would cancel out the decrease in solubility in the stomach in the fed state.

12.2.3.6   pH Change in the Small Intestine. A decrease in the small intestinal pH was also speculated to be a reason for the negative food effect in a base drug with low permeability, as it would decrease the intestinal epithelial membrane permeability of the drug [21]. However, the microclimate pH is maintained relatively constant even when the bulk fluid pH was changed between pH 6.0 and 8.0 (Fig. 6.16). In addition, if this speculation was true, this pH effect should result in a positive food effect for acid drugs with low permeability. However, this is not clinically observed [18, 19]. On the contrary, acid drugs with low permeability usually show no or negative food effect (e.g., pravastatin, furosemide). As discussed earlier, the negative food effect observed for bases with low permeability can be explained by bile micelle binding. At present, little evidence exists to support a negative food effect via the intestinal pH change. Further investigation is required to prove this hypothesis.

12.3   EFFECT OF FOOD TYPE

It is well known that the positive food effect largely depends on the fat content of the food. The oral absorption of atovaquone in humans was higher when

TABLE 12.6 The Stomach pH and Food Effects for Dissociable Drugs with Low Solubility

Drug	pK_a	Fa% Change[a] High/Low Gastric pH	Food Effect (Fed/Fasted)	References Gastric pH	Food
Free base					
Albendazole	4.2	0.71 (1400 mg)	5	46	47
Aprepitant	4.2	—	1.31 (125 mg)	—	48
Cinnarizine	7.5	0.13–0.27 (25 mg)	1.2–1.7 (50 mg)	49	50
Clofazimine	8.5	0.85 (200 mg)	1.45 (200 mg)	51	51
Dasatinib	6.8	0.4 (50 mg)	1.2 (100 mg)	52	52
Dipyridamole	6.2	0.63	1	53	54
Gefitinib	5.28, 7.17	0.53 (250 mg)	1.37	55	55
Ketoconazole	2.9, 6.5	0.08 (200 mg)	0.61 (200 mg)[b] 1.05 (200 mg) 1.34 (200 mg)[d] 1.59 (400 mg)[c] 1.45 (600 mg)[c] 1.02 (800 mg)[c]	56	—
Itraconazole	3.7	0.35 (200 mg)[e] 0.54 (200 mg)[f]	3 (100 mg)	—	57
Posaconazole	3.6 4.6	0.66 (400 mg)	5 (400 mg)	58	58
Triclabendazole	3.1	—	3.7 (600 mg)	—	59
Salt of base					
Amiodarone HCl	9.0	—	2.4 (600 mg)	—	60
Atazanavir sulfate	4.25	0.25 (300 mg)	1.7 (400 mg)	61	62
Darunavir (ethanolate)	2.2	1 (400 mg)	1.4–1.8 (400 mg)	63	63
Dabigatran etexilate mesylate	4.0, 6.7	0.35 (200 mg)	1.42 (200 mg)	64	64
Delavirdine mesylate	4.6	0.52 (300 mg)	0.74 (300 mg)[g]	65	65
Erlotinib HCl	5.6	0.51 (150 mg)	2.9 (150 mg)	66	66
Halofantrine HCl	8.2	0.5 (250 mg in dogs)	3–5 (250–500 mg)[h] 13 (250 mg in dogs)[i]	67	—
Indinavir sulfate	3.8, 6.2	0.53 (800 mg)	0.57 (800 mg)[g,j] 0.88 (800 mg) (+RTV)[k]	68	—
Lapatinib tosylate	4.6, 6.7	—	4.25 (1500 mg)	—	69
Nelfinavir sulfate	6.0	0.36 (1250 mg)	2.4 (500 mg) 5.2 (1250 mg)	70	71

TABLE 12.6   *(Continued)*

Drug	pK_a	Fa% Change[a] High/Low Gastric pH	Fa% Change[a] Food Effect (Fed/Fasted)	References Gastric pH	References Food
Nilotinib HCl monohydrate	5.4	0.66 (400 mg)	1.8 (400 mg)	72	73
Saquinavir mesylate	7.0	—	6.7 (600 mg)	70, 74	75
Ticlopidine HCl	7.6	0.8 (250 mg)	1.2 (250 mg)	76	76
Ziprasidone HCl	6.5	—	2 (80 mg)	—	77
Salt of acid					
Raltegravir potassium	6.6	3.1 (400 mg)	Variable (Table 12.6)	78	79

[a] AUC ratio.
[b] Reference 80.
[c] Reference 81.
[d] Reference 56.
[e] Reference 82.
[f] Reference 83.
[g] Suggested to be due to desaturation of the hepatic first-pass effect.
[h] Reference 84.
[i] Reference 24.
[j] Reference 85.
[k] Reference 86.

TABLE 12.7   Effect of Food Type on Atovaquone (500-mg Tablet) Absorption in Humans[a]

	AUC, µgh/ml	C_{max}, µg/ml
Fasted	121 ± 74	1.5 ± 1.3
Two slices of toast	147 ± 144	1.7 ± 0.6
Two slices of toast + butter (23 g fat)	356 ± 165	5.7 ± 1.3
Two slices of toast + butter (56 g fat)	469 ± 152	8.3 ± 2.0
Fasted/CCK-OP (i.v.)	180 ± 47	1.7 ± 0.9

[a] Reference 141.

the fat content was higher (Table 12.7) [141]. To investigate the sole effect of endogenous bile micelles, cholecystokinin octapeptide (CCK-OP) was infused to induce gallbladder shrinkage. Compared to meals that are low and high in fat, CCK-OP had a smaller effect, suggesting that fat and/or digested fat affected the solubilization of atovaquone. This evidence support the advantage of FeSSIFv2 (which contains fatty acids and monoglycerides) compared to the original FeSSIF [142] as a surrogate for the real *in vivo* fluid in the fed state. The oral absorption of phenytoin in dogs (300 mg) was increased by casein and oleate (ca. 1.5- and

TABLE 12.8 Effect of Food Type on LY303366 (250 mg) Absorption in Dogs[a]

	AUC, μgh/ml	C_{max}, μg/ml
Fasted	21.2 ± 5.84	1.1 ± 0.27
Mixed meal (Ensure, 250 kcal)	8.9 ± 2.56	0.5 ± 0.17
Lipid meal (20% Intralipid, 250 kcal)	7.5 ± 1.84	0.4 ± 0.13
Protein meal (CASEC, 125 kcal)	8.9 ± 2.77	0.5 ± 0.20
Carbohydrate meal (Moducal, 125 kcal)	25.2 ± 5.13	1.6 ± 0.30

[a]Reference 144.

TABLE 12.9 Food Effect on Oral Absorption of Raltegravir Potassium (400 mg) in Humans[a]

	C_{max}, μM (90% CI)	AUC 0–12 (μM h) (90% CI)
Fasted	2.71 (1.80–4.08)	10.0 (7.20–14.0)
Low fat	1.31 (0.87–1.97)	5.38 (3.86–7.50)
Moderate fat	2.85 (1.89–4.29)	11.3 (8.12–15.8)
High fat	5.32 (3.53–8.01)	21.2 (15.2–29.6)

[a]Reference 79.

2-fold, respectively), but not by glucose and saline [143]. The positive food effect was reversed by coadministration of CCK antagonist. These results may suggest that the bile secretion is necessary, but not sufficient, for the positive food effect via increased solubility.

The extent of the negative food effect is also affected by the type of food. The oral absorption of LY303366 was reduced by lipid and protein meals, but not by carbohydrate meal (Table 12.8) [144]. Coadministration of CCK antagonist did not reverse the negative food effect.

Raltegravir is an interesting example [79]. With food low in fat, the food effect is negative, whereas with a meal high in fat, it is positive (Table 12.9).

12.4 BIOPHARMACEUTICAL MODELING OF FOOD EFFECT

12.4.1 Simple Flowchart and Semiquantitative Prediction

It is empirically well established that when the dose number (Do) of a drug is larger than 1, the food effect, when it occurs, would be positive [18, 19, 31]. In addition, the drugs with high lipophilicity also tend to show a positive food effect. These empirical classifications are theoretically supported by the GUT framework and would suggest that bile micelle binding/solubilization is the most frequent and significant reason for the positive food effect. The positive food effect is often observed for SL-U cases, sometimes as well as for DL cases.

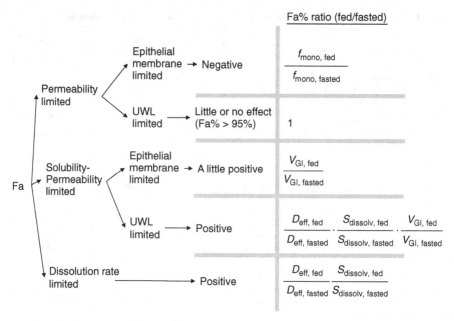

Figure 12.15 Mechanism-based flowchart to estimate the food effect by bile micelles.

On the other hand, for Do $<$ 1 and drugs with low permeability, a negative food effect would be observed.[2] As discussed, based on the GUT framework, the food effect by bile micelles will be (Fig. 12.15)

- permeability-limited case: negative food effect
- dissolution-rate-limited case: positive food effect
- solubility–epithelial membrane permeability limited case: no or a little positive food effect
- solubility–UWL permeability limited case: positive food effect.

12.4.2 More Complicated Cases

Food intake simultaneously changes various physiological factors. Theoretically, biopharmaceutical modeling can handle this complicated situation. However, as the first step, we should first confirm that the effect of each physiological factor is well simulated by biopharmaceutical modeling. Prospective prediction of the food effects on intestinal metabolism and a carrier-mediated transport are challenging. As a prerequisite for this, the effect of these factors on Fa% in the fasted state should be well predicted. However, this has not been achieved yet (Chapter 14).

---

[2]Telmisartan [44] and zafirlukast [45] show negative food effect, although these compounds have low solubility, probably because these drugs are formulated using a solubilization technique.

Predictions for the effects of various meal types are also a challenging area. The first step will be characterizing the GI physiology after taking various types of meals.

Meanwhile, the applicable area of biopharmaceutical modeling will be limited to some simple factors such as bile micelles, GET, and gastric pH.

REFERENCES

1. Dressman, J. (1986). Comparison of canin and human gastrointestinal physiology. *Pharm. Res.*, 3, 123–130.
2. Klein, S., Butler, J., Hempenstall, J.M., Reppas, C., Dressman, J.B. (2004). Media to simulate the postprandial stomach I. Matching the physicochemical characteristics of standard breakfasts. *J. Pharm. Pharmacol.*, 56, 605–610.
3. Scholz, A., Abrahamsson, B., Diebold, S.M., Kostewicz, E., Polentarutti, B.I., Ungell, A.L., Dressman, J.B. (2002). Influence of hydrodynamics and particle size on the absorption of felodipine in labradors. *Pharm. Res.*, 19, 42–46.
4. Mudie, D.M., Amidon, G.L., Amidon, G.E. (2010). Physiological parameters for oral delivery and in vitro testing. *Mol. Pharm.*, 7, 1388–1405.
5. Carver, P.L., Fleisher, D., Zhou, S.Y., Kaul, D., Kazanjian, P., Li, C. (1999). Meal composition effects on the oral bioavailability of indinavir in HIV-infected patients. *Pharm. Res.*, 16, 718–724.
6. Farkas, D., Greenblatt, D.J. (2008). Influence of fruit juices on drug disposition: discrepancies between in vitro and clinical studies. *Expert Opin. Drug Metab. Toxicol.*, 4, 381–393.
7. Penzak, S.R., Acosta, E.P., Turner, M., Edwards, D.J., Hon, Y.Y., Desai, H.D., Jann, M.W. (2002). Effect of Seville orange juice and grapefruit juice on indinavir pharmacokinetics. *J. Clin. pharmacol.*, 42, 1165–1170.
8. De Castro, W.V., Mertens-Talcott, S., Rubner, A., Butterweck, V., Derendorf, H. (2006). Variation of flavonoids and furanocoumarins in grapefruit juices: a potential source of variability in grapefruit juice-drug interaction studies. *J. Agric. Food. Chem.*, 54, 249–255.
9. Lennernas, H. (2009). Ethanol-drug absorption interaction: potential for a significant effect on the plasma pharmacokinetics of ethanol vulnerable formulations. *Mol. Pharm.*, 6, 1429–1440.
10. FDA, www.fda.gov/downloads/Drugs/GuidanceComplianceRegulatoryInformation/ Guidances.
11. Franke, A., Teyssen, S., Harder, H., Singer, M.V. (2004). Effect of ethanol and some alcoholic beverages on gastric emptying in humans. *Scand. J. Gastroenterol.*, 39, 638–644.
12. Walden, M., Nicholls, F.A., Smith, K.J., Tucker, G.T. (2007). The effect of ethanol on the release of opioids from oral prolonged-release preparations. *Drug Dev. Ind. Pharm.*, 33, 1101–1111.
13. Sathyan, G., Sivakumar, K., Thipphawong, J. (2008). Pharmacokinetic profile of a 24-hour controlled-release OROS formulation of hydromorphone in the presence of alcohol. *Curr. Med. Res. Opin.*, 24, 297–305.

14. Kalantzi, L., Reppas, C., Dressman, J.B., Amidon, G.L., Junginger, H.E., Midha, K.K., Shah, V.P., Stavchansky, S.A., Barends, D.M. (2006). Biowaiver monographs for immediate release solid oral dosage forms: acetaminophen (paracetamol). *J. Pharm. Sci.*, 95, 4–14.

15. Rostami-Hodjegan, A., Shiran, M.R., Ayesh, R., Grattan, T.J., Burnett, I., Darby-Dowman, A., Tucker, G.T. (2002) A new rapidly absorbed paracetamol tablet containing sodium bicarbonate. I. A four-way crossover study to compare the concentration-time profile of paracetamol from the new paracetamol/sodium bicarbonate tablet and a conventional paracetamol tablet in fed and fasted volunteers. *Drug Dev. Ind. Pharm.*, 28, 523–531.

16. Stillings, M., Havlik, I., Chetty, M., Clinton, C., Schall, R., Moodley, I., Muir, N., Little, S. (2000). Comparison of the pharmacokinetic profiles of soluble aspirin and solid paracetamol tablets in fed and fasted volunteers. *Curr. Med. Res. Opin.*, 16, 115–124.

17. Rawlins, M.D., Henderson, D.B., Hijab, A.R. (1977). Pharmacokinetics of paracetamol (acetaminophen) after intravenous and oral administration. *Eur. J. Clin. pharmacol.*, 11, 283–286.

18. Singh, B.N. (2005). A quantitative approach to probe the dependence and correlation of food-effect with aqueous solubility, dose/solubility ratio, and partition coefficient (Log P) for orally active drugs administered as immediate-release formulations. *Drug Dev. Res.*, 65, 55–75.

19. Gu, C.H., Li, H., Levons, J., Lentz, K., Gandhi, R.B., Raghavan, K., Smith, R.L. (2007). Predicting effect of food on extent of drug absorption based on physicochemical properties. *Pharm. Res.*, 24, 1118–1130.

20. Wu, C.Y., Benet, L.Z. (2005). Predicting drug disposition via application of BCS: transport/absorption/ elimination interplay and development of a biopharmaceutics drug disposition classification system. *Pharm. Res.*, 22, 11–23.

21. Marasanapalle, V.P., Crison, J.R., Ma, J., Li, X., Jasti, B.R. (2009). Investigation of some factors contributing to negative food effects. *Biopharm. Drug Dispos.*, 30, 71–80.

22. Poelma, F.G.J., Breaes, R., Tukker, J.J. (1990). Intestinal absorption of drugs. III. The influence of taurocholate on the disappearance kinetics of hydrophilic and lipophilic drugs from the small intestine of the rat. *Pharm. Res.*, 7, 392–397.

23. Etiretinate. Interview form.

24. Humberstone, A.J., Porter, C.J., Charman, W.N. (1996). A physicochemical basis for the effect of food on the absolute oral bioavailability of halofantrine. *J. Pharm. Sci.*, 85, 525–529.

25. Farnesil, I. Interview form.

26. Sugano, K., Kataoka, M., Mathews, C.C., Yamashita, S. (2010). Prediction of food effect by bile micelles on oral drug absorption considering free fraction in intestinal fluid. *Eur. J. Pharm. Sci.*, 40, 118–124.

27. Schwebel, H.J., van Hoogevest, P., Leigh, M.L., Kuentz, M. (2011). The apparent solubilizing capacity of simulated intestinal fluids for poorly water-soluble drugs. *Pharm. Dev. Technol.*, 16, 278–286.

28. Celecoxib. FDA approval document.

29. Shono, Y., Jantratid, E., Janssen, N., Kesisoglou, F., Mao, Y., Vertzoni, M., Reppas, C., Dressman, J.B. (2009). Prediction of food effects on the absorption of cele-coxib based on biorelevant dissolution testing coupled with physiologically based pharmacokinetic modeling. *Eur. J. Pharm. Biopharm.*, 73, 107–114.

30. Kaniwa, N., Ogata, H., Aoyagi, N., Ejima, A., Takahashi, T., Uezono, Y., Imazato, Y. (1991). Effect of food on the bioavailability of cyclandelate from commercial capsules. *Clin. Pharmacol. Ther.*, 49, 641–647.

31. Kawai, Y., Fujii, Y., Tabata, F., Ito, J., Metsugi, Y., Kameda, A., Akimoto, K., Takahashi, M. (2011). Profiling and trend analysis of food effects on oral drug absorption considering micelle interaction and solubilization by bile micelles. *Drug Metab. Pharmacokinet*, 26, 180–191.

32. Buch, P., Langguth, P., Kataoka, M., Yamashita, S. (2009). IVIVC in oral absorption for fenofibrate immediate release tablets using a dissolution/permeation system. *J. Pharm. Sci.*, 98, 2001–2009.

33. Guzzo, C.A., Furtek, C.I., Porras, A.G., Chen, C., Tipping, R., Clineschmidt, C.M., Sciberras, D.G., Hsieh, J.Y.K., Lasseter, K.C. (2002). Safety, tolerability, and phar-macokinetics of escalating high doses of ivermectin in healthy adult subjects. *J. Clin. Pharmacol.*, 42, 1122–1133.

34. Castro, N., Medina, R., Sotelo, J., Jung, H. (2000). Bioavailability of praziquantel increases with concomitant administration of food. *Antimicrob. Agents Chemother.*, 44, 2903–2904.

35. Telaprevir. FDA approval document.

36. Ivermectine, Interview form, in.

37. Okazaki, A., Mano, T., Sugano, K. (2008). Theoretical dissolution model of poly-disperse drug particles in biorelevant media. *J. Pharm. Sci.*, 97, 1843–1852.

38. Desai, K.G., Mallery, S.R., Holpuch, A.S., Schwendeman, S.P. (2011). Development and in vitro-in vivo evaluation of fenretinide-loaded oral mucoadhesive patches for site-specific chemoprevention of oral cancer. *Pharm. Res.*, 28, 2599–2609.

39. Abdel-Rahman, S.M., Kearns, G.L. (1998). Single-dose pharmacokinetics of a ple-conaril (VP63843) oral solution and effect of food. *Antimicrob. Agents Chemother.*, 42, 2706–2709.

40. Marasanapalle, V.P., Boinpally, R.R., Zhu, H., Grill, A., Tang, F. (2011). Correlation between the systemic clearance of drugs and their food effects in humans. *Drug Dev. Ind. Pharm.*, 37, 1311–1317.

41. Olanoff, L.S., Walle, T., Cowart, T.D., Walle, U.K., Oexmann, M.J., Conradi, E.C. (1986). Food effects on propranolol systemic and oral clearance: support for a blood flow hypothesis. *Clin. Pharmacol. Ther.*, 40, 408–414.

42. Masubuchi, Y., Hosokawa, S., Horie, T., Suzuki, T., Ohmori, S., Kitada, M., Nari-matsu, S. (1994). Cytochrome P450 isozymes involved in propranolol metabolism in human liver microsomes. The role of CYP2D6 as ring-hydroxylase and CYP1A2 as N-desisopropylase. *Drug Metab. Dispos.*, 22, 909–915.

43. Melander, A., Danielson, K., Schersten, B., Wahlin, E. (1977). Enhancement of the bioavailability of propranolol and metoprolol by food. *Clin. Pharmacol. Ther.*, 22, 108–112.

44. Olsson, B., Brynne, N., Johansson, C., Arnberg, H. (2001). Food increases the bioavailability of tolterodine but not effective exposure. *J. Clin. pharmacol.*, 41, 298–304.

45. Rizatriptan. Label information.

46. Schipper, H.G., Koopmans, R.P., Nagy, J., Butter, J.J., Kager, P.A., Van Boxtel, C.J. (2000). Effect of dose increase or cimetidine co-administration on albendazole bioavailability. *Am. J. Trop. Med. Hyg.*, 63, 270–273.

47. Albendazole. Interview form.

48. Aprepitant (2009). Aprepitant Interview form. ver. 3.

49. Ogata, H., Aoyagi, N., Kaniwa, N., Ejima, A., Sekine, N., Kitamura, M., Inoue, Y. (1986). Gastric acidity dependent bioavailability of cinnarizine from two commercial capsules in healthy volunteers. *Int. J. Pharm.*, 29, 113–120.

50. Guangli, W., Shuhua, X., Changxiao, L. (1997). Effect of food on bioavailabil ity of cinnarizine capsules. *Chin. J. Clin. Pharmacol. Ther.*, 2, 249–252.

51. Nix, D.E., Adam, R.D., Auclair, B., Krueger, T.S., Godo, P.G., Peloquin, C.A. (2004). Pharmacokinetics and relative bioavailability of clofazimine in relation to food, orange juice and antacid. *Tuberculosis (Edinb)*, 84, 365–373.

52. Dasatinib. FDA approval document.

53. Russell, T.L., Berardi, R.R., Barnett, J.L., O'Sullivan, T.L., Wagner, J.G., Dressman, J.B. (1994). pH-Related changes in the absorption of dipyridamole in the elderly. *Pharm. Res.*, 11, 136–143.

54. Dipyridamole. Interview form.

55. Gefitinib (2009). Gefitinib Interview form. ver. 3.

56. Lelawongs, P., Barone, J.A., Colaizzi, J.L., Hsuan, A.T.M., Mechlinski, W., Legendre, R., Guarnieri, J. (1988). Effect of food and gastric acidity on absorption of orally administered ketoconazole. *Clin. Pharm.*, 7, 228–235.

57. Itraconazole. Interview form.

58. Krishna, G., Moton, A., Ma, L., Medlock, M.M., McLeod, J. (2009). Pharmacokinetics and absorption of posaconazole oral suspension under various gastric conditions in healthy volunteers. *Antimicrob. Agents Chemother.*, 53, 958–966.

59. Lecaillon, J.B., Godbillon, J., Campestrini, J., Naquira, C., Miranda, L., Pacheco, R., Mull, R., Poltera, A.A. (1998). Effect of food on the bioavailability of triclabendazole in patients with fascioliasis. *Br. J. Clin. Pharmacol.*, 45, 601–604.

60. Meng, X., Mojaverian, P., Doedee, M., Lin, E., Weinryb, I., Chiang, S.T., Kowey, P.R. (2001). Bioavailability of amiodarone tablets administered with and without food in healthy subjects. *Am. J. Cardiol.*, 87, 432–435.

61. Zhu, L., Persson, A., Mahnke, L., Eley, T., Li, T., Xu, X., Agarwala, S., Dragone, J., Bertz, R. (2011). Effect of low-dose omeprazole (20mg daily) on the pharmacokinetics of multiple-dose atazanavir with ritonavir in healthy subjects. *J. Clin. pharmacol.*, 51, 368–377.

62. Atazanavir. Interview form.

63. Darunavir. Interview form.

64. Methanesulfonate, D.E. Approval document (Japan).

65. Delavirdine. Interview form.

66. Erlotinib. Interview form.

67. Ajayi, F.O., Brewer, T., Greenfield, R., Fleckenstein, L. (1999). Absolute bioavailability of halofantrine-HCl: effect of ranitidine and pentagastrin treatment. *Clin. Res. Regul. Aff.*, 16, 13–28.

68. Tappouni, H.L., Rublein, J.C., Donovan, B.J., Hollowell, S.B., Tien, H.C., Min, S.S., Theodore, D., Rezk, N.L., Smith, P.C., Tallman, M.N., Raasch, R.H., Kashuba, A.D. (2008). Effect of omeprazole on the plasma concentrations of indinavir when administered alone and in combination with ritonavir. *Am. J. Health Syst. Pharm.*, 65, 422–428.

69. Lapatinib. Approval document.

70. Falcon, R.W., Kakuda, T.N. (2008). Drug interactions between HIV protease inhibitors and acid-reducing agents. *Clin. Pharmacokinet*, 47, 75–89.

71. Nelfinavir. Interview form.

72. Yin, O.Q., Gallagher, N., Fischer, D., Demirhan, E., Zhou, W., Golor, G., Schran, H. (2010). Effect of the proton pump inhibitor esomeprazole on the oral absorption and pharmacokinetics of nilotinib. *J. Clin. pharmacol.*, 50, 960–967.

73. Nilotinib. FDA approval document.

74. Winston, A., Back, D., Fletcher, C., Robinson, L., Unsworth, J., Tolowinska, I., Schutz, M., Pozniak, A.L., Gazzard, B., Boffito, M. (2006). Effect of omeprazole on the pharmacokinetics of saquinavir-500mg formulation with ritonavir in healthy male and female volunteers. *AIDS*, 20, 1401–1406.

75. Saquinavir. Interview form.

76. Shah, J., Fratis, A., Ellis, D., Murakami, S., Teitelbaum, P. (1990). Effect of food and antacid on absorption of orally administered ticlopidine hydrochloride. *J. Clin. Pharmacol.*, 30, 733–736.

77. Miceli, J.J., Glue, P., Alderman, J., Wilner, K. (2007). The effect of food on the absorption of oral ziprasidone. *Psychopharmacol. Bull.*, 40, 58–68.

78. Iwamoto, M., Wenning, L.A., Nguyen, B.Y., Teppler, H., Moreau, A.R., Rhodes, R.R., Hanley, W.D., Jin, B., Harvey, C.M., Breidinger, S.A., Azrolan, N., Farmer, H.F. Jr, Isaacs, R.D., Chodakewitz, J.A., Stone, J.A., Wagner, J.A. (2009). Effects of omeprazole on plasma levels of raltegravir. *Clin. Infect. Dis.*, 48, 489–492.

79. Brainard, D.M., Friedman, E.J., Jin, B., Breidinger, S.A., Tillan, M.D., Wenning, L.A., Stone, J.A., Chodakewitz, J.A., Wagner, J.A., Iwamoto, M. (2011). Effect of low-, moderate-, and high-fat meals on raltegravir pharmacokinetics. *J. Clin. pharmacol.*, 51, 422–427.

80. Mannisto, P.T., Mantyla, R., Nykanen, S., Lamminsivu, U., Ottoila, P. (1982). Impairing effect of food on ketoconazole absorption. *Antimicrob. Agents Chemother.*, 21, 730–733.

81. Daneshmend, T.K., Warnock, D.W., Ene, M.D., Johnson, E.M., Potten, M.R., Richardson, M.D., Williamson, P.J. (1984). Influence of food on the pharmacokinetics of ketoconazole. *Antimicrob. Agents Chemother.*, 25, 1–3.

82. Jaruratanasirikul, S., Sriwiriyajan, S. (1998). Effect of omeprazole on the pharmacokinetics of itraconazole. *Eur. J. Clin. pharmacol.*, 54, 159–161.

83. Lange, D., Pavao, J.H., Wu, J., Klausner, M. (1997). Effect of a cola beverage on the bioavailability of itraconazole in the presence of H2 blockers. *J. Clin. pharmacol.*, 37, 535–540.

84. Halofantrin. FDA label.

85. Indinavir. Interview form.

86. Aarnoutse, R.E., Wasmuth, J.C., Fatkenheuer, G., Schneider, K., Schmitz, K., de Boo, T.M., Reiss, P., Hekster, Y.A., Burger, D.M., Rockstroh, J.K. (2003). Administration of indinavir and low-dose ritonavir (800/100mg twice daily) with food reduces nephrotoxic peak plasma levels of indinavir. *Antivir. Ther.*, 8, 309–314.

87. Lennernas, H. (2003). Clinical pharmacokinetics of atorvastatin. *Clin. Pharmacokinet*, 42, 1141–1160.

88. Form, I., Nisoldipine, in.

89. Bornemann, L.D., Crews, T., Chen, S.S., Twardak, S., Patel, I.H. (1986). Influence of food on midazolam absorption. *J. Clin. pharmacol.*, 26, 55–59.

90. Gammans, R.E., Mayol, R.F., LaBudde, J.A. (1986). Metabolism and disposition of buspirone. *Am. J. Med.*, 80, 41–51.

91. FDA, Buspirone Label, in.

92. Drabant, S., Nemes, K.B., Horvath, V., Tolokan, A., Grezal, G., Anttila, M., Gachalyi, B., Kanerva, H., Al-Behaisi, S., Horvai, G., Klebovich, I. (2004). Influence of food on the oral bioavailability of deramciclane from film-coated tablet in healthy male volunteers. *Eur. J. Pharm. Biopharm.*, 58, 689–695.

93. Cheng, K.L., Nafziger, A.N., Peloquin, C.A., Amsden, G.W. (1998). Effect of grapefruit juice on clarithromycin pharmacokinetics. *Antimicrob. Agents Chemother.*, 42, 927–929.

94. Gertz, M., Davis, J.D., Harrison, A., Houston, J.B., Galetin, A. (2008). Grapefruit juice-drug interaction studies as a method to assess the extent of intestinal availability: utility and limitations. *Curr. Drug Metab.*, 9, 785–795.

95. Kirby, B.J., Unadkat, J.D. (2007). Grapefruit juice, a glass full of drug interactions? *Clin. Pharmacol. Ther.*, 81, 631–633.

96. Becquemont, L., Verstuyft, C., Kerb, R., Brinkmann, U., Lebot, M., Jaillon, P., Funck-Brentano, C. (2001). Effect of grapefruit juice on digoxin pharmacokinetics in humans. *Clin. Pharmacol. Ther.*, 70, 311–316.

97. Parker, R.B., Yates, C.R., Soberman, J.E., Laizure, S.C. (2003). Effects of grapefruit juice on intestinal P-glycoprotein: evaluation using digoxin in humans. *Pharmacotherapy*, 23, 979–987.

98. Xu, J., Go, M.L., Lim, L.Y. (2003). Modulation of digoxin transport across Caco-2 cell monolayers by citrus fruit juices: lime, lemon, grapefruit, and pummelo. *Pharm. Res.*, 20, 169–176.

99. Bockbrader, N. (1995) Clinical pharmacokinetics of gabapentin. *Drugs Today*, 31, 613–619.

100. Chen, C., Cowles, V.E., Hou, E. (2011). Pharmacokinetics of gabapentin in a novel gastric-retentive extended-release formulation: comparison with an immediate-release formulation and effect of dose escalation and food. *J. Clin. pharmacol.*, 51, 346–358.

101. Ribavirin. Interview form.

102. Levy, G., Jusko, W.J. (1966). Factors affecting the absorption of riboflavin in man. *J. Pharm. Sci.*, 55, 285–289.

103. Patil, S.D., Ngo, L.Y., Glue, P., Unadkat, J.D. (1998). Intestinal absorption of ribavirin is preferentially mediated by the Na+-nucleoside purine (N1) transporter. *Pharm. Res.*, 15, 950–952.

104. Fujimura, M., Yamamoto, S., Murata, T., Yasujima, T., Inoue, K., Ohta, K.Y., Yuasa, H. (2010). Functional characteristics of the human ortholog of riboflavin transporter 2 and riboflavin-responsive expression of its rat ortholog in the small intestine indicate its involvement in riboflavin absorption. *J. Nutr.*, 140, 1722–1727.

105. Yamaguchi, T., Oida, T., Ikeda, C., Sekine, Y. (1986). Intestinal absorption of a b-adrenergic blocking agent nadolol. III. Nuclear magnetic resonance spectroscopic study on nadolol-sodium cholate micellar complex and intestinal absorption of nadolol derivatives in rats. *Chem. Pharm. Bull.*, 34, 4259–4264.

106. Yamaguchi, T., Ikeda, C., Sekine, Y. (1986). Intestinal absorption of a b-adrenergic blocking agent nadolol. II. Mechanism of the inhibitory effect on the intestinal absorption of nadolol by sodium cholate in rats. *Chem. Pharm. Bull.*, 34, 3836–3843.

107. Yamaguchi, T., Ikeda, C., Sekine, Y. (1986). Intestinal absorption of a b-adrenergic blocking agent nadolol. I. Comparison of absorption behavior of nadolol with those of other b-blocking agents in rats. *Chem. Pharm. Bull.*, 34, 3362–3369.

108. Lennernaes, H., Regaardh, C.G. (1993). Evidence for an interaction between the b-blocker pafenolol and bile salts in the intestinal lumen of the rat leading to dose-dependent oral absorption and double peaks in the plasma concentration-time profile. *Pharm. Res.*, 10, 879–883.

109. Ingels, F., Beck, B., Oth, M., Augustijns, P. (2004). Effect of simulated intestinal fluid on drug permeability estimation across Caco-2 monolayers. *Int. J. Pharmaceutics*, 274, 221–232.

110. Dongowski, G., Fritzsch, B., Giessler, J., Haertl, A., Kuhlmann, O., Neubert, R.H.H. (2005). The influence of bile salts and mixed micelles on the pharmacokinetics of quinine in rabbits. *Eur. J. Pharmaceutics Biopharm.*, 60, 147–151.

111. Persson, E.M., Nordgren, A., Forsell, P., Knutson, L., Oehgren, C., Forssen, S., Lennernaes, H., Abrahamsson, B. (2008). Improved understanding of the effect of food on drug absorption and bioavailability for lipophilic compounds using an intestinal pig perfusion model. *Eur. J. Pharm. Sci.*, 34, 22–29.

112. de Castro, B., Gameiro, P., Guimaraes, C., Lima, J.L., Reis, S. (2001). Partition coefficients of beta-blockers in bile salt/lecithin micelles as a tool to assess the role of mixed micelles in gastrointestinal absorption. *Biophys. Chem.*, 90, 31–43.

113. Davies, N.M., Takemoto, J.K., Brocks, D.R., Yanez, J.A. (2010). Multiple peaking phenomena in pharmacokinetic disposition. *Clin. Pharmacokinet*, 49, 351–377.

114. Schwarz, U.I., Seemann, D., Oertel, R., Miehlke, S., Kuhlisch, E., Fromm, M.F., Kim, R.B., Bailey, D.G., Kirch, W. (2005). Grapefruit juice ingestion significantly reduces talinolol bioavailability. *Clin. Pharmacol. Ther.*, 77, 291–301.

115. Maraviroc. Interview form.

116. Daneshmend, T.K., Roberts, C.J. (1982). The influence of food on the oral and intravenous pharmacokinetics of a high clearance drug: a study with labetalol. *Br. J. Clin. Pharmacol.*, 14, 73–78.

117. Barrett, J.S., Rohatagi, S., DeWitt, K.E., Morales, R.J., DiSanto, A.R. (1996). The effect of dosing regimen and food on the bioavailability of the extensively metabolized, highly variable drug eldepryl((R)) (Selegiline Hydrochloride). *Am. J. Ther.*, 3, 298–313.

118. Dresser, G.K., Bailey, D.G., Leake, B.F., Schwarz, U.I., Dawson, P.A., Freeman, D.J., Kim, R.B. (2002). Fruit juices inhibit organic anion transporting polypeptide-mediated drug uptake to decrease the oral availability of fexofenadine. *Clin. Pharmacol. Ther.*, 71, 11–20.

119. Ieiri, I., Doi, Y., Maeda, K., Sasaki, T., Kimura, M., Hirota, T., Chiyoda, T., Miyagawa, M., Irie, S., Iwasaki, K., Sugiyama, Y. (2011). Microdosing clinical study: pharmacokinetic, pharmacogenomic (SLCO2B1), and interaction (Grapefruit Juice) profiles of celiprolol following the oral microdose and therapeutic dose. *J. Clin. pharmacol.*, [Epub ahead of print]

120. Tapaninen, T., Neuvonen, P.J., Niemi, M. (2010). Grapefruit juice greatly reduces the plasma concentrations of the OATP2B1 and CYP3A4 substrate aliskiren. *Clin. Pharmacol. Ther.*, 88, 339–342.

121. Clancy, A., Locke-Haydon, J., Cregeen, R.J., Ireson, M., Ziemniak, J. (1987). Effect of concomitant food intake on absorption kinetics of fenoldopam (SK&F 82526) in healthy volunteers. *Eur. J. Clin. pharmacol.*, 32, 103–106.

122. Beique, L., Giguere, P., la Porte, C., Angel, J. (2007). Interactions between protease inhibitors and acid-reducing agents: a systematic review. *HIV Med.*, 8, 335–345.

123. Yeh, K.C., Deutsch, P.J., Haddix, H., Hesney, M., Hoagland, V., Ju, W.D., Justice, S.J., Osborne, B., Sterrett, A.T., Stone, J.A., Woolf, E., Waldman, S. (1998). Single-dose pharmacokinetics of indinavir and the effect of food. *Antimicrob. Agents Chemother.*, 42, 332–338.

124. Voriconazole. Interview form.

125. Purkins, L., Wood, N., Kleinermans, D., Greenhalgh, K., Nichols, D. (2003) Effect of food on the pharmacokinetics of multiple-dose oral voriconazole. *Br. J. Clin. Pharmacol.*, 56(Suppl 1), 17–23.

126. Purkins, L., Wood, N., Kleinermans, D., Nichols, D. (2003) Histamine H2-receptor antagonists have no clinically significant effect on the steady-state pharmacokinetics of voriconazole. *Br. J. Clin. Pharmacol.*, 56(Suppl 1), 51–55.

127. Pao, L.H., Zhou, S.Y., Cook, C., Kararli, T., Kirchhoff, C., Truelove, J., Karim, A., Fleisher, D. (1998). Reduced systemic availability of an antiarrhythmic drug, bidisomide, with meal co-administration: relationship with region-dependent intestinal absorption. *Pharm. Res.*, 15, 221–227.

128. Parojcic, J., Vasiljevic, D., Ibric, S., Djuric, Z. (2008). Tablet disintegration and drug dissolution in viscous media: paracetamol IR tablets. *Int. J. Pharm.*, 355, 93–99.

129. Gertz, B.J., Holland, S.D., Kline, W.F., Matuszewski, B.K., Freeman, A., Quan, H., Lasseter, K.C., Mucklow, J.C., Porras, A.G. (1995). Studies of the oral bioavailability of alendronate. *Clin. Pharmacol. Ther.*, 58, 288–298.

130. Aliskiren. Interview form.

131. Kindler, J., Ruegg, P.C., Neuray, M., Pacha, W. (1987). Effect of food intake on plasma levels and antihypertensive response during maintenance therapy with endralazine. *Eur. J. Clin. pharmacol.*, 32, 367–372.

132. Etidronate. Interview form.

133. Stoltz, M., Arumugham, T., Lippert, C., Yu, D., Bhargava, V., Eller, M., Weir, S. (1997). Effect of food on the bioavailability of fexofenadine hydrochloride (MDL 16455A). *Biopharm. Drug Dispos.*, 18, 645–648.

134. Eriksson, U.G., Bredberg, U., Hoffmann, K.J., Thuresson, A., Gabrielsson, M., Ericsson, H., Ahnoff, M., Gislen, K., Fager, G., Gustafsson, D. (2003). Absorption, distribution, metabolism, and excretion of ximelagatran, an oral direct thrombin inhibitor, in rats, dogs, and humans. *Drug Metab. Dispos.*, 31, 294–305.

135. Buice, R.G., Subramanian, V.S., Duchin, K.L., Uko-Nne, S. (1996). Bioequivalence of a highly variable drug: an experience with nadolol. *Pharm. Res.*, 13, 1109–1115.

136. Mitchell, D.Y., Heise, M.A., Pallone, K.A., Clay, M.E., Nesbitt, J.D., Russell, D.A., Melson, C.W. (1999). The effect of dosing regimen on the pharmacokinetics of risedronate. *Br. J. Clin. Pharmacol.*, 48, 536–542.

137. Terhaag, B., Palm, U., Sahre, H., Richter, K., Oertel, R. (1992). Interaction of talinolol and sulfasalazine in the human gastrointestinal tract. *Eur. J. Clin. pharmacol.*, 42, 461–462.

138. Zhou, H., Khalilieh, S., Lau, H., Guerret, M., Osborne, S., Alladina, L., Laurent, A.L., McLeod, J.F. (1999). Effect of meal timing not critical for the pharmacokinetics of tegaserod (HTF 919). *J. Clin. pharmacol.*, 39, 911–919.

139. Telmisartan. Interview form.

140. Zafirlukast. Interview form.

141. Rolan, P.E., Mercer, A.J., Weatherley, B.C., Holdich, T., Meire, H., Peck, R.W., Ridout, G., Posner, J. (1994). Examination of some factors responsible for a food-induced increase in absorption of atovaquone. *Br. J. Clin. Pharmacol.*, 37, 13–20.

142. Jantratid, E., Janssen, N., Reppas, C., Dressman, J.B. (2008). Dissolution media simulating conditions in the proximal human gastrointestinal tract: an update. *Pharm. Res.*, 25, 1663–1676.

143. Miles, C., Dickson, P., Rana, K., Lippert, C., Fleisher, D. (1997). CCK antagonist pre-treatment inhibits meal-enhanced drug absorption in dogs. *Regul. Pept.*, 68, 9–14.

144. Li, C., Fleisher, D., Li, L., Schwier, J.R., Sweetana, S.A., Vasudevan, V., Zornes, L.L., Pao, L.H., Zhou, S.Y., Stratford, R.E. (2001). Regional-dependent intestinal absorption and meal composition effects on systemic availability of LY303366, a lipopeptide antifungal agent, in dogs. *J. Pharm. Sci.*, 90, 47–57.

CHAPTER 13

BIOPHARMACEUTICAL MODELING FOR MISCELLANEOUS CASES

"The ability to simplify means to eliminate the unnecessary so that the necessary may speak."

—Hans Hofmann

A specific physiological condition of the GI tract can be changed by a coadministered drug. For example, a proton pump inhibitor (PPI) increases the stomach pH. These cases are clinically important. In addition, owing to its specific effect, the clinical data of such cases can be used to validate a specific feature of biopharmaceutical modeling. Some GI physiology of animals are different from that of humans. Biopharmaceutical modeling can be used to estimate and elucidate the behavior of a drug under such situations.

13.1 STOMACH pH EFFECT ON SOLUBILITY AND DISSOLUTION RATE

The pH shift in the stomach can affect Fa% of dissociable drugs with low solubility. The stomach pH can be altered by a coadministered drug, such as PPIs, H2 blockers, and acid neutralizers. In the elder Japanese, the number of hypoacid patients are significant (40% at >50 years old) [1]. Therefore, biopharmaceutical modeling for these cases would be of significant importance to drug development. The effect of gastric pH on Fa% of several drugs is summarized in Table 12.4.

Biopharmaceutics Modeling and Simulations: Theory, Practice, Methods, and Applications,
First Edition. Kiyohiko Sugano.
© 2012 John Wiley & Sons, Inc. Published 2012 by John Wiley & Sons, Inc.

13.1.1 Free Bases

In the case of free bases with low solubility, when the stomach pH is increased to a neutral pH, the oral absorption can be significantly reduced. Biopharmaceutical modeling for such cases is discussed in Section 8.6. To avoid variable oral absorption in patients, it is preferable to design an API and/or a formulation that gives high Fa% even with high stomach pH. For example, if Fa% with high stomach pH is 80%, the maximum variation caused by the stomach pH would be 20%. Fa% with high stomach pH can be easily estimated using Fa_{SS} equation (Section 8.5).

13.1.2 Free Acids and Undissociable Drugs

On the other hand, the effect of the stomach pH for free acids and undissociable drugs has not been clinically observed (to the best of the author's knowledge). No literature information about the effect of H_2 blocker and PPI on the oral absorption of NSAIDS (as free acids) is available. As the effect of the stomach pH can be negligible, Fa_{SS} equation can be used to estimate Fa% (Section 8.5).

13.1.3 Salts

The effect of gastric pH on Fa% of several salts is summarized in Table 12.4. Even when dosed as a salt form API, many bases with low solubility precipitate out as a free base in the stomach when the stomach pH is elevated by an acid-reducing agent, resulting in reduced Fa%.

In the case of a salt of an acid drug, the salt form might convert to a free form when in contact with the low pH fluid in the stomach. This conversion would not occur when the stomach pH is high. For example, the oral absorption of raltegravir potassium significantly increased when dosed with a PPI [2].

As discussed in Section 8.7, biopharmaceutical modeling for a salt is currently difficult.

13.1.4 Chemical and Enzymatic Degradation in the Stomach and Intestine

In the case of acid-degradable drugs such as triazolam [3], an increase in the stomach pH can increase Fa%. Other marketed drugs that undergo acid hydrolysis are erythromycin [4], omeprazole, lansoprazole, pantoprazole [5], etc. Usually, an acid-catalyzed degradation follows first-order kinetics (k_{deg}). Degradation % in the stomach can be estimated as

$$\text{Degraded} \% = \frac{k_{deg}}{k_{deg} + K_{t,\text{stomach}}} \tag{13.1}$$

where k_{deg} is the degradation rate constant.

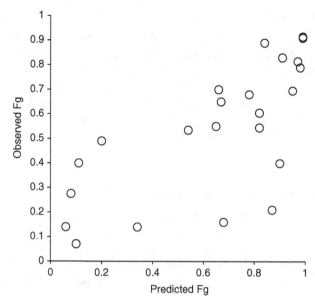

Figure 13.1 Fg prediction using *in vitro* metabolic clearance with the Q_{gut} method. In the original publication [6], PS_{perm} was calculated based on the linear $\log P_{app}-\log P_{eff}$ relationship. Log P_{app} was obtained in either Caco-2 or MDCK-MDR1 cells.

13.2 INTESTINAL FIRST-PASS METABOLISM

Prediction of the intestinal first-pass metabolism has been extensively investigated, mainly for CYP3A4 metabolism, and also for glucuronic and sulfonic conjugations. Figure 13.1 shows the prediction of Fg using the Q_{gut} model [6]. As discussed in Section 4.10, it is difficult to accurately predict Fg from *in vitro* data (Figs. 4.29 and 13.1).

Fg can be calculated from F, Fa, and Fh as $Fg = F/(Fa \cdot Fh)$. However, Fh estimation from CL_h and Q_h (Fh $= 1 - CL_h/Q_h$) could have some errors [7]. The use of intestinal CYP3A4-specific inhibitor, such as grape fruit juice, might be useful to evaluate clinical Fg for CYP3A4 [8].

Substantial sulfate conjugation has been reported for terbutaline and fenoterol (Fg < 0.3) [9–11]. These drugs are hydrophilic drugs, and the mechanism to access the enzymes in the enterocyte is not well known.[1] Glucuronization significantly reduces the bioavailability of some drugs that have planner phenolic groups such as raloxifen (BA 2%) [12, 13].

---

[1] As the surface area of the basolateral membrane is threefold larger than that of the apical membrane and the basolateral pH is ca. 1 unit higher than the apical pH, the passive membrane clearance of a base is ca. 30-fold higher in the basolateral membrane. Owing to the subepithelial diffusion resistance, removal of a drug from the basolateral membrane would not be infinitely fast. Therefore, it might be possible that a base drug that permeated through the paracellular pathway may diffuse into the cytosol. This point requires further investigation.

To predict the extent of DDI via intestinal first-pass metabolism, metabolic and escaping clearances have to be quantitatively predicted for both the victim and inhibitor drugs (Section 4.10). Even though a fully mechanistic simulation model is available, the estimation method for escaping clearance has not been thoroughly validated.

13.3 TRANSIT TIME EFFECT

13.3.1 Gastric Emptying Time

Gastric emptying pattern can be changed by the pharmacological effect of a drug. Propantheline increases gastric emptying, resulting in faster T_{max} of paracetamol, whereas metoclopramide had the opposite effect (Fig. 13.2) [14].

Alprazolam has the muscle relaxant effect and reduces the gastric motility, resulting in the double peaks in its plasma concentration profiles after oral administration in rats [15, 16]. However, the double peak phenomena was not observed in humans.

Avitriptan clearly showed a double peak in C_p–time profile conjugated with the stomach emptying simultaneously measured by Gamma scintigraphy in humans [17].

In dogs, celiprolol showed double peak C_p–time profile, which is associated with MMC [18]. Interestingly, faster gastric emptying resulted in the increased bioavailability. The most likely explanation was that an increase in intestinal concentration (caused by faster gastric emptying) saturated the P-gp efflux. However, in rats, the double peak was observed even after duodenum administration [19], suggesting that another reason might also be involved.

Ranitidine and cimetidine also change the gastric motility [20]. The double peak phenomena were observed in humans [21].

13.3.2 Intestinal Transit Time

Cisapride reduces the intestinal transit time of a drug. When dosed with cisapride, the bioavailabilities of drugs with low permeability were reduced, for example, sotalol [22], cimetidine [23], ranitidine [24], and digoxin [25] (decreased by 30%, 18%, 26% and 12%, respectively). Figure 13.3 shows the effect of cisapride on the C_p–time profile of sotalol [22]. T_{max} of sotalol was shortened from 2.8 to 1.2 h, and the AUC was decreased by 30%.

13.4 OTHER CHEMICAL AND PHYSICAL DRUG–DRUG INTERACTIONS

13.4.1 Metal Ions

Tetracyclines, quinolones, and bisphosphonates make complexes with metal ions in the GI tract. Antacids ($Mg(OH)_2$, etc.) and milk (contains Ca^{2+}) should not

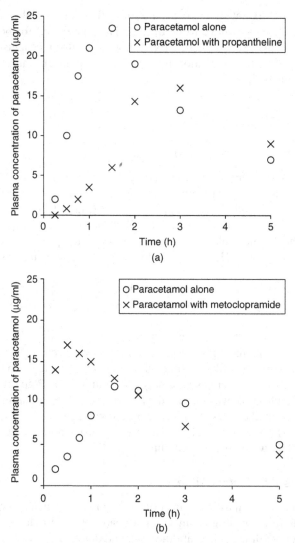

Figure 13.2 The effect of (a) propantheline and (b) metoclopramide on the C_p–time profile of acetaminophen. *Source:* Adapted from Reference 14 with permission.

be taken simultaneously [26–28]. Biopharmaceutical modeling for this kind of DDI has not been reported.

13.4.2 Cationic Resins

Resin-based drugs, such as chorestylamine and sevelamer, can bind to various drugs and reduce oral absorption of the drug [29, 30]. Biopharmaceutical modeling for this kind of DDI has not been reported.

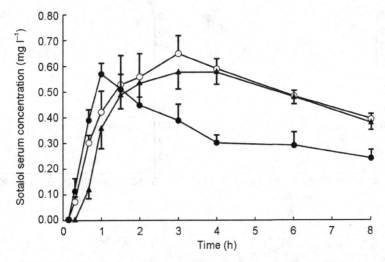

Figure 13.3 Mean (±S.E.) sotalol serum concentrations of seven healthy subjects after the administration of 80 mg sotalol as an oral solution (open circles), as an oral solution also containing 20 mg cisapride (closed circles), and as a sublingual tablet (triangles). *Source:* Adapted from Reference 22 with permission.

13.5 SPECIES DIFFERENCE

13.5.1 Permeability

Figure 13.4 shows the relationship of Fa% among human, rat, dog, and monkeys [31–33]. All of the drugs plotted are drugs with high solubility. This data suggests that the intestinal epithelial membrane permeability is comparable among human, rats, and monkeys, but not dogs. In dogs, Fa% of paracellular pathway permeants was higher than that in humans, whereas that of transcellular permeants were comparable. This is due to the larger paracellular pore size in dogs. Therefore, for permeability-limited absorption drugs (BCS III), rats and monkeys would be the appropriate species to predict human Fa%. The dog data should be carefully interpreted, especially for base or neutral drugs with MW < 500.

The good correlation of Fa% in rats and humans (Fig. 13.4) looks as if it contradicts to the experimental data that P_{eff} in rats is 6- to 15-fold lower than that in humans (Table 8.1) [34]. However, as the radius of the rat intestine is smaller than that of the human intestine, the permeation rate and Fa% in rats and humans becomes similar.

$$k_{perm} = \frac{2DF}{R_{GI}} P_{eff} \left(= \frac{SA_{GI}}{V_{GI}} P_{eff} \right) \qquad (13.2)$$

The difference in P_{eff} and the similarity of Fa% between rats and humans are well captured by the GUT framework as it considers the difference in plicate and villi structure (Figs. 8.9 and 13.5) [35]. For dogs, the GUT framework also well

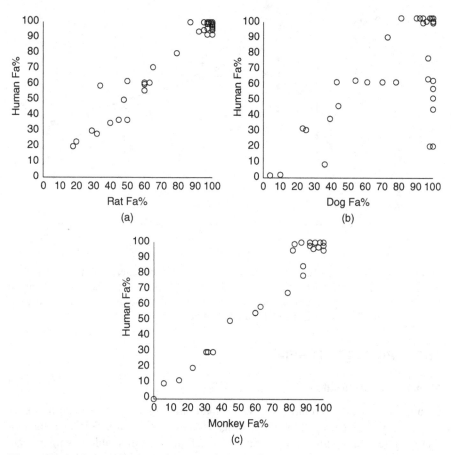

Figure 13.4 Comparison of Fa% in humans with that in (a) rats, (b) dogs, and (c) monkeys. *Source:* Replotted from References 31–33.

captures the difference of Fa% for the paracellular permeants and the similarity of Fa% for the others. The paracellular pathway model is necessary to simulate the species difference for dogs.[2]

13.5.2 Solubility/Dissolution

Species differences in solubility/dissolution perspectives have not been well characterised. As the bile concentration in rats is fivefold higher than that in fasted state humans because of continuous secretion of bile (rats lack the gallbladder), Fa% of drugs with low solubility would be overestimated. This is in good

---

[2]In one commercial software (as of 2011), the dog P_{eff} value of any drug is assumed to be threefold larger than the human P_{eff} values regardless of the permeation pathway of a drug. However, this assumption is not valid for the transcellular- and UWL-controlled cases. For these cases, the dog P_{eff} should be threefold lower than the human P_{eff}.

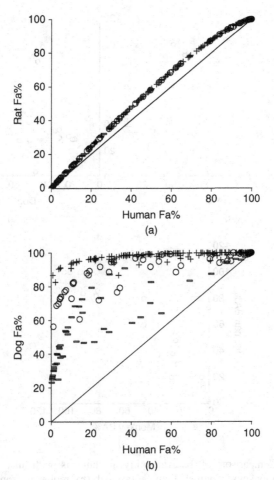

Figure 13.5 Theoretical prediction of Fa% correlation between rats, dogs, and humans by the GUT framework.

agreement with real-life experiences in drug research that as the animal species becomes larger, Fa% of drugs with low solubility becomes lower.

From a practical perspective, dogs are most frequently used as an animal species for the investigation of the performance of drug formulation. However, dogs have a little higher bile concentration, higher agitation strength, and shorter intestinal transit time compared to humans. The stomach pH of dogs should be controlled to mimic that of humans (Sections 6.3.2.1 and 7.10.3). Dogs are also appropriate for investigating the food effect [36] (Section 7.10.3).

13.5.3   First-Pass Metabolism

It is well known that there are significant species differences in the intestinal and liver first-pass metabolism.

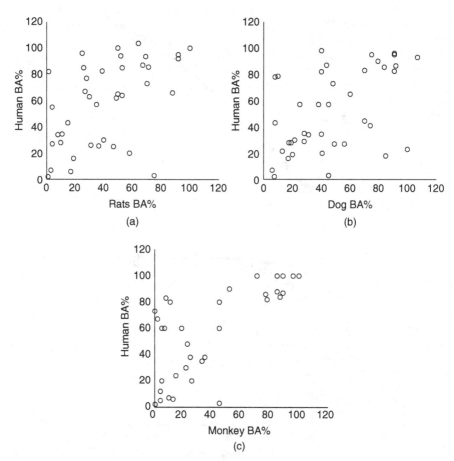

Figure 13.6 Comparison of bioavailability in humans with that in (a) rats, (b) dogs, and (c) monkeys. *Source:* Figures (a) and (b) replotted from References 32 and 43.

Figure 13.6 shows the comparison of bioavailability (F) in humans, with that in rats, dogs, and monkeys. All of the drugs plotted are drugs with high solubility. As Fa is rather consistent among rats, monkeys, and humans, Fg · Fh is suggested to have significant species differences. The oral bioavailability of CYP3A4 and UDT substrates, is markedly lower in monkeys than in humans [37], due to extensive first-pass metabolism in the monkey intestine [38–40]. On the other hand, pharmacokinetics after intravenous administration in humans is closer to that in monkeys than that in rats and dogs [41, 42].

Figure 13.7 shows the comparison of the biliary excretion percentages of drugs in humans with that in rats and dogs. Rats tend to overestimate biliary excretion in humans [44, 45]. Existence of MW cutoffs for biliary excretion has been reported. Minimum MW cutoffs for rats, guinea pigs, rabbits, dogs, and humans were reported to be 325, 400, 475, 400, and 500, respectively [44, 45].

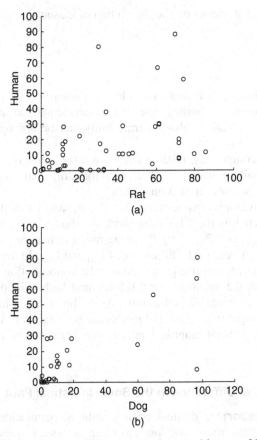

Figure 13.7 Biliary excretion in rats, dogs, and humans [44, 45].

These cutoffs were determined for organic anions and may not be applied for other types of drugs.

13.6 VALIDATION OF GI SITE-SPECIFIC ABSORPTION MODELS

Considering the significant physiological difference, the stomach, the small intestine, and the colon should be separately considered.

13.6.1 Stomach

The stomach has a much smaller surface area and shorter transit time compared to the small intestine. It is often suggested that its low pH is also a disadvantage for permeability of a basic drug (however, this would be arguable as the microclimate pH at the surface is higher [46]). Therefore, the permeability of a drug in the stomach is often neglected in biopharmaceutical modeling. However, the stomach pH has a significant impact on the dissolution of dissociable drugs (Sections 8.6 and 13.1).

13.6.2 Colon

The colon also has a much smaller surface area compared to the small intestine. For epithelial-membrane-limited cases, by the shape and surface parameters for colon (PE, VE, and DF), colonic permeability can be appropriately expressed (Section 6.1.2).

For BCS III compounds, relative BA% from the colon is ca. 20% compared to that in the small intestine [47]. The preferable drug characteristics for colonic absorption are discussed in Section 11.8.5.2.

The general relationships between P_{oct}, P_{eff}, k_a, and Fa in the small intestine and colon predicted by the GUT framework are shown in Figure 13.8. Since the estimations of K_{bm} and $P_{trans,0}$ by P_{oct} were rough estimations, this figure should be taken as general trends. The difference of P_{eff} and k_{perm} in log $P_{oct} > 1.5$ region is due to the difference of h_{UWL} and bile-micelle concentration. It was suggested that, compared to the small intestine, 0.5 log unit higher lipophilicity would be required to have a similar Fa in the colon. As the lipophilicity increased, the rate-limiting step changes from epithelial membrane permeation to UWL permeation, resulting in a superficial empirical relationship between the permeability ratio and log P_{oct}.

13.6.3 Regional Difference in the Small Intestine: Fact or Myth?

13.6.3.1 Transporter. A site-specific membrane permeation of a drug in the small intestine ("absorption window") is often discussed in the literature, especially for transporter substrates. There are many reports investigating the GI position dependency of membrane permeability of drugs using *ex vivo* and *in situ* methods such as the Ussing chamber and intestinal perfusion methods (Table 13.1, Fig. 13.9). However, a significant difference (>2-fold) in permeability is rarely observed. As discussed in Section 6.4, the transporters such as P-gp, PEP-T1, and OATP are expressed more or less all along with the small intestine.

There is little *in vivo* and clinical evidence that shows more than twofold difference in permeability or Fa% caused by possible regional differences in the small intestine. From a C_p–time curve, it is perhaps nearly impossible to conclude the site-specific absorption of a drug in the small intestine. The bimodal peak in a C_p–time profile can be explained by an erratic gastric emptying and bile-micelle binding for many cases.

13.6.3.2 Bile-Micelle Binding and Bimodal Peak Phenomena. Pafenolol shows a double peak C_p–time profile in both humans and rats. Bile-micelle binding was suggested as the reason (Fig. 12.10) [56]. Owing to the site-specific reabsorption of bile acids, the unbound fraction increases at the end of the ileum. Especially, in the case of an efflux transporter substrate, a decrease in unbound

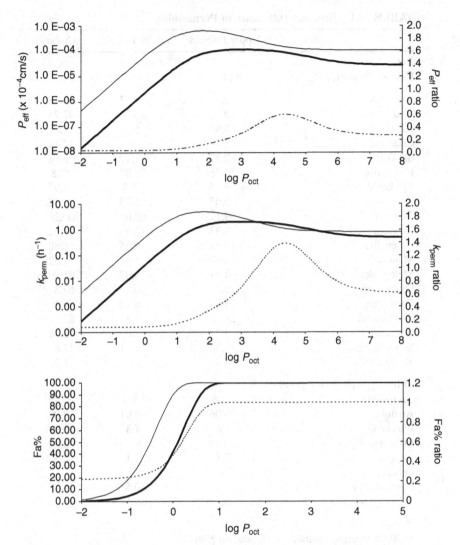

Figure 13.8 Comparison of the general relationship between P_{oct}, P_{eff}, k_a, and Fa in the small intestine and the colon. Solid line, small intestine; bold line, colon; dotted line, ratio of small intestine/colon.

drug concentration by bile-micelle binding can desaturate the efflux transporter in the proximal and middle small intestine.

Weitschies reported that talinolol showed double peak phenomena, whereas coadministered acetaminophen did not [57], suggesting that the bimodal peak was not caused by the irregular gastric emptying. It is interesting that when a food was taken after 1 h administration of talinolol, the double peak phenomena disappeared. One possible explanation would be that the two peaks collapsed as the intestinal transit time of the chymes already residing in the small intestine

TABLE 13.1 Regional Difference in Permeability

	Upper Intestine	Lower Intestine	Colon
Rat			
Ussing chambers (P_{app} (10^{-6} cm/s)) [48]			
Almokalant	11.4	16.23	30.18
Antipyrine	39.74	43.07	92.74
Atenolol	5.95	5.08	1.7
Creatinine	7.74	7.63	2.54
dDAVP	2.37	1.12	0.88
D-Glucose	56.75	51.93	2.8
Erythritol	8.25	5.7	2.02
Foscarnet	5.05	3.33	2.37
Gemfibrozil	59.12	69.65	100.26
Inogatran	3.33	3.95	1.32
L-Leucine	71.32	19.64	8.88
Mannitol	5.88	3.68	1.32
Metoprolol	34.91	78.07	85.09
Omeprazole	29.6	40.7	69.3
Phenytoin	24.04	46.13	66.1
Propranolol	28.95	41.3	87.9
Raffinose	4.37	2.63	2.48
Salicylic acid	19.74	19.51	17.6
Terbutaline	3.4	2.9	1.2
SPIP (P_{eff} (10^{-4} cm/s)) [49]			
Antipyrine	1.6	1.3	0.75
Atenolol	0.06	0.01	0.02
Fluvastatin	1.6	1.3	0.99
Metoprolol	0.33	0.53	0.09
Naproxen	2.1	2.1	2.5
Others			
Fexofenadine[a]	1	0.5	—
Bepotastine[b]	83	27	6
Rabbit			
SPIP permeation clearance (ml/min/cm) [50]			
Gancyclovir	0.44	0.63	0.47
Lobucavir	1.1	1.5	0.46
Human			
Talinolol[c]	1	0.52	—
Gabapentin[d]	29.6	15.2	7.9

[a] Perfusion/serum AUC ratio [51].
[b] % absorbed at 30 min in closed loop at 2 mM [52].
[c] Ratio of AUC in human intestinal perfusion study (upper intestine = 1) [53].
[d] AUC after regional dose in humans (μg h/ml) [54].

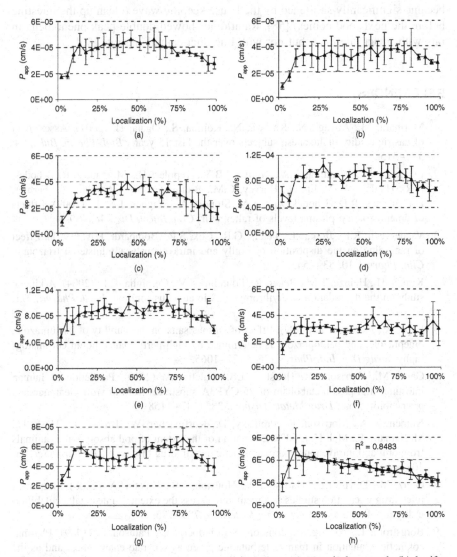

Figure 13.9 P_{app} (cm/s) along the rat small intestine. (a) mannitol, neutral; (b) lucifer yellow, anionic; (c) ranitidine, cationic: passive paracellular diffusion; (d) Testosterone; (e) antipyrine: passive transcellular diffusion; (f) L-Dopa; (g) glycylsarcosine: influx transporters LAT2 and PepT1, respectively; and (h) Digoxin: efflux transporter (P-glycoprotein). Each figure shows the P_{app} values (cm/s) plotted against the localization of each everted sac as percentage of the total length of the small intestine. The points are the means $\pm$ S.D ($n = 3$). Source: Adapted from Reference 55 with permission.

became significantly shortened by the house keeping wave (clean up the intestine before the next food comes) [58]. Ranitidine showed double peak phenomena in rats with intact bile duct, but not with bile duct-cannulated rats [59].

REFERENCES

1. Morihara, M., Aoyagi, N., Kaniwa, N., Kojima, S., Ogata, H. (2001). Assessment of gastric acidity of Japanese subjects over the last 15 years. *Biol. Pharm. Bull.*, 24, 313–315.

2. Iwamoto, M., Wenning, L.A., Nguyen, B.Y., Teppler, H., Moreau, A.R., Rhodes, R.R., Hanley, W.D., Jin, B., Harvey, C.M., Breidinger, S.A., Azrolan, N., Farmer, H.F., Isaacs, R.D., Chodakewitz, J.A., Stone, J.A., Wagner, J.A. Jr. (2009). Effects of omeprazole on plasma levels of raltegravir. *Clin. Infect. Dis.*, 48, 489–492.

3. Vanderveen, R.P., Jirak, J.L., Peters, G.R., Cox, S.R., Bombardt, P.A. (1991). Effect of ranitidine on the disposition of orally and intravenously administered triazolam. *Clin. Pharm.*, 10, 539–543.

4. Kim, Y.H., Heinze, T.M., Beger, R., Pothuluri, J.V., Cerniglia, C.E. (2004). A kinetic study on the degradation of erythromycin A in aqueous solution. *Int. J. Pharm.*, 271, 63–76.

5. Ekpe, A., Jacobsen, T. (1999). Effect of various salts on the stability of lansoprazole, omeprazole, and pantoprazole as determined by high-performance liquid chromatography. *Drug Dev. Ind. Pharm.*, 25, 1057–1065.

6. Gertz, M., Harrison, A., Houston, J.B., Galetin, A. (2010). Prediction of human intestinal first-pass metabolism of 25 CYP3A substrates from *in vitro* clearance and permeability data. *Drug Metab. Dispos.*, 38, 1147–1158.

7. Nomeir, A.A., Morrison, R., Prelusky, D., Korfmacher, W., Broske, L., Hesk, D., McNamara, P., Mei, H. (2009). Estimation of the extent of oral absorption in animals from oral and intravenous pharmacokinetic data in drug discovery. *J. Pharm. Sci*, 98, 4027–4038.

8. Gertz, M., Davis, J.D., Harrison, A., Houston, J.B., Galetin, A. (2008). Grapefruit juice-drug interaction studies as a method to assess the extent of intestinal availability: utility and limitations. *Curr. Drug Metab.*, 9, 785–795.

9. Borgstrom, L., Nyberg, L., Jonsson, S., Lindberg, C., Paulson, J. (1989). Pharmacokinetic evaluation in man of terbutaline given as separate enantiomers and as the racemate. *Br. J. Clin. Pharmacol.*, 27, 49–56.

10. Hochhaus, G., Mollmann, H. (1992). Pharmacokinetic/pharmacodynamic characteristics of the beta-2-agonists terbutaline, salbutamol and fenoterol. *Int. J. Clin. Pharmacol. Ther. Toxicol.*, 30, 342–362.

11. Mizuma, T., Kawashima, K., Sakai, S., Sakaguchi, S., Hayashi, M. (2005). Differentiation of organ availability by sequential and simultaneous analyses: intestinal conjugative metabolism impacts on intestinal availability in humans. *J. Pharm. Sci*, 94, 571–575.

12. Kemp, D.C., Fan, P.W., Stevens, J.C. (2002). Characterization of raloxifene glucuronidation *in vitro*: contribution of intestinal metabolism to presystemic clearance. *Drug Metab. Dispos.*, 30, 694–700.

13. Mizuma, T. (2009). Intestinal glucuronidation metabolism may have a greater impact on oral bioavailability than hepatic glucuronidation metabolism in humans: a study with raloxifene, substrate for UGT1A1, 1A8, 1A9, and 1A10. *Int. J. Pharm.*, 378, 140–141.

14. Nimmo, J., Heading, R.C., Tothill, P., Prescott, L.F. (1973). Pharmacological modification of gastric emptying: effects of propantheline and metoclopromide on paracetamol absorption. *Br. Med. J.*, 1, 587–589.

15. Wang, Y., Roy, A., Sun, L., Lau, C.E. (1999). A double-peak phenomenon in the pharmacokinetics of alprazolam after oral administration. *Drug Metab. Dispos.*, 27, 855–859.

16. Metsugi, Y., Miyaji, Y., Ogawara, K., Higaki, K., Kimura, T. (2008). Appearance of double peaks in plasma concentration-time profile after oral administration depends on gastric emptying profile and weight function. *Pharm. Res.*, 25, 886–895.

17. Marathe, P.H., Sandefer, E.P., Kollia, G.E., Greene, D.S., Barbhaiya, R.H., Lipper, R.A., Page, R.C., Doll, W.J., Ryo, U.Y., Digenis, G.A. (1998). *In vivo* evaluation of the absorption and gastrointestinal transit of avitriptan in fed and fasted subjects using gamma scintigraphy. *J. Pharmacokinet Biopharm*, 26, 1–20.

18. Lipka, E., Lee, I.D., Langguth, P., Spahn-Langguth, H., Mutschler, E., Amidon, G.L. (1995). Celiprolol double-peak occurrence and gastric motility: nonlinear mixed effects modeling of bioavailability data obtained in dogs. *J. Pharmacokinet Biopharm*, 23, 267–286.

19. Uesawa, Y., Mohri, K. (2008). Hesperidin in orange juice reduces the absorption of celiprolol in rats. *Biopharm Drug Dispos.*, 29, 185–188.

20. Parkman, H.P., Urbain, J.L., Knight, L.C., Brown, K.L., Trate, D.M., Miller, M.A., Maurer, A.H., Fisher, R.S. (1998). Effect of gastric acid suppressants on human gastric motility. *Gut*, 42, 243–250.

21. Yin, O.Q., Tomlinson, B., Chow, A.H., Chow, M.S. (2003). A modified two-portion absorption model to describe double-peak absorption profiles of ranitidine. *Clin. Pharmacokinet*, 42, 179–192.

22. Deneer, V.H., Lie, A.H.L., Kingma, J.H., Proost, J.H., Kelder, J.C., Brouwers, J.R. (1998). Absorption kinetics of oral sotalol combined with cisapride and sublingual sotalol in healthy subjects. *Br. J. Clin. Pharmacol.*, 45, 485–490.

23. Kirch, W., Janisch, H.D., Ohnhaus, E.E., van Peer, A. (1989). Cisapride-cimetidine interaction: enhanced cisapride bioavailability and accelerated cimetidine absorption. *Ther. Drug Monit.*, 11, 411–414.

24. Rowbotham, D.J., Milligan, K., McHugh, P. (1991). Effect of single doses of cisapride and ranitidine administered simultaneously on plasma concentrations of cisapride and ranitidine. *Br. J. Anaesth.*, 67, 302–305.

25. Kirch, W., Janisch, H.D., Santos, S.R., Duhrsen, U., Dylewicz, P., Ohnhaus, E.E. (1986). Effect of cisapride and metoclopramide on digoxin bioavailability. *Eur. J. Drug Metab. Pharmacokinet*, 11, 249–250.

26. Akagi, Y., Sakaue, T., Yoneyama, E., Aoyama, T. (2011). Influence of mineral water on absorption of oral alendronate in rats. *Yakugaku Zasshi*, 131, 801–807.

27. Ogawa, R., Echizen, H. (2011). Clinically significant drug interactions with antacids: an update. *Drugs*, 71, 1839–1864.

28. Porras, A.G., Holland, S.D., Gertz, B.J. (1999). Pharmacokinetics of alendronate. *Clin. Pharm.acokinet*, 36, 315–328.

29. Prescrire Int. (2009). Sevelamer reduces the efficacy of many other drugs. *Prescrire Int.*, 18, 164–165.

30. Walker, J.R., Brown, K., Rohatagi, S., Bathala, M.S., Xu, C., Wickremasingha, P.K., Salazar, D.E., Mager, D.E. (2009). Quantitative structure-property relationships modeling to predict *in vitro* and *in vivo* binding of drugs to the bile sequestrant, colesevelam (Welchol). *J. Clin. Pharmacol.*, 49, 1185–1195.

31. Chiou, W.L., Jeong, H.Y., Chung, S.M., Wu, T.C. (2000). Evaluation of using dog as an animal model to study the fraction of oral dose absorbed of 43 drugs in humans. *Pharm. Res.*, 17, 135–140.

32. Chiou, W.L., Buehler, P.W. (2002). Comparison of oral absorption and bioavailability of drugs between monkey and human. *Pharm. Res.*, 19, 868–874.

33. Chiou, W.L., Barve, A. (1998). Linear correlation of the fraction of oral dose absorbed of 64 drugs between humans and rats. *Pharm. Res.*, 15, 1792–1795.

34. Zakeri-Milani, P., Valizadeh, H., Tajerzadeh, H., Azarmi, Y., Islambolchilar, Z., Barzegar, S., Barzegar-Jalali, M. (2007). Predicting human intestinal permeability using single-pass intestinal perfusion in rat. *J. Pharm. Pharm. Sci.*, 10, 368–379.

35. Sugano, K. (2009). Theoretical investigation of passive intestinal membrane permeability using Monte Carlo method to generate drug-like molecule population. *Int. J. Pharm.*, 373, 55–61.

36. Lentz, K.A., Quitko, M., Morgan, D.G., Grace, J.E. Jr, Gleason, C., Marathe, P.H. (2007). Development and validation of a preclinical food effect model. *J. Pharm. Sci.*, 96, 459–472.

37. Takahashi, M., Washio, T., Suzuki, N., Igeta, K., Yamashita, S. (2010). Investigation of the intestinal permeability and first-pass metabolism of drugs in cynomolgus monkeys using single-pass intestinal perfusion. *Biol. Pharm. Bull.*, 33, 111–116.

38. Sakuda, S., Akabane, T., Teramura, T. (2006). Marked species differences in the bioavailability of midazolam in cynomolgus monkeys and humans. *Xenobiotica*, 36, 331–340.

39. Ogasawara, A., Kume, T., Kazama, E. (2007). Effect of oral ketoconazole on intestinal first-pass effect of midazolam and fexofenadine in cynomolgus monkeys. *Drug Metab. Dispos.*, 35, 410–418.

40. Nishimura, T., Amano, N., Kubo, Y., Ono, M., Kato, Y., Fujita, H., Kimura, Y., Tsuji, A. (2007). Asymmetric intestinal first-pass metabolism causes minimal oral bioavailability of midazolam in cynomolgus monkey. *Drug Metab. Dispos.*, 35, 1275–1284.

41. Ward, K.W., Smith, B.R. (2004). A comprehensive quantitative and qualitative evaluation of extrapolation of intravenous pharmacokinetic parameters from rat, dog, and monkey to humans. I. Clearance. *Drug Metab. Dispos.*, 32, 603–611.

42. Ward, K.W., Smith, B.R. (2004). A comprehensive quantitative and qualitative evaluation of extrapolation of intravenous pharmacokinetic parameters from rat, dog, and monkey to humans. II. Volume of distribution and mean residence time. *Drug Metab. Dispos.*, 32, 612–619.

43. Sietsema, W.K. (1989). The absolute oral bioavailability of selected drugs. *Int. J. Clin. Pharmacol. Ther. Toxicol.*, 27, 179–211.

44. Yang, X., Gandhi, Y.A., Morris, M.E. (2010). Biliary excretion in dogs: evidence for a molecular weight threshold. *Eur. J. Pharm. Sci.*, 40, 33–37.

45. Yang, X., Gandhi, Y.A., Duignan, D.B., Morris, M.E. (2009). Prediction of biliary excretion in rats and humans using molecular weight and quantitative structure-pharmacokinetic relationships. *AAPS J.*, 11, 511–525.

46. Chu, S., Tanaka, S., Kaunitz, J.D., Montrose, M.H. (1999). Dynamic regulation of gastric surface pH by luminal pH. *J. Clin. Invest.*, 103, 605–612.

47. Tannergren, C., Bergendal, A., Lennernas, H., Abrahamsson, B. (2009). Toward an increased understanding of the barriers to colonic drug absorption in humans: implications for early controlled release candidate assessment. *Mol. Pharm.*, 6, 60–73.

48. Ungell, A.L., Nylander, S., Bergstrand, S., Sjoberg, A., Lennernas, H. (1998). Membrane transport of drugs in different regions of the intestinal tract of the rat. *J. Pharm. Sci.*, 87, 360–366.

49. Fagerholm, U., Lindahl, A., Lennernas, H. (1997). Regional intestinal permeability in rats of compounds with different physicochemical properties and transport mechanisms. *J. Pharm. Pharmacol.*, 49, 687–690.

50. Yang, Z., Manitpisitkul, P., Sawchuk, R.J. (2006). *In situ* studies of regional absorption of lobucavir and ganciclovir from rabbit intestine and predictions of dose-limited absorption and associated variability in humans. *J. Pharm. Sci.*, 95, 2276–2292.

51. MacLean, C., Moenning, U., Reichel, A., Fricker, G. (2010). Regional absorption of fexofenadine in rat intestine. *Eur. J. Pharm. Sci.*, 41, 670–674.

52. Ohashi, R., Kamikozawa, Y., Sugiura, M., Fukuda, H., Yabuuchi, H., Tamai, I. (2006). Effect of P-glycoprotein on intestinal absorption and brain penetration of antiallergic agent bepotastine besilate. *Drug Metab. Dispos.*, 34, 793–799.

53. Gramatte, T., Oertel, R., Terhaag, B., Kirch, W. (1996). Direct demonstration of small intestinal secretion and site-dependent absorption of the beta-blocker talinolol in humans. *Clin. Pharmacol. Ther.*, 59, 541–549.

54. Bockbrader, N. (1995). Clinical pharmacokinetics of gabapentin. *Drugs Today*, 31, 613–619.

55. Lacombe, O., Woodley, J., Solleux, C., Delbos, J.M., Boursier-Neyret, C., Houin, G. (2004). Localisation of drug permeability along the rat small intestine, using markers of the paracellular, transcellular and some transporter routes. *Eur. J. Pharm. Sci.*, 23, 385–391.

56. Lennernaes, H., Regaardh, C.G. (1993). Evidence for an interaction between the b-blocker pafenolol and bile salts in the intestinal lumen of the rat leading to dose-dependent oral absorption and double peaks in the plasma concentration-time profile. *Pharm. Res.*, 10, 879–883.

57. Weitschies, W., Bernsdorf, A., Giessmann, T., Zschiesche, M., Modess, C., Hartmann, V., Mrazek, C., Wegner, D., Nagel, S., Siegmund, W. (2005). The talinolol double-peak phenomenon is likely caused by presystemic processing after uptake from gut lumen. *Pharm. Res.*, 22, 728–735.

58. Fadda, H.M., McConnell, E.L., Short, M.D., Basit, A.W. (2009). Meal-induced acceleration of tablet transit through the human small intestine. *Pharm. Res.*, 26, 356–360.

59. Suttle, A.B., Brouwer, K.L. (1994). Bile flow but not enterohepatic recirculation influences the pharmacokinetics of ranitidine in the rat. *Drug Metab. Dispos.*, 22, 224–232.

CHAPTER 14

INTESTINAL TRANSPORTERS

"How wonderful we have met with a paradox. Now we have some hope of making progress."

—Neils Bohr

Biopharmaceutical modeling of carrier-mediated CM) transport processes is still under extensive investigation. At present, an apparent K_m value is used for kinetic analysis in many cases. However, as discussed in Section 4.8, the effect of UWL and differences of apical and cytosolic concentrations have to be taken into account when calculating the intrinsic K_m value, which is required for mechanistic modeling. In addition, the expression levels of transporters in the human intestine have not been quantified with sufficient accuracy. CM transports have been mainly investigated *in vitro*, and the results have been well summarized in many excellent review articles [1]. However, knowledge about the role of CM transport in *in vivo* oral absorption is limited. Even though many drugs have been identified as substrates for transporters *in vitro*, nonlinearity in AUC has been rarely reported, probably because the K_m values are often very high (>1 mM) [2] or contribution of CM transport is insignificant *in vivo* [3, 4].[1] This point is further discussed in Section 14.4. In this chapter, the literature information about

---

[1]A cellular or vehicle uptake assay does not reflect the paracellular permeation, resulting in underestimation of the contribution of passive permeation.

Biopharmaceutics Modeling and Simulations: Theory, Practice, Methods, and Applications, First Edition. Kiyohiko Sugano.
© 2012 John Wiley & Sons, Inc. Published 2012 by John Wiley & Sons, Inc.

430

in vivo CM transports is mainly reviewed as the starting point for the development of biopharmaceutical modeling.

14.1   APICAL INFLUX TRANSPORTERS

Theoretically, as the dissolved drug concentration in the GI tract exceeds the K_m value, the main permeation route could change from CM transport to passive transport (Fig. 7.31). To appropriately simulate this change, not only the K_m and V_{max} values but also the contribution of passive permeation should be appropriately estimated. In the literature, the following equation is sometimes used to analyze the apparent dose–Fa% relationship [5]:

$$\text{Fa} = \frac{X_{abs}}{\text{Dose}} = \frac{X_{abs,max,CM}}{K_{dose} + \text{Dose}} + \text{Fa}_{passive} \tag{14.1}$$

where X_{abs} is the amount of the absorbed drug and K_{dose} is the half of the maximum absorbable dose ($X_{abs,max,CM}$) via CM transport.

14.1.1   Case Example 1: Antibiotics

Several antibiotics permeate the intestinal epithelial membrane via PEP-T1. It was demonstrated that Fa% of PEP-T1 substrates in humans can be predicted from the CM uptake clearance in Caco-2 [6] (Fig. 14.1).

Amoxicillin shows the subproportionality in dose–AUC profile (Fig. 14.2) [5, 7–9]. The dose–AUC data suggested that *in vivo* K_{dose} value at 2500-mg dose would be [ca. 55 mM (20 mg/ml) in the intestinal fluid] in the clinical dose range. After i.v. administration, the dose–AUC profile was linear. Several *in vitro* assays suggested that PEP-T1 plays a dominant role in cellular uptake of amoxicillin. The K_m value measured by the rat SPIP study was found to be 0.058 mM [10]. In the same report, significant contribution of passive transport was also noted (ca. 50%). In another report, no transmembrane permeation was observed in MDCK-PEP-T1 cells [11]. The solubility curve of amoxicillin is U shaped, with a minimum at pH 5, 5.5 mg/ml at 37°C [12], which is lower than the apparent K_m value in the clinical situation.

Cefatrizine also shows a dose-subproportional AUC increase between 500 and 1000 mg [8 and 17 mM (3.8 and 6.9 mg/ml) in the human small intestine[2]][13]. The K_m for the rat PEP-T1 was 0.6 mM [14]. The solubility of cefatrizine is 4.6 mg/ml.

The rate of oral absorption of cefadroxil was reduced by ca. 50% as the dose was increased from 5 to 30 mg/kg [7.4 to 44.5 mM, K_i (hPEP-T1, GlySar) = 7.2 mM, K_m (rPEP-T1) = 5.9 mM] [2, 14]. Coadministration of cephalexin [45 mg/kg (70 mM), K_i (hPEP-T1, GlySar) = 14.4 mM] decreased the oral

---

[2]Based on $V_{GI} = 130$ ml. In this section, the intestinal concentration of a drug is calculated in the same manner.

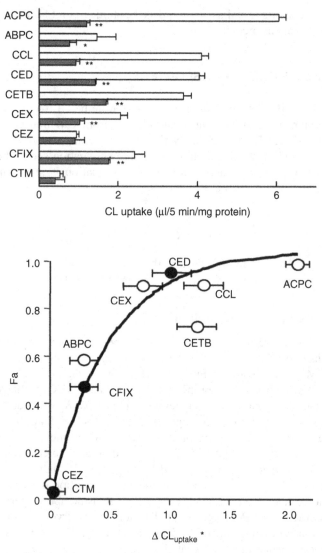

Figure 14.1   Prediction of clinical Fa% from Caco-2 uptake clearance (*$P < 0.05$, **$P < 0.01$). *Source*: Adapted from Reference 6 with permission.

absorption rate of cefadroxil by 50% [15]. As the amount of urinary excretion remained the same, it was suggested that Fa% was not changed as cefadroxil was completely absorbed even at a high dose or in the presence of cephalexin. Therefore, the contribution of PEP-T1 to the oral absorption rate of cefadroxil would likely to be ca. 50%, but the other process(es) is fast enough to give a sufficient oral absorption. However, in the other two reports, dose-subproportionality in the absorption rate was not observed in the 250- to 1500-mg dose range [16, 17].

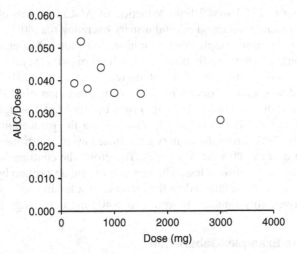

Figure 14.2 Dose−normalized AUC of amoxicillin [5, 7−9].

14.1.2 Case Example 2: Valacyclovir

Valacyclovir is a prodrug of acyclovir and has been suggested to be absorbed via PEP-T1 [18, 19]. The K_m value for human PEP-T1 is 1.6 mM [20]. Valacyclovir is rapidly converted to acyclovir in the body. The dose-normalized AUC (as of acyclovir) after dosing valacyclovir is plotted in Figure 14.3. In this dose range

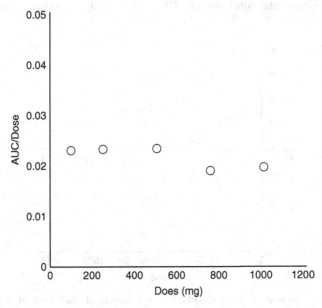

Figure 14.3 Dose−normalized AUC of acyclovir after dosing valacyclovir [21].

[100–1000 mg (2.1–21 mM)] little reduction of AUC/dose was observed [21]. In addition, moderate reduction of total urinary excretion (ca. 40%) was observed in this dose range after single-dose administration (but not after multiple-dose administration). The therapeutic dose is 500–1000 mg. The acyclovir AUC after dosing valacyclovir (500 mg) did not correlate with the PEP-T1 expression level [22] and was affected only a little by coadministration of PEP-T1 inhibitor [cephalexin 500 mg (11 mM)] [6, 23]. From the molecular weight of valacyclovir free base (=324) and pK_a (=7.47), Fa% via the paracellular pathway is predicted to be 39%. From the urinary excretion, Fa% was estimated to be from 50% (at high dose) to 80% (at low dose). Therefore, the contribution of PEP-T1 would likely to be ca. 50% or less. The increase of oral absorption by the prodrug approach may be partly explained by the increase in solubility, as acyclovir shows solubility-permeability-limited absorption at >400-mg dose range (Section 8.5).

14.1.3 Case Example: Gabapentin

Gabapentin is a substrate of LAT-1. The dose dependency of Fa% of gabapentin in humans is shown in Figure 14.4). Fa% is 74% at <400-mg dose and decreases to 36% at higher doses. Fa% of gabapentin in humans was appropriately predicted from rat P_{eff} data [24]. From the dose–Fa% relationship, it can be suggested that passive transport contributes ca. 50% of total permeability at <400-mg dose. In *in situ* and *ex vivo* studies in rats (perfusion and chamber methods, respectively), permeability of gabapentin is about twofold higher than that of mannitol (a paracellular marker) at 0.01 mM concentration [25]. In the presence of an inhibitor, the permeability of gabapentin was reduced to a value similar to that of mannitol. Considering the similarity of MW (171 vs 180) and charge (neutral), data

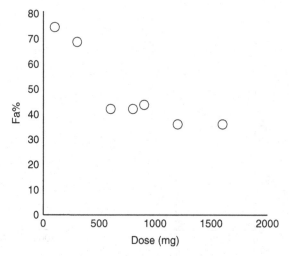

Figure 14.4 Fraction of dose absorbed as a function of oral dose of gabapentin to humans [24].

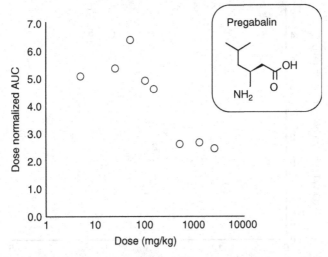

Figure 14.5 Dose-normalized AUC of pregabalin in rats [26]

from rats suggest that paracellular permeation explains about half of the total permeability. From the molecular weight of gabapentin and pK_a [3.68 (acid) and 10.70 (base)], Fa% via the paracellular pathway is predicted to be 70%. This is in good agreement with the clinical data of gabapentin. The contribution of CM and passive transport is likely to be ca. 50:50 to the net permeability of gabapentin at <400-mg dose.

Pregabalin has a chemical structure similar to gabapentin; however, the contribution of CM transport to its oral absorption was suggested to be more significant than that for gabapentin [26]. However, the oral PK is linear in the 50–300 mg range in humans. The oral absorption in rats was nonlinear in the 50 ~ 500 mg/kg range (Fig. 14.5) [27].

14.2 EFFLUX TRANSPORTERS

14.2.1 Effect of P-gp

Prediction of the effect of P-gp on *in vivo* oral absorption of drugs from *in vitro* data has not been investigated for humans, partly because there is little quantitative evaluation of data of the P-gp effect in humans. A specific inhibitor for P-gp would be of great help to progress in this area.

By using knockout (KO) mice, the predictability of the Caco-2 cells for the P-gp effect was investigated. The bioavailability ratio of KO and wild-type mice was found to correlate with the absorption quotient obtained by the Caco-2 cell assay (Fig. 14.6) [28].

The oral absorption of maraviroc was suggested to be reduced by P-gp (Fig. 14.7; Fig. 12.12). The exposure after oral administration was found to be dose-supraproportional, whereas it was dose-linear after i.v. administration

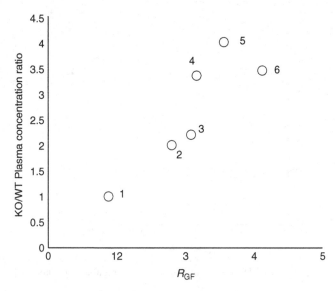

Figure 14.6 Correlation of R_{GF} ($P_{app,inhibitor}/P_{app,no\ inhibitor}$ in Caco-2) with oral plasma concentration in P-gp KO and wild-type mice after i.v. correction for effects of P-gp on drug clearance. Data points are 1, verapamil; 2, digoxin; 3, paclitaxel; 4, S09788; 5, saquinavir; and 6, tacrolimus. *Source:* Replotted from Reference 28.

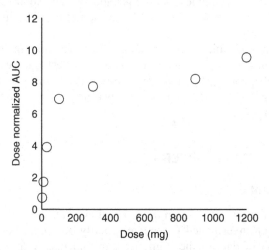

Figure 14.7 Dose–AUC dependency of maraviroc.

[29, 30]. The K_m value for P-gp is 37 µM [31]. Maraviroc is mainly metabolized by CYP3A4 ($K_m = 21$ µM) [31]. The intrinsic hepatic clearance is 44 ml/min/kg, suggesting that Fg is 0.91 (Section 4.10.2). The unbound drug concentration in the portal vein is estimated to be less than 1 µM (=dose $\times k_{abs} \times$ Fg $\times f_{u,p}/Q_h$). Therefore, the dose supralinearity was suggested to be due to the P-gp efflux in the oral absorption process, rather than first-pass metabolisms and systemic

clearance processes. Considering that the cytosolic unbound drug concentration would be one-tenth of that on the apical side (see next section), the dose strength that saturates P-gp efflux can be estimated as 25 mg from the *in vitro* K_m value (assuming $V_{GI} = 130$ ml). This value is in good agreement with the clinical observation.

14.2.2   Drug–Drug Interaction (DDI) via P-gp

Drug–drug interaction (DDI) via P-gp has been extensively discussed in the literature [32]. As an empirical rule, the following criteria has been proposed to determine the possible DDI via intestinal efflux transporters [33].

$$\frac{[I]_2}{IC50} \geq 10$$

$$[I]_2 = \frac{\text{Dose}}{250 \text{ ml}} \tag{14.2}$$

Theoretically, owing to the concentration gradient across the epithelial membrane, the concentration of a drug in the cytosol is lower than that in the intestinal fluid (Section 4.9). The following criteria would be useful to diagnose the DDI and saturation of efflux transport [34]:

$$\text{Undissociable } C_{\text{dissolv}} f_{\text{mono}} \times 1/3 > K_m, K_i$$

$$\text{Base (pK}_a > 7.5) C_{\text{dissolv}} f_{\text{mono}} \times 1/10 > K_m, K_i$$

$$\text{Acid (pK}_a < 5.5) C_{\text{dissolv}} f_{\text{mono}} \times 1/2 > K_m, K_i$$

where $C_{\text{dissolv}} f_{\text{mono}} = \text{Dose} f_{\text{mono}}/V_{GI}$ (Do < 1) or $C_{\text{dissolv}} f_{\text{mono}} = S_{\text{dissolv}} f_{\text{mono}}$ ($= S_{\text{blank}}$) (Do > 1) [35]. It should be noted that here K_m and K_i are the intrinsic values (Section 4.9.5). Owing to the asymmetry of apical and basolateral membranes and difference of apical and cytosolic pH, when the permeation of the drug is epithelial membrane limited, the unbound drug concentration in the cytosol is roughly 1/2, 1/3, and 1/10 of the apical unbound concentration for acid, undissociable, and base drugs, respectively. For the UWL-limited case, the cytosolic concentration becomes smaller further. These theoretical results are in good agreement with the empirical rule of $[I]_2/IC50 > 10$ as the rule is obtained mainly based on the DDI with base drugs.

The K_m values for P-gp are usually less than 100 μM for many drugs. For the MW = 400 and $K_m = 100$ μM case, the doses for >50% saturation would be at ca. 20, 50, and 3 mg for undissociable, base, and acid drugs, respectively.

Figure 14.8 shows the relationship between $[I]_2/IC50$ and the digoxin AUC and C_{max} ratio with/without inhibitor [36]. Even though the DDI via an intestinal transporter has been extensively discussed in the literature, clinical evidences seem to be sparse. Compared to the DDI via intestinal CYP3A4, the DDI via intestinal P-gp was reported to be milder, usually less than two- to three-fold change in AUC [35, 36]. From the theoretical perspective, as discussed in

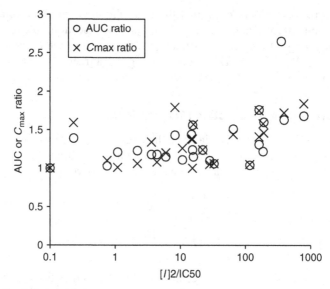

Figure 14.8 Relationship between $[I]_2/IC_{50}$ of various inhibitors and clinical AUC and C_{max} ratios of digoxin (with/without an inhibitor) [36].

Section 4.9, the maximum difference in Fa% with and without P-gp inhibition (ca. sevenfold) would be observed for moderately lipophilic basic drugs (Fig. 4.22).

Digoxin has most often been used as a probe compound for P-gp in clinical studies. However, the appropriateness of digoxin as a probe has been questioned [37, 38]. The effect of P-gp on Fa of a target drug in humans is difficult to quantify, as there is no appropriate specific inhibitor for intestinal P-gp. P-gp not only affects the intestinal absorption but also affects the biliary and renal eliminations.

Induction of P-gp also causes DDI. After repeated dose of rifampin, the AUC of digoxin after oral administration was significantly reduced, whereas after i.v. administration, it was unchanged (Fig. 14.9) [39]. The AUC of talinolol was also reduced by rifampin [40], but it is not conclusive whether this is via intestinal P-gp or change in drug disposition [41].

14.3 DUAL SUBSTRATES

14.3.1 Talinolol

Talinolol is a substrate of both P-gp and OATP in the small intestine. As the metabolism of talinolol is negligible, it is a suitable substrate for transport studies. Figure 14.10 shows the dose-normalized AUC change of talinolol in humans [42]. This dose dependency was suggested to be due to the saturation of P-gp.

The effect of naringin, a component of grapefruit juice, on the oral absorption of talinolol in rats is shown in Figure 14.11 [43]. Naringin has an IC_{50} of 12.7 μM for OATP (rat Oatp 1a5) and 604 μM for P-gp. Therefore it was suggested that

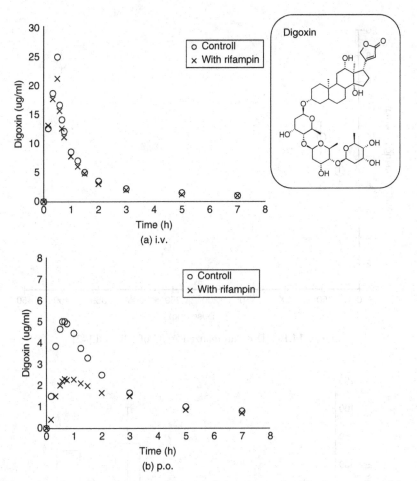

Figure 14.9 Mean ($n = 8$) plasma concentration (mean $\pm$ SD) time curves of intravenously (a) and orally (b) administered digoxin (1 mg) before and during coadministration of rifampin (600 mg). *Source:* Replotted from Reference 39.

at a low dose of naringin, only OATP was inhibited and AUC was decreased, whereas at a high dose, P-gp was inhibited and AUC was increased.

In a clinical study, 300 ml of grapefruit juice decreased the talinolol AUC and C_{max} values to 56% and 57% (Fig. 12.11), respectively, of those of water at 50-mg dose strength (1 mM) [44]. Talinolol T_{max} and $T_{1/2}$ were not affected. The 48-h cumulative excretion of talinolol into urine was reduced to 56% of that observed with water without alteration in renal clearance. The amounts of grapefruit juice constituents, naringin, dihydroxybergamottin, and bergamottin, were 712, 492, and 45 μM, respectively. K_m of talinolol for human OATP is 600–700 μM [45] and that for human P-gp is 74 μM [46].

The grapefruit juice effect in rats is different from that in humans. The K_m value of naringin is 604 μM for rat P-gp (Mdr1a), whereas it is >2000 μM

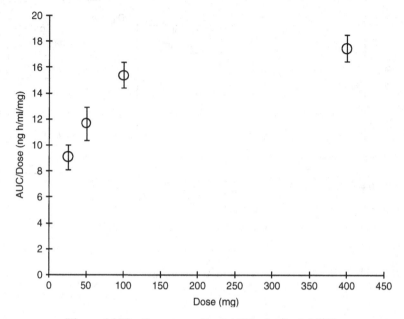

Figure 14.10   Dose-normalized AUC of talinolol [42].

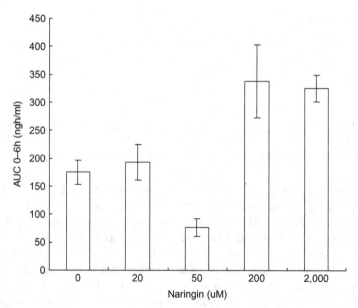

Figure 14.11   Effect of naringin on AUC of talinolol in rats [43]. Area under plasma concentration-time curve from 0 to 6 h is plotted against naringin concentration. Talinolol was administered as a racemic mixture at 10 mg/kg; 5 ml/kg. Data are represented as means $\pm$ SEM ($n = 4$).

for human P-gp (MDR1). Therefore, naringin in grapefruit juice of ca. 700 μM inhibited the rat P-gp but did not inhibit the human P-gp. In a clinical study, oral coadministration of the antibiotic erythromycin (2 g), a known P-gp inhibitor, significantly increased the talinolol serum AUC [47]. However, another P-gp substrate, verapamil, decreased the AUC of talinolol by 25% [48].

14.3.2 Fexofenadine

Fexofenadine is a well-established substrate for P-gp and OATP [49, 50]. The jejunum P_{eff} in humans is low ($0.1-0.2 \times 10^{-4}$ cm/s) and variable. According to the BCS, the drug is classified as a compound with low permeability (BCS class III) [51]. Fexofenadine has MW = 468 and is a zwitter ion. Therefore, the contribution of the paracellular pathway was estimated to be minimal.

The plasma exposure of fexofenadine was found to be linear over a wide clinical dose range of 40–800 mg (0.7–13 mM) [52]. In addition, fexofenadine had similar bioavailability (40% vs 28%) when given orally as a microdose (<100 μg) and at a higher dose of 120 mg [53]. P-gp inhibition by coadministration of verapamil and itraconazole was shown to increase AUC by threefold (so that BA% was increased to nearly 100%), whereas the elimination half-life was not changed [54, 55].

On the other hand, fruit juice (grapefruit, orange, and apple) significantly decreased the AUC of fexofenadine after oral administration (Fig. 12.13). Inhibition of OATP is suggested to be the mechanism behind these fruit juice effects. The estimated drug concentration at 120-mg dose is 1.8 mM. K_m for human OATP was 6 μM [50] and rat Oatp was 59 μM [56].

Fexofenadine displayed polarized transport in Caco-2 cells, with the $P_{app,BA}$ (apparent basolateral to apical permeability) being 28- to 85-fold higher than the $P_{app,AB}$ in the concentration range of 10–1000 μM [49]. $P_{app,BA}$ decreased with increasing concentration ($V_{max} = 5.21$ nmol/cm^2/s and apparent $K_m = 150$ μM). In addition, *in vitro* data obtained using Caco-2 cells suggest that the *in vitro* permeability was increased in the apical to basolateral direction by approximately two- to threefold in the presence of various P-gp inhibitors, such as verapamil, ketoconazole, and GF 120918 [49, 50, 57]. However, the $P_{app,AB}$ was independent of the concentration applied (10 μM–1000 μM range) (cf. drug concentration in the cytosol is lower than that in the apical side). This is in good agreement with the above-described dose-linear clinical PK.

Most reported clinical DDIs of fexofenadine, including those for verapamil and ketoconazole, partly resulting in increase in plasma levels (AUC), were explained by inhibition of intestinal efflux by P-gp [54]. However, it was recently found that there was no or a little acute effect of any of these two P-gp inhibitors, verapamil and ketoconazole, on the jejunum P_{eff} of fexofenadine in humans and rats [51, 56]. A recent *in vivo* perfusion study with simultaneous assessment of intestinal transport and plasma pharmacokinetics suggested that liver uptake of fexofenadine was mediated by OATP1B1 and/or OATP1B3, which could also be inhibited by verapamil and ketoconazole [58]. In addition, by using double transfected cells expressing OATP1B1/multidrug-resistance-associated protein 2 (MRP2) and OATP1B3/MRP2, it was shown that OATP1B1 and OATP1B3 are involved in hepatic uptake of fexofenadine [59]. Therefore, this evidence suggested that the DDI could occur in the liver uptake process rather than in the intestinal membrane permeation process, which is also supported by a recent physiological-based pharmacokinetic model [60].

14.4   DIFFICULTIES IN SIMULATING CARRIER-MEDIATED TRANSPORT

As discussed in the previous sections, many drugs have been identified as substrates for a transporter(s). However, the contribution of a transporter to the net permeability of a drug *in vivo* is often difficult to estimate. Furthermore, it is difficult to predict the dose-nonlinearity *in vivo* from the *in vitro* K_m values. As examples of this fact, gabapentin, valacyclovir, cefadoxil, talinolol, and fexofenadine have already been discussed in Section 14.1.

14.4.1   Absorptive Transporters

14.4.1.1   Discrepancies Between In Vitro and In Vivo K_m Values. Simulation of dose dependency for CM transport is of great interest. However, as exemplified below, it is currently difficult to estimate the *in vivo* dose dependency from an *in vitro* K_m value.

Considering the K_m and dose strength, cyclacillin (Fa% = 95%, hPEP-T1K_m or $K_i = 1.15$ mM, hereafter the same), cephradine (94%, 8.3 mM), cefaclor (90%, 7.6 mM), cephalexin (90%, 2.9–7.5 mM), and ceftibuten (70%, 0.5–1.0 mM) [6] should be good examples to show a dose-subproportional oral absorption in humans. The AUC of cefaclor in humans was dose-linear between 250 mg (5.2 mM) and 500 mg (10.4 mM), but the C_{max} was slightly nonlinear (20% reduction) [61]. The AUC of ceftibuten in humans was dose-linear between 25 mg (0.43 mM) and 200 mg (3.4 mM), but the C_{max} was slightly nonlinear between 25 and 100 mg (26% reduction) [62]. The AUC and C_{max} of cephalexin in humans were dose-linear between 250 (5.5 mM) and 1000 mg (22 mM) [61]. On the other hand, in studies on rats, these compounds showed clear evidences for CM transports [10, 14, 63]. Cyclacillin (1500 mg) delayed the T_{max} of amoxicillin, but AUC was changed only slightly [64]. However, cyclacillin had only slight effect on the PK profiles of ampicillin and bacampicillin [64].

The oral absorption of celiprolol at 100-mg dose was significantly reduced by grapefruit juice [65]. In addition, its AUC was reduced by 50% in an OAPT2B1 gene mutant [65]. However, the K_m for humans was 21 μM [66] and the estimated intestinal concentration at 100 mg was 2.8 mM. Interestingly, when coadministered, the AUC of celiprolol correlated with that of atenolol [65]. In a mouse *ex vivo* study, the permeability of celiprolol was found to be similar to that of FITC-4000 (a paracellular marker) [66].

Pravastatin and oseltamivir were suggested to be predominantly absorbed by transporters (OATP and PEP-T1, respectively) from *in vitro* and rat data [67, 68]. The oral absorption of pravastatin in rats (100 mg/kg, 127 mM) was found to be decreased by more than 10-fold under the coexistence of naringin (1 mM, IC50 0.03 mM). The K_m of pravastatin for rat Oatp1a5 is 0.12 mM. The oral absorption of oseltamivir (30 mg/kg in rats, ca. 52 mM) was decreased by more than 10-fold under the coexistence of an inhibitor (125 mM GlySar), suggesting that PEP-T1 plays a predominant role in its oral absorption. *In vitro* (HeLa cell/PEP-T1), K_m was 8.59 mM. However, these substantial effects were not observed in humans [69, 70].

Ribavirin and riboflavin were also substrates for influx transporters [71, 72]. These compounds show dose-subproportional absorption in humans (600– 2400 mg [71] and 5–30 mg [73]). The intestinal concentration estimated from the clinical dose is significantly higher than the K_m values obtained in *in vitro* experiments [5–10 μM (Na$^+$ nucleoside purine transporter) and <1 μM] [71, 72].

All in all, these extensive gaps between *in vitro* and *in vivo* observations suggest that further investigation is required to fully understand the role of transporters in oral absorption of drugs.

14.4.1.2 *Contribution of Other Pathways.*

The contributions of PEP-T1 in *in vivo* oral absorption are reported to be ca. 60% for cefixime (by normal/KO mice comparison) [74], ca. 50% for cephalexin (from rat *in situ* permeability) [75], and 30–60% for GlySar (by normal/KO mice comparison) [76]. For ampicillin and ceftibuten, it was suggested that the paracellular component was significant [3, 4].

A similar aspect was also demonstrated for ACE inhibitors [77, 78], some of which are historically claimed to be substrates for PEP-T1. Of the 14 ACE inhibitors investigated, the majority displayed weak or no CM transport. Very low transports were observed *in vitro* only for four of the inhibitors, including enalapril, which has previously been cited as a drug that is transported by PEP-T1. Considering the low affinities, low transport activities, relatively moderate to high lipophilicity (log $D_{oct} > 0$ in 10 of 14 drugs), and daily dose (higher concentration would be achieved in the intestine at a clinical dose, compared to the concentration used in an *in vitro* study), it was suggested that it is highly unlikely that the peptide transporters dominantly controlled *in vivo* intestinal absorption of any of the ACE inhibitors.

14.4.2 Efflux Transporters

Even though many drugs have been diagnosed as substrates of P-gp in an *in vitro* model, its effect on *in vivo* oral absorption is minimal for many cases. This point has been clearly demonstrated by using P-gp KO animals (Table 14.1 and Table 14.2) [79–81].[3] Four reasons have been proposed to explain this

---

[3]This is in good contrast to the P-gp effect on the distribution of a drug in the brain.

TABLE 14.1   P-gp Knockout Data of Mice[a]

Drug	Plasma AUC or Concentration Ratio		BA Ratio	Brain to Plasma ratio
	i.v.	p.o.		
Amprenavir	NA	1.3	<1.3	21
Asimadoline	1.0	1.1	1.1	9.1
Benzo(a)pyrene	0.8	0.8	1.0	1.6
Cyclosporine A	1.1	0.6–0.9	0.5–0.8, 1.6	11–29
Digoxin	NA	2.4	2	4–28
Dihydroergocryptine	1.8	1.8	1.0	1.1
Erythromycin	1.5	3.4	2.3	1.2
Fexofenadine	1.0, 4.6	4.6, 6.5	1.0, 6.5	1.9
Fluconazole	1.2	1.2	1.0	0.9
Indinavir	0.7	2.0	2.9	3–10
Ivermectin	NA	1.9–3.7	<1.9–3.7	17–27
Loperamide	2.0	2.0	1.0	6.7
Nelfinavir	1.3	4.8	3.7	31
Paclitaxel	1.1–2	5.0–6.0	2.5–5.5, 3.18–6.71	7.9
Reserpine	1.2	1.2	1.0	2.4
Retinoic acid	1.0	1.1	1.1	1.0
Ritonavir	1.0	1.0	1.0	6.9
S 09788	NA	2.4	3.4	NA
Salinomycin	NA	NA	1.5	NA
Saquinavir	0.7–1.1	6.5	1.55, 5.9–9.3	2.2–6.8
Tacrolimus	2.3	8.2	3.5, 3.6	6
Topotecan	NA	2.3	<2.3	2.0
UK-224,671	1.1	>40	>36	NA
Verapamil	NA	1	1	8.3
Vinorelbine	NA	NA	1.5	NA
Rifampicin	NA	3.5	NA	NA
Talinolol	NA	2.9	NA	NA

Abbreviation: NA, not available.
[a]References 28, 84 and 85

discrepancy: (i) at a clinical dose, the concentration of a drug in the intestinal fluid is high enough to saturate P-gp [a low concentration (2–10 μM) is often used in an *in vitro* assay), (ii) the passive permeability of the drug is fast enough to overcome the effect of efflux transporter and to give 100% absorption, (iii) paracellular permeants are not prone to be affected by P-gp,[4] and (iv) no addition of plasma proteins in the basolateral side results in higher unbound

---

[4]As the surface area of the basolateral membrane is three-fold larger than that of the apical membrane and the basolateral pH is ca. 1 unit higher than the apical pH, the passive membrane clearance of a base is ca. 30-fold higher in the basolateral membrane. Owing to the subepithelial diffusion resistance, removal of a drug from the basolateral membrane would not be infinitely fast. Therefore, it might be possible that a base drug, which permeated through the paracellular pathway, may diffuse into the cytosol. This point requires further investigation.

TABLE 14.2   P-gp Knockout Data of Dogs[a]

Drug	Dose mg/kg	P-gp Expression	C_{max}	AUC
Fexofenadine	0.1	Wild type ($n = 5$)	53.9 ± 13.4 ng/ml	392 ± 77 ng h/ml
	0.1	P-gp null ($n = 6$)	90.7 ± 23.1 ng/ml	881 ± 249 ng h/ml
Quinidine	0.1	Wild type ($n = 5$)	16.5 ± 3.4 ng/ml	58.8 ± 12.8 ng h/ml
	0.1	P-gp null ($n = 6$)	20.0 ± 7.9 ng/ml	89.3 ± 21.8 ng h/ml
Loperamide	0.01	Wild type ($n = 5$)	80.8 ± 9.0 pg/ml	467 ± 85 pg h/ml
	0.01	P-gp null ($n = 6$)	101 ± 15 pg/ml	556 ± 91 pg h/ml

Drug	Dose (mg/kg)		BA%	
Quinidine	0.1	Wild type ($n = 3$)	41 ± 24	
	0.1	P-gp null ($n = 3$)	32 ± 13	
Loperamide	0.2	Wild type ($n = 2$)	67 (38–96)	
	0.2	P-gp null ($n = 3$)	46 ± 36	
Nelfinavir	2	Wild type ($n = 2$)	4.5 (4.4–4.6)	
	2	P-gp null ($n = 3$)	3.6 ± 2.6	
Cyclosporin	4	Wild type ($n = 2$)	40 (32–48)	
	4	P-gp null ($n = 3$)	44 ± 10	

[a]References 79 and 80.

fraction in an *in vitro* assay [82]. Considering the vacuum cleaner mechanism of P-gp, hydrophilic compounds would not be efficiently carried by P-gp (Section 4.9). Therefore, the effect of P-gp on the oral absorption of a drug can be significant only for drugs with low to moderate passive permeability. The clinical evidences suggested that this DDI via intestinal transporters is usually mild [83], compared to that via CYP3A4.

P-gp-CYP3A4 interplay has been under extensive investigation (Section 4.10.4). However, recent simulation study suggested that this interplay would occur only in limited conditions with K_m and passive permeability [86].

14.5 SUMMARY

In this chapter, the contributions of intestinal transporters to the oral absorption of drugs were reviewed focusing on the clinical data. In the literature, many drugs have been identified as substrates for transporters by using a highly sensitive *in vitro* assay (e.g., overexpression cells, use of low concentration, etc.). However, even though extensive literature survey was performed, it was difficult to find a case in which a CM transport contributed predominantly (>75%) to oral absorption of a drug in humans. There are several cases in which a drug diagnosed as a transporter substrate by an *in vitro* study is later questioned on contribution in *in vivo* pharmacokinetics. This situation illustrates the difficulties in predicting the contribution of CM transports from *in vitro* data. Biopharmaceutical modeling for CM transports is still challenging and requires further investigations in the future.

REFERENCES

1. Tsuji, A., Tamai, I. (1996). Carrier-mediated intestinal transport of drugs. *Pharm. Res.*, 13, 963–977.

2. Bretschneider, B., Brandsch, M., Neubert, R. (1999). Intestinal transport of beta-lactam antibiotics: analysis of the affinity at the H+/peptide symporter (PEPT1), the uptake into Caco-2 cell monolayers and the transepithelial flux. *Pharm. Res.*, 16, 55–61.

3. Lafforgue, G., Arellano, C., Vachoux, C., Woodley, J., Philibert, C., Dupouy, V., Bousquet-Melou, A., Gandia, P., Houin, G. (2008). Oral absorption of ampicillin: role of paracellular route vs. PepT1 transporter. *Fundam. Clin. Pharmacol.*, 22, 189–201.

4. Menon, R.M., Barr, W.H. (2003). Comparison of ceftibuten transport across Caco-2 cells and rat jejunum mounted on modified Ussing chambers. *Biopharm. Drug Dispos.*, 24, 299–308.

5. Sjovall, J., Alvan, G., Westerlund, D. (1985). Dose-dependent absorption of amoxycillin and bacampicillin. *Clin. Pharmacol. Ther.*, 38, 241–250.

6. Shimizu, R., Sukegawa, T., Tsuda, Y., Itoh, T. (2008). Quantitative prediction of oral absorption of PEPT1 substrates based on *in vitro* uptake into Caco-2 cells. *Int. J. Pharm.*, 354, 104–110.

7. Chulavatnatol, S., Charles, B.G. (1994). Determination of dose-dependent absorption of amoxycillin from urinary excretion data in healthy subjects. *Br. J. Clin. Pharmacol.*, 38, 274–277.

8. Sjovall, J., Alvan, G., Akerlund, J.E., Svensson, J.O., Paintaud, G., Nord, C.E., Angelin, B. (1992). Dose-dependent absorption of amoxicillin in patients with an ileostomy. *Eur. J. Clin. Pharmacol.*, 43, 277–281.

9. Spyker, D.A., Rugloski, R.J., Vann, R.L., O'Brien, W.M. (1977). Pharmacokinetics of amoxicillin: dose dependence after intravenous, oral, and intramuscular administration. *Antimicrob. Agents Chemother.*, 11, 132–141.

10. Oh, D.M., Sinko, P.J., Amidon, G.L. (1992). Characterization of the oral absorption of several aminopenicillins: determination of intrinsic membrane absorption parameters in the rat intestine in situ. *Int. J. Pharm.*, 85, 181–187.

11. Faria, T.N., Timoszyk, J.K., Stouch, T.R., Vig, B.S., Landowski, C.P., Amidon, G.L., Weaver, C.D., Wall, D.A., Smith, R.L. (2004). A novel high-throughput pepT1 transporter assay differentiates between substrates and antagonists. *Mol. Pharm.*, 1, 67–76.

12. Tsuji, A., Nakashima, E., Hamano, S., Yamana, T. (1978). Physicochemical properties of amphoteric beta-lactam antibiotics I: stability, solubility, and dissolution behavior of amino penicillins as a function of pH. *J. Pharm. Sci.*, 67, 1059–1066.

13. Pfeffer, M., Gaver, R.C., Ximenez, J. (1983). Human intravenous pharmacokinetics and absolute oral bioavailability of cefatrizine. *Antimicrob. Agents Chemother.*, 24, 915–920.

14. Sinko, P.J., Amidon, G.L. (1988). Characterization of the oral absorption of beta-lactam antibiotics. I. Cephalosporins: determination of intrinsic membrane absorption parameters in the rat intestine *in situ*. *Pharm. Res.*, 5, 645–650.

15. Garrigues, T.M., Martin, U., Peris-Ribera, J.E., Prescott, L.F. (1991). Dose-dependent absorption and elimination of cefadroxil in man. *Eur. J. Clin. Pharmacol.*, 41, 179–183.

16. Barbhaiya, R.H. (1996). A pharmacokinetic comparison of cefadroxil and cephalexin after administration of 250, 500 and 1000mg solution doses. *Biopharm. Drug Dispos.*, 17, 319–330.

17. Marino, E.L., Dominguez-Gil, A. (1980). Influence of dose on the pharmacokinetics of cefadroxil. *Eur. J. Clin. Pharmacol.*, 18, 505–509.

18. Han, H.K., Oh, D.M., Amidon, G.L. (1998). Cellular uptake mechanism of amino acid ester prodrugs in Caco-2/hPEPT1 cells overexpressing a human peptide transporter. *Pharm. Res.*, 15, 1382–1386.

19. Ganapathy, M.E., Huang, W., Wang, H., Ganapathy, V., Leibach, F.H. (1998). Valacyclovir: a substrate for the intestinal and renal peptide transporters PEPT1 and PEPT2. *Biochem. Biophys. Res. Commun.*, 246, 470–475.

20. Guo, A., Hu, P., Balimane, P.V., Leibach, F.H., Sinko, P.J. (1999). Interactions of a nonpeptidic drug, valacyclovir, with the human intestinal peptide transporter (hPEPT1) expressed in a mammalian cell line. *J. Pharmacol. Exp. Ther.*, 289, 448–454.

21. Weller, S., Blum, M.R., Doucette, M., Burnette, T., Cederberg, D.M., de Miranda, P., Smiley, M.L. (1993). Pharmacokinetics of the acyclovir pro-drug valaciclovir after escalating single- and multiple-dose administration to normal volunteers. *Clin. Pharmacol. Ther.*, 54, 595–605.

22. Landowski, C.P., Sun, D., Foster, D.R., Menon, S.S., Barnett, J.L., Welage, L.S., Ramachandran, C., Amidon, G.L. (2003). Gene expression in the human intestine and correlation with oral valacyclovir pharmacokinetic parameters. *J. Pharmacol. Exp. Ther.*, 306, 778–786.

23. Phan, D.D., Chin-Hong, P., Lin, E.T., Anderle, P., Sadee, W., Guglielmo, B.J. (2003). Intra- and interindividual variabilities of valacyclovir oral bioavailability and effect of coadministration of an hPEPT1 inhibitor. *Antimicrob. Agents Chemother.*, 47, 2351–2353.

24. Stewart, B.H., Kugler, A.R., Thompson, P.R., Bockbrader, H.N. (1993). A saturable transport mechanism in the intestinal absorption of gabapentin is the underlying cause of the lack of proportionality between increasing dose and drug levels in plasma. *Pharm. Res.*, 10, 276–281.

25. Jezyk, N., Li, C., Stewart, B.H., Wu, X., Bockbrader, H.N., Fleisher, D. (1999). Transport of pregabalin in rat intestine and Caco-2 monolayers. *Pharm. Res.*, 16, 519–526.

26. Piyapolrungroj, N., Li, C., Bockbrader, H., Liu, G., Fleisher, D. (2001). Mucosal uptake of gabapentin (neurontin) vs. pregabalin in the small intestine. *Pharm. Res.*, 18, 1126–1130.

27. Regulatory submission data (common technical document), form, P.i.

28. Collett, A., Tanianis-Hughes, J., Hallifax, D., Warhurst, G. (2004). Predicting P-glycoprotein effects on oral absorption: Correlation of transport in Caco-2 with drug pharmacokinetics in wild-type and mdr1a(-/-) mice in vivo. *Pharm. Res.*, 21, 819–826.

29. Abel, S., Russell, D., Whitlock, L.A., Ridgway, C.E., Nedderman, A.N., Walker, D.K. (2008). Assessment of the absorption, metabolism and absolute bioavailability of maraviroc in healthy male subjects. *Br. J. Clin. Pharmacol.*, 65 Suppl 1, 60–67.

30. Abel, S., van der Ryst, E., Rosario, M.C., Ridgway, C.E., Medhurst, C.G., Taylor-Worth, R.J., Muirhead, G.J. (2008). Assessment of the pharmacokinetics, safety and tolerability of maraviroc, a novel CCR5 antagonist, in healthy volunteers. *Br. J. Clin. Pharmacol.*, 65 Suppl. 1, 5–18.

31. Hyland, R., Dickins, M., Collins, C., Jones, H., Jones, B. (2008). Maraviroc: *in vitro* assessment of drug-drug interaction potential. *Br. J. Clin. Pharmacol.*, 66, 498–507.

32. Giacomini, K.M., Huang, S.M., Tweedie, D.J., Benet, L.Z., Brouwer, K.L., Chu, X., Dahlin, A., Evers, R., Fischer, V., Hillgren, K.M., Hoffmaster, K.A., Ishikawa, T., Keppler, D., Kim, R.B., Lee, C.A., Niemi, M., Polli, J.W., Sugiyama, Y., Swaan, P.W., Ware, J.A., Wright, S.H., Yee, S.W., Zamek-Gliszczynski, M.J., Zhang, L. (2010). Membrane transporters in drug development. *Nat. Rev. Drug Discov.*, 9, 215–236.

33. Zhang, L., Zhang, Y.D., Zhao, P., Huang, S.M. (2009). Predicting drug-drug interactions: an FDA perspective. *AAPS J.*, 11, 300–306.

34. Sugano, K., Shirasaka, Y., Yamashita, S. (2011). Estimation of Michaelis-Menten constant of efflux transporter considering asymmetric permeability. *Int. J. Pharm.*, 8, 8.

35. Tachibana, T., Kato, M., Watanabe, T., Mitsui, T., Sugiyama, Y. (2009). Method for predicting the risk of drug-drug interactions involving inhibition of intestinal CYP3A4 and P-glycoprotein. *Xenobiotica*, 39, 430–443.

36. Fenner, K.S., Troutman, M.D., Kempshall, S., Cook, J.A., Ware, J.A., Smith, D.A., Lee, C.A. (2009). Drug-drug interactions mediated through P-glycoprotein: clinical relevance and *in vitro-in vivo* correlation using digoxin as a probe drug. *Clin. Pharmacol. Ther.*, 85, 173–181.

37. Ma, J.D., Tsunoda, S.M., Bertino, J.S. Jr., Trivedi, M., Beale, K.K., Nafziger, A.N. (2010). Evaluation of *in vivo* P-glycoprotein phenotyping probes: a need for validation. *Clin. Pharmacokinet.*, 49, 223–237.

38. Shi, J.G., Zhang, Y., Yeleswaram, S. (2011). The relevance of assessment of intestinal P-gp inhibition using digoxin as an *in vivo* probe substrate. *Nat. Rev. Drug Discov.*, 10, 75. author reply 75.

39. Greiner, B., Eichelbaum, M., Fritz, P., Kreichgauer, H.P., von Richter, O., Zundler, J., Kroemer, H.K. (1999). The role of intestinal P-glycoprotein in the interaction of digoxin and rifampin. *J. Clin. Invest.*, 104, 147–153.

40. Zschiesche, M., Lemma, G.L., Klebingat, K.J., Franke, G., Terhaag, B., Hoffmann, A., Gramatte, T., Kroemer, H.K., Siegmund, W. (2002). Stereoselective disposition of talinolol in man. *J. Pharm. Sci*, 91, 303–311.

41. Chiou, W.L., Ma, C., Wu, T.C., Jeong, H.Y. (2003). Unexpected lack of effect of the rifampin-induced P-glycoprotein on the oral bioavailability of its substrate, talinolol, in humans: implication in phenotyping. *J. Pharm. Sci.*, 92, 4–7; discussion 8–9.

42. Wetterich, U., Spahn-Langguth, H., Mutschler, E., Terhaag, B., Rosch, W., Langguth, P. (1996). Evidence for intestinal secretion as an additional clearance pathway of talinolol enantiomers: concentration- and dose-dependent absorption *in vitro* and *in vivo*. *Pharm. Res.*, 13, 514–522.

43. Shirasaka, Y., Li, Y., Shibue, Y., Kuraoka, E., Spahn-Langguth, H., Kato, Y., Langguth, P., Tamai, I. (2009). Concentration-dependent effect of naringin on intestinal absorption of beta(1)-adrenoceptor antagonist talinolol mediated by p-glycoprotein and organic anion transporting polypeptide (Oatp). *Pharm. Res.*, 26, 560–567.

44. Schwarz, U.I., Seemann, D., Oertel, R., Miehlke, S., Kuhlisch, E., Fromm, M.F., Kim, R.B., Bailey, D.G., Kirch, W. (2005). Grapefruit juice ingestion significantly reduces talinolol bioavailability. *Clin. Pharmacol. Ther.*, 77, 291–301.

45. Shirasaka, Y., Kuraoka, E., Spahn-Langguth, H., Nakanishi, T., Langguth, P., Tamai, I. (2010). Species difference in the effect of grapefruit juice on intestinal absorption of talinolol between human and rat. *J. Pharmacol. Exp. Ther.*, 332, 181–189.

46. Doppenschmitt, S., Langguth, P., Regardh, C.G., Andersson, T.B., Hilgendorf, C., Spahn-Langguth, H. (1999). Characterization of binding properties to human P-glycoprotein: development of a [3H]verapamil radioligand-binding assay. *J. Pharmacol. Exp. Ther.*, 288, 348–357.

47. Schwarz, U.I., Gramatte, T., Krappweis, J., Oertel, R., Kirch, W. (2000). P-glycoprotein inhibitor erythromycin increases oral bioavailability of talinolol in humans. *Int. J. Clin. Pharmacol. Ther.*, 38, 161–167.

48. Schwarz, U.I., Gramatte, T., Krappweis, J., Berndt, A., Oertel, R., von Richter, O., Kirch, W. (1999). Unexpected effect of verapamil on oral bioavailability of the beta-blocker talinolol in humans. *Clin. Pharmacol. Ther.*, 65, 283–290.

49. Petri, N., Tannergren, C., Rungstad, D., Lennernaes, H. (2004). Transport characteristics of fexofenadine in the Caco-2 cell model. *Pharm. Res.*, 21, 1398–1404.

50. Cvetkovic, M., Leake, B., Fromm, M.F., Wilkinson, G.R., Kim, R.B. (1999). OATP and P-glycoprotein transporters mediate the cellular uptake and excretion of fexofenadine. *Drug Metab. Dispos.*, 27, 866–871.

51. Tannergren, C., Knutson, T., Knutson, L., Lennernas, H. (2003). The effect of ketoconazole on the *in vivo* intestinal permeability of fexofenadine using a regional perfusion technique. *Br. J. Clin. Pharmacol.*, 55, 182–190.

52. Russel, T., Stoltz, M., Weir, S. (1998). Pharmacokinetics, pharmacodynamics, and tolerance of single- and multiple-dose fexofenadine hydrochloride in healthy male volunteers. *Clin. Pharmacol. Ther.*, 64, 612–621.

53. Lappin, G., Shishikura, Y., Jochemsen, R., Weaver, R.J., Gesson, C., Houston, B., Oosterhuis, B., Bjerrum, O.J., Rowland, M., Garner, C. (2010). Pharmacokinetics of fexofenadine: evaluation of a microdose and assessment of absolute oral bioavailability. *Eur. J. Pharm. Sci.*, 40, 125–131.

54. Yasui-Furukori, N., Uno, T., Sugawara, K., Tateishi, T. (2005). Different effects of three transporting inhibitors, verapamil, cimetidine, and probenecid, on fexofenadine pharmacokinetics. *Clin. Pharmacol. Ther.*, 77, 17–23.

55. Uno, T., Shimizu, M., Sugawara, K., Tateishi, T. (2006). Lack of dose-dependent effects of itraconazole on the pharmacokinetic interaction with fexofenadine. *Drug Metab. Dispos.*, 34, 1875–1879.

56. Kikuchi, A., Nozawa, T., Wakasawa, T., Maeda, T., Tamai, I. (2006). Transporter-mediated intestinal absorption of fexofenadine in rats. *Drug Metab. Pharmacokinet.*, 21, 308–314.

57. Glaeser, H., Bailey, D.G., Dresser, G.K., Gregor, J.C., Schwarz, U.I., McGrath, J.S., Jolicoeur, E., Lee, W., Leake, B.F., Tirona, R.G., Kim, R.B. (2007). Intestinal drug transporter expression and the impact of grapefruit juice in humans. *Clin. Pharmacol. Ther.*, 81, 362–370.

58. Tannergren, C., Petri, N., Knutson, L., Hedeland, M., Bondesson, U., Lennernas, H. (2003). Multiple transport mechanisms involved in the intestinal absorption and first-pass extraction of fexofenadine. *Clin. Pharmacol. Ther.*, 74, 423–436.

59. Matsushima, S., Maeda, K., Ishiguro, N., Igarashi, T., Sugiyama, Y. (2008). Investigation of the inhibitory effects of various drugs on the hepatic uptake of fexofenadine in humans. *Drug Metab. Dispos.*, 36, 663–669.

60. Swift, B., Tian, X., Brouwer, K. L. R. (2009). Integration of preclinical and clinical data with pharmacokinetic modeling and simulation to evaluate fexofenadine as a probe for hepatobiliary transport function. *Pharm. Res.*, 26, 1942–1951.

61. Barbhaiya, R.H., Shukla, U.A., Gleason, C.R., Shyu, W.C., Wilber, R.B., Pittman, K.A. (1990). Comparison of cefprozil and cefaclor pharmacokinetics and tissue penetration. *Antimicrob. Agents Chemother.*, 34, 1204–1209.

62. Nakashima, M., Uematsu, T., Takiguchi, Y., Mizuno, A., Iida, M., Yoshida, T., Yamamoto, S., Kitagawa, K., Oguma, T., Ishii, H., Yamada, H. (1988). Phase I clinical studies of 7432-S, a new oral cephalosporin: safety and pharmacokinetics. *J. Clin. Pharmacol.*, 28, 246–252.

63. Tsuji, A., Nakashima, E., Kagami, I., Yamana, T. (1981). Intestinal absorption mechanism of amphoteric beta-lactam antibiotics II: michaelis-menten kinetics of cyclacillin absorption and its pharmacokinetic analysis in rats. *J. Pharm. Sci.*, 70, 772–777.

64. Sjovall, J., Alvan, G., Westerlund, D. (1985). Oral cyclacillin interacts with the absorption of oral ampicillin, amoxycillin, and bacampicillin. *Eur. J. Clin. Pharmacol.*, 29, 495–502.

65. Ieiri, I., Doi, Y., Maeda, K., Sasaki, T., Kimura, M., Hirota, T., Chiyoda, T., Miyagawa, M., Irie, S., Iwasaki, K., Sugiyama, Y. (2011). Microdosing clinical study: pharmacokinetic, pharmacogenomic (SLCO2B1), and interaction (Grapefruit Juice) profiles of celiprolol following the oral microdose and therapeutic dose. *J. Clin. Pharmacol.* [Epub ahead of print].

66. Kato, Y., Miyazaki, T., Kano, T., Sugiura, T., Kubo, Y., Tsuji, A. (2009). Involvement of influx and efflux transport systems in gastrointestinal absorption of celiprolol. *J. Pharm. Sci.*, 98, 2529–2539.

67. Shirasaka, Y., Suzuki, K., Nakanishi, T., Tamai, I. (2010). Intestinal absorption of HMG-CoA reductase inhibitor pravastatin mediated by organic anion transporting polypeptide. *Pharm. Res.*, 27, 2141–2149.

68. Ogihara, T., Kano, T., Wagatsuma, T., Wada, S., Yabuuchi, H., Enomoto, S., Morimoto, K., Shirasaka, Y., Kobayashi, S., Tamai, I. (2009). Oseltamivir (tamiflu) is a substrate of peptide transporter 1. *Drug Metab. Dispos.*, 37, 1676–1681.

69. Lilja, J.J., Kivisto, K.T., Neuvonen, P.J. (1999). Grapefruit juice increases serum concentrations of atorvastatin and has no effect on pravastatin. *Clin. Pharmacol. Ther.*, 66, 118–127.

70. Fukazawa, I., Uchida, N., Uchida, E., Yasuhara, H. (2004). Effects of grapefruit juice on pharmacokinetics of atorvastatin and pravastatin in Japanese. *Br. J. Clin. Pharmacol.*, 57, 448–455.

71. Patil, S.D., Ngo, L.Y., Glue, P., Unadkat, J.D. (1998). Intestinal absorption of ribavirin is preferentially mediated by the Na+-nucleoside purine (N1) transporter. *Pharm. Res.*, 15, 950–952.

72. Fujimura, M., Yamamoto, S., Murata, T., Yasujima, T., Inoue, K., Ohta, K.Y., Yuasa, H. (2010). Functional characteristics of the human ortholog of riboflavin transporter 2 and riboflavin-responsive expression of its rat ortholog in the small intestine indicate its involvement in riboflavin absorption. *J. Nutr.*, 140, 1722–1727.

73. Levy, G., Jusko, W.J. (1966). Factors affecting the absorption of riboflavin in man. *J. Pharm. Sci.*, 55, 285–289.

74. Kato, Y., Sugiura, T., Nakadera, Y., Sugiura, M., Kubo, Y., Sato, T., Harada, A., Tsuji, A. (2009). Investigation of the role of oligopeptide transporter PEPT1 and sodium/glucose cotransporter SGLT1 in intestinal absorption of their substrates using small GTP-binding protein Rab8-null mice. *Drug Metab. Dispos.*, 37, 602–607.

75. Hironaka, T., Itokawa, S., Ogawara, K.-I., Higaki, K., Kimura, T. (2009). Quantitative evaluation of PEPT1 contribution to oral absorption of cephalexin in rats. *Pharm. Res.*, 26, 40–50.

76. Jappar, D., Hu, Y., Smith, D.E. (2011). Effect of dose escalation on the *in vivo* oral absorption and disposition of glycylsarcosine in wild-type and Pept1 knockout mice. *Drug Metab. Dispos.*, 39(12), 2250–2257.

77. Brandsch, M., Knutter, I., Bosse-Doenecke, E. (2008). Pharmaceutical and pharmacological importance of peptide transporters. *J. Pharm. Pharmacol.*, 60, 543–585.

78. Knutter, I., Wollensky, C., Kottra, G., Hahn, M., Fischer, W., Zebisch, K., Neubert, R., Daniel, H., Brandsch, M. (2008). Transport of angiotensin-converting enzyme inhibitors by H+/Peptide transporters revisited. *J. Pharmacol. Exp. Ther.*, 327, 432–441.

79. Kitamura, Y., Koto, H., Matsuura, S., Kawabata, T., Tsuchiya, H., Kusuhara, H., Tsujimoto, H., Sugiyama, Y. (2008). Modest effect of impaired P-glycoprotein on the plasma concentrations of fexofenadine, quinidine, and loperamide following oral administration in collies. *Drug Metab. Dispos.*, 36, 807–810.

80. Mealey, K.L., Waiting, D., Raunig, D.L., Schmidt, K.R., Nelson, F.R. (2010). Oral bioavailability of P-glycoprotein substrate drugs do not differ between ABCB1-1Delta and ABCB1 wild type dogs. *J. Vet. Pharmacol. Ther.*, 33, 453–460.

81. Sugano, K., Kansy, M., Artursson, P., Avdeef, A., Bendels, S., Di, L., Ecker, G.F., Faller, B., Fischer, H., Gerebtzoff, G., Lennernaes, H., Senner, F. (2010). Coexistence of passive and carrier-mediated processes in drug transport. *Nat. Rev. Drug Discov.*, 9, 597–614.

82. Neuhoff, S., Artursson, P., Zamora, I., Ungell, A.-L. (2006). Impact of extracellular protein binding on passive and active drug transport across Caco-2 cells. *Pharm. Res.*, 23, 350–359.

83. Lee, C.A., Cook, J.A., Reyner, E.L., Smith, D.A. (2010). P-glycoprotein related drug interactions: clinical importance and a consideration of disease states. *Expert Opin. Drug Metab. Toxicol.*, 6, 603–619.

84. Chen, C., Liu, X., Smith, B.J. (2003). Utility of Mdr1-gene deficient mice in assessing the impact of P-glycoprotein on pharmacokinetics and pharmacodynamics in drug discovery and development. *Curr. Drug Metab.*, 4, 272–291.

85. del Amo, E.M., Heikkinen, A.T., Moenkkoenen, J. (2009). *In vitro-in vivo* correlation in p-glycoprotein mediated transport in intestinal absorption. *Eur. J. Pharm. Sci.*, 36, 200–211.

86. Darwich, A.S., Neuhoff, S., Jamei, M., Rostami-Hodjegan, A. (2010). Interplay of metabolism and transport in determining oral drug absorption and gut wall metabolism: a simulation assessment using the "Advanced Dissolution, Absorption, Metabolism (ADAM)" model. *Curr. Drug Metab.*, 11, 716–729.

CHAPTER 15

STRATEGY IN DRUG DISCOVERY AND DEVELOPMENT

"Science finds, industry applies, and man conforms."

—Anonymous

Biopharmaceutical modeling will be an effective tool to improve the productivity of drug discovery and development if we use it appropriately [1]. At present, several software packages are commercially available [2]. Biopharmaceutical modeling will also be useful for the quality-by-design strategy [3–6].

Drugs with low bioavailability tend to show variable Cp-time profiles [7]. (Fig. 15.1). Therefore, to increase the success rate of drug development, it is preferable to have a drug candidate with high bioavailability. Therefore, it would be preferable to have a strategy to design and select a candidate drug with appropriate BA% from the early stages of drug discovery.

15.1 LIBRARY DESIGN

The quality of a compound library directly affects the quality of a lead compound and may impact the quality of a clinical candidate compound and the success rate of drug development. Therefore, a lead compound with a reasonable biopharmaceutical profile had better be discovered from the compound library. Generally, during the lead optimization stage, the average solubility of a compound series decreases because the average of molecular weight (MW) and lipophilicity would increase to achieve a high pharmacological potency and selectivity [8, 9]. The

Biopharmaceutics Modeling and Simulations: Theory, Practice, Methods, and Applications,
First Edition. Kiyohiko Sugano.
© 2012 John Wiley & Sons, Inc. Published 2012 by John Wiley & Sons, Inc.

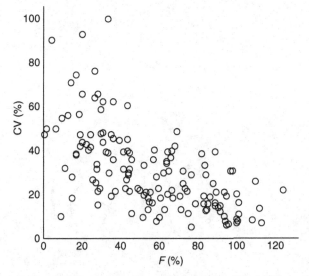

Figure 15.1   Relationship between absolute bioavailability (F) and intersubject variability (CV) in absolute bioavailability. *Source:* Replotted from Reference 7.

large number of hydrogen bonds and high lipophilicity might cause high crystalline energy and high hydrophobicity, leading to low solubility (Section 2.2.1).

In order to find a high quality lead compound, "drug-likeness" [10, 11] and structural diversity should be considered in library design. "Drug-likeness" can be assessed by a simple rule such as the "rule of five," which calculates the molecular weight, the number of hydrogen bond donors and acceptors, and the lipophilicity [10–12]. These factors also affect the biopharmaceutical profiles. High MW might cause either or both of ADME property and synthetic complexity issues and might lead to a development candidate with a low success rate. Therefore, it is preferred that the MW of the library compounds is set as low as possible (e.g., <400) [13]. In addition to oral absorption of a drug, lipophilicity also affects the volume of distribution [14–16], renal clearance (renal reabsorption) [17, 18], etc.

For library design, an *in silico* approach is ordinary (Section 5.1) [19]. However, at present, the prediction accuracy of *in silico* tools is not completely satisfactory. If one keeps in mind its limitations, it can be used for the purpose of library design.

Even though the concept of "drug-likeness" would be the baseline for library design, it should also be remembered that there are many exceptions (Fig. 15.2) [20]. It is important to be flexible so as not to fail the chance.

15.2   LEAD OPTIMIZATION

In the lead optimization stage, medium- to high throughput screening data will become available. An apparent solubility screening with PLM crystallinity

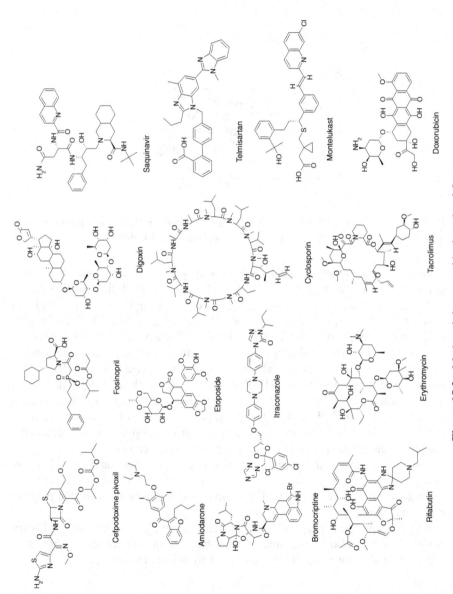

Figure 15.2 Marketed drugs outside the rule of five.

assessment [21] can be performed in parallel with a membrane permeability assay such as PAMPA. These information can be used for the initial assessment of the BCS category for the chemical series [22]. These data are usually stored into an in-house database. Biopharmaceutical modeling can be integrated to the in-house database and automatically run in the background.

At the late optimization stage, in addition to the basic physicochemical data, the solubility data in biorelevant media such as FaSSIF would be available.

15.3 COMPOUND SELECTION

Compounds that passed *in vitro* assays would then be evaluated by *in vivo* assays. Apparent solubility assay with powder material accompanied with crystallinity evaluation should take place at this stage. These data can be used to run detailed biopharmaceutical modeling. Biopharmaceutical modeling can be useful to select an appropriate formulation for *in vivo* studies (such as early toxicology studies) and also to interpret the *in vivo* results.

15.4 API FORM SELECTION

A detailed solubility profile (the pH–solubility profile and the effect of bile) should be studied at this stage as part of preformulation studies [23, 24]. The effect of bile should also be evaluated to assess the effect of food on oral absorption. If the candidate compounds (may be 1–3 compounds from a project) have low solubility, salt formation, cocrystal formation, and/or particle size reduction would be investigated to improve the dissolution profile. Miniscale dissolution tests can be used at this stage [25, 26].

In addition to the biopharmaceutical performance, developability of the API (stability, production suitability, production facility, ease of quality control, etc.) should be simultaneously evaluated [23, 24].

15.5 FORMULATION SELECTION

If the API form optimization was not successful to give sufficient exposure, particle size reduction would be the next measure. In the case of the dissolution-rate-limited absorption, particle size reduction may be effective to increase Fa%. The effectiveness of particle size reduction can be assessed by biopharmaceutical modeling. Usually, the initial dissolution rate is reciprocal to the particle size. It is worth mentioning that a milling process can change the solid form, especially to an amorphous state. Therefore, the milling feasibility should be simultaneously studied.

If the API form selection and standard particle size reduction (ca. 5–10 μm) was not successful to improve Fa%, special formulations such as nanoparticle, solid dispersion, and SEDDS could be the next option to achieve a target *in vivo* exposure. The mechanism-based flow chart (Fig. 11.18) may be a useful guide.

However, the successful development of special formulations is not always guaranteed. Therefore, we suppose that the primary solution to the low solubility issue would be to fix it in chemistry (compound structure or API form) [27]. If low solubility is inevitable, we should then challenge special formulations. To reduce the risk of the special formulations while exploring the possibilities, it is preferable to experimentally examine these special formulations as early as possible in the drug discovery and development process. At the same time as the assessment of oral absorption, developability and market competitiveness (compliance, cost of goods, development speed, etc.) should be addressed. The development of special formulations is always expensive with respect to time and man power. The maximum loading dose in special formulations is often smaller than that of the standard formulations. To avoid over and under expectation on special formulations, sufficient accountability for the project team is necessary. It is important to have a decision tree before the *in vivo* oral absorption study, because a discovery project team can be fascinated by the significant enhancement of oral absorption by a special formulation and developability and market competitiveness are put aside.

15.6   STRATEGY TO PREDICT HUMAN FA%

It is important to validate biopharmaceutical modeling by comparing with the real experimental data. A step-by-step cross validation strategy is shown in Figure 15.3. If there is a discrepancy between simulated and observed data,

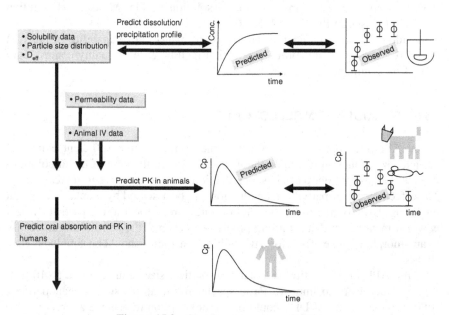

Figure 15.3   Step-by-step cross validation.

the reason for the discrepancy should be investigated by independent mechanistic experiments, rather than solely estimated by parameter fitting. "All-in-all" validation and compound by compound parameter optimization should not be taken [28]. The parameter responsible for the simulation error cannot be selected simply by try and error curve fitting. For example, the degree of flatness (DF) in the $P_{eff}-k_{perm}$ equation might be selected and optimized, even though the real reason was an error in P_{eff}. If this DF is used for humans and dose dependency is simulated, the prediction would fail.

REFERENCES

1. Kuentz, M., Nick, S., Parrott, N., Rothlisberger, D. (2006). A strategy for preclinical formulation development using GastroPlus(TM) as pharmacokinetic simulation tool and a statistical screening design applied to a dog study. *Eur. J. Pharm. Sci.*, **27**, 91–99.
2. Parrott, N., Lave, T. (2002). Prediction of intestinal absorption: comparative assessment of GASTROPLUS and IDEA. *Eur. J. Pharm. Sci.*, **17**, 51–61.
3. Jiang, W., Kim, S., Zhang, X., Lionberger, R. A., Davit, B. M., Conner, D. P., Yu, L. X. (2011). The role of predictive biopharmaceutical modeling and simulation in drug development and regulatory evaluation. *Int. J. Pharm.*, **418**, 151–160.
4. Yu, L. X. (2008). Pharmaceutical quality by design: product and process development, understanding, and control. *Pharm. Res.*, **25**, 781–791.
5. Lionberger, R. A., Lee, S. L., Lee, L., Raw, A., Yu, L. X. (2008). Quality by design: concepts for ANDAs. *AAPS J.*, **10**, 268–276.
6. Henck, J. O., Byrn, S. R. (2007). Designing a molecular delivery system within a preclinical timeframe. *Drug Discovery Today*, **12**, 189–199.
7. Hellriegel, E. T., Bjornsson, T. D., Hauck, W. W. (1996). Interpatient variability in bioavailability is related to the extent of absorption: implications for bioavailability and bioequivalence studies. *Clin. Pharmacol. Ther.*, **60**, 601–607.
8. Sugano, K., Obata, K., Saitoh, R., Higashida, A., Hamada, H., Processing of Biopharmaceutical Profiling Data in Drug Discovery, in: B. Testa, S., Krämer, H., Wunderli-Allenspach, G., Folkers (eds) *Pharmacokinetic Profiling in Drug Research*, Wiley-VCH, Zurich, 2006, pp. 441–458.
9. Wenlock, M. C., Austin, R. P., Barton, P., Davis, A. M., Leeson, P. D. (2003). A comparison of physiochemical property profiles of development and marketed oral drugs. *J. Med. Chem.*, **46**, 1250–1256.
10. Lipinski, C. A., Lombardo, F., Dominy, B. W., Feeney, P. J. (1997). Experimental and computational approaches to estimate solubility and permeability in drug discovery and development settings. *Adv. Drug Delivery Rev.*, **23**, 3–25.
11. Lipinski, C. A. (2004). Lead- and drug-like compounds: the rule-of-five revolution. *Drug Discovery Today Technol.*, **1**, 337–341.
12. Leeson, P. D., Springthorpe, B. (2007). The influence of drug-like concepts on decision-making in medicinal chemistry. *Nat. Rev. Drug Discovery*, **6**, 881–890.
13. Oprea, T. I., Davis, A. M., Teague, S. J., Leeson, P. D. (2001). Is there a difference between leads and drugs? A historical perspective. *J. Chem. Inf. Comput. Sci.*, **41**, 1308–1315.

14. Lombardo, F., Obach, R. S., Shalaeva, M. Y., Gao, F. (2002). Prediction of volume of distribution values in humans for neutral and basic drugs using physicochemical measurements and plasma protein binding data. *J. Med. Chem.*, **45**, 2867–2876.

15. Rodgers, T., Rowland, M. (2006). Physiologically based pharmacokinetic modelling 2: predicting the tissue distribution of acids, very weak bases, neutrals and zwitterions. *J. Pharm. Sci.*, **95**, 1238–1257.

16. Rodgers, T., Rowland, M. (2007). Mechanistic approaches to volume of distribution predictions: understanding the processes. *Pharm. Res.*, **24**, 918–933.

17. Barza, M., Brown, R. B., Shanks, C., Gamble, C., Weinstein, L. (1975). Relation between lipophilicity and pharmacological behavior of minocycline, doxycycline, tetracycline, and oxytetracycline in dogs. *Antimicrob. Agents Chemother.*, **8**, 713–720.

18. Varma, M. V., Feng, B., Obach, R. S., Troutman, M. D., Chupka, J., Miller, H. R., El-Kattan, A. (2009). Physicochemical determinants of human renal clearance. *J. Med. Chem.*, **52**, 4844–4852.

19. Lombardo, F., Gifford, E., Shalaeva, M. Y. (2003). In silico ADME prediction: data, models, facts and myths. *Mini-Rev. Med. Chem.*, **3**, 861–875.

20. Sakaeda, T., Okamura, N., Nagata, S., Yagami, T., Horinouchi, M., Okumura, K., Yamashita, F., Hashida, M. (2001). Molecular and pharmacokinetic properties of 222 commercially available oral drugs in humans. *Biol. Pharm. Bull.*, **24**, 935–940.

21. Sugano, K., Kato, T., Suzuki, K., Keiko, K., Sujaku, T., Mano, T. (2006). High throughput solubility measurement with automated polarized light microscopy analysis. *J. Pharm. Sci.*, **95**, 2115–2122.

22. Obata, K., Sugano, K., Machida, M., Aso, Y. (2004). Biopharmaceutics classification by high throughput solubility assay and PAMPA. *Drug Dev. Ind. Pharm.*, **30**, 181.

23. Fiese, E. F. (2003). General pharmaceutics-the new physical pharmacy. *J. Pharm. Sci.*, **92**, 1331–1342.

24. Balbach, S., Korn, C. (2004). Pharmaceutical evaluation of early development candidates "the 100mg-approach". *Int. J. Pharmaceutics*, **275**, 1–12.

25. Takano, R., Sugano, K., Higashida, A., Hayashi, Y., Machida, M., Aso, Y., Yamashita, S. (2006). Oral absorption of poorly water-soluble drugs: computer simulation of fraction absorbed in humans from a miniscale dissolution test. *Pharm. Res.*, **23**, 1144–1156.

26. Avdeef, A., Tsinman, O. (2008). Miniaturized rotating disk intrinsic dissolution rate measurement: effects of buffer capacity in comparisons to traditional wood's apparatus. *Pharm. Res.*, **25**, 2613–2627.

27. Lipinski, C. (2004). Solubility in the design of combinatorial libraries. *Chem. Anal.*, **163**, 407–434.

28. Jones, H. M., Parrott, N., Jorga, K., Lave, T. (2006). A novel strategy for physiologically based predictions of human pharmacokinetics. *Clin. Pharmacokinet*, **45**, 511–542.

CHAPTER 16

EPISTEMOLOGY OF BIOPHARMACEUTICAL MODELING AND GOOD SIMULATION PRACTICE

"The greatest obstacle to discovering the shape of the earth, the continents and the ocean was not ignorance but the illusion of knowledge."

—Daniel J. Boorstin

16.1 CAN SIMULATION BE SO PERFECT?

In the literature, accurate predictions of the C_p-time profile by using a commercial software package have been often advocated. However, as discussed in Section 8.1, considering the uncertainty and variations in the input data and the model equations (as well as the variation in *in vivo* data), such accurate predictions should be unattainable.

It is often assumed without judgment that a commercial software package should have been fully validated. However, it would be a good practice to investigate the software package before using it. Appropriateness of the equations should be thoroughly investigated, for example, equations for the solid surface pH, the common ion effect, the paracellular pathway, the pH-partition theory with microclimate pHs, the UWL permeation, the nucleation, and the unbound fraction. In addition, appropriateness of physiological parameters should be thoroughly investigated, for example, the intestinal fluid volume and the degree of

---

Biopharmaceutics Modeling and Simulations: Theory, Practice, Methods, and Applications,
First Edition. Kiyohiko Sugano.
© 2012 John Wiley & Sons, Inc. Published 2012 by John Wiley & Sons, Inc.

flatness (or SA_{GI}/V_{GI} ratio). In several reports, the intestinal fluid volume of 600–1500 ml was used (should be 100–250 ml) and the SA_{GI}/V_{GI} ratio was set to be ca. 1.3 (should be ca. 2.3).[1] Furthermore, the drug data used in a report should also be carefully checked. All experimental scientists know that the results of an *in vitro* assay have variations, which often become more than twofold. Artificial intestinal fluids (such as FaSSIF) and *in vitro* membrane assays (such as Caco-2) cannot be a perfect surrogate for corresponding *in vivo* factors. Incorrect drug parameters were sometimes used in the literature. For example, in one report, instead of the true density of the drug, the tap density was used for surface area calculation. In another report, a pK_a value for an acid was used for a base. In many cases, because the details of simulation were not fully disclosed, it is not clear why accurate simulation results were obtained despite the insufficiency of equations and/or the use of incorrect input data.

As discussed in Chapter 8, even for the simplest cases, the current average simulation error of the GUT framework (all of which is constructed by public scientific knowledge), is ca. twofold. A scientific progress of this area should start with admitting this reality.

16.2   PARAMETER FITTING

Probably, drug-by-drug parameter fitting is one of the most frequent reasons to give a superficially good simulation.

Parameter fitting is sometimes performed unwittingly. For example, when we have four different P_{eff} values estimated from the PAMPA, Caco-2, MDCK, rat *in situ* perfusion, and *in silico* methods, we might select one method, on a drug-by-drug basis, which gives the best fitting to *in vivo* results. This is mathematically equivalent to doing a parameter fitting for each drug. If we were to select a suitable assay, it should be based on an independent reason (e.g., because the drug is a transporter substrate, rat *in situ* perfusion data is used). In some cases, as clinical i.v. data was not available, CL and Vd were obtained by fitting to p.o. data. In one report, different CL and Vd values were used for i.v. and p.o. simulations, respectively.

However, parameter fitting is sometimes necessary when a physiological parameter cannot be directly obtainable and have to be back-estimated from the clinical PK data of drugs. For this purpose, the drugs that are free from

---

[1] In some reports, $V_{GI} = 600$ ml was used with the surface area of 800 cm^2, that is, $SA_{GI}/V_{GI} = 1.3$, which is equal to the cylindrical tube shape. Compared to the current most credible values of $V_{GI} = 130$ ml and $SA_{GI}/V_{GI} = 2.3$, the previous V_{GI} is larger and the previous SA_{GI}/V_{GI} is smaller. These errors worked in opposite directions and were coincidently canceled out, resulting in semiquantitative Fa% prediction for solubility-permeability-limited cases. However, with $V_{GI} = 600$ ml, the inflation point in the dose–AUC curve would be upshifted (Fig. 10.1). In addition, with $SA_{GI}/V_{GI} = 1.3$, for permeability-limited cases, human Fa% is underestimated by ca. twofold from the experimental P_{eff} values in humans (Fig. 8.2).

the uncertainty in the other factors should be used for parameter fitting. The number of model drugs should be sufficient to avoid overlearning ($>5-10$ data points per parameter). From a single C_p–time profile, only a little information is identifiable [1]. For example, the one-compartment model with three parameters, that is, k_a, k_{el}, and Vd, is usually sufficient to describe the oral PK profile of a drug. On the other hand, a mechanistic biopharmaceutical model contains dozens to hundreds of parameters. It is often difficult to identify a correct parameter for optimization solely from the C_p–time profile (Section 15.6).

16.3 GOOD SIMULATION PRACTICE

In modeling and simulation, transparency is a paramount requisite [2]. We have to exert every effort to improve the transparency of simulation processes. It is the cost we must pay for a healthy development of sciences.

16.3.1 Completeness

All the model equations and physiological parameters used in a simulation should be fully disclosed in a report or appropriate references should be cited so that independent readers can check the report. It is often the case that only the name of a commercial software package is described and mentioned as "the default setting was used." In this case, it is often difficult for the readers to judge the scientific rigor,[2] especially for the ones who do not have access to the commercial software package. The details of mechanistic equations and physiological parameters are usually described in the user's manual. However, the user's manual is not disclosed for public readers (even for journal referees). The transparency should be provided not only for the users but also for the public readers.

In addition, experimental conditions to obtain the drug parameters should be fully described in a report or appropriate references should be added Table 16.1. The API information such as solid form (free/salt, crystalline/amorphous, hydrate/anhydrate) and particle size should be reported. When simulating the C_p–time profile, the method to obtain CL, Vd, Fg, and Fh should be fully described.

A failed simulation should be reported. It is not a failure but a clue for progresses in the future. When parameter optimization is performed,[3] the simulation results before and after optimization should be reported.

---

[2]This is the reason why publications using commercial software packages are not used as scientific references in this book.

[3]As discussed above, drug-by-drug parameter optimization is not recommended.

16.3.2 Comprehensiveness

When a complicated model is used, the essence of the biopharmaceutical profile of a drug can be lost in complicated description. Even if all the simulation details were disclosed, it would be practically impossible for a third party to trace all simulation processes. To increase the comprehensiveness, the dose number, the dissolution number, and the permeation number should be at least reported. These dimensionless parameters can be used to capture the regime of oral absorption of a drug. This helps us to focus on the most important part of biopharmaceutical modeling of the drug. The use of a simpler model should be considered when it is sufficient (the Occam's razor, or parsimony principle). Even when all the factors are automatically calculated by a program, it would be helpful to describe which factor is/is not important. For example, a description like "because MW = 600, the contribution of the paracellular pathway is negligible" would be helpful for readers. When showing C_p–time profiles for the purpose of investigating the absorption phase, a log-normal plot should not be used. The use of support lines in a figure (Fig. 16.1) should be kept minimal. Even when calculating the C_p–time profile, Fa% data should be also reported.

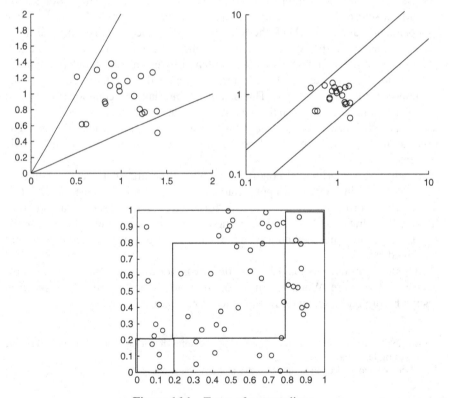

Figure 16.1 Types of support lines.

TABLE 16.1   List of Drug Parameters to be Reported (An Example)

Data	Comments
MW	Free form/salt/cocrystal/hydrate
Chemical structure	If possible to disclose
Chemical formula	If possible to disclose
pK_a	Experimental value is preferable
$\log P_{oct}$	Experimental value is preferable
API solid form	Free form/salt/cocrystal/hydrate Crystalline/amorphous [lot number (for internal report)]
Particles	Size (D50, D90, SD, etc.) Shape
True density	Not tap and bulk density
Solubility	Final pH
	Final solid form
	Buffer species
	Bile micelle composition and concentration
	Solid separation method (filtration, centrifuge)
	Quantification method (HPLC, LC-MS, UV, etc.)
Permeability	Membrane type (Caco-2, MDCK, PAMPA, etc)
	pH
	Other additives in the media (bile micelles, BSA, etc)
	Agitation condition (or UWL thickness) for $P_{app} > 20 \times 10^{-6}$ cm/s cases
	Validity indicator (TEER, permeability standards (e.g., metoprolol))

REFERENCES

1. Yates, J.W., Jones, R.D., Walker, M., Cheung, S.Y. (2009). Structural identifiability and indistinguishability of compartmental models. *Expert Opin. Drug Metab. Toxicol.*, **5**, 295–302.

2. Williams, P., Kim, Y., Ette, E., The epistemology of pharmacometrics, in: *Pharmacometrics*, P. Williams, E. Ette (Eds.) John Wiley & Sons, Inc., Hoboken, New Jersey, 2007, pp. 223–244.

APPENDIX A

GENERAL TERMINOLOGY

Following are the definitions of some major terms used in this book. Other terms are defined as required in each section.

A.1 BIOPHARMACEUTIC

"Biopharmaceutic" is originally used to mean the sciences related to the performance of a pharmaceutical product in a biological system (e.g., human body). Recently, the same word has been used to represent biological molecules (proteins, siRNA, etc.). In this book, "biopharmaceutic" is used as of its original meaning.

A.2 BIOAVAILABILITY (BA% OR *F*)

The bioavailability of a drug product is the fraction of an administered drug reaching the systemic circulation. Bioavailability is expressed as BA% or *F* in this book. In the case of oral absorption, *F* is usually defined based on the total amount of a drug that reached the systemic circulation after oral administration. This definition is used in this book unless otherwise noted. However, the bioavailability of a drug is essentially a time-dependent value. For example, the bioavailability is 10% until 1 h, 20% until 2 h, and so on.

Biopharmaceutics Modeling and Simulations: Theory, Practice, Methods, and Applications,
First Edition. Kiyohiko Sugano.
© 2012 John Wiley & Sons, Inc. Published 2012 by John Wiley & Sons, Inc.

The oral bioavailability of a drug is expressed as $F = Fa \times Fg \times Fh$, where Fa is the fraction of a dose absorbed, Fg is the fraction of a drug passing though the gut wall without metabolism, and Fh is the fraction of a drug passing though the liver without metabolism and biliary excretion.

A.3 DRUG DISPOSITION

Drug disposition is the fate of a drug after entering the systemic circulation. Drug disposition includes distribution to each body part, renal excretion, hepatic metabolism and elimination (except first-pass metabolism), etc.

A.4 FRACTION OF A DOSE ABSORBED (FA)

The fraction of a dose absorbed is the fraction of an administered drug that permeated the first biological barrier, for example, the apical membrane of the intestinal epithelial membrane (or the tight junction). Similar to bioavailability, in the case of oral administration, Fa is usually defined as the absorbed amount after oral administration. However, Fa is essentially a time-dependent value. For example, Fa is 15% until 1 h, 30% until 2 h, and so on.

A.5 MODELING/SIMULATION/*IN SILICO*

Modeling and simulation refers to a mathematical calculation of a more complex phenomenon from simpler phenomena, for example, from *in vitro* data to *in vivo* data. In this book, "*in silico*" means the prediction of a drug property solely from chemical structural information, for example, calculation of octanol–water partition coefficient (log P_{oct}) from chemical structure.

A.6 ACTIVE PHARMACEUTICAL INGREDIENT (API)

Active pharmaceutical ingredient is the raw material of a drug. It is usually in solid crystalline form, but could also be in amorphous or liquid states.

A.7 DRUG PRODUCT

Drug products are the formulated drugs such as tablets or capsules.

A.8 LIPOPHILICITY

As the scale of lipophilicity of a drug, octanol–water distribution coefficient (log D_{oct}) at a pH is employed in this book. The following classification is used in this book:

- Low lipophilicity: log $D_{oct} < -0.5$
- Moderate lipophilicity: $-0.5 < $ log $D_{oct} < 0.5$
- High lipophilicity: $0.5 < $ log D_{oct}.

A.9 ACID AND BASE

When a drug is more than 50% dissociable at a neutral pH in aqueous media, it is called *dissociable* and *acid* or *base* unless otherwise noted. Acids have $pK_a < 6.0\text{--}7.4$ and bases have $pK_a > 6.0\text{--}7.4$.

A.10 SOLUBILITY

Solubility refers to *equilibrium solubility* in this book. The terminology related to solubility is discussed in Section 7.6.1. The following categorization is used in this book:

- Low solubility: <100 µg/ml (ca. 250 µM)
- Moderate solubility: >100 µg/ml, <1 mg/ml (ca. 0.25–2.5 mM)
- High solubility: >1 mg/ml (ca. 2.5 mM).

Unless otherwise noted, the solubility of a drug refers to that measured at a neutral pH of interest (e.g., pH 6.5 for oral absorption). However, the solubility of dissociable drugs largely depends on the pH of the media. For example, a base drug can have a high solubility at a low pH even though its solubility is low at a neutral pH.

A.11 MOLECULAR WEIGHT (MW)

The molecular weight of the free form of a drug, but not a salt or solvate, is used unless otherwise noted. The following categorization is used in this book:

- Small molecule: <250
- Moderate size molecule: >250, <450
- Large molecule: >450.

A.12 PERMEABILITY OF A DRUG

The permeability of a drug has a dimension of length per time. This value changes depending on the morphology of the surface area. As there is no unified scale, the permeability range of a drug is defined based on the permeability of a drug in the Caco-2 or MDCK assay (at pH 6.5). The following categorization is used in this book:

- Low permeability: $<1 \times 10^{-6}$ cm/s
- Moderate permeability: $>1 \times 10^{-6}$ cm/s, $<10 \times 10^{-6}$ cm/s
- High permeability: $>10 \times 10^{-6}$ cm/s

Unless otherwise noted, the permeability of a drug refers to that measured at a neutral pH of interest (e.g., pH 6.5 for oral absorption). Roughly speaking, each category of permeability corresponds to those of lipophilicity (i.e., a drug with low lipophilicity tends to have low permeability).

APPENDIX B

FLUID DYNAMICS

This section is a brief introduction to fluid dynamics. Historically, a simplified concept of the boundary layer, "the unstirred water layer," has been operationally used in the pharmaceutical sciences. However, to raise up biopharmaceutical modeling to the next level, it is necessary to understand the essential concepts of fluid dynamics. Unfortunately, fluid dynamics is usually not introduced in the textbooks of the pharmaceutical sciences. Therefore, a brief introduction to fluid dynamics is provided in this book.

B.1 NAVIER–STOKES EQUATION AND REYNOLDS NUMBER

The first principle of fluid dynamics is described by the Navier–Stokes (NS) equation (Fig. B.1). The NS equation is derived from Newton's second law (conservation of momentum) in mechanics. The NS equation is a nonlinear partial differential equation.

The Reynolds number characterizes the relative importance of each term in the NS equation. The Reynolds number (Re) is defined as

$$Re = \frac{U \rho_f L}{\mu} = \frac{UL}{\nu}$$

where U is the flow speed around an object, ρ_f is the density of the fluid, μ is the viscosity of the fluid, and ν is the kinematic viscosity of the fluid ($\nu = \mu/\rho_f$). The

Biopharmaceutics Modeling and Simulations: Theory, Practice, Methods, and Applications,
First Edition. Kiyohiko Sugano.
© 2012 John Wiley & Sons, Inc. Published 2012 by John Wiley & Sons, Inc.

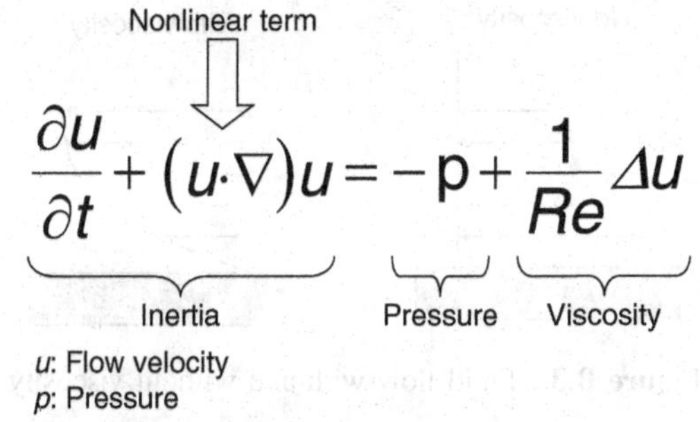

Nonlinear term

$$\frac{\partial u}{\partial t} + (u \cdot \nabla)u = -p + \frac{1}{Re}\Delta u$$

$\underbrace{\qquad\qquad}_{\text{Inertia}}$ $\underbrace{\quad}_{\text{Pressure}}$ $\underbrace{\quad}_{\text{Viscosity}}$

u: Flow velocity
p: Pressure

Figure B.1 Navier–Stokes equation (for noncompressive fluid).

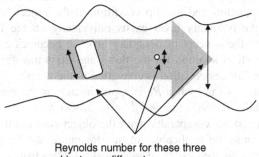

Reynolds number for these three
objects are different.

Figure B.2 Reynolds numbers of a particle, tablet, and intestinal tube.

Reynolds number can be interpreted as the balance between inertia and viscosity. The Reynolds number determines the flow regimen, "laminar" or "turbulence." When viscosity exceeds inertia ($Re < 1$), the flow pattern becomes laminar, whereas when inertia exceeds viscosity ($R \gg 1000$), the flow pattern becomes turbulent.

The representative length of an object is the length that mainly characterizes the flow pattern around the object. Therefore, even though two objects, for example, API particle (μm scale) and tablet (mm), are put in the same flow, the Reynolds numbers are different (Fig. B.2).

B.2 BOUNDARY LAYER APPROXIMATION

As shown in Figure B.3, on the fluid–object interface, there is a thin fluid layer where the fluid sticks to the object surface by its viscosity. As the distance from the object surface becomes larger, the effect of viscosity gradually becomes smaller and the flow begins to be governed by inertia, eventually becoming a potential flow. The layer within which the effect of viscosity cannot be neglected is called *the boundary layer*.

No viscosity   With viscosity

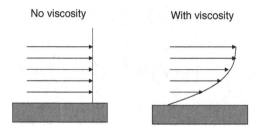

Figure B.3   Fluid flow with and without viscosity.

The concept of the boundary layer was introduced by Prandtl in 1904. The existence of a boundary layer on the object surface is concluded from the Navier–Stokes equation and no-slip condition at the object surface. In a fluid with viscosity, the boundary layer exists universally on the fluid–solid interface. By applying the concept of boundary layer, it becomes easier to obtain an approximate analytical solution for the flows and mass transfer in the boundary layer (the Navier–Stokes equation is converted to the boundary layer equations). This approximation is valid when *Re* is approximately in the range of 1–4 digits. When *Re* is smaller (called *creeping flow* or *Stokes flow*), the thickness of the boundary layer becomes comparable with the object size and the boundary layer approximation cannot be applicable. In this *Re* range, the Stokes' and Oseen's approximations can be used to derive analytical solutions from the Navier–Stokes equation. On the other hand, when *Re* is greater than 3–4 digits, the flow regimen becomes turbulent and the boundary layer approximation is not applicable.

B.3 THE BOUNDARY LAYER AND MASS TRANSFER

On the object surface ($\delta = 0$ in Fig. B.3), there is no convection by fluid flow and solute molecules have to self-diffuse. As the distance from the surface increases, the mass transfer by convection also increases. The diffusion resistance by the boundary layer is represented as a distance. In many textbooks of pharmaceutical science, it is described as if there is a distinct region where there is no flow (called *unstirred water layer*), and this region becomes the diffusion barrier for mass transfer (Fig. 3.4). However, this description is a conventional one.

B.4 THE THICKNESS OF THE BOUNDARY LAYER

Figure B.2 shows a plane in parallel to the flow from the left to the right. After the flow senses the head of the plane, the boundary layer starts to grow. Because of the fluid viscosity, the flow speed near the surface is slower than that of the main flow (U). At the surface of the plane, there is no flow (no-slip condition).

There are a few methods to define the thickness of the boundary layer (δ). δ is usually expressed in the form of

$$\delta \propto LRe^{-1/2}$$

By applying the boundary layer approximation, an approximate equation to calculate δ can be obtained. The boundary layer approximation is valid when $\delta < L$, $Re > 10-100$, and the flow regimen is laminar.

B.4.1   99% of Main Flow Speed

δ is defined as the distance from the plane at which the flow speed becomes 99% of the main stream flow speed (U_∞).

$$\delta_{99\%}(x) \approx 5.0\sqrt{\frac{\nu x}{U_\infty}} = 5.0xRe_x^{-1/2}$$

where Re_x is the Reynolds number defined based on the distance from the head of the plane, x as $\text{Re}_x = xU_\infty/\nu$.

B.4.2   Displacement Thickness

Owing to the boundary layer where the flow speed becomes slower than the main stream, the flux becomes smaller compared to a flow without the boundary layer (Fig. B.3). This looks similar to the thickness of the plane being increased. This thickness is called *displacement thickness* and expressed as

$$\delta_{\text{displacement}}(x) \approx 1.73\sqrt{\frac{\nu x}{U_\infty}} = 1.73x\text{Re}_x^{-1/2}$$

B.4.3   Momentum Thickness

The thickness of the boundary layer can be defined based on the loss of momentum in the boundary layer.

$$\delta_{\text{m}}(x) \approx 0.664\sqrt{\frac{\nu x}{U_\infty}} = 0.664xRe_x^{-1/2}$$

B.5   SHERWOOD NUMBER

As discussed above, the boundary layer is the resistance for mass transfer. In the boundary layer, as the position of the fluid approaches the object surface, the mass transfer by convection becomes smaller and the molecular diffusion begins to be dominant. At the object surface, there is no flow and the mass transfer is only by molecular diffusion. On the other hand, in the outside of the boundary layer, the mass transfer is dominated by convection. The concentration boundary layer ($\delta_c(x)$), where a concentration gradient exists is usually much smaller than that of the flow momentum boundary layer ($\delta_m(x)$) in aqueous media. The ratio of the $\delta_c(x)/\delta_m(x)$ is related to the Schmidt number (Sc).

$$\frac{\delta_c(x)}{\delta_m(x)} = Sc^{-1/3} = \left(\frac{\nu}{D_{\text{eff}}}\right)^{-1/3}$$

where D_{eff} is the diffusion coefficient of a solute. By rearranging this equation,

$$\delta_c(x) = \delta_m(x)Sc^{-1/3} = 0.664xRe_x^{-1/2}Sc^{-1/3} = xSh_x^{-1}, \quad Sh_x = \frac{1}{0.664}Re_x^{1/2}Sc^{1/3}$$

The local Sherwood number and local δ_c at a point (x) on the object surface varies point-by-point (Fig. B.4). Therefore, to calculate the mass transfer from/to the object, the average Sherwood number for the object is often used. In this book, the Sherwood number means the average Sherwood number of an object unless otherwise indicated.

For a plate with a length (L), the Sh becomes

$$Sh_{\text{plane}} = 0.66Re_{\text{plane}}^{1/2}Sc^{1/3}, \quad \delta_c(x) = \frac{L_{\text{plane}}}{Sh_{\text{plane}}}$$

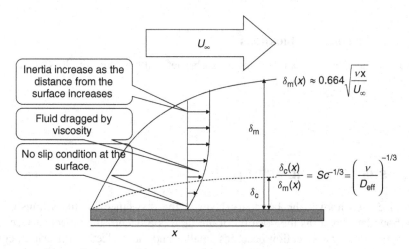

Figure B.4   Boundary layer on a plate placed in parallel to flow.

where Re_{plane} is the Reynolds number defined based on the length of the plane (L_{plane}). The mass transfer from/into the plane is then expressed as

$$\frac{\mathrm{d}X}{\mathrm{d}t} = SA_{\text{plane}} \frac{D_{\text{eff}}}{\delta_{\text{C}}(x)} \Delta C$$

In general, when the boundary layer concept is applied, the Sherwood number becomes

$$Sh \propto Re^{1/2} Sc^{1/3}$$

These equations are valid in a laminar flow. However, even in turbulent flow, the boundary layer exists (which is called *viscous sublayer*).

B.6 TURBULENCE

As *Re* increases from a single digit to 3–6 digit order, the flow regimen gradually changes from laminar to turbulent. The turbulent flow is characterized as the assemblage of fluid dynamical eddies (vortex) of variable scales. Large-scale eddies are introduced when the fluid flow contacts with the object. The large eddies cascade down to smaller-scale eddies until their energy is dissipated by viscosity. For understanding the essence of turbulence, Lewis Fry Richardson expressed the essence of turbulence as (a parody of On Poetry, A Rhapsody (Swift,1733)),

Big whirls have little whirls

That feed on their velocity,

And little whirls have lesser whirls

And so on to viscosity

(in the molecular sense.)[1]

Even though the large-scale eddy is not isotropic, the small size eddies produced by the crumbling of large eddies have isotropic energy distribution. Regardless of the way a large eddy is produced, the structure of the small eddy becomes the same. This is called *hypothesis of local isotropy* introduced by Kolmogorov. The minimum scale of Kolmogorov (η) is

$$\eta = \left(\frac{\nu^3}{\varepsilon} \right)^{1/4}$$

where ε is the energy per fluid weight introduced by the large eddy. When the minimum scale of eddy is close to the drug particle size, the mass transfer by this eddy becomes significant (Fig. 3.10).

[1]Lewis Fry Richardson, Weather prediction by numerical process, Cambridge, 1922.

B.7 FORMATION OF EDDIES

The flow pattern behind a cylinder is the best example to understand the mechanism of a vortex formation. When a cylinder is put in flow (such as a pier column in a river), a street of vortex is observed (Figs. B.5 and B.6). This is called *Karman vortex street*. Near the cylinder wall, owing to the viscosity of the fluid, the fluid tend to stick to the wall (viscosity wins here), whereas at the distance from the cylinder, the flow becomes uniform and the flow speed becomes close to that of the main flow (inertia wins here). The change of the flow speed in the boundary layer causes a shear force and introduces an eddy (Figure B.6).

B.8 COMPUTATIONAL FLUID DYNAMICS

The Navier–Stokes equation is a nonlinear partial differential equation. As discussed above, for simple (but important) situations, the NS equation can

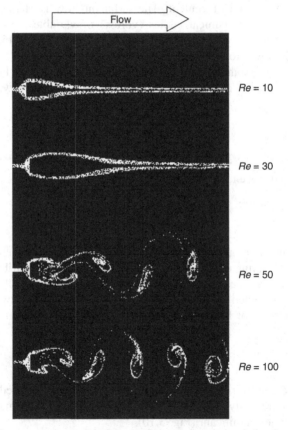

Figure B.5 Kerman vortex street. *Source:* Computational simulation by a program provided in Reference 1.

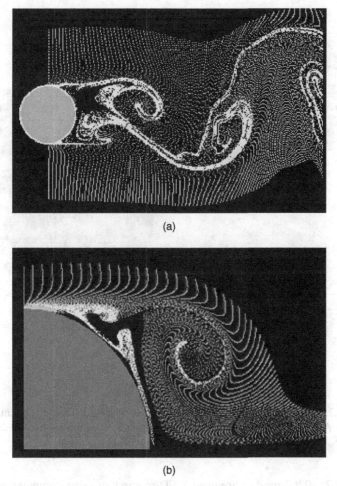

(a)

(b)

Figure B.6 Formation of eddy at the cylinder surface. *Source:* Computational simulation by a program provided in Reference 1.

be analytically solved by applying an approximation. However, for most situations, it is impossible to derive an analytical solution from the NS equation. The Computational Fluid Dynamics (CFD), which numerically solves the Navier–Stokes equation using a high speed computer, can be used for such cases.

The finite element method is widely used to solve the NS equation. The space is separated by meshes and the flow at each grid is calculated. Figure B.7 shows the mesh system used for the CFD calculation of the USP II paddle method [2]. The mesh size determines the minimum size of flow patterns captured by the CFD simulation. For example, the mesh system of Figure B.7 can capture the flow pattern around the paddle ($d = 10$ cm), but not the API particles (<0.1 cm). In

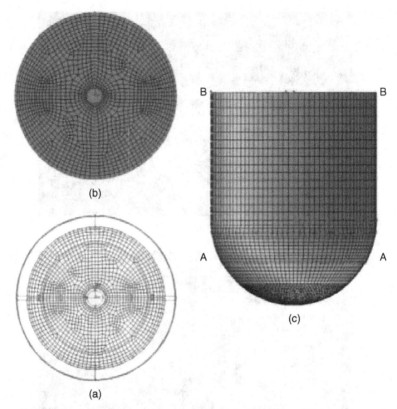

Figure B.7   Mesh used in the CFD simulation for the USP paddle apparatus: (a) iso-surface at A–A; (b) iso-surface at B–B; and (c) axial, side view. *Source*: Adapted from Reference 2 with permission.

Figure B.7, 80262 meshes are used. CFD requires massive computational power so that it cannot be directly used for biopharmaceutical modeling at present.

REFERENCES

1. Genki, Y., The sciences of flow visualized by computer, Kodan-sha, Tokyo, 2001.
2. Bai, G., Armenante, P.M., Plank, R.V., Gentzler, M., Ford, K., Harmon, P. (2007). Hydrodynamic investigation of USP dissolution test apparatus II. *J. Pharm. Sci*., 96, 2327–2349.

INDEX

Biopharmaceutics Modeling and Simulations: Theory, Practice, Methods, and Applications,
First Edition. Kiyohiko Sugano.
© 2012 John Wiley & Sons, Inc. Published 2012 by John Wiley & Sons, Inc.

Printed in the United States
By Bookmasters

Printed in the United States
By Bookmasters